Methods in Cartilage Research

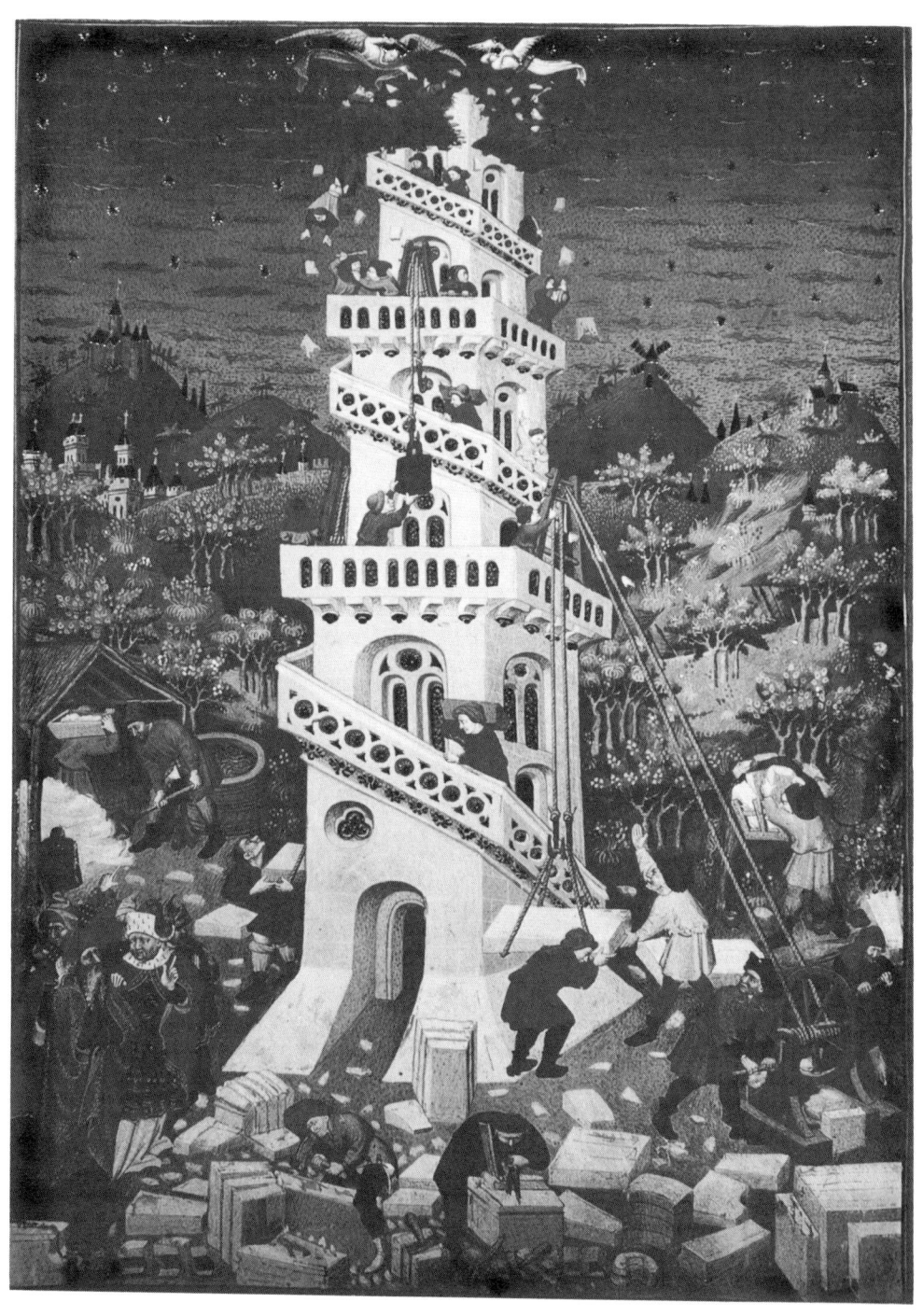

The Tower of Babel, from a fifteenth century French manuscript.
Reproduced with permission of Terra Sancta Arts.

Methods in Cartilage Research

Edited by

A. MAROUDAS

Department of Biomedical Engineering
Technion—Israel Institute of Technology
Haifa, Israel

K. KUETTNER

Department of Biochemistry, Rush Medical College
Rush-Presbyterian-St. Luke's Medical Center
Chicago, USA

ACADEMIC PRESS
Harcourt Brace Jovanovich, Publishers
LONDON SAN DIEGO NEW YORK BOSTON
SYDNEY TOKYO TORONTO

ACADEMIC PRESS LIMITED
24/28 Oval Road
London NW1 7DX

United States Edition published by
ACADEMIC PRESS INC.
San Diego, CA 92101

Copyright © 1990 by
ACADEMIC PRESS LIMITED

This book is printed on acid-free paper ∞

All rights Reserved

No part of this book may be reproduced in any form by photostat, microfilm, or any other means, without written permission from the publishers

British Library Cataloguing in Publication Data

Methods in cartilage research.
 1. Man. Cartilage. Physiology
 I. Maroudas, A. II. Kuettner, K.
 611.0183

 ISBN 0-12-473280-1

Typeset in Great Britain by EJS Chemical Composition, Midsomer Norton, Bath, Avon
Printed and bound in Great Britain by M & A Thomson Litho Ltd, East Kilbride

Contents

Contributors xi
Preface xvii
Introduction: Summary of the Batsheva Seminar xxi

SECTION 1 SAMPLING, CHARACTERIZATION AND HANDLING *EX VIVO* OF TISSUE SPECIMENS
Collated by *M.T. Bayliss*

1. Overview
   M.T. Bayliss 1
2. Articular cartilage samples
   D.L. Gardner 4
3. Selection and classification of human articular cartilage
   T.R. Oegema 7
4. Choice of specimens in comparative studies involving human femoral head cartilage
   A. Maroudas, R. Schneiderman, C. Weinberg and G. Grushko 9
5. Sampling of the intervertebral disc
   S. Roberts 17
6. Tissue sampling and preservation for morphological studies
   E.B. Hunziker 19
   References 23

SECTION 2 EXTRACTION, SEPARATION AND ANALYSIS OF MATRIX CONSTITUENTS
Collated by *D.R. Eyre*

7. Overview
   D.R. Eyre 27
8. The cartilage collagens: analysis of their cross-linking interactions and matrix organization
   D.R. Eyre, J.J. Wu, C. Niyibizi and L. Chun 28
9. Mammalian cartilage collagens: identification of their forms *in vivo*
   S. Ayad, A. Marriott, K. Morgan, C. Cummings, A.P.L. Kwan, A.P. Mould and M.E. Grant 33
10. Extraction and purification of proteoglycan and hyaluronan from human articular cartilage
    M. Bayliss 36
11. Composite agarose–acrylamide electrophoresis of proteoglycans and large protein complexes
    C.A. McDevitt 40
12. Analytical and preparative electrophoresis of proteoglycan monomers in agarose submerged gels
    V. Stanescu 44

13. Centrifugal methodologies to study the proteoglycans from articular cartilage
    J.C. Pita and F.J. Müller 46
14. Microsequencing of cartilage components
    M. van der Rest, E. de Miguel, Q. Nguyen, B. Dublet, J.S. Mort and P.J. Roughley .. 50
15. Summary review
    H. Muir 56
    References 57

SECTION 3 MORPHOLOGY OF CARTILAGE
Collated by *R.A. Stockwell*

16. Overview
    R.A. Stockwell 61
17. Methods for the study of cartilage by low temperature scanning electron microscopy and related techniques
    D.L. Gardner, K. Oates, D.M. Lawton, J.G. Pidd and J.F.S. Middleton 63
18. Electron-microscopic study of the articular surface using cationized ferritin labeling
    R. Stanescu 67
19. New experimental approaches to the understanding of structure–function relationships in articular cartilage
    N.D. Broom 70
20. The application of recent stereological methods in articular cartilage research
    E.B. Hunziker 74
21. Chondrons extracted from articular cartilage: methods and applications
    C.A. Poole 78
    References 81

SECTION 4 CHONDROCYTE CULTURE
Collated by *P.D. Benya*

22. Introduction and survey of techniques
    P.D. Benya 85
23. Subpopulations of articular chondrocytes cultured in agarose gel
    M.B. Aydelotte, B.L. Schumacher and K.E. Kuettner 90
24. A three-dimensional culture model for studying human chondrocytes
    C. Bassleer, Y. Henrotin, R. Bassleer and P. Franchimont 93
25. Immortalization of chondrocytes in culture
    S. Thenet and M. Adolphe 95
26. Culturing chondrocytes for implantation
    Z. Nevo, D. Robinson, N. Halperin and S. Edelstein 98
    References 100

SECTION 5 SHORT- AND LONG-TERM EXPLANT CULTURE OF CARTILAGE
Collated by *C.J. Handley*

27. Introduction
    C.J. Handley, C.K. Ng and A.J. Curtis 105
28. Steady-state metabolism of proteoglycans in bovine articular cartilage
    V.C. Hascall, F.P. Luyten, A.H.K. Plaas and J.D. Sandy 108

29. Cartilage explant cultures: a model system for the analysis of matrix degradation
    J. Tyler and Y. Sawyer 112
30. The effect of mechanical compression on cartilage metabolism
    R.L.Y. Sah, Y.-J. Kim and A.J. Grodzinsky 116
31. Effects of mechanical and osmotic pressure on the rate of glycosaminoglycan synthesis in the human adult femoral head cartilage
    A. Maroudas and R. Schneiderman 119
32. Explant culture of the intervertebral disc
    B. Johnstone 123
References 126

SECTION 6 USE OF RADIOISOTOPES TO STUDY METABOLISM OF MATRIX MACROMOLECULES
Collated by *V.C. Hascall*

33. Introduction
    V.C. Hascall 131
34. The use of radiolabeled glucosamine as a precursor for measuring hyaluronan synthesis
    V.C. Hascall, M. Yanagishita, A. Salustri and T.I. Morales 132
35. Assessment of turnover of proteoglycans *in vivo*
    R.M. Mason 137
36. *In vivo* measurement of collagen metabolism in cartilage and bone
    R.J. McAnulty and G.J. Laurent 140
37. Determination of the rate of glycosaminoglycan synthesis *in vivo* using radioactive sulfate as tracer: comparison with *in vitro* results
    A. Maroudas 143
38. Biosynthesis of cartilage proteoglycan: an analysis of posttranslational events by different *in vitro* labeling protocols
    L.S. Lohmander 148
References 152

SECTION 7 IMMUNOCHEMICAL METHODS IN CARTILAGE RESEARCH
Collated by *T. Hardingham*

39. Introduction
    T. Hardingham 155
40. Immunochemical methods and their use in characterizing cartilage proteoglycans
    T. Hardingham 156
41. Methods for the production and characterization of monoclonal antibodies to connective-tissue proteoglycans
    B. Caterson, T. Calbro, T. Blankenship-Paris, M. Adams, R. Pearce and A. Malcolm . 164
42. Characterization and use of polyclonal antibodies to collagen
    D.J. Hartmann 168
43. Measurement of antigenic keratan sulfate by an enzyme-linked immunosorbant assay
    E.J.M.A. Thonar, M.E. Lenz, B. Maldonado, L. Otten, T. Glant and K.E. Kuettner . 170

viii CONTENTS

44. Quantitation of keratan sulfate epitope in bovine and human cartilage proteoglycans: comparison of immunoassay procedures and antikeratan sulfate antibodies
M. Seibel, R. Jelsma, F. Saed-Nejad and A. Ratcliffe 173
45. Antigen-specific T-lymphocyte clone as a new tool in proteoglycan research
T.T. Glant 177
References 181

SECTION 8 RECOMBINANT DNA AND CARTILAGE MATRIX
Collated by *M. Tanzer*

46. Overview
M. Tanzer 185
47. Domain structure and sequence homologies in cartilage proteoglycan
T.E. Hardingham, J. Dudhia and A.J. Fosang 187
48. From the gene to the protein: the discovery of type XII collagen
M. van der Rest 190
49. The source of lysozyme in chick embryo cartilage
S.J. Keating and K.P.H. Pritzker 194
50. Approaches to studying the regulation of chondrocyte gene expression
W.E. Horton, Jr and S. Chandrasekhar 196
51. Detection of type II collagen gene mutations in familial osteoarthritis
S.A. Jimenez 199
References 206

SECTION 9 TISSUE COMPOSITION AND ORGANIZATION
Collated by *A. Maroudas*

52. Introduction
A. Maroudas 209
53. Different ways of expressing concentration of cartilage constituents with special reference to the tissue's organization and functional properties
A. Maroudas 211
54. Age-related changes in the stoichiometry of human articular cartilage proteoglycan aggregates
M.T. Bayliss 220
55. The use of enzyme-modified tissues to study selected aspects of tissue structure and function
F.A. Meyer 222
56. Characterization of the packing of collagen in cartilage using X-ray scattering
E. Wachtel and A. Maroudas 227
57. Low-angle X-ray diffraction analysis of cartilaginous tissues
C. Berthet-Colominas, M-C. Ronziere and D. Herbage 232
58. Cell compartment in articular cartilage
R.A. Stockwell 235
References 237

SECTION 10 SOLUTE TRANSPORT BETWEEN TISSUE AND ENVIRONMENT
Collated by *J.P.G. Urban*

59. Introduction and review of general principles and procedures
    J.P.G. Urban 241
60. Determining the elemental composition of articular cartilage: a comparison between human and non-human primates
    M.D. Grynpas, J.M.D. Chateauvert and K.P.H. Pritzker 248
61. Measurement of partition coefficient by gel chromatography
    B.N. Preston, M-P. I. Van Damme and W.H. Murphy 251
62. Measurement of diffusion coefficients in biopolymer solutions and gels
    C.P. Winlove and K.H. Parker 255
63. Techniques for studying membrane transport
    A.C. Hall 258
64. Characterization of networks by the use of molecular probes: static and dynamic methods
    A. Silberberg 263

References 270

SECTION 11 MECHANICAL AND ELECTRICAL PROPERTIES AND THEIR RELEVANCE TO PHYSIOLOGICAL PROCESSES
Collated by *A.J. Grodzinsky*

65. Overview
    A.J. Grodzinsky 275
66. Pressure measurement in the human hip joint using Fujifilm
    A. Afoke, W.C. Hutton and P.D. Byers 281
67. Physical properties of articular cartilage from uniaxial confined compression
    S.R. Eisenberg 287
68. Unconfined compression for studying cartilage creep
    J. Mizrahi, A. Maroudas and E. Benaim 293
69. Measurement of swelling pressure of cartilage
    A. Maroudas and G. Grushko 298
70. Osmometer for rapid measurement of swelling pressure of nucleus pulposus from the intervertebral disc
    A.R. Hargens 302
71. Measurement of the compressive properties of thin cartilage slices: evaluating tissue inhomogeneity
    P.A. Torzilli 304

References 308

SECTION 12 ARTICULAR CARTILAGE REPAIR AND REMODELING
Collated by *B. Caterson*

72. Overview
    B. Caterson and J. Buckwalter 313
73. Reflections on the repair of articular cartilage
    P.D. Byers and R.A. Brown 318

74. Fluorescent–tracer labeling for measuring remodeling in the zone of calcified cartilage
    T.R. Oegema, Jr and R.C. Thompson, Jr 322
75. Spongialization and cartilage healing in the human
    C. Ficat 324
76. Use of cultured chondrocytes as implants for repairing cartilage defects
    D. Robinson, N. Halperin and Z. Nevo 327
References 329

SECTION 13 OSTEOARTHRITIS: MAN, MODELS AND MOLECULAR MARKERS
Collated by *L.S. Lohmander*

77. Introduction
    L.S. Lohmander 337
78. Studies of naturally occurring degenerative arthritis in rhesus macaques as a model for degenerative arthritis in man
    K.P.H. Pritzker, J. Chateauvert, M.D. Grynpas and M.J. Kessler 341
79. Proteoglycan components in synovial fluid as markers of experimental and natural joint disease
    T.E. Hardingham 342
80. Measurement of serum keratan sulfate provides important information about the metabolism of cartilage proteoglycans *in vivo*
    E.J.M.A. Thonar, J. William, M.E. Lenz, M.B. Sweet, L. Otten, G. Campion, T.J. Schnitzer and K.E. Kuettner 345
81. Collagen markers in urine in human arthritis
    S.R. Robins, M.J. Seibel and A.M. McLaren 348
82. The 'clearance' of macromolecular substances such as cartilage markers from synovial fluid and serum
    J.R. Levick 352
References 358

Index 363

Contributors

Mark E. Adams Department of Medicine, University of Calgary, 3330 Hospital Drive NW, Calgary, Alberta T2N 4N1, Canada

Monique Adolphe Laboratoire de Pharmacologie Cellulaire de l'Ecole Pratique des Hautes Etudes, 15 rue de l'Ecole de Medecine, 75006 Paris, France

Andrew Afoke Polytechnic of Central London, 115 New Cavendish Street, London W1M 8JS, UK

Shirley Ayad Departments of Biochemistry and Molecular Biology, University of Manchester Medical School, Stopford Building, Manchester M13 9PT, UK

Margaret B. Aydelotte Department of Biochemistry, Rush-Presbyterian-St. Luke's Medical Center, 1653 West Congress Parkway, Chicago, IL 60612, USA

Corinne Bassleer Laboratory of Radioimmunology and Endocrinology CHU, Bat. B23, 4000-Sart-Tilman/Liege 1, Belgium

R. Bassleer Laboratory of Histology, 20 rue de Pitteurs B-4020 Liege, Belgium

Michael T. Bayliss Kennedy Institute of Rheumatology, Bute Gardens, Hammersmith, London W6 7DW, UK

E. Benaim Department of Biomedical Engineering, Technion — Israel Institute of Technology, Haifa 32000, Israel

Paul D. Benya Bone and Connective Tissue Research Program Department of Orthopaedics, University of Southern California Orthopaedic Hospital, Los Angeles, CA 90007-2697 USA

Carmen Berthet-Colominas European Molecular Biology Laboratory, Grenoble Outstation, 38042 Grenoble Cedex, France

Terry Blankenship-Paris Department of Biochemistry, University of West Virginia, Morgantown, West Virginia, USA

Neil D. Broom Biomechanics Laboratory, School of Engineering, University of Auckland, Private Bag, Auckland, New Zealand

Robert A. Brown Experimental Pathology Department, Institute of Orthopaedics, Royal National Orthopaedic Hospital, Brockley Hill, Stanmore, Middlesex HA7 4LP, UK

Joseph Buckwalter Department of Orthopaedic Surgery, The University of Iowa Hospitals and Clinics, Iowa City, Iowa, USA

Paul Byers Reader Emeritus in Morbid Anatomy, University of London (Institute of Orthopaedics), London WC1E 7HU, UK

Tony Calbro Department of Biochemistry, University of West Virginia, Morgantown, West Virginia, USA

Giles Campion Departments of Biochemistry and Medicine, Rush-Presbyterian-St. Luke's Medical Center, 1653 W. Congress Parkway, Chicago, IL 60612, USA

Bruce Caterson Division of Orthopaedics, School of Medicine, University of North Carolina at Chapel Hill, Burnett Womack Building CB#7055 Chapel Hill, NC 27599-7055, USA

Srinivasan Chrandrasekhar Lilly Research Laboratories, Department of Connective Tissue Research, Lilly Corporate Center, Indianapolis, IN 46285, USA

Joanne Chateauvert Department of Pathology, Mount Sinai Hospital, 600 University Avenue, Toronto, Ontario M5G 1X5, Canada

L. Chun Orthopaedic Research Laboratories, University of Washington, Seattle, WA 98195, USA

Christine Cummings Department of Medical Biophysics, University of Manchester Medical School, Stopford Building, Manchester M13 9PT, UK

Andrea J. Curtis Department of Biochemistry, Monash University, Clayton, Victoria 3168, Australia

E. De Miguel Genetics Unit, Shriners Hospital, 1529 Cedar Avenue, Montreal, QC H3G 1A6, Canada

B. Dublet Genetics Unit, Shriners Hospital, 1529 Cedar Avenue, Montreal, QC H3G 1A6, Canada

Jayesh Dudhia Kennedy Institute of Rheumatology, Bute Gardens, Hammersmith, London W6 7DW, UK

S. Edelstein Department of Biochemistry, The Weizmann Institute of Science, Rehovot 76100, Israel

Sol Eisenberg Department of Biomedical Engineering, Boston University, Room 410, 44 Cummington Street, Boston, MA 02215, USA

David R. Eyre Department of Orthopaedics, RK-10, University of Washington, Seattle, WA 98195 USA

Christian Ficat Department of Orthopaedics, Hopital Beaujon, Universite Paris VIII, 92 Clichy, France

Amanda J. Fosang Kennedy Institute of Rheumatology, Bute Gardens, Hammersmith, London W6 7DW, UK

P. Franchimont Laboratory of Radioimmunology and Endocrinology, CHU Bat. B23, 4000-Sart-Tilman/Liege 1 Belgium

Dugald Gardner Department of Pathology, University of Edinburgh, Medical School, Teviot Place, Edinburgh EH8 9AG, UK

Tibor Glant Department of Biochemistry, Rush-Presbyterian-St. Luke's Medical Center, 1653 W. Congress Parkway, Chicago, IL 60612, USA

Michael E. Grant Department of Biochemistry and Molecular Biology, University of Manchester Medical School, Stopford Building, Manchester M13 9PT, UK

Alan J. Grodzinsky Department of Electrical Engineering and Computer Science, Massachusetts Institute of Technology, Room 38–377, Cambridge, MA 02139, USA

Galina Grushko Department of Biomedical Engineering, Technion — Israel Institute of Technology, Haifa 32000, Israel

Marc D. Grynpas Department of Pathology, Mount Sinai Hospital, 600 University Avenue, Room 609, Toronto, Ontario, M5G 1X5, Canada

Andrew C. Hall University Laboratory of Physiology, University of Oxford, Parks Road, Oxford OX1 3PT, UK

N. Halperin Department of Orthopaedic Surgery, Assaf Harofeh Medical Center, Zeriffin 70300, Israel

Christopher Handley Department of Biochemistry, Monash University, Clayton, Melbourne, Victoria 3168, Australia

Timothy Hardingham Kennedy Institute of Rheumatology, Bute Gardens, Hammersmith, London W6 7DW, UK

Alan R. Hargens Life Science Division, NASA-Ames Research Center (239–17), Moffett Field, CA 94035, USA

Daniel J. Hartmann Centre de Radioanalyse Institut Pasteur de Lyon, 13–15 rue Domer, Lyon Cedex 07 69366, France

Vincent Hascall Bone Research Branch, National Institute of Dental Research, The National Institutes of Health, Building 30, Room 106, Bethesda, MD 20892, USA

Yves Henrotin Laboratory of Radioimmunoassy, Universite de Liege, CHU Sart-Tilman, Tower of Pathology (-1), B23 4020 Liege, Belgium

Daniel Herbage, Laboratoire de Biologie et Chimie des Proteines, CNRS UPR 412, Cytologie Moleculaire, Universite Claude Bernard, 69622 Villeurbanne Cedex, France

W.E. Horton Department of Connective Tissue and Monoclonal Antibody Research, Lilly Research Laboratories, Indianapolis, Indiana 46286, USA

Ernst B. Hunziker H.E. Muller Institute for Biomechanics, University of Bern, P.O. Box 130, 3010 Bern, Switzerland

W.C. Hutton Department of Orthopaedics, Emory University Medical School, Atlanta, GA 30303, USA

R. Jelsma Orthopaedic Research Laboratory, Columbia University, New York, NY 10032, USA

Sergio Jimenez Department of Medicine, Thomas Jefferson University, Room M-46 Jefferson Alumni Hall, 1020 Locust Street, Philadelphia, PA 19107, USA

Brian Johnstone Division of Orthopaedics, University of North Carolina at Chapel Hill, CB#7055 Burnett-Womack Building, Chapel Hill, NC 27599–7055, USA

Sarah J. Keating Department of Pathology, Mount Sinai Hospital, 600 University Avenue, Toronto, Ontario M5G 1X5, Canada

Matt J. Kessler DVM, Caribbean Primate Research Centre, Sebana Seca, Puerto Rico

Young-Jo Kim Continuum Electromechanics Group, Laboratory for Electromagnetic and Electronic Systems, Department of Electrical Engineering and Computer Science, Massachusetts Institute of Technology, Cambridge, MA 02139, USA

Klaus E. Kuettner Department of Biochemistry, Rush Medical College, Rush-Presbyterian-St. Luke's Medical Center, 1653 West Congress Parkway, Chicago, IL 60612, USA

Alvin P.L. Kwan Department of Biochemistry and Molecular Biology, University of Manchester Medical School, Stopford Building, Manchester M13 9PT, UK

Michael K. Kwan University of California, San Diego, Division of Orthopaedic Surgery, M-030, La Jolla, CA 92092, USA

Geoffrey John Laurent Biochemistry Unit, Department of Thoracic Medicine, National Heart and Lung Institute, University of London, Dovehouse Street, London SW3 6LY, UK

D.M. Lawton Department of Pathology, University of Manchester Medical School, Stopford Building, Manchester M13 9PT, UK

Mary Ellen Lenz Department of Biochemistry, Rush-Presbyterian-St. Luke's Medical Center, 1653 West Congress Parkway, Chicago, IL 60612, USA

J. Rodney Levick George's Hospital Medical School, University of London, Department of Physiology, Cranmer Terrace, Tooting, London SW17 0RE, UK

Stefan Lohmander Department of Orthopaedics, University Hospital at Lund, S-22185 Lund, Sweden

Frank P. Lund Bone Research Branch, National Institute of Dental Research, The National Institutes of Health, Bethesda, MD 20892, USA

Frank P. Luyten Bone Cell Biology Section, National Institute of Dental Research, The National Institutes of Health, Bethesda, MD 20892, USA

Andrew Malcolm Department of Pathology, University of British Columbia, Vancouver, B.C., Canada

Brian Maldonado Department of Biochemistry, Rush-Presbyterian-St. Luke's Medical Center, 1653 West Congress Parkway, Chicago, IL 60612, USA

Alice Maroudas Department of Biomedical Engineering, Technion — Israel Institute of Technology, Haifa 32000, Israel

Anne Marriott Departments of Biochemistry and Molecular Biology, University of Manchester Medical School, Stopford Building, Manchester M13 9PT, UK

Roger Mason Department of Biochemistry, Charing Cross and Westminster Medical School, University of London, Fulham Palace Road, London W6 8RF, UK

R.J. McAnulty Biochemistry Unit, Department of Thoracic Medicine National Heart and Lung Institute, University of London, Dovehouse Street, London SW3 6LY, UK

Cahir McDevitt Cleveland Clinic Foundation Research Institute, Department of Musculoskeletal Research (Wb-3), 9500 Euclid Avenue, Cleveland, OH 44195, USA

Alison M. McLaren Department of Orthopaedics, Columbia University, New York, NY, USA

Frank Meyer Arthritis Research Unit, Ichilov Hospital, Tel Aviv, Israel

James F.S. Middleton Strangeways Research Laboratory, Worts Causeway, Cambridge CN1 4RN, UK

Joseph Mizrahi Department of Biomedical Engineering, Technion — Israel Institute of Technology, Haifa 32000, Israel

Teresa I. Morales Bone Research Branch, National Institute of Dental Research, National Institutes of Health, Bethesda, MD 20892, USA

Keith Morgan Departments of Biochemistry and Molecular Biology, University of Manchester Medical School, Manchester M13 9PT, UK

J.S. Mort Joint Diseases Laboratory, Shriners Hospital, 1529 Cedar Avenue Montreal, QC H3G 1A6, Canada

A. Paul Mould Departments of Biochemistry and Molecular Biology, University of Manchester Medical School, Manchester M13 9PT, UK

Helen Muir Kennedy Institute of Rheumatology, Bute Gardens, Hammersmith, London W6 7DW, UK

Francisco J. Müller Arthritis Division, School of Medicine, University of Miami, Veterans Administration Medical Center, Miami, Florida, USA

William H. Murphy Department of Biochemistry, Monash University, Clayton, Victoria 3168, Australia

Zvi Nevo Department of Chemical Pathology, Sackler School of Medicine, Tel Aviv University, Tel Aviv 69978, Israel

Chee Keng Ng Department of Biochemistry, Monash University, Clayton, Victoria 3168, Australia

Q. Nguyen Joint Diseases Laboratory, Shriners Hospital, 1529 Cedar Avenue, Montreal, QC, H3G 1A6 Canada

C. Niyibizi Orthopaedic Research Laboratories, University of Washington, Seattle, WA 98195, USA

K. Oates Department of Biological Sciences, University of Lancaster, Lancaster LA1 4YR, UK

Theodore, Oegema University of Minnesota, Department of Orthopaedic Surgery and Biochemistry, Box 310 UMHC, 420 Delaware Street, SE Minneapolis, MN 55455, USA

Lori Otten Department of Biochemistry, Rush-Presbyterian-St. Luke's Medical Center, 1653 West Congress Parkway, Chicago, IL 60612, USA

K.H. Parker Physiological Flow Studies Unit, Imperial College, Prince Consort Road, London, SW7 2AZ, UK

Richard Pearce Department of Pathology, University of British Columbia, Vancouver, BC, Canada

J.G. Pidd Department of Pathology, University of Manchester Medical School, Stopford Building, Manchester M13 9PT, UK

Julio C. Pita Arthritis Division, Department of Medicine, University of Miami, P.O. Box 016960, Miami, FL 35101, USA

Anna Plaas Orthopaedic Research Laboratories, Shriners Hospital for Crippled Children, Tampa Unit, 12502 North Pine Drive, Tampa, FL 33612–9499, USA

C. Anthony Poole Department of Surgery, University of Auckland, Private Bag, Auckland 1, New Zealand

Barry N. Preston Department of Biochemistry, Monash University, Clayton, Victoria 3168, Australia

Kenneth Pritzker Connective Tissue Research Group, Mount Sinai Hospital, Room 609, 600 University Avenue, Toronto, Ontario M5G 1X5, Canada

Anthony Ratcliffe Head of Biochemistry Section, Orthopaedic Research Laboratory, Columbia University, 630 West 168th Street, Balck Building, Room 1412, New York, NY 10032, USA

Sally Roberts Charles Salt Research Centre, Robert Jones & Agnes Hunt Orthopaedic Hospital, Oswestry, Shropshire 8710 0AH, UK

Simon Robins Rowett Research Institute, Greenburn Road, Bucksburn, Aberdeen AB2 98B, UK

Dror Robinson Department of Orthopaedic Surgery, Assaf Harofeh Medical Center, Haamoraim Street 13, Tel Aviv 69207, Israel

Marie-Claire Ronziere Experimental Histology Laboratory, Claude Bernard University, 69622 Villeurbanne Cedex, France

P.J. Roughley Joint Diseases Laboratory, Shriners Hospital, 1529 Cedar Avenue, Montreal, QC H3G 1A6 Canada

F. Saed-Nejad Orthopaedic Research Laboratory, Columbia University, New York, NY 10032, USA

Robert L.Y. Sah Continuum Electromechanics Group, Laboratory for Electromagnetic and Electronic Systems, Department of Electrical Engineering and Computer Science, Massachusetts Institute of Technology, Cambridge, MA 02139, USA

Antonietta Salustri Department of Sanita Pubblica e Biologia Cellulare, Faculty of Medicine, 2nd University of Rome, via O. Raimondo, Rome, Italy

John David Sandy Shriners Hospital for Crippled Children, Tampa Unit, 12502 North Pine Drive, Tampa, FL 33612–9499, USA

Y. Sawyer Strangeways Research Laboratory, Worts' Causeway, Cambridge CB1 4RN, UK

Rosa Schneiderman Department of Orthopaedics, State University of New York at Stony Brook, Stony Brook, New York 11794-8181, USA

Thomas J. Schnitzer Department of Medicine, Rush-Presbyterian-St. Luke's Medical Centre, 1653 West Congress Parkway, Chicago, IL 60612, USA

Barbara L. Schumacher Department of Biochemistry, Rush Medical College, Rush-Presbyterian-St. Luke's Medical Center, 1653 West Congress Parkway, Chicago, IL 60612, USA

M.J. Seibel Orthopaedic Research Laboratory, Columbia University, New York, NY 10032, USA

Alexander Silberberg Polymers Department, Weizmann Institute of Science, Rehovot 76100, Israel

Ritta Stanescu Inserm Unite de Recherches de Genetique Medicale, Hopital des Enfants Malades (UIZ), 149 Rue de Sevres, Paris 75015, France

Victor Stanescu Inserm Unite de Recherches de Genetique Medicale, Hopital des Enfants Malades (UIZ), 149 Rue de Sevres, Paris 75015, France

Robin A. Stockwell Department of Anatomy, University of Edinburgh, Medical School, Teviot Place, Edinburgh EH8 9AG, UK

M. Barry Sweet Department of Orthopaedic Surgery, Witwatersrand University, Johannesburg, South Africa

Marvin Tanzer Department of Biostructure and Function, University of Connecticut Health Center, Farmington, CT 06032, USA

Sophie Thenet Laboratoire de Pharmacologie Cellulaire de l'EPHE, 15 rue de l'Ecole de Medecine, 75006 Paris, France

R.C. Thompson Jr. Departments of Orthopaedic Surgery and Biochemistry, University of Minnesota, Box 310 UMHC, 420 Delaware Street, SE, Minneapolis, MN 55455, USA

Eugene J.M.A. Thonar Department of Biochemistry and Medicine, Rush-Presbyterian-St. Luke's Medical Center, 1647 Highland, Berwyn, IL 60402, USA

Peter A. Torzilli Department of Biomechanics, Hospital for Special Surgery, 535 East 70th Street, New York, NY 10021, USA

Jenny Tyler Strangeways Research Laboratory, Worts Causeway, Cambridge CB1 4RN, UK

Jill P.G. Urban University Laboratory of Physiology, Oxford University, Oxford OX1 3PT, UK

Marie-Paule I. Van Damme Department of Biochemistry, Monash University, Clayton, Victoria 3168, Australia

Michael Van der Rest Institut de Biologie et Chimie des Proteines, CNRS UPR 412, Cytologie Moleculaire, Universite Claude Bernard, 43 Boulevard du 11 Novembre 1918, 69622 Villeurbanne Cedex, France

Ellen Wachtel Polymers Department, Weizmann Institute of Science, P.O. Box 26, Rehovot 76100, Israel

Claude Weinberg Department of Biomedical engineering, Technion — Israel Insitute of Technology, Haifa 32000, Israel

Charles P. Winlove Imperial College, Physiological Flow Studies Unit, Prince Consort Road, London, SW7, UK

James Williams Departments of Biochemistry, Anatomy and Medicine, Rush-Presbyterian-St. Luke's Medical Center, 1653 West Congress Parkway, Chicago, IL 60612, USA

J.J. Wu Orthopaedic Research Laboratories, University of Washington, Seattle, WA 98195, USA

Masaki Yanagishita Bone Research Branch, National Institute of Dental Research, The National Institutes of Health, Bethesda, MD 20892, USA

Preface

The studies of joints and the spine form a major part of the research into the musculo-skeletal system and are par excellence an interdisciplinary endeavor. It is now generally accepted that the interactions between the physicochemical, biochemical and cellular elements lie at the basis of the intricate function of cartilaginous tissues, and that a disturbance in the balance between these constituents is likely to play a major part in the pathogenesis of degenerative diseases. Indeed, the fact that articular cartilage and the intervertebral disc are primarily involved in two major degenerative diseases, viz. osteoarthritis and low-back pain, has undoubtedly given impetus to cartilage research over the recent years. Furthermore, the relevance of cartilage research to the understanding of other connective tissues has stimulated more general interest in these areas. The net result has been a remarkable expansion in the whole field of cartilage research. This can be illustrated, for instance, by the fact that, whilst in 1969 there had been some 40 publications dealing with articular cartilage, in 1989 the number rose to more than 200.

This rapid growth has been accompanied by a parallel increase in the numbers and the diversity of the methods being used. In addition to the more classical methodologies which have been painstakingly developed over the years, new procedures are being introduced through interactions of different disciplines. Also new expertises have entered the field, bringing with them entirely new techniques. We thus felt that the time was ripe for assembling the various methodologies in a single volume which, on the one hand, would reflect the sophistication of each aspect of the field, and, on the other hand, would be written so as to be comprehensible to investigators from other disciplines. Different approaches are described, compared, discussed and assessed: our aim is to show the researcher various choices and possibilities and to discuss the appropriateness of the different experimental designs, without ignoring their inherent shortcomings, limitations and difficulties.

The book is made up of thirteen sections, each dealing with a different methodology. Each section starts with an overview by the main author, who has wide expertise in the field. The overview is followed by short chapters dealing with specific topics within the general area of the section. Throughout the book the main authors worked in close concert with the editors. A special effort was made to show the multiple connections between methodologies in different areas by providing frequent cross-references. A comprehensive bibliography was compiled, including titles, in order to facilitate its use.

One of the first and major problems confronting the researcher in the cartilage field is the selection of experimental material and its characterization. Since so many variables are involved, it is essential to describe precisely the type of sample one is handling and to have objective criteria for its characterization. Otherwise, no matter how sensitive and precise the methods of analysis or testing, few objectively valid and communicable results will be derived and the old saying '*quod duo faciunt idem non est idem*' will often be the only significant conclusion of the research. Because of this, it was felt that the first section of the book should deal in depth with the problems of sample selection, classification and preservation, as well as with the broader question of communication between scientists.

Once one has a 'macroscopically' well defined specimen in hand one can proceed to characterize it biochemically. Section 2 deals with the procedure for the extraction and separation of collagens and proteoglycan components, a major concern being to preserve as far as possible their native polymeric structure and in situ composition.

Section 3 describes modern morphological techniques for elucidating cartilage structure, with special reference to the study of the articular surface, the collagen fibril organization and the chondrocytes and their immediate environment.

The subject of the next three sections is the chondrocyte and its metabolism. Section 4 is concerned with the isolated chondrocyte and deals with different methods of culture and their special features, discussing their advantages and limitations, as well as their fields of application.

Section 5 deals with explant culture of tissue segments, both short- and long-term, with special reference to the procedures for the study of matrix synthesis and degradation. Techniques for investigating the effects of extracellular factors, be they biochemical (e.g. hormones) or mechanical, are also included. A separate chapter is devoted to the special problems encountered during the handling and culture of the intervertebral disc.

Since most of the studies of the metabolism of cartilage macromolecules rely on the use of radioisotopes, mostly as metabolic precursors, Section 6 is entirely devoted to such methods, dealing with various aspects of both *in vivo* and *in vitro* studies in relation to both proteoglycans and collagen.

Section 7 explores the area of immunochemistry applied to cartilage, an area which has immensely expanded over the last few years. Various immunochemical techniques used for the characterization of cartilage proteoglycans are described; procedures for the production and characterization of monoclonal antibodies to the proteoglycans are given, as well as those involved in the characterization and use of polyclonal antibodies to collagen. In view of the major interest in detecting traces of cartilage-derived substances in body fluids as a measure of cartilage damage in joint disease, immunoassays for detecting keratan sulfate epitopes are described and discussed.

Section 8 explores the possibility of using various contemporary molecular biological approaches to the study of cartilage matrix and provides a sample of some of the applications of recombinant DNA technology and molecular biology to the study of cartilage.

Section 9 deals with the quantiative aspects of cartilage composition, and discusses the different ways in which the concentrations of consituents can be expressed, with special reference to the tissue's organization, functional properties and metabolism. Various methods for studying tissue organization and for distinguishing between the roles of the different components are also described. As in Section 1, one of the aims of this section is to explore the use of an appropriate 'common language' for investigators in the field of cartilage — this time in a quantitative, rather than a qualitative sense.

Solute transport (Section 10) is not only involved in a fundamental manner in most of the physiological processes, such as cellular nutrition, metabolism and matrix turnover, but it also plays an important — though often unrecognized — part in many of the experimental methods used throughout the cartilage field, from extraction procedures to immunochemical techniques. The general principles governing solute transport and the standard procedures for measuring transport parameters are reviewed. In addition, some of the more recent and more specialized techniques are described.

The main purpose of articular cartilage and the intervertebral disc is load-bearing and both these tissues are characterized by a number of material properties (physicochemical, mechanical and electromechanical) which make them eminently suitable to fulfill this role. In Section 11 recent developments in measuring some of these properties are described and compared. Since understanding how a joint functions requires, in addition, a knowledge of the pressure distribution at the cartilage surface, this aspect of methodology is also included, with particular reference to the hip joint.

The book ends with two sections, relevant to physiological processes. Section 12 deals with the processes of cartilage repair, under what circumstances and to what extent they can take place, and if and how they can be controlled and stimulated. Current experimental and clinical approaches are described, and some hypotheses as to the basic mechanisms involved are also discussed.

Section 13 concentrates on the discussion of the utilization of different degradation products of joint cartilage matrix detectable in body fluids — synovial fluid, serum and urine — as markers of cartilage metabolism and disease processes. The use of proteoglycan components detectected in synovial fluid, keratan sulfate in serum and pyridinoline in urine as markers is described and discussed.

The chapters in this book do not purport to provide a comprehensive record of all the existing procedures. They do, however, seek to present a balanced selection of the methodologies available across the whole spectrum of cartilage research, from biophysics and biomechanics to classic biochemistry and molecular biology, with special emphasis on areas which are common to all the disciplines. We trust that the book will not only help the researcher to be aware of the wide range of existing methods, but will also enable him or her to avoid artifacts and to ensure that the techniques he or she uses are objectively valid, up to date and correctly applied for the purposes intended. This will, hopefully, lead to a more efficient use of research time and resources.

Finally, we hope that one of the outcomes of the book will be the emergence of new, testable hypotheses and fresh research directions which may eventually provide some answers to the fundamental problems of cartilage physiology, disease and repair.

Our gratitude is extended to the Technion — Israel Institute of Technology, and in particular to the Julius Silver Institute of Biomedical Engineering in Haifa, and to Rush Medical College at Rush-Presbyterian-St. Luke's Medical Center in Chicago for their unstinting cooperation and support throughout this endeavor.

We wish to thank Jennifer Thonar for her very efficient help in copy editing. Last, but not least, Alice Maroudas wishes to extend her deepest appreciation to her secretary, Cecily Hyams, for her most capable assistance in all the aspects and at all the stages of planning and editing the present book.

ALICE MAROUDAS AND KLAUS KUETTNER

Introduction

The idea for this book arose as a result of an international seminar — The Bat Sheva Seminar on Methods Used in Research on Cartilaginous Tissues — which was held in Israel in March 1989.

This was the first conference ever to be devoted entirely to methodology developed and used in cartilage research. We felt that in this interdisciplinary field, with its multiplicity of methods, there has been too little attempt in the past at any in-depth discussion of the experimental techniques and associated problems. We thus thought that the time was ripe for getting together in order to exchange views about procedures in an informal workshop environment. Our aim was to assemble at the Seminar the experts who had developed the existing procedures, as well as the colleagues who are applying them now and will modify them later.

We were fortunate to obtain for the Seminar the sponsorship of the Bat-Sheva de Rothschild Foundation for the Advancement of Science in Israel. We were also helped by a number of generous contributions from various organizations.

Because communication between scientists is of such vital importance and because the Meeting took place in the Holy Land, we chose the Tower of Babel as the emblem for our Seminar, with the following quotation from the Bible.

> And the Lord said, Behold, the people is one, and they have all one language; and this they begin to do: and now nothing will be restrained from them, which they have imagined to do.
>
> Genesis XI, 6

The Seminar opening took place in Jerusalem, but the main scientific program was held at Nof Ginossar, a kibbutz on the northern shores of the Sea of Galilee. The Seminar closed in Herzliya, a seaside resort in central Israel. Apart from the scientific program, visits were organised to various sites to give all participants a taste of the rich history of Israel and its natural beauty.

The scientific program consisted of sixteen sessions, spanning more or less the same area of cartilage research as has been covered in this book. The emphasis of the whole meeting was on discussion; however, each session started with a 15 minute formal overview by the 'Discussion Leader', in which the overall goals, approaches and methods, as well as the problems associated with them, were presented. The invited members of the 'Session Panel' then gave a brief summary and evaluation of their methods, comparing them with related techniques. These brief presentations laid the framework for extensive general discussion. In addition, each participant was invited to exhibit a poster containing the description of a specific technique, illustrative results and a critical appraisal. The standard of the posters was very high and endless deliberations took place in front of them, accompanied by cool drinks at all times of day and night.

The formal sessions were held during the mornings and the evenings. The participants had the afternoons free for informal discussions whilst exploring the Galilee or strolling along the lovely gardens of the kibbutz and the neighbouring fields, filled with wild flowers and the scent of orange blossom. The distinctive mark of the Seminar was an exceptionally friendly, relaxed and uncompetitive atmosphere. Old channels of communication amongst many participants were revived and many new ones were formed.

Many participants have said that the Seminar consitutes an important precedent and that too much time should not elapse before another one is held. We do indeed hope that the Bat Sheva Seminar was the first step in promoting future efforts by the international research community at reviewing regularly the methodology being developed in cartilage research.

We are very happy to be able to offer this book as a brainchild of the Seminar and wish particularly to thank Academic Press for their enthusiastic and efficient help in bringing the book into the world.

We wish to thank the Discussion Leaders for taking upon themselves the task of compiling and organizing the different sections of the book. Without their hard work this book would not have been possible.

Our gratitude is extended to the Bat-Sheva de Rothschild Foundation for the Advancement of Science in Israel for their sponsorship of the Meeting and to the following organizations for their generous contributions: Carl Zeiss, FRG, Ciba-Geigy Corporation, USA, EI Du Pont Nemours & Company, USA, Eldan Electronic Instrument Co. Ltd., Israel, Glaxco Inc., USA, Hoechst AG. Aktiengesellschaft, FRG, ICI Pharmaceuticals Group, UK, Ministry of Health, Israel, Lilly Research Laboratories, USA, Merck Sharp & Dohme Research Laboratories, USA, Miles Inc., USA, Natterman & Cie GmbH, FRG, Pfizer Laboratories Division, USA, Rhone-Poulenc Sante, France, Robapharm AG, Switzerland, Roussel UCLAF, France, Schering-Plough Corporation, USA, Searle Research & Development, USA, Syntex Laboratories Inc., USA, The Technion — Israel Institute of Technology, Israel, Teva Pharmaceuticals Industries, Israel.

We also wish to thank the members of the local Organizing Committee — Frank Meyer, Joe Mizrahi, Menachem Nahir, Zvi Nevo and Israel Ziv — as well as members of the Technion Cartilage Research Laboratory for their invaluable cooperation and assistance, both before and during the Meeting.

Special thanks are due to Pat Bridges, Shirin and Yaakov Scheimann, Cecily Hyams and Dalia Zalmon for their tireless help in preparing the Meeting, and especially to Shirin and Yaakov for their unstinting assistance to participants with all their problems at the Meeting, and for helping in the organization of the extensive social program.

ALICE MAROUDAS AND KLAUS KUETTNER

1

SAMPLING, CHARACTERIZATION AND HANDLING *EX VIVO* OF TISSUE SPECIMENS

COLLATED BY M.T. BAYLISS

1

Overview

M.T. BAYLISS

Genesis II,
Chapter XI, Verses 1–9

[1] And the whole earth was of one language, and of one speech.

[2] And it came to pass, as they journeyed from the east, that they found a plain in the land of Shinar; and they dwelt there.

[3] And they said one to another, go to, let us make brick, and burn them throughly. And they had brick for stone, and slime had they for morter.

[4] And they said, go to, let us build us a city and a tower, whose top may reach unto heaven; and let us make us a name, lest we be scattered abroad upon the face of the whole earth.

[5] And the lord came down to see the city and the tower, which the children of men builded.

[6] And the lord said, Behold, the people is one, and they have all one language; and this they begin to do: and now nothing will be restrained from them, which they have imagined to do.

[7] Go to. Let us go down. And there confound their language, that they may not understand one another's speech.

[8] So the Lord scattered them abroad from thence upon the face of all the earth: and they left off to build the city.

[9] Therefore, is the name of it called babel; because the Lord did there confound the language of all the earth: and from thence did the Lord scatter them abroad upon the face of all the earth.

A friend of mine has a theory that the Tower of Babel story is not really about man's presumption, as one usually thinks, but is far more to do with God's feeling threatened and fearing what mankind might achieve if it practiced mutual cooperation. Indeed, a cursory glance at the relevant passage in Genesis bears this out; 'And they said, Go to, let us build us a city and a tower, whose top may reach unto heaven; and let us make us a name, lest we be scattered abroad upon the face of the whole earth.' The motives of the builders seem fairly unexceptional and will be familiar to any scientist: Noah's descendants wanted to achieve something that had never been done before and, less nobly perhaps, they sought recognition.

Everyone will be familiar with the punishment of course — God decided to, 'confound their language, that they may not understand one another's speech', but the reasoning behind this punishment is perhaps less well known. God fears that if they have one language, 'nothing will be restrained from them which they have imagined to do'. The words I should like to focus on in this introduction are 'one language' and 'imagined'. To start with 'imagined': Einstein tells us that 'imagination is more important than knowledge' and certainly we all exercise our imaginations as well as rigorous scientific method in our work; it is this link, between vision and method, which I shall be considering. The 'language' that we share is science. We assume that when we talk about our work we understand each other. Like the old inhabitants of Shinar, we hope that by sharing our knowledge and speaking the same language we shall make scientific progress — metaphorically, we shall build a tower of knowledge.

Having put this introduction rather fancifully into a religio-scientific context, I should like to move on to the difficulties that God has placed in the path of the modern tower builder/scientist and one of these (only at the level of finding the right consistency of mortar — let us not be too presumptuous) is to develop a common language for methods used in research on cartilaginous tissues. Since it is impossible to cover every aspect in this review, I shall limit myself to discussing a few aspects which I personally find interesting and I shall illustrate these with the tissue with which I am most familiar, but that is not to say that my remarks may not apply equally to other sources of tissue.

The problem confronting the ancient people of Shinar prompted a consideration of our own problems. My title, 'Sampling, characterization and handling *ex vivo* of tissue specimens', seemed fairly obvious at first glance, for surely everybody takes these factors into account when designing their experimental protocol, but a little personal soul-searching forced me to admit that there had been occasions when I had accepted less than the best and used tissue that did not necessarily fit the stringent criteria one hopes to set oneself. There are usually very good reasons for this. For example, most of my work is concerned with the biosynthesis of matrix components in human articular cartilage and I always measure the rate of proteoglycan (PG) synthesis on a representative piece of cartilage from the specimen (within 1–2 h of operation), regardless of the experiment, and I use this value as a measure of tissue well-being. I look to see if the rate is within the range I expect for that age based on the extensive analysis of the samples I have accumulated over the years. However, there are occasions when I wait for an amputation and, for one reason or another, I receive it late in the day. I cannot drive back to Hammersmith to start the experiment, so I put the tissue into culture overnight at source, collect it the next morning and start the experiment approximately 16 h after the operation. It is important to remember that by the time I calculate a rate of PG synthesis the experiment is well under way, and often complete, with all the time and money (isotopes) committed to it. So I am under great psychological and economic pressure to accept the results, especially if they confirm my starting hypothesis. If the rate of synthesis is acceptable, I use the tissue and subsequent experimental results! Am I correct in doing this? Is ^{35}[S]sulfate incorporation the correct marker to use to assess how the tissue has survived its ordeal? Should I be using some other criteria as well and, if so, what? This is really no trivial matter and the principle is an important one, especially in trying to compare results from different laboratories. In other words, to go back to the opening analogy, has my 'language' changed without my realizing it and how does it now compare with that of other laboratories? For example, I am now very reluctant to use postmortem tissue for my work unless I can get it within 18–24 h of death, even though in the past I have analyzed a number of specimens 4–5 days after death and obtained respectable rates of PG synthesis. You may wonder what the arbitrary time of 18–24 h is based on. What makes tissue obtained within this period any better than that obtained 36 h or 48 h after death? Well, I do not have an answer to that, other than to say that it is the earliest possible time I can get the tissue and I am convinced this is often the main factor constraining most people who use postmortem material. If they cannot get tissue within 24 h, they raise their time limit to 36 or 48 h. I am not saying that I think postmortem tissue should not be used for metabolic studies, rather that the influence of time after death has not been investigated as fully as it might have been and may significantly affect results.

As an example, I have been singularly unsuccessful in getting interleukin-1 to stimulate degradation of fresh human articular cartilage, although it will inhibit PG synthesis very rapidly and effectively. Yet, I know of a number of studies that have demonstrated degradation and release of PG. These have all been carried out on postmortem tissue of unknown or varying times after death! This problem of timing is even more pertinent when it comes to handling the intervertebral disc, which, if anything, seems to be even more sensitive to *ex vivo* handling, both in terms of storage and cutting; the argument applies equally well to animal tissue obtained from abattoirs.

We should also remember that those of us who study the biochemistry and biomechanical properties of these tissues do not apply anything like the stringent conditions upon which a morphologist would insist. I am sure there would be no question of Dugald Gardner or Ernst Hunziker accepting the postmortem or late operative tissue that I have described for their studies. I think it is extremely important for us to remember that even if it were impractical for us to apply the same criteria to biochemical and biomechanical studies, we should be aware that *ex vivo* tissue becomes abnormal very rapidly.

Now we come to the selection of tissue in studies comparing normal and pathological cartilage. What do we mean by normal? I have written about that topic to some extent already, but I am more concerned with what we consider to be an acceptable 'control'. For example, it has been common practice in the past, when studying osteoarthritic hips, to use fractured neck of femur cartilage as the control, and many characteristics of this cartilage do compare favorably with fresh normal amputation tissue of this age. However, the only extensive study that I know of is that by Roberts *et al.* (1986) who found considerable differences in the biochemical and biomechanical properties of this cartilage. It is, after all, a pathological tissue and of an older age group than most osteoarthritics. But, is it any less acceptable as a control than fresh postmortem hips which are the only other readily available source of cartilage of the same age? A similar problem arises with animal models. There are three possibilities. One may use the non-operated joint of the animal as the control; 'normal' tissue (whatever one considers that to be) from the operated joint; or even normal cartilage from different sites within the same or different animals. Each has its advantages and disadvantages, depending on the particular model and animal.

Selection of diseased cartilage is even more of a problem. For instance many of the laboratories that I am familiar with select their specimens of human cartilage on the basis of whether the jar they receive from the operating theater has osteoarthritis or rheumatoid arthritis written on it. At best, they will look at the patient's notes, but these are notoriously unreliable. The very best will collaborate with the resident rheumatologist and in that way try to make some correlation between clinical and laboratory findings. But which clinical data and which laboratory data should we use to enable us to assess the stage of the disease? Are we being naive in expecting criteria based on totally different measurements and evaluations to show a correlation? And, if they do, are the correlations worth anything? Surely it is better to accept that these are specimens from the end of the disease and as such reflect a common end result of different primary events. I think that it would be very presumptuous to assume that data obtained from analysis of this cartilage will help to define the etiological factors relating to individual specimens. Furthermore, how do we decide which tissue to take? At least with animal models we have the advantage of knowing where the lesion will develop. We cannot wait for a histological evaluation and I am not sure that would be the most valuable marker anyway. So how do people choose their tissue? And once it has been chosen, how representative is it of the diseased cartilage? A histological and biochemical examination of multiple sites from a single resected femoral head will give as many, if not more, different analyses as an examination of single samples from a large number of joints and, in any case, do we have to worry about this morphological and biochemical variability? Can we not just overcome it by pooling and randomizing the tissue, or would that procedure introduce further problems and mask important changes?

There are two other aspects of choosing tissue that apply equally to both normal and diseased cartilage and to both human and animal studies. First, site variations. We know that there is considerable variation in the biochemical and metabolic properties of cartilage, depending on the area of the joint surface that is sampled. This must be a potential source of error given the focal loss of cartilage that is characteristic of osteoarthritis. Second, zonal variation. To my mind, this is the most important single factor that could influence any comparison of normal and diseased cartilage. There is no point in comparing full-thickness normal cartilage with partial-thickness diseased cartilage even from a comparable site (see Chapter 4). However, site and zonal variations generate only minor problems in articular cartilage compared with the nightmare they impose on any analysis of intervertebral disc. In an adult, what is normal disc tissue? Which piece of 'crabmeat' should one choose? When it comes to classifying disc syndromes, we are just as badly, if not worse, off than we are with our attempts at clinical classification of articular cartilage pathology.

I could continue to highlight areas where we seem to be discussing the same thing, but owing to inevitable constraints on our selection criteria, we are, in fact, in a Tower of Babel, and these 'language' differences are only one aspect of our problems in the sampling, characterization and handling *ex vivo* of tissue specimens. Other factors do need to be discussed and what follows is a valuable compilation of various contributions which consider a variety of approaches to this issue.

2

Articular cartilage samples

D.L. GARDNER

This paper defines some of the desirable criteria to be considered when specimens of hyaline articular cartilage are required for biological, biochemical or biomechanical testing. The properties of hyaline cartilage that dictate the character of selection and collection techniques are widely known (Gardner, 1990) and sequences of preferred methods for the preparation of cartilage have been described (Gardner *et al.*, 1987).

HISTORY

It is only too easy to omit critical aspects of the information that should accompany all selection procedures. It is necessary to record the clinical, social and dietary history of human and animal subjects from whom cartilage has been collected and a note of the physical activity of the donor is also highly relevant. The precise identity, quantity and duration of all forms of therapy require documentation. It is essential that species, age, sex and stature are recorded.

ANATOMICAL ASPECTS

Hyaline articular cartilage is highly non-homogeneous. A minimum requirement in controlled studies is to define the identity and laterality of the joint to be dissected. The region, area and zone from which samples will be taken are verified. There are large anatomical differences between the many bearing surfaces of the 187 synovial joints of the average adult human. In a single joint surface such as that of the medial tibial condyle, there are corresponding variations in microscopic structure and in macromolecular composition between *regions* (parts designated in the sagittal plane), *areas* (parts designated in the coronal plane), and *zones* (parts defined in a plane perpendicular to the bearing surface), (Stockwell, 1979).

ASEPSIS

Cartilage is subject to bacterial degradation (putrefaction) just as it is to autolysis. Many collection procedures must therefore be carried out under the same conditions of surgical asepsis as those used in tissue culture. Articular cartilage is tolerant of low oxygen partial pressures: individual chondrocytes remain alive long after clinical death, but autolysis ultimately prevails. The ambient temperature influences the rate of autolysis but, in human cartilage studies, there is seldom opportunity for determining core temperatures in joints. It is therefore desirable to work with material obtained within 3 h of cessation of circulation. In experiments based on retrieving human surgical material, it is relevant to note that orthopedic surgeons often apply a tourniquet to a limb before amputation. When tissue from such limbs is to form the basis of a chemical or mechanical experiment, it is necessary to remember that the total time (t_a) between ischemia (a time approximating to onset of autolysis) is the surgical tourniquet time (t_s) *plus* the time taken to transport tissue to the laboratory and to effect its efficient freezing or preservation (t_p). The total time (t_a) may be in excess of 3 h.

DISSECTION

Like all biological tissues, cartilage is sensitive to distortion. The abnormal pressures caused by handling and cutting create artifact and may prejudice or invalidate some microscopic tests. Gentle dissection, the avoidance of forceps and the use of very sharp instruments with large, plane cutting surfaces are desirable.

HYDRATION

The most important physiological and mechanical properties of hyaline articular cartilage depend upon the retention in this tissue of normal water content and distribution. Ideally, therefore, specimens required for culture, for metabolic study, for chemical analysis or for physical tests should remain fully hydrated (Figure 2.1). Large specimens retain water for long periods and human hip joint *postmortem* tissue, stored at 4°C, displays no measurable change in proteoglycan (PG) concentration over 48 h. Small samples are quickly prejudiced by their high surface area : volume ratio. The rate of water loss by evaporation, which may be extremely rapid in microscopic samples, is influenced by both the ambient temperature and by atmospheric humidity. Studies by techniques such as low-temperature scanning electron microscropy (Lawton *et al.*, 1989) demand the retention of ≥99% normal tissue water in very small specimens. To achieve this aim, it has proved necessary to construct a hydration chamber within the artificially humidified atmosphere in which joints can be opened and cartilage blocks prepared. The dissected samples are then transferred to a culture medium or quenched in a liquid such as nitrogen slush ($-210°C$) in vessels positioned within the hydration chamber.

CONCLUSIONS

In most cartilage studies, the race, species, age, sex, stature and therapeutic profile of the source individual/animal should be defined and samples, selected from laterally identified joints, taken from demarcated regions, areas and zones by very sharp, plane blades. In many circumstances, collection under conditions of surgical asepsis is desirable. Small samples quickly lose water by evaporation at ambient temperatures. The

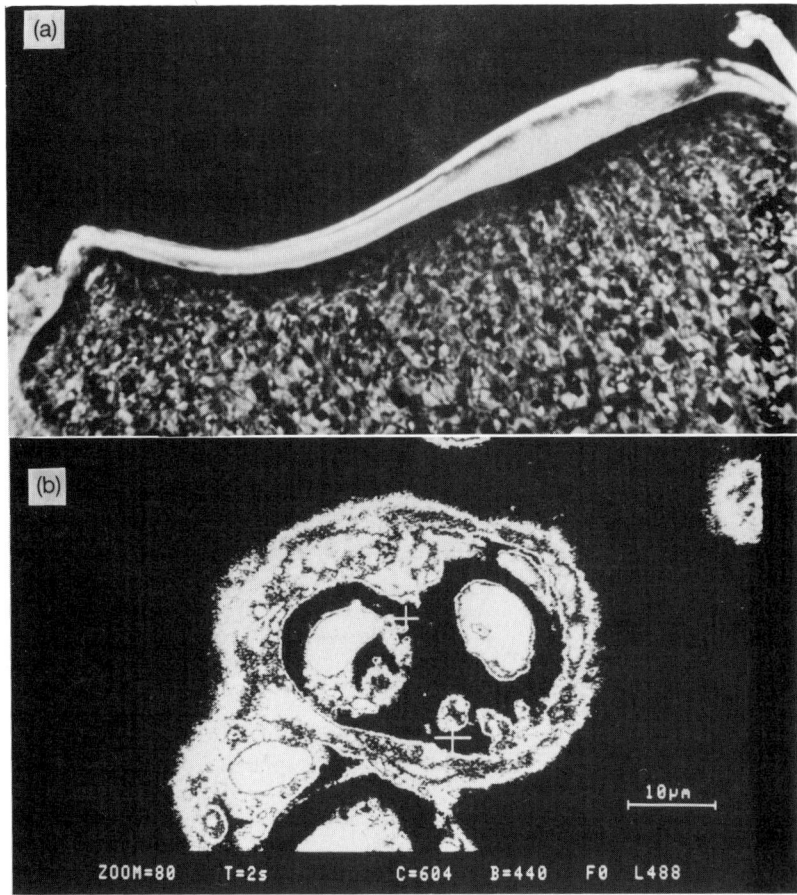

Figure 2.1 (a) Hydrated, unfixed articular cartilage: dog tibial condyle. A circular, diamond-edged saw has been used to cut a 200 μm thick slice of upper end of tibia from dog. Viewed without staining, in plane-polarized light, slice displays varied thickness of hyaline cartilage and non-homogeneity of structure. Darker and lighter parts correspond approximately to orientation of collagen fiber bundles. Divided anterior cruciate ligament lies top right. (b) Chondrons in hydrated, unfixed human tibial condylar cartilage. Slice of hyaline cartilage, cut tangential to bearing surface, is viewed in a c. 1 μm thick optical plane 'cut' by confocal scanning fluorescence microscopy (Gardner et al., 1990). Two chondrocytes, each c. 12 μm in diameter and each with a single ovoid nucleus, lie within a lacuna in which they are surrounded by (black) pericellular matrix. The lacuna is outlined by its thin (white) pericellular capsule (Poole et al., 1988). The paired cells and their pericellular matrix constitute a 'double chondron'. Another chondron is transected at the bottom of the figure. Both chondrons are surrounded by a territorial matrix, the rim or 'border zone' (Stockwell, 1979) of which is the inner edge of the black background which forms the remainder of the confocal image.

collection of very small pieces of tissue is, therefore, best accomplished in an artificially humidified atmosphere. After dissection, the prepared blocks or slices are immediately placed in a sterile culture medium or quenched in a low-temperature liquid or gas.

ACKNOWLEDGMENTS

The support of the Arthritis and Rheumatism Council for Research and of the Scottish Home and Health Department is gratefully acknowledged.

3

Selection and classification of human articular cartilage

T.R. OEGEMA

Animal models have given new insight into the early changes in cartilage associated with degenerative joint disease. However, there is a continuing need to analyze normal and osteoarthritic human cartilage, especially to correlate this data with the changes seen in animal models and also to obtain end-stage tissue that is frequently not available in the models. The ability to interpret the results obtained from such tissues is often limited by inadequate knowledge of the histology of the samples. There is also a need to classify adequately the tissues so that the results can be compared among laboratories or within the same laboratory over time. Unified cartilage classification would allow comparison of tissues with similar pathology. The protocol for tissue collection and classification and the collection of patient data should be agreed upon in advance so that information can be readily exchanged between the orthopedic surgeon, biochemist, biomechanical engineer, histologist and pathologist. *Pro forma* should be standardized and three concise areas need to be addressed: (i) patient history, (ii) anatomical location, and (iii) cartilage morphology. Since human-derived tissue can be obtained under a wide variety of circumstances, including at autopsy or from the operating room, it is advantageous to have a previously prepared checklist available.

PATIENTS' RECORDS

Although patients' records will be later coded to provide confidentiality, the initial record should contain the patient's name, hospital number, clinical diagnosis, clinical stage of disease (especially duration and presence or absence of an inflammatory component), age, sex and any mechanical alteration of the joint. The chart should also document relevant drug usage. Drugs that should be specifically examined include nonsteroidal anti-inflammatory drugs, where the generic name of the drug should be noted since recent studies have shown that nonsteroidals may exhibit drug-specific effects on cartilage metabolism. Recording past treatment with interarticular injections of steroids is also important and for postmenopausal women it is particularly important to know if they are on supplementary estrogen or estrogen–progesterone regimens. It should also be determined whether the patient has undergone chemotherapy or received radiation to the joint. The latter two are particularly relevant because many 'controls' available from the operating room are from amputations for distal tumors. In the case of samples derived from postmortem, it is much more difficult to evaluate these key factors, but as much information as practical should be obtained. There is a wide variety of currently marketed database systems that would allow this information to be cataloged in a form easily retrievable for correlation with results of the histological, biochemical or biomechanical analyses.

ANATOMICAL LOCATION

It is convenient to use an anatomical sketch so that the position of the samples collected in the operating room or at the time of autopsy can be marked anatomically. Photographs of the joints before and after sample removal are useful. Furthermore, the need to document location is vital since the position within the joint has been shown to play a key role in determining many of the metabolic parameters of normal tissues and it is also suspected that it has a role in osteoarthritic (OA) tissues.

TISSUE CLASSIFICATION

Classification of cartilage can play a key role in the interpretation of results and in establishing correlations among groups of samples, among patients, among samples from the same patient and between human and animal disease. The simplest and most useful classification, because it involves the least amount of work, is the definition of surface integrity and the degree of fibrillation (Freeman and Meachim, 1979). In this protocol, samples are stained with diluted Indian ink which is applied with a paint brush and gently washed to remove nonadherent ink. The method readily allows identification of smooth, slightly rough, partial- and deeply-fibrillated cartilagenous surfaces. Several variations of this classification system have been proposed (Goldberg et al., 1984). The method has even been applied semiquantitatively for evaluating changes in fibrillation in response to treatment in a rabbit, partial-meniscectomy model (Rosner et al., 1982). Since the staining can be done under sterile conditions and Indian ink is nontoxic to the cells, it provides an excellent preliminary classification especially of tissue with only a slightly abnormal surface cartilage.

At the other end of the spectrum of cartilage classification, Mankin et al. (1971) have proposed the most in depth histological classification of cartilage using histologic samples that were stained with Safranin O-fast green (Kiviranta et al., 1985), although a wide variety of other proteoglycan (PG) stains are possible (Kincaid et al., 1972). The Mankin et al. classification has additional advantages because, by obtaining histologic samples, a large number of parameters can be assessed. The major advantage of this system is the evaluation of sample homogeneity. OA lesions change rapidly and, within a small region of tissue, vast differences in pathology can occur. The presence of nonhomogenous samples can greatly affect the biomechanical, biochemical and metabolic studies. Cells in a relatively 'normal' region could contribute significantly different products to those in immediately adjacent, highly-fibrillated tissue. Additionally, the PG-rich regions would dominate the analysis for PG structure, while those that have lost PG would contribute significantly to water changes. Therefore, it is important to know the nature of the tissue tested.

The Mankin et al. system is based on combining scores for several different parameters. The first parameter is the degree of surface fibrillation ranging from smooth to clefts through the tidemark. The next parameter is the integrity of the tidemark and its violation by vascular ingrowth. The third level is the degree of cellularity ranging from normal, hypercellularity, cloning and hypocellularity. The last level and dominant feature of the grading system is degree of Safranin O staining of the matrix. A composite score is obtained ranging from 0 (for completely normal tissue) to 12 (almost completely disrupted tissue). One of the drawbacks of the scale is that, while it is abundantly clear that there are differences between normal and grossly affected tissue, it is not clear that the gradations, as measured by this score, are related in a linear fashion to the disease process. In addition, one set of parameters may be highly dependent on another. For example, smooth surface, partial clefts may be very closely related to the value for Safranin O staining. Thus, the parameters are not an independent measure of the disease process. However, the information provided does allow grouping of tissues into broad categories. This has proved to be helpful in a number of studies (Martel-Pelletier et al., 1984). Once the parameters have been agreed upon by the various observers, interobserver differences are relatively small: of the order of one grade or less when scoring over a wide variety of samples. It is important to obtain proper histology for correlation with other parameters, such as magnetic resonance imaging (MRI) scans, and biomechanical and biochemical properties of the tissue.

4

Choice of specimens in comparative studies involving human femoral head cartilage

A. MAROUDAS, R. SCHNEIDERMAN,
C. WEINBERG and G. GRUSHKO

INTRODUCTION

Cartilage composition, and morphology, as well as biochemical and biophysical characteristics show considerable variations with species, age, joint, location on the joint and distance from the surface. These differences, apart from being of interest in themselves, are essential to recognize if valid conclusions are to be drawn from studies such as those relating to pathological change *or* ageing, *or* to the choice of suitable animal models for the study of human joint disease, *or*, in more general terms, if any objective comparison between the results of different laboratories is to be made.

This article presents some recently studied examples of such variations for the case of the human femoral head cartilage (Weinberg, 1987; Grushko *et al.*, 1989; Maroudas *et al.*, 1990).

VARIATIONS IN FIXED CHARGE DENSITY AND H$_2$O CONTENT OF INTACT CARTILAGE WITH POSITION ON THE FEMORAL HEAD FOR DIFFERENT AGE GROUPS

A systematic decrease in fixed charge density (FCD) is observed in going from the superior to the inferior region in all age groups, though the difference between the cartilage from the superior region and that from the anterior and posterior region is not significant, particularly in the young age groups. A systematic increase in the mean FCD of full depth plugs with ageing is observed in all four regions of the femoral head. The relative increases with age appear to be approximately the same in all regions (Fig. 4.1).

In *intact* cartilage, the water content decreases somewhat with age and this occurs throughout the joint surface. In all age groups there is a small increase in passing from the superior to the inferior region. It can be seen that after the age of approximately 30 years the differences in the water content between the different age groups are less clear-cut than the differences in FCD (Fig. 4.1).

Apart from the inherent interest of the site-related variations, it is necessary to take these into account when planning many types of comparative experiments. Sometimes it is possible to side-step the problem by taking random samples of finely diced cartilage pooled from the whole area of the femoral head (e.g. Yaron *et al.*, 1989). However, this method cannot always be used validly, as for instance in the case of the comparison between normal and osteoarthritic (OA) cartilage (see example below). The method obviously cannot be used when larger specimens are needed, as in the

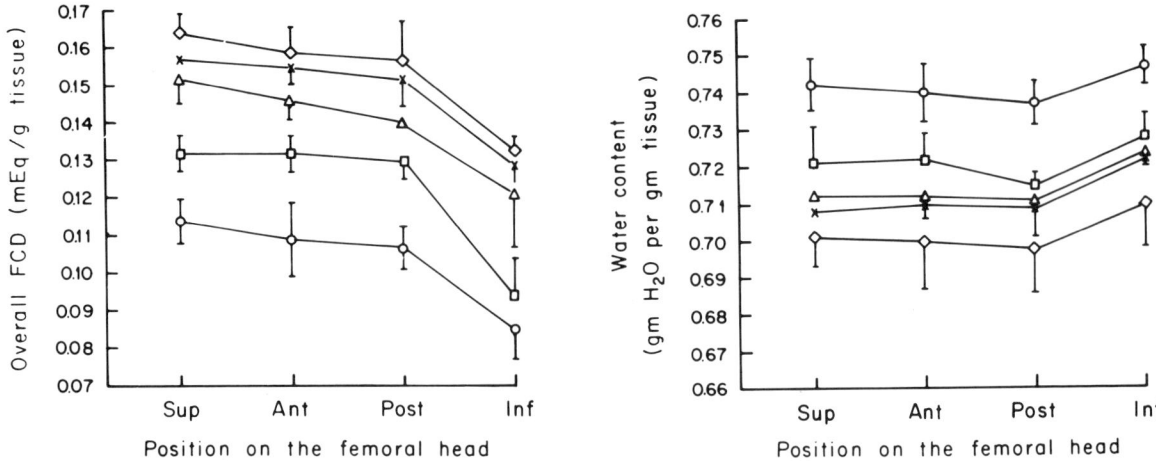

Figure 4.1 Variations in fixed charge density (FCD) and water content for intact cartilage with position on the femoral head for different age groups. (○) 17–20 years old; (□) 21–30 years old; (△) 30–45 years old; (X) 50–65 years old; (◇) 70–81 years old.

studies of transport or mechanical properties. Furthermore, the use of pooled material may in certain cases actually hide important site-related specific effects. The only alternative in all of the above cases is to employ carefully matched controls from adjacent sites (e.g. Schneiderman et al., 1986).

VARIATION IN FIXED CHARGE DENSITY AND H₂O CONTENT WITH DEPTH FOR DIFFERENT AGE GROUPS

Curves of FCD and H_2O content versus fractional cartilage depth are shown for specimens from the superior region for four ages, viz. < 20, 30–40, 60–70 and 82 years, in Fig. 4.2. A curve representing superficially fibrillated cartilage from one individual (age 82 years) is included for comparison (Fig. 4.2).

The specimens showing superficial fibrillation have a distinctly different FCD profile from the intact samples. In the superficial zone, to which the fibrillation was limited, the FCD is much lower than that of intact cartilage in any age group except the youngest; in the middle zone the FCD rises steeply, in the deep zone reaching the level of intact tissue characteristic of the same age group.

The fibrillated specimens also have a higher water content than the intact cartilage from the same age groups. Moreover, the profile is different, with a characteristically increased hydration in the middle zone (Maroudas, 1976; Maroudas and Venn, 1977).

It is thus clear that if one wishes to distinguish age-related changes in normal cartilage from those caused by degenerative changes, it is necessary to make sure that all fibrillated tissue is excluded from the experimental material. If fibrillated material is not excluded, one obtains a composite result of changes with ageing, superimposed on changes with increasing degeneration. Since the two trends are in fact in opposite directions (Grushko et al., 1989), a confused picture is obtained.

Furthermore, in degenerate cartilage, wear has often led to partial thickness loss so that one may no longer be dealing with a specimen in which all the original zones are fully represented. One needs to take into account the possible absence of the superficial layer if one is to carry out a meaningful

4. SPECIMENS FOR COMPARATIVE STUDIES: FEMORAL HEAD CARTILAGE 11

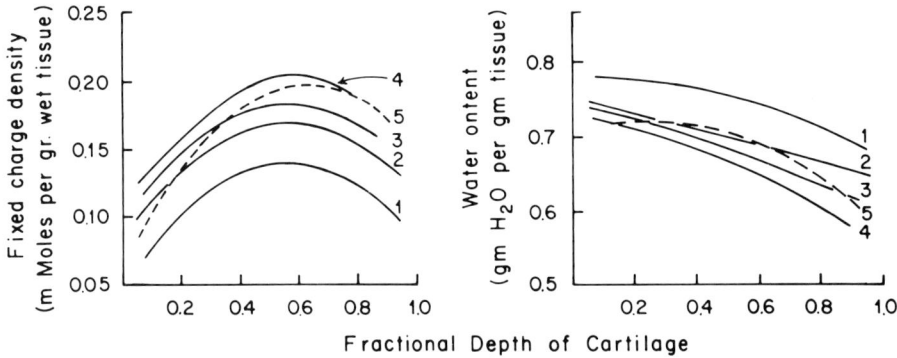

Figure 4.2 Variation in fixed charge density and water content with depth below the articular surface for cartilage samples from the superior region for different age groups. (1) 17–20 years old; (2) 30–40 years old; (3) 60–70 years old; (4) 82 years old; (5) 81 years old, fibrillated.

comparison between the properties of the so-called 'full depth' plugs or if one is to compare their respective profiles as a function of distance from the articular surface.

TOPOGRAPHICAL VARIATIONS OVER THE JOINT SURFACE IN THE RATE OF SULFATE UPTAKE, FIXED CHARGE DENSITY AND THICKNESS IN NORMAL FEMORAL HEADS

Typical variations in sulfate uptake, thickness and FCD over the surface of a normal femoral head, age 75 years, are shown in Fig. 4.3(a–c). It can be seen that there is a significant systematic increase in sulfate uptake from position 120° (the supero-anterior region) to position 0 (or 360°) below the fovea. The gradient is steepest in the regions 60–0° and 300–360°. There is also a steep gradient in sulfate uptake on passing from the central region towards the margins. On the whole, the profiles of sulfate incorporation are inversely related to cartilage thickness as well as to glycosaminoglycan (GAG) content.

The values of sulfate uptake vs. location for six femoral heads in the age range 55–85 years are given in Fig. 4.3(d). This age range was chosen because it corresponds to that of the majority of OA specimens.

PROFILES OF SULFATE UPTAKE VS. DEPTH FROM ARTICULAR SURFACE IN OSTEOARTHRITIC CARTILAGE COMPARED WITH NORMAL CARTILAGE UNDER SHORT-TERM CULTURE CONDITIONS

Figure 4.4 shows profiles of sulfate uptake, expressed on a dry weight basis, versus fractional distance from the articular surface for both osteoarthritic cartilage and normal cartilage sampled from the same regions of the femoral head and the same age group and cultured for less than 8 h in minimal medium. A graph is also included in the figure for comparison of cartilage from normal joints, pooled from the whole surface of the femoral head.

The OA cartilage was divided into three groups: (i) plugs with a visually intact surface and a usual water content in the range 2.5–3.4 g/g dry weight; (ii) plugs showing mild fibrillation, water content in the range 3.4–4.3 g/g dry weight; and (iii) coarsely fibrillated cartilage, water content in the range 4.3–4.7 g/g dry weight.

It is clear that, whilst the rate of sulfate uptake is actually either the same or decreased in cartilage derived from OA joints as compared with the rate in cartilage from the same region of normal joints, this is not the case when comparison is made with

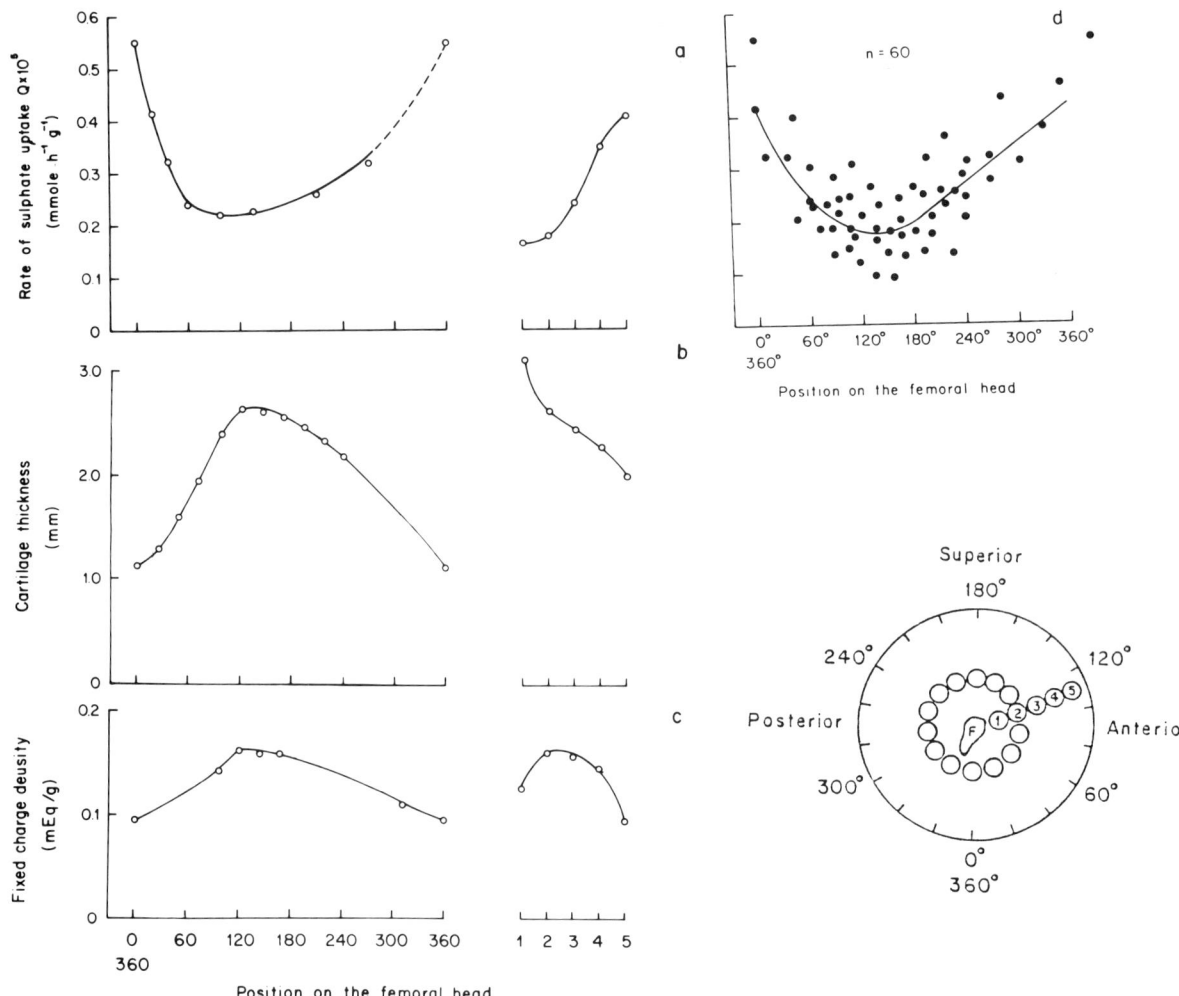

Figure 4.3 Typical topographical variations in (a) sulfate uptake (Q), (b) thickness, and (c) FCD over the surface of a normal femoral head, age 75 years. (d) Topographical variations in sulfate uptake for six femoral heads, age range 55–85 years.

pooled cartilage from all the regions of the normal femoral heads (Byers et al., 1977). The reason for this is obvious. When one is dealing with OA femoral heads, some of the cartilage is no longer present. The area of cartilage that has usually been worn away is the whole of the superior surface, an area that in fact corresponds to the regions with the lowest rate of ^{35}S incorporation in normal specimens, particularly in the older age groups. If this area is not specifically excluded from the results to be used for comparison and if, instead, cartilage from all areas of a normal femoral head is pooled (as has been done by most researchers in the past), it is clear that one will necessarily obtain a lower overall figure for the ^{35}S uptake on a normal head than for cartilage from an OA head from which the superior surface is missing. This may be one of the reasons that has given rise to the observations reported in the literature of a higher sulfate uptake in OA cartilage than in normal human cartilage (e.g. Mankin et al., 1971).

4. SPECIMENS FOR COMPARATIVE STUDIES: FEMORAL HEAD CARTILAGE

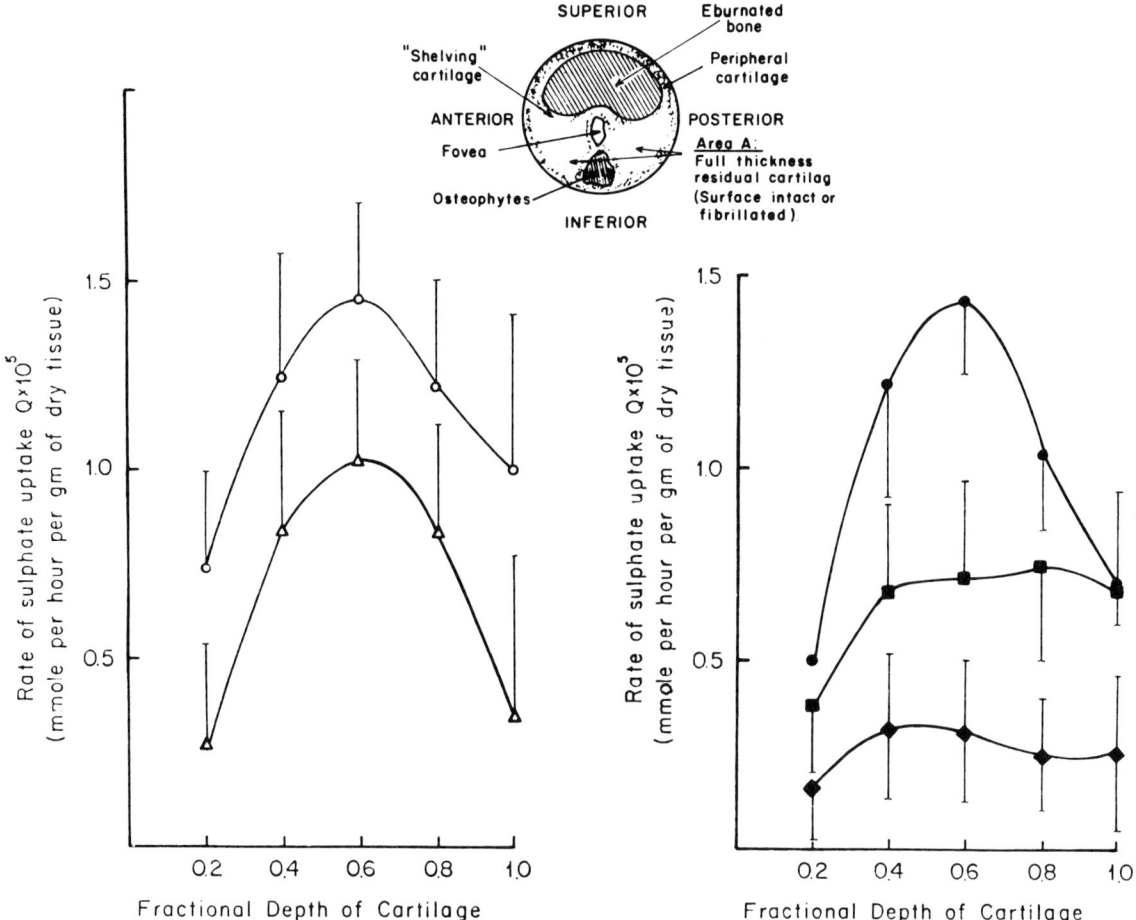

Figure 4.4 Profiles of sulfate uptake vs. depth from articular surface in osteoarthritic cartilage compared with normal cartilage. (△) Intact cartilage from the *whole surface* of normal femoral heads; (○) intact cartilage obtained from area A of normal femoral heads; (●) intact cartilage obtained from osteoarthritic femoral heads; (■) superficially fibrillated cartilage obtained from osteoarthritic femoral heads; (◆) coarsely fibrillated cartilage obtained from osteoarthritic femoral heads.

AGE CHANGES IN SULFATE UPTAKE

Figure 4.5 shows the variation in sulfate uptake with age for cartilage from (a) the superior region (120–240°) and (b) the posterior and anterior regions (40–100° and 260–320°). This latter region was specifically chosen and the results within it were pooled in order to facilitate comparison between cartilage from OA and normal femoral heads. It can be seen that there is a significant decrease in sulfate uptake with age in the superior region, whilst the posterior and anterior regions show hardly any systematic variation with age, although there is possibly a very small increase. In order to eliminate the scatter due to variations in sulfate uptake (Q) from joint to joint, we have also examined the variation in the ratio (Q superior)/(Q anterior, posterior) versus age, each point representing one femoral head (Fig. 4.5(b)). The

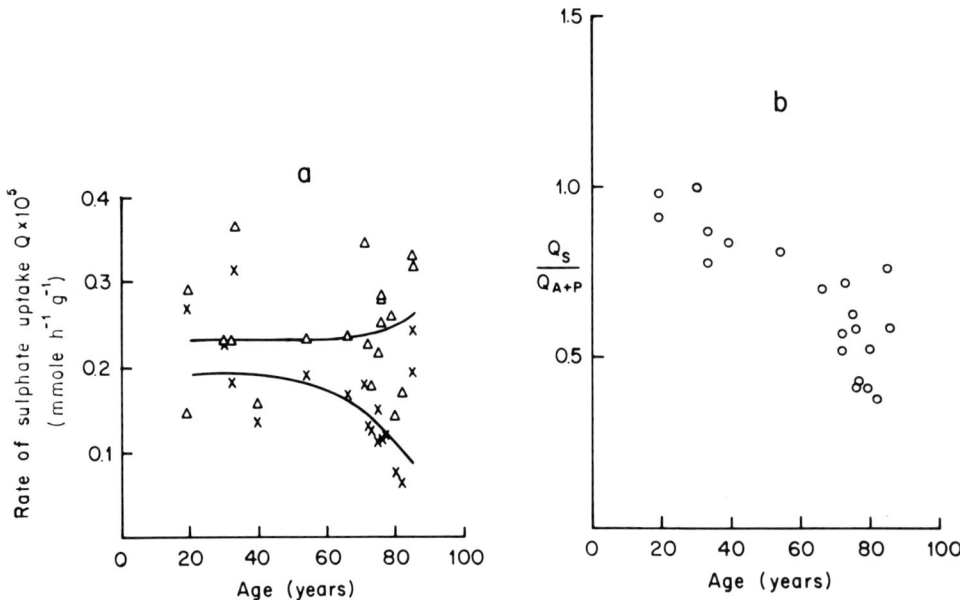

Figure 4.5 (a) Variation in the rate of sulfate uptake with age for cartilage from the superior region (120–240°), and the posterior (260–320°) and anterior (40–100°) regions. (△) Cartilage samples from anterior and posterior regions; (X) cartilage samples from superior region. (b) Variation with age in the ratio of the rate of sulfate uptake by cartilage samples from the superior (Q_s) to the rate of sulfate uptake by cartilage samples from the anterior and posterior regions (Q_{A+P}). Each value of the ratio refers to the one femoral head.

decrease in the ratio, from values very close to unity in the 20–30 year old age group to around 0.5 at 80 years is very clear.

ZONAL VARIATIONS IN SULFATE INCORPORATION UNDER 'LONG-TERM' CULTURE CONDITIONS: INFLUENCE OF FETAL CALF SERUM AND INSULIN

Preliminary remarks

For plugs incubated in medium alone (Dulbecco's modified eagle's medium, DMEM), there was an increase of 50–100% in the rate of sulfate incorporation after one day of culture. It is likely that the conditions prevailing during the interval between operation or death and the start of the incubation have a temporarily adverse effect on proteoglycan (PG) synthesis (Bayliss *et al.*, 1988), which disappears with time in culture. This is consistent with the fact that the values of Q_o (i.e. the rate of sulfate uptake at time zero), obtained when the above interval was fairly long (10–24 h) are lower than those previously obtained when the 'storage' interval was shorter (4–5 h) (Schneiderman *et al.*, 1986). Thus, the rise in sulfate uptake (Q) from time zero to one day after the start of the culture could simply represent the return to the value in the immediate *ex vivo* condition. This would provide one explanation for the observed initial rise in sulfate uptake. A second reason could be a general adaptation of the cells to culture conditions which may differ from those *in vivo* (e.g. nutritional supply).

From day one to day nine, Q_t/Q_o remained approximately constant, at about 1.75 times the initial values.

Comparison between sulfate incorporation in medium with and without fetal calf serum

For cartilage incubated as full-depth plugs, we observed that fetal calf serum (FCS) produced a time-dependent increase in sulfate incorporation similar to that reported by other workers (see Chapter 5). However, slicing of these plugs after incorporation showed that by far the greatest increase occurs in the sulfate zone. After approximately 12–20 h, this zone has the highest rate of incorporation, whereas in DMEM controls it has the lowest. At 'steady state' the surface layer has an incorporation rate more than five times its initial value. The deeper layers show a two-fold increase in sulfate uptake *with* or *without* FCS in the incubation medium (Fig. 4.6). There are a number of possible causes for this variation in the effect of FCS with depth. Firstly, serum growth factors may transform the relatively numerous but low-activity chondrocytes of the surface zone into a higher activity type. Secondly, the high PG

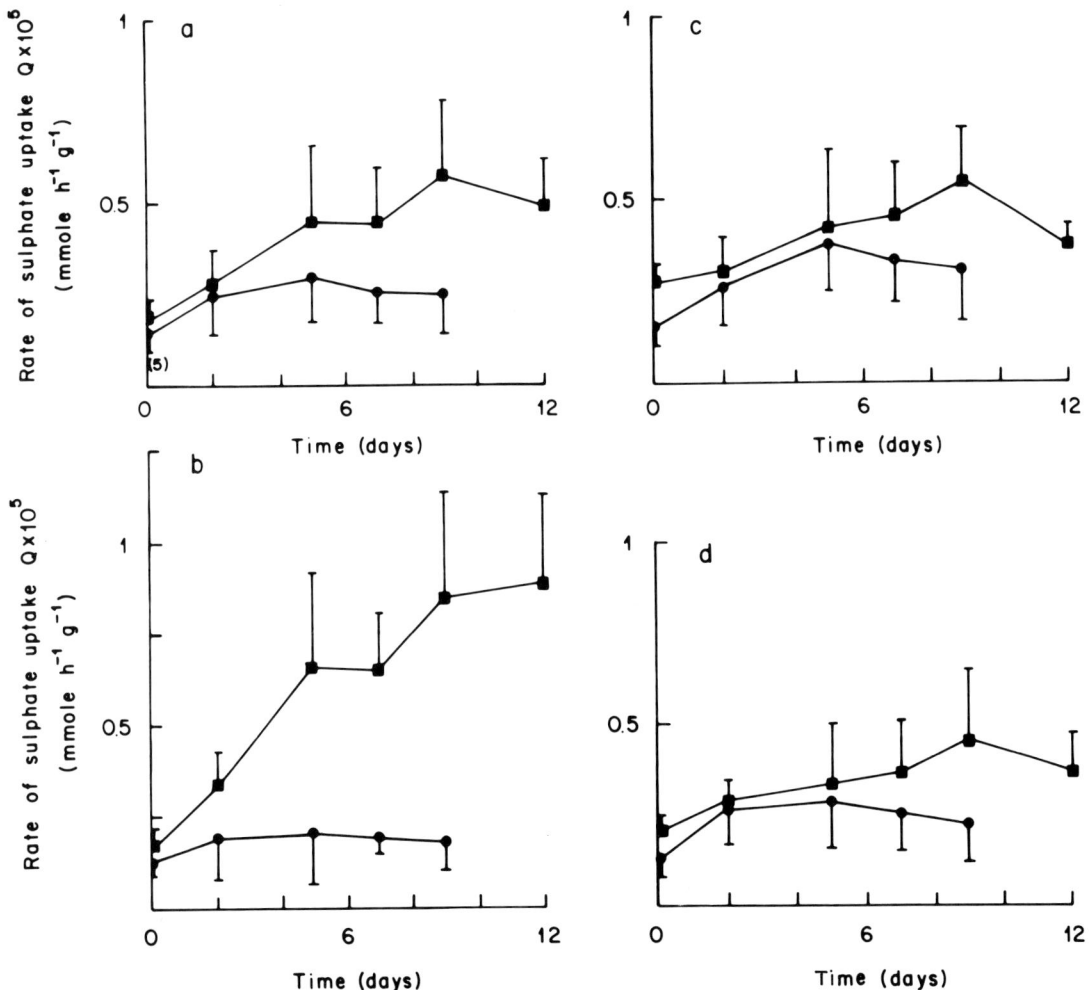

Figure 4.6 Comparison between sulfate uptake in different zones of cartilage and different media as a function of culture time. (●) Pure DMEM; (■) DMEM + 10% FCS; (a) full-depth plug; (b) superficial zone; (c) middle zone; (d) deep zone.

content of the middle and deep zones results in a low partition coefficient for large molecules (Snowden and Maroudas, 1976), and this may limit the concentration of growth factors present in the pericellular environment (see Chapter 10). Thirdly, the steady-state consumption of growth factors by chondrocytes in the middle zones may be limited by the inability of such factors to diffuse rapidly enough into the layers further removed from the source of supply. However, the latter does not appear likely as slicing the plugs prior to culture does not alter the profile.

Comparison between effects of fetal calf serum and insulin

Figure 4.7 shows a comparison between sulfate uptake up to five days in culture into the superficial

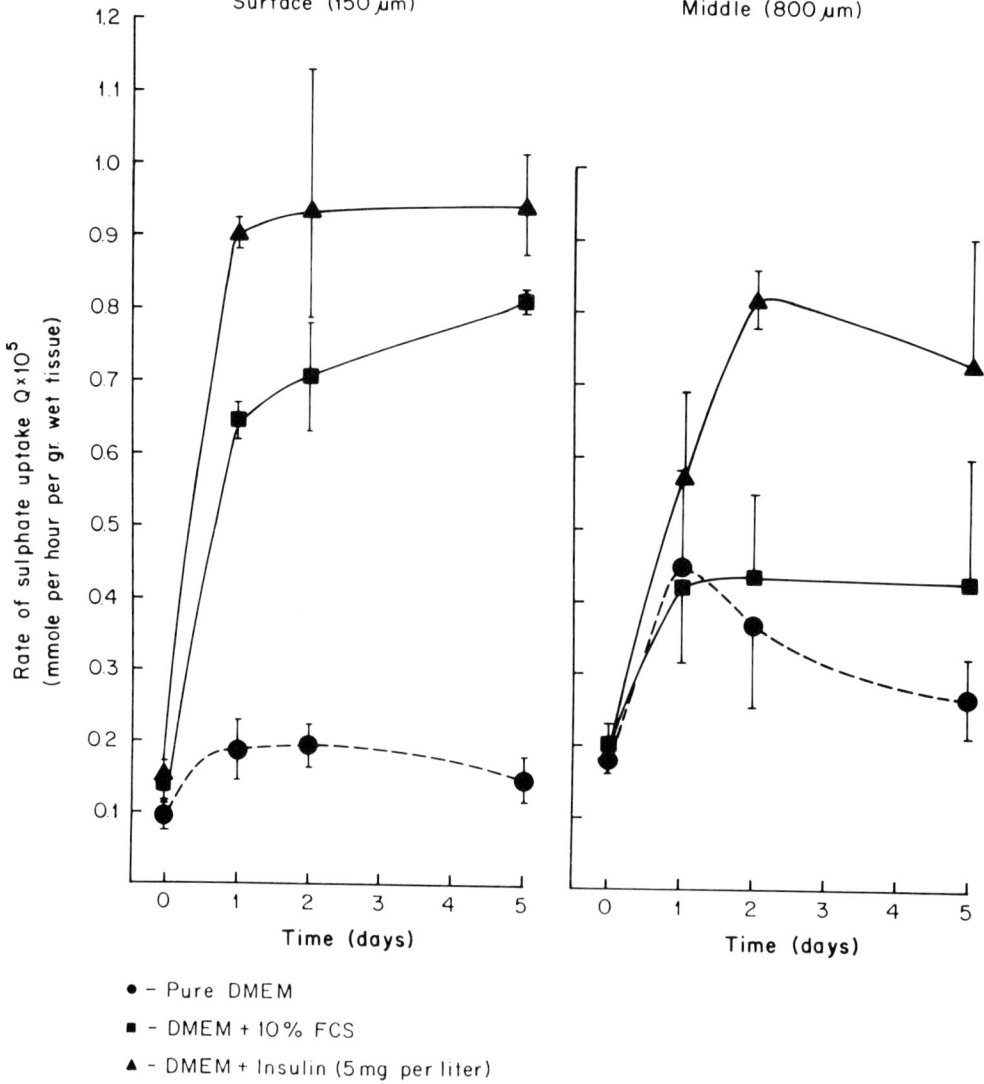

Figure 4.7 Comparison between the effects of FCS and insulin on sulfate uptake in the superficial and middle zones of cartilage as a function of time. (●) Pure DMEM; (■) DMEM + 10% FCS; (▲) DMEM + insulin (5 mg l^{-1}).

and the middle zones of cartilage in the presence of (i) DMEM alone, (ii) DMEM + 10% FCS, and (iii) DMEM + insulin (5 mg l^{-1}).

It can be seen that, whilst insulin at the concentration employed has only a slightly higher enhancing effect on the sulfate uptake in the superficial zone than 10% FCS, its effect in the middle zone is much larger than that of 10% FCS. This, we think, is because insulin penetrates without difficulty throughout the tissue, whereas the much larger IGF–I protein complex, as it probably exists in the serum, has very limited access to areas of higher PG content found within the middle and deep zones of cartilage (Snowdon and Maroudas, 1976).

Summary

Whilst insulin stimulates more or less equally the sulfate uptake into GAG in the different zones of cultured human adult cartilage, the effect of 10% FCS is mainly limited to the surface zone.

The dramatic increase in the activity of the cells from the superficial zone in long-term culture in medium containing FCS as compared with the far smaller increases observed in the remainder of the tissue should be borne in mind when the effects of various factors and drugs are tested in organ culture systems, in particular when comparisons are made between systems employing different media.

CONCLUSIONS

The above examples illustrate the importance of trying to select appropriate samples in any comparative studies of cartilage.

ACKNOWLEDGMENT

This research was supported by a grant from the United States–Israel Binational Science Foundation (BSF), Jerusalem, Israel.

5

Sampling of the intervertebral disc

S. ROBERTS

The intervertebral disc is made up of two regions: the inner nucleus pulposus and the outer, more fibrous, annulus fibrosus. They have different embryological origins; the nucleus is derived from endoderm, being in part a remnant of the notochord, whilst the annulus is derived from mesoderm (Coventry et al., 1945) and the two regions differ in composition and organization, particularly in early life. The nucleus contains more water and proteoglycan (PG) than the annulus, but less collagen (Fig. 5.1) (Roberts et al., 1982). Furthermore, some of the water is actually inside the collagen fibrils (approximately 1.2 cm/g dry collagen in tendon) and hence is inaccessible to the PGs (Maroudas and Urban, 1980). Since this extrafibrillar water content is important to the physiological functioning of the PGs within the tissue, the difference in water content between the two regions of the disc is even greater, due to the proportional difference in collagen content.

There is also a difference in the type of collagen present. Type I and II collagen are present generally in the outer layers of the annulus, whilst type II is the predominant collagen in the nucleus (Eyre and Muir, 1976; Beard et al., 1981). In addition, collagen types III, VI, IX and XI have

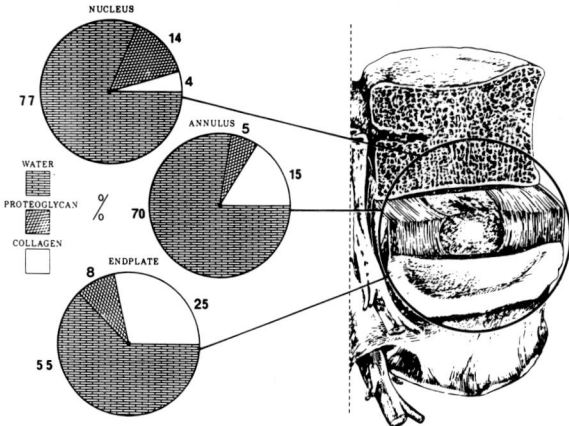

Figure 5.1 The relative proportions of the three main components of the human disc and end plate.

been found in the nucleus and III, V, VI, IX and XI in the annulus (Eyre, 1988). The organization of the collagen also varies with location. In the nucleus there are individual fibrils of approximately 30 nm diameter which are randomly dispersed and do not appear to be organized into a more complex structure (Inoue, 1981). This is in contrast to the annulus where the collagen is highly organized and the fibrils, also approximately 30 nm in diameter (Hickey and Hukins, 1982), are aligned into bundles to make up the fibrous concentric annular lamellae. Each lamella tilts with respect to the axis of the spine, the direction of tilt alternating by approximately 70° in successive lamellae in the human lumbar spine.

In addition, the cell shape, number and activity are different in the annulus and nucleus. In the nucleus the cells are rounded and resemble chondrocytes, unlike those of the annulus which are smaller, elongated and more fibroblast like. The cell number is highest closest to the nutrient supply, i.e. near the cartilage endplate and the periphery of the annulus (Maroudas et al., 1975). However, it is the cells of the mid-annulus in the human adult which show the greatest metabolic activity, at least for sulfate incorporation (Bayliss et al., 1988). Furthermore, the structure of these macromolecules also varies between the two regions. The nucleus has a high proportion of PGs that are nonaggregating and have a higher content of keratan sulfate chains compared with those from the annulus (Humzah and Soames, 1988).

There are other tissues adjacent to the disc which inadvertently might be sampled as 'disc tissue' and could lead to erroneous data. Above and below the disc is a thin layer of hyaline cartilage, the endplate, which is less hydrated but more collagenous than either the annulus or nucleus (Fig. 5.1). In addition, there are longitudinal ligaments running anterior and posterior to the disc which also have different properties and composition.

Unfortunately, the boundaries between the different tissues and areas of the disc are not always distinct and it is often difficult to differentiate between these regions. The tissue type can usually be identified if care is taken, although the actual junction is often unclear and can pose considerable sampling problems. The clarity of the boundary between the annulus and nucleus depends, to some extent, on the species of

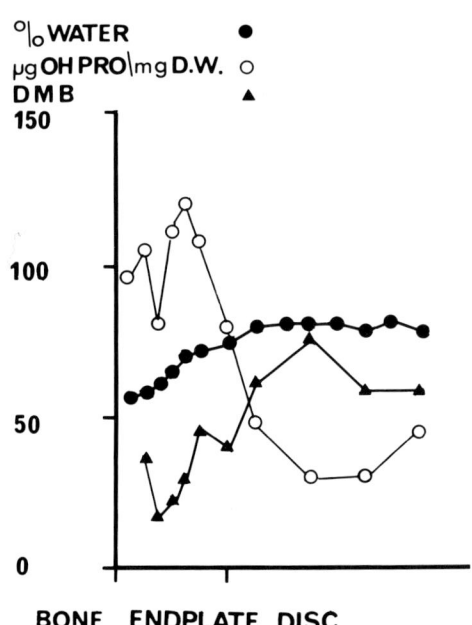

Figure 5.2 Vertical profile of water, collagen (μg hydroxyproline/mg dry weight) and proteoglycan (degree of dimethylmethylene blue binding/mg dry weight) contents in the human end plate and disc.

the animal used and, to a large extent, on the age of the specimen. In young humans (less than 20 years old) the nucleus is a distinct gelatinous area, but with increasing age this becomes more fibrous, rendering the two regions increasingly difficult to differentiate.

Even with the same region of tissue, there can be considerable topographical variations in composition. Within the cartilaginous endplate there is a marked increase in the water and glycosaminoglycan content of cartilage sampled adjacent to the bone compared with that adjacent to the nucleus/annulus (Fig. 5.2). The distance involved is little more than 1 mm (Roberts *et al.*, 1989), but the results demonstrate how the tissue properties can vary over a relatively small distance at any one site within any one specimen. Similarly, there are concentration gradients from the inner annulus through to the outer annulus; PG and water contents decrease whilst collagen increases (Roberts *et al.*, 1982).

The manner in which the sample is stored *ex vivo* may also affect profoundly the subsequent biochemical analysis. For assessment of water content, or any procedure that is dependent on water content, such as matrix turnover measurements, the tissue must be handled very carefully. To avoid dehydration, disc tissue should be collected into a sealed, 100% humidity chamber and must not be allowed to come into contact with water, or the hydrophilic nature of the PG will cause swelling of the tissue. Bayliss *et al.* (1986) found that the rate of sulfate incorporation in swollen disc tissue was less than that in tissue maintained at an *in vivo* water content. Moreover, even if hydration was controlled *ex vivo*, there was a finite period over which the cells within the matrix were viable biosynthetically.

The selection of sampling sites is of utmost importance in all studies of cartilaginous tissues, but particularly so for intervertebral disc which exhibits such a heterogeneous structure. If analyses from different laboratories are to be meaningfully compared, then a procedure for sampling and storage of this complex structure has to be established.

6

Tissue sampling and preservation for morphological studies

E.B. HUNZIKER

The initial practical steps of any morphological, stereological or immunohistochemical study involve the excision of tissue blocks and sampling of specimens; the thorough planning of an appropriate sampling strategy is of paramount importance to the success of such projects (Gundersen, 1984; Cruz-Orive and Hunziker, 1986; Hunziker and Schenk, 1987). For any quantitative and stereological study, one of the most efficient and powerful sampling procedures is the 'systematic random sampling' protocol (Fig. 6.1). Within the structure of interest (for example, an organ, the articular cartilage of a joint), tissue blocks are sampled systematically and the pattern adopted is varied among animals (Hunziker *et al.*, 1987). In each case (i.e. each animal), the position of the initial cut made as part of a regular series during tissue subdivision is varied randomly within a narrow dimensional limit (Fig. 6.1). Further subdivision into tissue slices and then into tissue

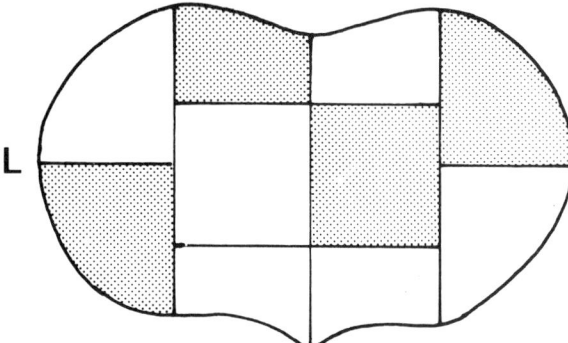

Figure 6.1 A systematic scheme of growth-plate subdivision. Random variation of this systematic sampling pattern is obtained by varying the depth at which the first tissue slice is cut (e.g. on the left) in a random manner within about 1/5 of the width of the tissue slice. All subsequent slices are cut at a fixed distance from the first. After cutting and numbering of blocks from the tissue slices, those chosen for analysis are also selected in a systematic way from animal to animal. (From Cruz-Orive and Hunziker (1986), with permission of the authors and the publisher.)

blocks is always carried out at regular intervals, according to a systematic protocol (Cruz-Orive and Hunziker, 1986).

In the case of cartilage, it is also important to pay attention to the tissue excision technique itself. The use of scalpels or razor blades is always associated with unphysiologically high, local compression forces which lead to cell collapse at scattered intervals throughout tissue blocks. The use of a *gentle sawing* technique is essential to obtain good tissue slices. In our laboratory, fine dental saws are used routinely for this purpose. Further cutting of tissue slices into small blocks may thereafter be performed using well-sharpened, thin razor blades (Hunziker *et al.*, 1984). Prior to fixation, tissue slices or blocks are frequently subjected to experimental procedures, such as testing of biomechanical properties or tissue culture, and it is important to bear in mind that whenever cartilage tissue is immersed in a buffer solution or culture medium, extraction of proteoglycan (PG) (and other) molecules will begin to take place immediately (Hunziker and Graber, 1986). In addition, within the first 20–30 min about 10% of tissue PGs have usually been lost from the cartilage matrix. Although the precise origin of the PGs lost is not known, the pericellular matrix compartment, representing only approximately 2–4% of the cartilage matrix volume, is a very sensitive morphological indicator of this loss, even when it only occurs in minute amounts. Loss of PGs from this region leads to immediate cell shrinkage or even collapse (Fig. 6.2), since this interface has been destroyed and hence 'empty' pericellular rings or spaces become apparent. This optically 'empty' pericellular space was previously referred to as the lacuna, and is now known to be an artifact caused by PG loss.

Such losses and cell shrinkage also occur under routine aldehyde chemical fixation conditions (Hunziker *et al.*, 1983); the extent to which these phenomena occur can, however, be considerably

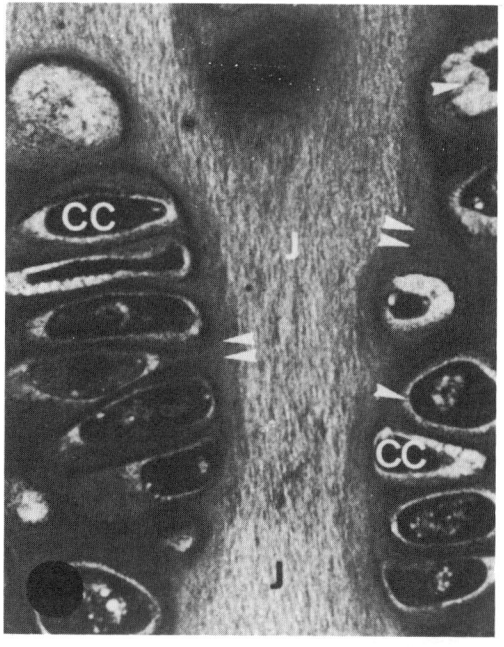

Figure 6.2 Rat growth-plate cartilage (proliferative zone), proximal tibia. Photomicrograph of a 1-μm thick section, stained with toluidine blue 0, showing shrunken/collapsed chondrocytes (CC), surrounded by a PG depleted pericellular matrix compartments ($\triangle$), called 'lucauna'. ($\triangle\triangle$) Territorial matrix compartment. (J) Interterritorial matrix. (From Hunziker and Graber (1986), with permission of the authors and the publisher.)

reduced or even prevented by including an appropriate cationic dye in the fixation solution (Fig. 6.3).

This problem of PG extraction, which occurs under conventional chemical fixation conditions, also need to be borne in mind during the planning of immunohistochemical studies involving so-called 'mild' chemical fixation followed by pre-embedding immunostaining. Due to the inherent properties of cartilage PGs, namely, their extremely high water solubility and existence in an underhydrated state, significant losses of these molecules are incurred and the dramatic molecular shifts taking place in the cartilage matrix significantly reduce the lateral resolution potential of the immunostaining results (Hunziker and Herrmann, 1987). These are reduced further when enzymatic matrix treatment (for example with hyaluronidase) is performed in order to render the cartilage matrix penetrable to the antibodies used. Tissue fixed and immunostained in such a manner is thus structurally altered to such a degree that electron-microscopic examination serves little purpose. Light-microscopic analysis is, however, still useful, but only to a limited degree (Hunziker and Herrmann, 1987).

Proper *chemical* fixation of cartilage tissue without PG loss or cell-shape changes can be achieved only when carried out in the presence of cationic dyes. Examples of such dyes, which diffuse readily through cartilage (even when thick layers up to 3 mm in diameter are fixed), include

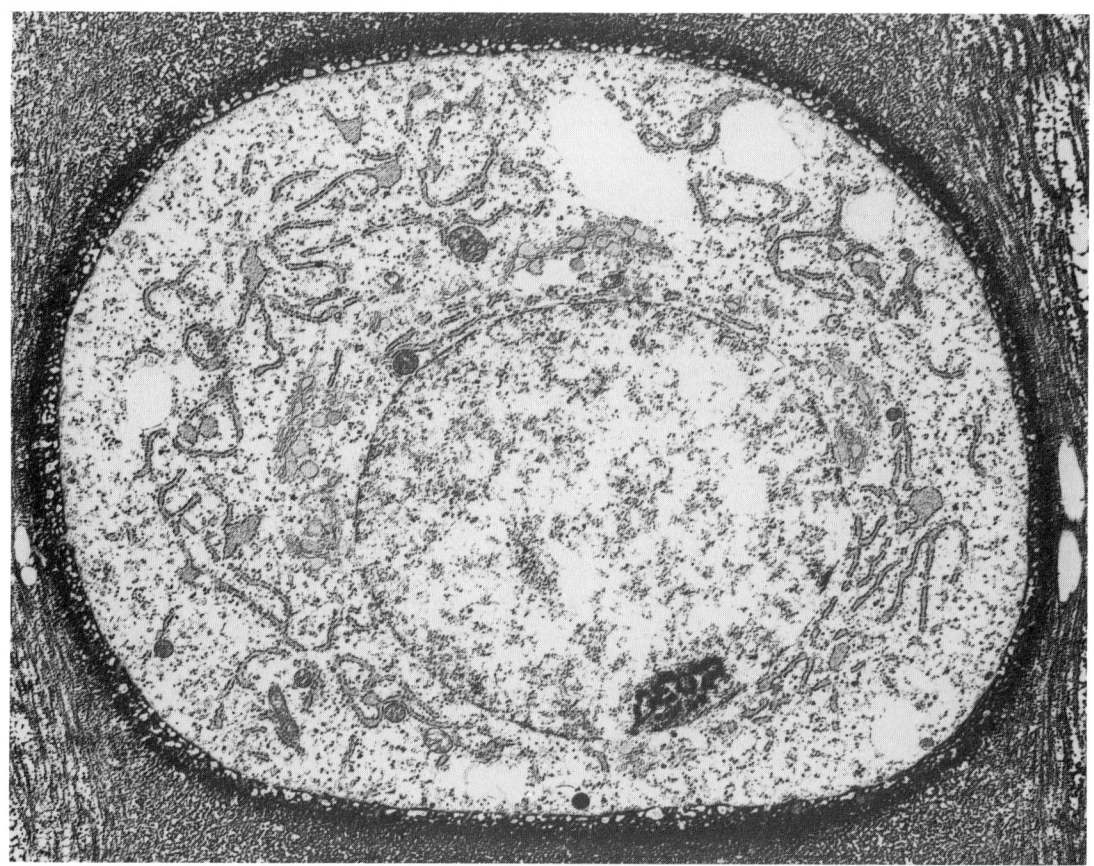

Figure 6.3 Electron micrograph of a hypertrophic chondrocyte after chemical fixation in the presence of RHT. The cell membrane is intact and contacting the pericellular matrix along the whole cell surface. (From Hunziker *et al.* (1983), with permission of the authors and the publisher.)

ruthenium hexammine trichloride (RHT), ruthenium red, alcian blue, toluidine blue, cobalt hexammine trichloride, trisbipyridyl ruthenium(II) chloride (TRC) and pentamin-ruthenium N-dimethylphenylen-diimine trichloride (PRT) (Hunziker, 1990). Dyes exhibiting limited diffusion and precipitation capacities leading to suboptimal preservation results when using thick tissue specimens (in the order of millimeters) include Safranin O, Acridine Orange and Cuprolinic Blue (Hunziker, 1990). Recently we have found that whenever an osmium tetroxide post-fixation is included in the fixation procedure, PG precipitates are disrupted and extracted, even when the cationic dye initially introduced during aldehydic pre-fixation is present. In consequence, 'lacuna' formations, together with cell shrinkage and collapse, occur and any quantitative analysis, for example by counting PG precipitates (matrix granules), will obviously yield unreliable results. The only two dyes which we have so far found to be capable of preventing PG loss and cell shrinkage/collapse during osmium tetroxide post-fixation in the presence of the dye, are RHT and PRT (Hunziker, 1990).

A disadvantage of these chemical-fixation procedures is the loss of antigenicity incurred by the molecules involved in these complexing processes, and hence their very limited usefulness for immunohistochemical investigations.

When tissue is processed according to cryotechnical procedures, it is possible to preserve both cell and matrix structure close to the native state and to prevent macromolecular loss or shifts within or from the extra cellular space and to maintain antigencity (Hunziker *et al.*, 1984; Hunziker and Herrmann, 1987). This approach involves rapid freezing of tissue (to liquid nitrogen temperature ($-196°C$)), followed by freeze substitution (at $-90°C$) and low-temperature embedding (in Lowicryl®) and polymerization (at -50 to $-35°C$). Under these conditions, both cells

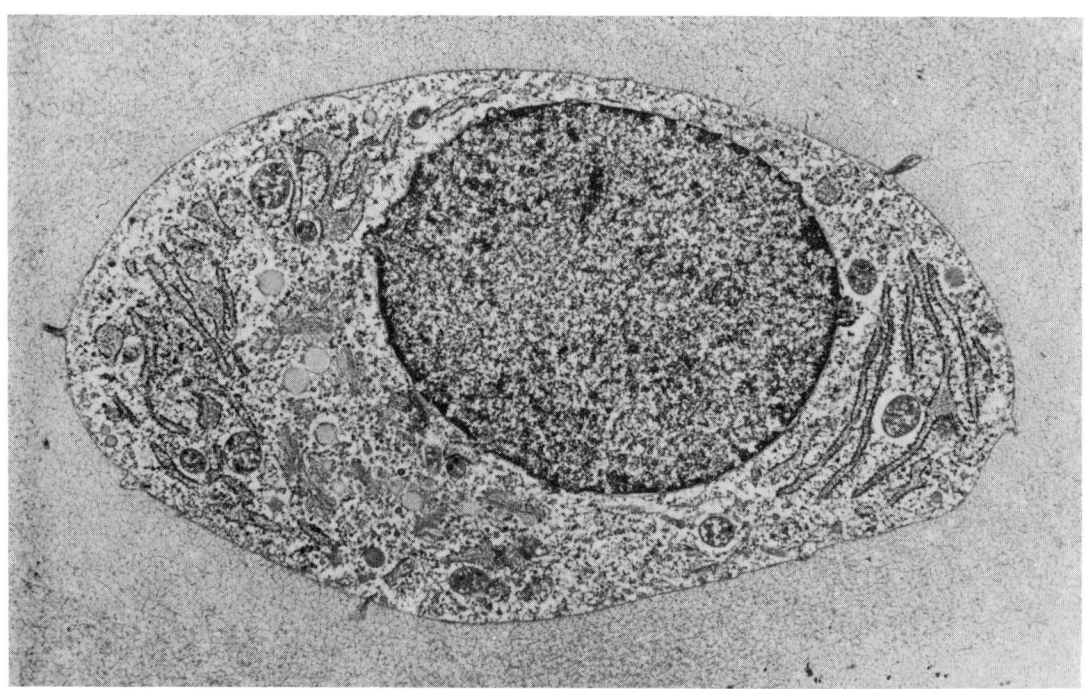

Figure 6.4 Electron micrograph of a growth-plate proliferating chondrocyte. Tissue was processed by high-pressure freezing, freeze substitution and low-temperature embedding. The chondrocyte is preserved in an expanded (i.e. unshrunken) state with the absence of PG loss from the pericellular matrix compartment. (From Hunziker and Herrmann (1987), with permission of the authors and the publisher.)

and matrix PGs are preserved close to the native state (Fig. 6.4). Moreover, the approach permits immunoelectron-microscopic investigations of cartilage tissue matrix to be carried out at a molecular level with respect to lateral resolution (Hunziker and Herrmann, 1987). The crucial step in the whole cryotechnical preparation procedure is the initial freezing process. Most methods used, such as slam- and copper-block freezing will give a superficial well-frozen tissue layer (i.e. free of large ice crystals) of no more than $c.$ 10 μm in depth. High-pressure freezing is still the only method capable of yielding tissue successfully frozen to a deeper level (i.e. down to $c.$ 300 μm).

References

Bayliss, M.T., Urban, J.P.G., Johnstone, B. and Holms, S. (1986). *In vitro* method for measuring synthesis rates in the intervertebral disc. *J. Orthop. Res.* **4**, 10–17

Bayliss, M.T., Johnstone, B. and O'Brien, J.P. (1988). Proteoglycan synthesis in the human disc: variation with age, region and pathology. *Spine* **13**, 972–981

Beard, H.K., Roberts, S. and O'Brien, J.P. (1981) Immunoflourescent staining for collagen and proteoglycan normal and scoliotic intervertebral discs. *J. Bone Joint Surg.* **63B**, 529–534

Byers, P., Maroudas, A., Oztop, F., Stockwell, R.A. and Venn, M.F. (1977) Histological and biochemical studies on cartilage from osteoarthritic femoral heads with special reference to surface characteristics. *Conn. Tiss. Res.* **5**, 41–49

Coventry, M.B., Ghormley, R.K. and Kernohan, J.W. (1945). The intervertebral disc; its microscopic anatomy and pathology. Part I. Anatomy, development and physiology. *J. Bone Joint Surg.* **27**, 105–112.

Cruz-Orive, L.M. and Hunziker, E.B. (1986). Steriology for anisotropic cells: application to growth cartilage. *J. Microsc.* **143**, 47–80

Eyre, D. (1988). Collagens of the disc. In *The Biology of the Intervertebral Disc*, Vol. 1 (P. Ghosh, ed.), pp. 171–188. CRC Press Inc., Boca Raton, FL

Eyre, D. and Muir, H. (1976). Types I and II collagens in intervertebral disc. Interchanging radial distribution in annulus fibrosus. *Biochem. J.* **157**, 267–270

Freeman, M.A.R. and Meachim, G. (1979). Ageing, degeneration and remodelling of articular cartilage. In *Adult Articular Cartilage*, 2nd edn (M.A.R. Freeman, ed.), pp. 487–543. Pitman Medical, Kent

Gardner, D.L. (1990). *Pathological Basis of the Connective Tissue Diseases*. Edward Arnold, London (in press)

Gardner, D.L., Mazuryk, R., O'Conner, P. and Orford, C.R. (1987). Anatomical changes and pathogenesis of OA in man, with particular reference to the hip and knee joints. In *Studies in Osteoarthrosis: Pathogenesis, Intervention, Assessment* (D.J. Lott, M.K. Jasani and G.F.B. Birdwood, eds), pp. 21–48. Wiley, Chichester

Gardner, D.L., Elliot, D. and Simpson, R. (1990). Rapid bone morphometry with blocks, not sections. Application of confocal scanning microscopy to the diagnosis of metabolic bone disease. *J. Pathol.* **160**, pp. 166a

Goldberg, V.M., Norby, D.P., Sacks, B.L., Moskowitz, R.W. and Malemud, G.J. (1984). Correlation of histopathology and sulphated proteoglycan in human osteoarthritic hip cartilage. *J. Orthop. Res.* **1**, 302–312

Grushko, G., Schneiderman, R. and Maroudas, A. (1989). Some biochemical and biophysical parameters for the study of the pathogenesis of osteoarthritis. A comparison between the process of ageing and degeneration in human hip cartilage. *Conn. Tiss. Res.* **19**, 149–176

Gunderson, H.J.G. (1984). In *Analysis of Organic and Biological Substances*) P. Echlin, ed.), p. 477. Wiley, New York

Hickey, D.S. and Hukins, D.W.L. (1982). Ageing changes in the macromolecular organisation of the intervertebral disc: an X-ray diffraction and electron microscopic study. *Spine* **7**, 235–242

Humzah, M.D. and Soames, R.W. (1988). Human intervertebral disc: structure and function. *Anat. Rec.* **220**, 337–356

Hunziker, E.B. (1990). *Transactions of 36th Meeting ORS*, Vol. 15, p. 16, New Orleans

Hunziker, E.B. and Graber, W. (1986). Differential extraction of proteoglycans from cartilage tissue matrix compartments in isotonic buffer salt solutions and commercial tissue-culture media. *J. Histochem. Cytochem.* **34**, 1149–1153

Hunziker, E.B. and Herrmann, W. (1987). *In situ* localisation of cartilage extracellular matrix components by immunoelectron microscopy after cryotechnical tissue processing. *J. Histochem. Cytochem.* **35**, 647–655

Hunziker, E.B. and Schenk, R.K. (1987). In *Biology of Proteoglycans* (T. Whight and R. Mecham, eds), p. 155. Academic Press, San Diego

Hunziker, E.B., Herrmann, W. and Schenk, R.K. (1983). Ruthenium hexammine trichloride (RHT)-mediated interaction between plasma lemmal components and pericellular matrix proteoglycans is responsible for the preservation of chondrocytic plasma membranes *in situ* during cartilage fixation. *J. Histochem. Cytochem.* **31**, 717–727

Hunziker, E.B., Herrmann, W., Schenk, R.K., Mueller, M. and Moor, H. (1984). Cartilage ultrastructure after high pressure freezine, freeze substitution, and low temperature embedding. (1) chondrocyte ultrastructure. Implications for the theories of mineralisation and vascular invasion. *J. Cell Biol.* **98**, 267–276

Hunziker, E.B., Schenk, R.K. and Cruz Orive, L.M. (1987). Quantitation of chondrocyte performance in growth-plate cartilage during longitudinal bone growth. *J. Bone Joint Surg.* **69A**, 162–173

Inoue, H. (1981). Three dimensional architecture of lumbar intervertebral discs. *Spine* **6**, 139–146

Kincaid, S.A., VanSickle, D.C. and Wilsman, N.J. (1972). Histochemical evidence of a functional heterogeneity of the chondrocytes of adult canine articular cartilage. *Histochem. J.* **4**, 237–243

Kiviranta, I., Jorvelin, J., Tammi, M., Saamanen, A.M. and Helminen, H.J. (1985). Microspectrophotometric quantitation of glycosaminoglycans in articular cartilage sections stained with Safranin O. *Histochemistry* **82**, 249–255

Lawton, D.M., Lamaletie, M.D.J. and Gardner, D.L. (1989). Biocompatibility of hydroxyapatite ceramic: response of chondrocytes in a test system using low temperature scanning electron microscopy. *J. Dent.* **17**, 21–27

Mankin, H.J., Dorfman, H.O., Lippiello, L. and Zarins, A. (1971). Biochemical and metabolic abnormalities in articular cartilage from osteoarthritic human hip. *J. Bone Joint Surg.* **53A**, 523–537

Martel-Pelletier, J., Pelletier, J.P., Cloutier, J.M., Howell, D.S., Ghander-Monaymreh, L. and Woessner, J.F. (1984). Neutral proteases capable of proteoglycan digesting activity in osteoarthritis and normal human articular cartilage. *Arth. Rheum.* **27**, 305–312

Maroudas, A. (1976). Balance between swelling pressure and collagen tension in normal and degenerate cartilage. *Nature* **260**, 808–809

Maroudas, A. and Urban, J.P.G. (1980). Swelling pressures of cartilaginous tissues. In *Studies in Joint Disease*, Vol. 1 (A. Maroudas and E.J. Holborow, eds), pp. 87–116. Pitman Medical, London

Maroudas, A. and Venn, M. (1977). Swelling of normal and osteoarthritic femoral head cartilage. *Ann. Rheum. Dis.* **36**, 399–406

Maroudas, A., Nachemson, A., Stockwell, R.A. and Urban, J.P.G. (1975) Factors involved in the nutrition of the intervertebral disc. *J. Anat.* **120**, 113–130

Maroudas, A., Schnaiderman, R. and Weinberg, C. (1990). Comparison between enhancing effects of serum and insulin on GAG synthesis in different zones of cultured human articular cartilage. *Trans. 36th Annual Meeting, Orthopaedic Research Society*, Vol. 15, p. 315. Louisiana

Poole, C.A., Ayad, S. and Schofield, J.R. (1988). Chondrons from articular cartilage: I. Immunolocalisation of type VI collagen in the pericellular capsule of isolated tibial chondrons. *J. Cell Sci.* **90**, 635–643

Roberts, S., Beard, H.K. and O'Brien, J.P. (1982). Biochemical changes of intervertebral discs in patients with spondylolisthesis or with tears of the posterior annulus fibrosus. *Ann. Rheum. Dis.* **41**, 78–85

Roberts, S., Weightman, B., Urban, J. and Chappell, D. (1986). Mechanical and biochemical properties of human articular cartilage from femoral head after subcapital fracture. *J. Bone Joint Surg.* **68B**, 418–422

Roberts, S., Menage, J. and Urban, J.P.G. (1989). Biochemical and structural properties of the cartilage end plate and its relation to the intervertebral disc. *Spine* **14**, 166–174

Rosner, I.A., Malemud, G.J., Goldberg, V.M., Papay, R.S., Getzy, L. and Moskowitz, R.W. (1982). Pathological and metabolic responses of experimental osteoarthritis to Estradiol and an Esstradiol antagonist. *Clin. Orthop. Rel. Res.* **171**, 280–286

Schneiderman, R., Keret, D. and Marudas, A. (1986). Effects of mechanical and osmotic pressure on the rate of glycosaminoglycan synthesis in the human adult femoral head cartilage. An *in vitro* study. *J. Orth. Res.* **4**, 393–408

Snowden, J. and Maroudas, A. (1976). The distribution of serum albumin in human normal and degenerate cartilage. *Biochem. Biophys. Acta* **428**, 726–733

Stockwell, R.A. (1979). *Biology of Cartilage Cells*, pp. 67–69. Cambridge University Press, Cambridge

Weinberg, C. (1987). Effects of serum on the rate of proteoglycan production by human articular cartilage in long term culture. MSc Thesis, Department of Biomedical Engineering, Technion – Israel Institute of Technology, Israel

Yaron, I., Meyer, F.A., Dayer, J-M., Bleiberg, I. and Yaron, M. (1989). Some recombinant human cytokines stimulate glycosaminoglycan synthesis in human synovial fibroblast cultures and inhibit it in human articular cartilage cultures. *Arthr. Rheum.* **32**, 173–180

2

EXTRACTION, SEPARATION AND ANALYSIS OF MATRIX CONSTITUENTS

COLLATED BY D.R. EYRE

7

Overview

D.R. EYRE

The articles in this section present methods aimed at defining the native polymeric structure and hence function of the collagens and proteoglycans (PGs) as they exist *in situ* in cartilage. New approaches are needed to understand the native polymeric states and the specific interactions of the various types of collagen molecule in cartilage. What is their spatial distribution (with respect to each other, to the cells and to other matrix ingredients) and to what degree are they polymerized into homopolymers and heteropolymers? The methods reported by Eyre *et al.* (Chapter 8), Ayad *et al.* (Chapter 9) and van der Rest *et al.* (Chapter 14) address these questions.

PGs present unique difficulties of extraction and analysis. Bayliss (Chapter 10) reviews the problems of extraction and recommends optimum methods for human tissue. Once extracted, proteoglycan molecules resist clean fractionation by traditional biochemical methods, in part because of their inherent posttranslational heterogeneity, making it difficult to distinguish genetically distinct molecules from post-translational variants and degradation products. McDevitt (Chapter 11) and Stanescu (Chapter 12) describe their latest large-pore gel electrophoresis systems for resolving PG subtypes and Pita *et al.* (Chapter 13) summarize their elegant micromethods for studying proteoglycan aggregation by ultracentrifugation. Finally, Helen Muir (Chapter 15) comments with insight on the significance of these methods in relation to the overall technical difficulties and outstanding questions in cartilage matrix biochemistry.

8

The cartilage collagens — analysis of their cross-linking interactions and matrix organization

D.R. EYRE, J.J. WU, C. NIYIBIZI and L. CHUN

INTRODUCTION

The material strength of cartilage rests on the tensile properties of its collagen fibril network. Collagen fibril strength depends on the formation of covalent bonds between its polymerized collagen molecules. In cartilage, these collagen cross-linking bonds are derived almost exclusively by the reactions of hydroxylysine side-chains with the aldehyde residues made from telopeptide hydroxylysines by lysyl oxidase (Eyre et al., 1984b). Methods are available to quantify the initial ketoamine and ensuing hydroxypyridinium cross-links (Eyre, 1987), of which hydroxylysyl pyridinoline (HP) is the predominant structure in mature cartilage collagen. This naturally fluorescent, trivalent cross-linking amino acid can be measured with great sensitivity (down to 1 pmol) in acid hydrolysates of whole cartilage or derived collagen fractions by an established procedure that uses reverse-phase high performance liquid chromatography (HPLC) and fluorescence detection (Eyre et al., 1984a).

All three cartilage-specific collagens, types II, IX and XI, contain such hydroxylysine-aldehyde based cross-links (Wu and Eyre, 1984). Isolation and analysis of tryptic peptides containing HP from type IX collagen showed that most of these cross-links form by an interaction between telopeptide domains of type II collagen and one or more helical domains in type IX collagen (Eyre et al., 1987a; van der Rest and Mayne, 1988). In mature bovine articular cartilage, the main site of HP in type IX collagen was traced to a tryptic peptide consisting of two $\alpha 1(II)$ carboxytelopeptides linked to a helical fragment (COL2) of the collagen type IX molecule, with a lesser amount in a peptide derived from two $\alpha 1(II)$ N-telopeptides linked to a type IX helical site (Eyre et al., 1987a). In embryonic chick cartilage, only $\alpha 1(II)$N-telopeptide to type IX helical sites have so far been identified (Van der Rest and Mayne, 1988).

The function of the covalent bonds between type IX collagen molecules and type II collagen molecules on the surface of fibrils (a location confirmed by immunogold localization analyses (Müller-Glaser et al., 1986; Vaughan et al., 1988) is not known. The bivalent bonding potential of type IX molecules could provide a mechanism for strengthening the collagen network by direct interfibrillar links, or such matrix reinforcement might occur simply because of increased frictional resistance to shear between the type-IX-coated collagen fibrils and their surrounding PGs. Whatever the function, it is becoming clear that heterotypic cross-linking between different types of collagen molecule, and perhaps between collagen and other matrix proteins, is a common occurrence in the extracellular matrix. Methods for identifying and quantifying such covalent interactions are clearly important in understanding how cartilage functions mechanically, how its matrix is assembled and maintained and how its collagen architecture fails in osteoarthritis.

MATERIALS AND METHODS

Cartilage was sampled from 2-year steer femoral condyles and from the growing ends of the long bones of 4–5 month old fetal calves. PGs were extracted from the cartilage slices using 4 M guanidine HCl, 0.05 M tris/HCl, pH 7.5 for 48 h at 4°C or by chondroitinase-ABC, trypsin and streptomyces hyaluronidase in sequence at 37°C (Chun et al., 1986) and the residues were washed exhaustively with water and minced with an Ultra-Turrax homogenizer. Collagen was solubilized from the residue by pepsin (1/50 w/w) at 4°C and fractionated by precipitation step-wise with increasing NaCl concentrations (0.7, 0.9, 1.2 and 2.2 M NaCl), essentially as described previously (Eyre et al., 1984c).

Individual collagen types were suspended in 0.1 M sodium phosphate, pH 7.4, and reacted with [^{3}H]-NaBH$_4$ (10 mCi mmol^{-1}) to reduce and label the borohydride reducible cross-linking residues (Eyre, 1987). After 1 h at 25°C, the collagen suspension was acidified, dialyzed against 0.1 M acetic acid and freeze dried. Individual collagen chains and derived tryptic peptides were resolved by reverse-phase HPLC (25 cm × 4.6 mm, C18 Vydac 218TP54 or Brownlee C8 Aquapore RP-300) (Eyre and Wu, 1983; Eyre et al., 1987a). Figure 8.1 outlines the strategy for locating cross-linking sites within a collagen molecule that is applicable to trivalent or divalent residues. Trivalent, pyridinoline cross-links are monitored during chromatography by their natural fluorescence (297-nm excitation at pH < 4, 330-nm excitation at pH > 6, 390-nm emission) and reduced divalent, ketoamine cross-links by their tritium activity incorporated from NaB^{3}H$_4$ (Eyre et al., 1984b).

Purified collagen molecules, individual α-chains and other chain fragments were reacted with sodium metaperiodate (NaIO$_4$), which will selectively cleave the borohydride reduced cross-links, dihydroxylysinonorlencine (DHLN) and hydroxylysinonorleucine (HLN) that are derived from hydroxylysine aldehydes (Eyre and Glimcher, 1973). The telopeptides released by this cleavage were resolved by reverse-phase HPLC and identified by protein microsequencing (see

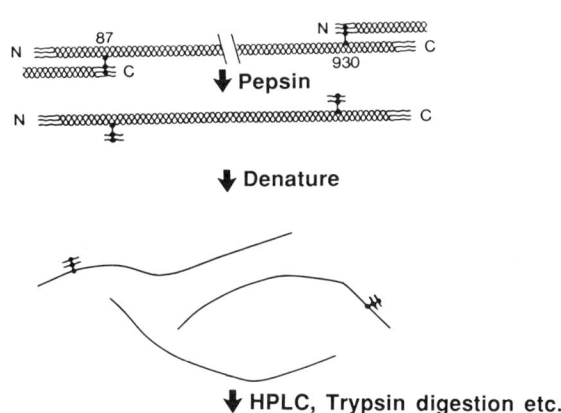

Figure 8.1 Strategy for defining sites of intermolecular cross-linking in collagen. An example of a trivalent cross-linking residue is shown (in reality the two telopeptides probably originate in two different collagen molecules, not one as shown here (Eyre et al., 1984b)). Divalent cross-links can also be located after NaB^{3}H$_4$ reduction.

Chapter 13 for other applications) on a Porton 2090E gas-phase sequencer with on-line phenylthiohydantoin (PTH) analysis. Figure 8.2 shows the reaction scheme that allows telopeptide sequences linked by ketoamine cross-links to be isolated from pepsin solubilized collagen chains. Tritium from NaB^{3}H$_4$ remains with the aldehyde donor residue (so far found only in telopeptide sequences of collagen) which is converted to the newly-created amino acid, δ-hydroxynorvaline, still in peptide linkage. The method therefore allows the originating peptide sequences that bear the aldehyde forming hydroxylysine and the reacting hydroxylysine ε-amino side-chain to be defined.

Pyridinoline cross-links were quantified in protein fractions by reverse-phase HPLC using a fluorescence detector (Eyre et al., 1984a). Both forms of pyridinoline (hydroxylysyl pyridinoline (HP) and lysyl pyridinoline (LP)) and the borohydride reduced DHLN and HLN were also quantified after enrichment by molecular sieving on a column of Bio-Gel P2 by ion exchange chromatography and ninhydrin detection (Eyre, 1987).

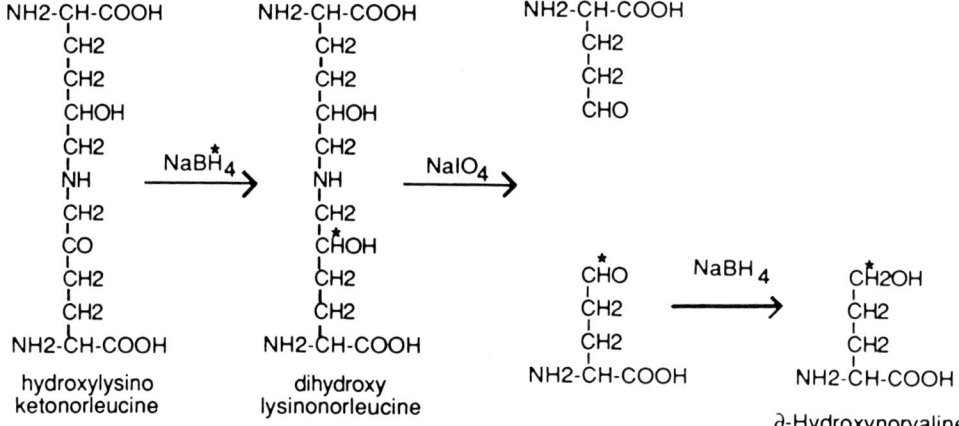

Figure 8.2 Reaction scheme whereby NaB^{3}H$_4$ reduced ketoamine cross-links in peptide linkage are cleaved by periodate oxidation. Tritiated δ-hydroxynorvaline is produced from the half of the cross-link which was originally an hydroxylysine aldehyde.

RESULTS AND DISCUSSION

After extraction with 4 M guanidine HCl (Eyre et al., 1987b; see also Chapter 9) or the enzymes, chondroitinase-ABC, trypsin and streptomyces hyaluronidase in sequence (Chun et al., 1986; unpublished data), the collagenous residue of bovine articular cartilage gives three collagen types by pepsin digestion at 4°C, types II, IX and XI. Only a small fraction of any of these collagens is extracted by protein denaturants (e.g. 4 M guanidine HCl) or by the glycosidase and trypsin combination, whereas the small amount of type VI collagen in cartilage is fully extracted (see Chapter 9). The recovered ratios of type II : type IX : type XI collagens are about 80 : 10 : 10 for fetal calf

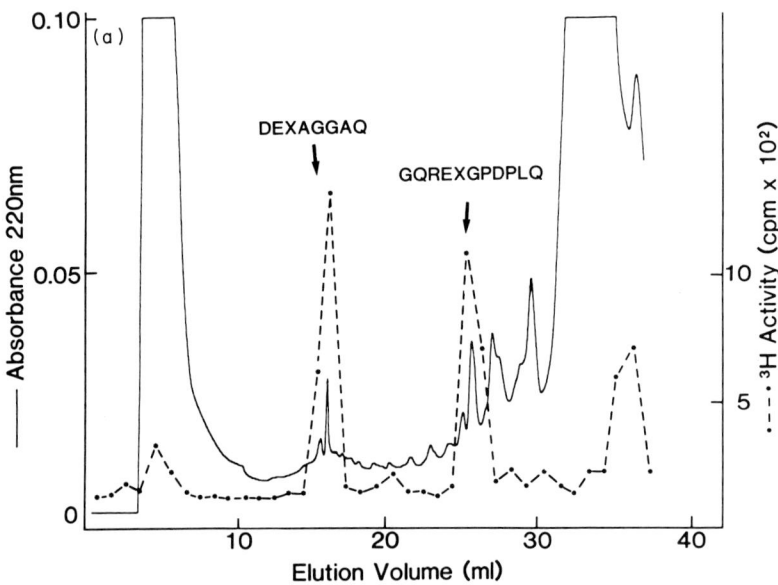

8. CARTILAGE COLLAGENS: INTERACTIONS AND ORGANIZATION   31

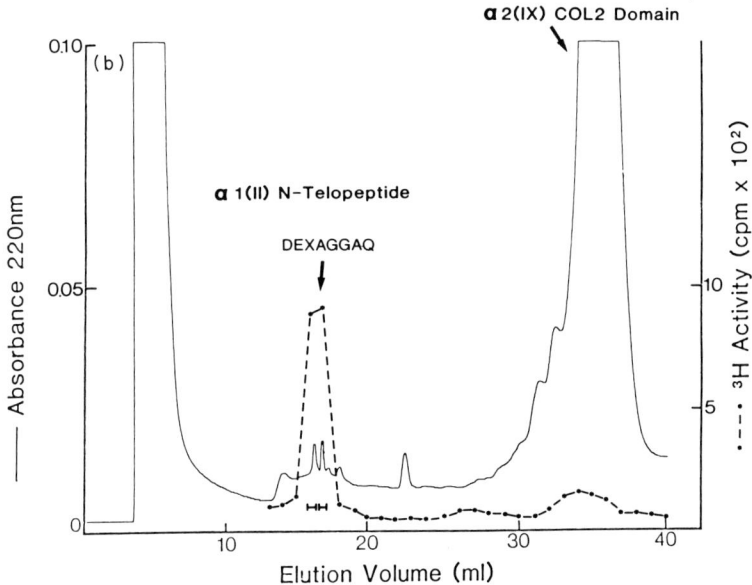

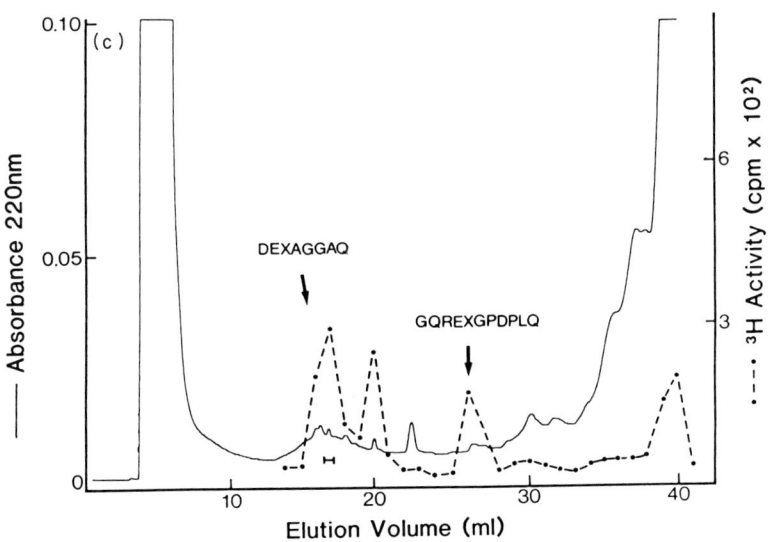

Figure 8.3 Fractionation by reverse-phase HPLC of tritiated telopeptide sequences released from bovine fetal cartilage type II and IX collagen preparations by periodate oxidation. (a) Isolated $\alpha1$(II) chains, (b) $\alpha2$(IX)COL2 fragment, (c) $\alpha1$(IX)COL2 plus $\alpha3$(IX)COL2 fragments.

cartilage (long-bone articular plus epiphyseal) and 96 : 1 : 3 for 18-month steer articular cartilage.

Cross-link analyses on the individual collagen types II, IX and XI, purified by salt precipitation from 3% (v/v) acetic acid at 0.7 M (type II), 1.2 M (type XI) and 2.2 M NaCl (type IX, HMW plus LMW fragments of type IX), showed borohydride reducible (largely dehydro-DHLN which gives DHLN after reduction) and mature pyridinoline (largely HP) residues in all three types (results not shown). In fetal cartilage, the reducible cross-links dominated over mature in all three collagen types but pyridinolines were dominant over reducibles (> 10 : 1 molar ratio) in collagen types II and IX of the adult tissue. Type IX collagen was distinguished from the other collagens by containing a significant amount of LP, the HP : LP ratio in type IX collagen from 18-month steer cartilage being about 8 : 1.

Figure 8.3, as an example, shows the results of applying the periodate method for isolating cross-linking telopeptides from type II and IX collagens of fetal bovine cartilage. The tritiated peptides released by the periodate reaction scheme (Fig. 8.2) were resolved from each other and from the helical chain fragment by reverse-phase HPLC. Their sequences, including the location of the tritiated δ-hydroxynorvaline residue, were determined by gas-phase microsequencing. The δ-hydroxynorvaline residue was identified both

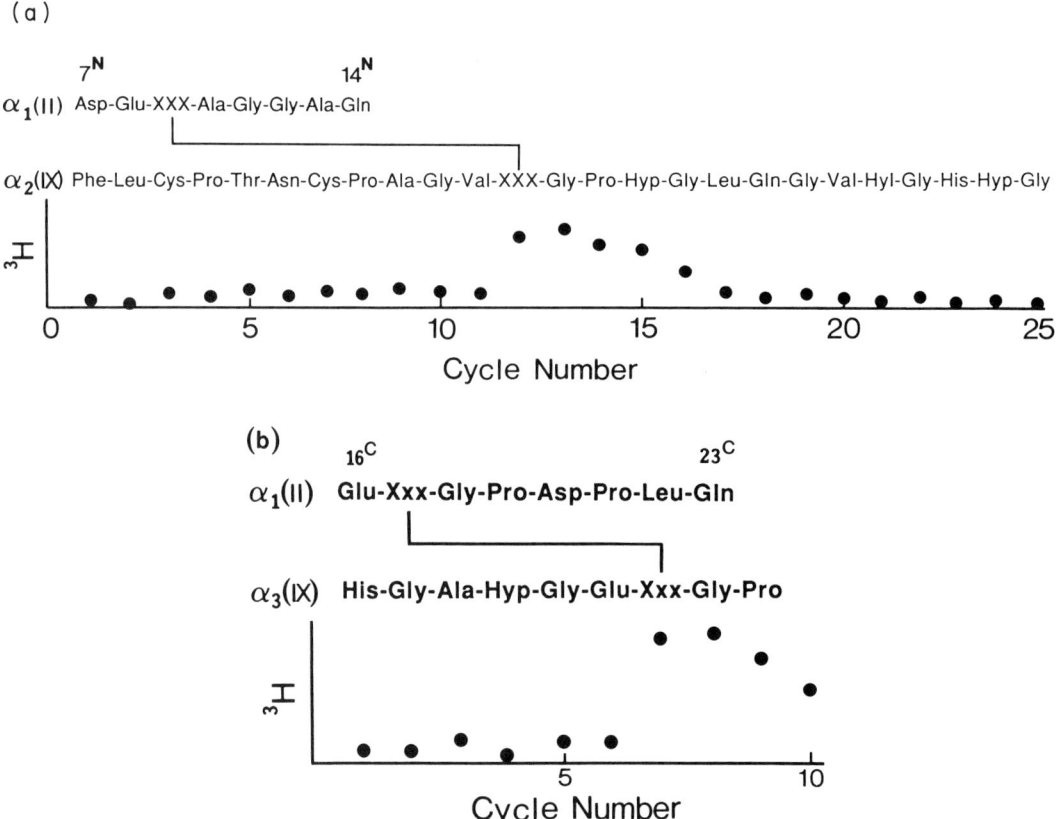

Figure 8.4 Results of protein microsequencing on two tryptic peptides purified from bovine fetal cartilage type IX collagen. (a) Site of $\alpha 2(IX)$ linkage to an $\alpha 1(II)$ N-telopeptide. (b) Site of $\alpha 3(IX)$ linkage to an $\alpha 1(II)$ C-telopeptide. A portion of each Edman degradation product (PTH derivative) was collected for tritium assay. In these two examples, counts appear at the cycle corresponding to the release of the second half of the cross-linking residue which was originally a hydroxylysine in the triple helical sequence.

as a PTH derivative in the HPLC chromatogram and as tritium activity measured in the portion of each cycle from the sequencer directed to a fraction collector. Sequences are shown using the single-letter amino acid code; X is used for the δ-hydroxynorvaline residue.

Figure 8.4 shows microsequencing results on highly purified tryptic peptides that were derived from fetal bovine cartilage type IX collagen. The peptide in Fig. 8.4(a) came from the site of the DHLN cross-link in the $\alpha 2(IX)$ chain (an hydroxylysine at residue 3 of the COL2 domain linked to an $\alpha 1(II)N$-telopeptide). In Fig. 8.4(b) the peptide was derived from one of the two sites of DHLN in the $\alpha 3(IX)COL2$ domain (and was formed by reaction with an $\alpha 1(II)C$-telopeptide).

Such methods are now being applied to collagen type XI and to the various cross-linked collagen polymers of other connective tissues in order to explore their original intermolecular bonding patterns and hence native organization in the extracellular matrix.

ACKNOWLEDGMENTS

This work was supported in part by USPHS grants from the NIH, AR37318 and AR36794.

9

Mammalian cartilage collagens: identification of their forms *in vivo*

SHIRLEY AYAD, ANNE MARRIOTT, KEITH MORGAN, CHRISTINE CUMMINGS, ALVIN P.L. KWAN, A. PAUL MOULD and MICHAEL E. GRANT

INTRODUCTION

The original concept that cartilage is a homogeneous tissue, comprising a network of type II collagen fibrils inflated by hydrated proteoglycans (PGs), has been modified in recent years. The chondrocytes and matrix macromolecules are not randomly disposed but exhibit a high degree of organization and compartmentalization which is related to the type and anatomical site of the cartilage, as well as to the species and age of the organism. Most types of cartilage contain two quantitatively minor collagens, types IX and XI, whereas type X collagen is present specifically in cartilage which calcifies and is replaced by bone. Our understanding of the intact forms of these collagens *in vivo* is based largely on biosynthetic studies using cell or organ culture and on the amino acid sequences deduced from cDNA/genomic DNA clones encoding the different collagen chains. Moreover, most studies have used avian cartilage. We have, therefore, developed a non-hydrolytic procedure to extract the collagens in an intact form from mammalian cartilage and have demonstrated that type VI collagen is also present in cartilage, confirming previous immuno-fluorescence studies (Ayad *et al.*, 1984).

METHODS

The protocol for the extraction and characterization of intact collagens from fetal bovine epiphysial and growth-plate cartilage is outlined in Fig. 9.1. The tissue was powdered in a stainless-steel mill under liquid nitrogen and then extracted twice with 4 M guanidine hydrochloride (GuHCl), 50 mM tris/HCl, pH 7.4 in the presence of proteinase inhibitors at 4°C for 24–48 h. The GuHCl extracts were dialyzed against 7 × vol. 50 mM tris/HCl, pH 7.4, and subjected to CsCl density gradient centrifugation under associative conditions (starting density 1.5–1.6 g cm^{-3}; 100 000 g for 72 h at 20°C). The collagens and other proteins concentrated as a gel at the top of the gradient. The gel was suspended in, and dialyzed exhaustively against, either 0.5 M acetic acid (HAc) or 1 M NaCl, 50 mM tris/HCl, pH 7.4 (NS), and the solubilized collagens fractionated by differential salt precipitation at acid or neutral pH, respectively. Fractions containing type II and IX collagens were diluted with 0.5 M ammonium acetate (final collagen concentration 2.6 μg ml^{-1}), glycerol dried and rotary shadowed with platinum and tungsten at an angle of 3° (Mould et al., 1985). The collagens and other proteins remaining in the HAc/NS-insoluble material were fractionated either: (i) in the native state on diethylamino-ethyl-cellulose (DEAE-cellulose) using 7 M urea, 50 mM tris/HCL, pH 8.3, containing 0.2% Triton X-100 and proteinase inhibitors and a NaCl gradient 0–0.5 M; or (ii) on Sepharose CL-4B using the 4 M GuHCl extraction buffer, after

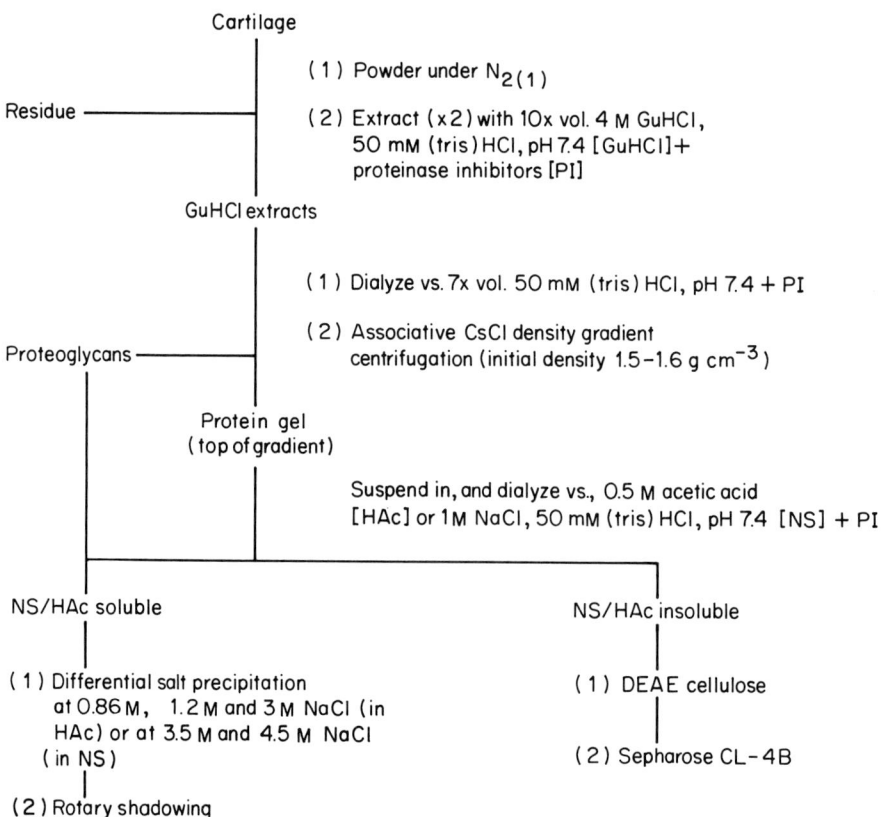

Figure 9.1 Extraction and characterization of the intact forms of mammalian cartilage collagens.

heating the sample at 60°C for 1 h. Aliquots of the unfractionated GuHCl extracts were also equilibrated in 0.5 M acetic acid, digested with pepsin and fractionated according to the procedure of Trueb et al. (1987) in which a high ionic strength is maintained throughout to prevent the aggregation of the pepsinized type VI collagen. Antisera were raised to the pepsinized forms of types II, IX and XI collagens from bovine cartilage (Evans et al., 1983) to the pepsinized form of type VI collagen from bovine uterus (Ayad et al., 1984; Poole et al., 1988) and to the intact form of type X collagen from chick chondrocyte culture medium (Kwan et al., 1986). The antisera were then used to identify the intact collagens in the GuHCl extracts before and after fractionation: fractions were analyzed by SDS/PAGE, transferred to nitocellulose and immunoblotted with the specific antisera using the method of Blake et al. (1984).

RESULTS AND APPLICATIONS

The collagens extracted using GuHCl accounted for approximately 10% of the total collagen present in fetal cartilage. The collagens regained their native conformations after removal of this reagent as shown by the presence of intact rod-like molecules on rotary shadowing (Fig. 9.2) and also by the recovery of their characteristic triple-helical domains following pepsin digestion. The M_r values of their component α-chains estimated using sodium dodecyl sulfate–polyacrylamide gel electrophoresis (SDS–PAGE) indicated that the chains were intact. Type II collagen was present as the processed form with chains of M_r 100 kDa. The extracted forms of type VI and IX collagen were similar to the procollagen forms observed in biosynthetic studies, indicating that little or no processing occurred before deposition in the

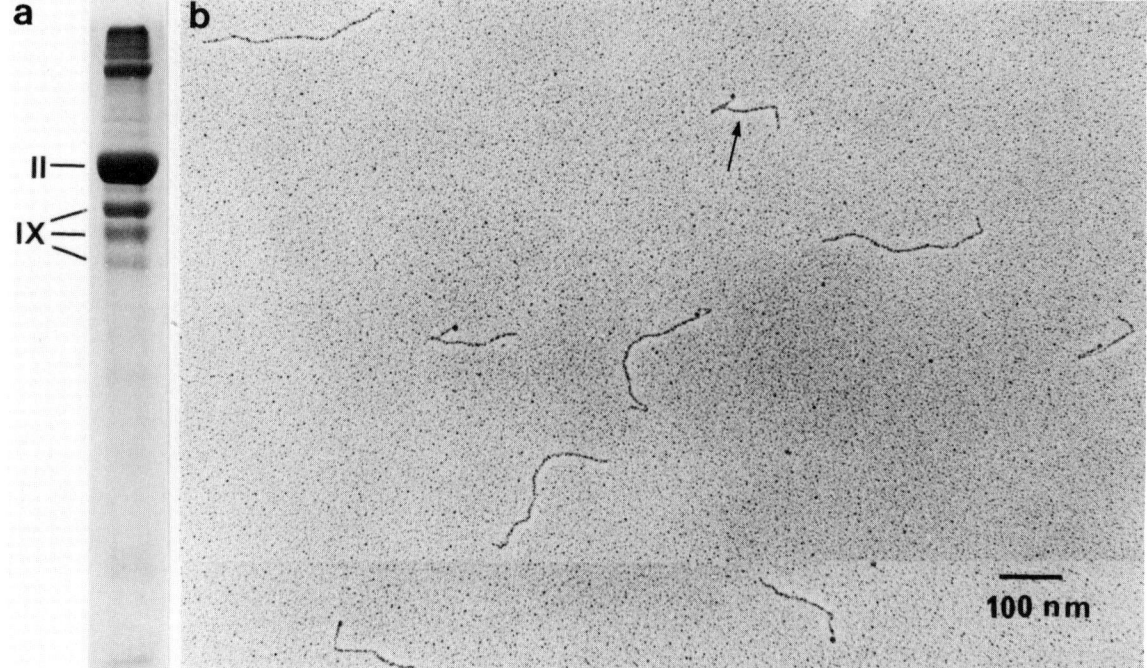

Figure 9.2 Electron micrograph of rotary-shadowed type II and IX collagen extracted from bovine cartilage. The 4.5 M NaCl precipitate from the NS-soluble fraction (Figure 9.1) comprising type II and IX collagen (a) was rotary shadowed with platinum and tungsten (b). Note the globular N-terminal domain and characteristic kinks in the linear structures of type IX collagen (arrowed). Scale bar 100-nm.

cartilage matrix. Cartilage type VI collagen was isolated as a large M_r disulfide bonded aggregate comprised of $\alpha 1(VI)$ and $\alpha 2(VI)$ chains of M_r 140 kDa and a heterogeneous $\alpha 3(VI)$ chain of M_r 200–240 kDa, similar to type VI collagen isolated from non-cartilaginous tissues. It eluted in the void volume of the Sepharose CL-4B column but tended to aggregate and remain bound to DEAE-cellulose if Triton X-100 was not included in the elution buffer. Type IX collagen consisted of three components of M_r 84, 72 and 66 kDa that were assigned to the $\alpha 1(IX)$, $\alpha 3(IX)$ and $\alpha 2(IX)$ chains respectively, on the basis of their behavior on DEAE-cellulose. At least 95% of this collagen did not bind to DEAE-cellulose and was unaffected by treatment with chondroitinase-ABC. Therefore, most of the extracted bovine type IX collagen (in contrast to the newly-synthesized chick collagen) (van der Rest and Mayne, 1987) had no covalently-bound glycosaminoglycan attached to the $\alpha 2(IX)$ chain. Type X collagen was extracted specifically from the calcifying growth-plate cartilage and occurred largely as the processed form with chains of M_r 49 kDa, although low levels of procollagen X with chains of M_r 59 kDa could be detected (Ayad et al., 1987). The antiserum to type XI collagen was specific for the pepsinized form and did not detect the intact form of this collagen in the GuHCl extracts.

In summary, cartilage collagens can be analyzed in their native state following extraction with 4 M GuHCl. In the case of types II, IX, X and XI collagens, only a small proportion of the total collagen is extractable as these collagens become cross-linked in the extracellular matrix. In contrast, type VI collagen is extracted completely by GuHCl and explains why this collagen has not been observed previously in pepsin digests of cartilage following the extraction of PGs by GuHCl (Ayad et al., 1984). The methods described are now being applied in studies on human articular cartilage to assess both qualitative and quantitative changes in the different collagens with age and disease.

ACKNOWLEDGEMENT

The financial support of the Arthritis and Rheumatism Council of Great Britain is gratefully acknowledged.

10

Extraction and purification of proteoglycan and hyaluronan from human articular cartilage

M. BAYLISS

The characteristic mechanical and physicochemical properties of articular cartilage are determined by the highly organized assembly of extracellular matrix components. Proteoglycans (PGs) have a large hydrodynamic size and they overlap and entangle with themselves and with the collagen. Collagen in articular cartilage has a fine spacing (of the order of 100 nm) and this is further subdivided by PGs into pore sizes of less than 5 nm (Maroudas, 1979). Diffusion of PG through these fine pores will be slowed down considerably because of this entanglement, and the larger PGs will move more slowly than the smaller ones. For example, Klein and Meyer (1982) have shown that it takes several weeks for hyaluronic acid to move through connective tissues (see also Chapters 55 and 64). Thus, the barrier to diffusion, imposed by the dense collagenous network, can be a serious problem when attempting to purify PG from some sources of cartilage. This has proved to be the case for human articular cartilage.

EXTRACTION

Attempts to isolate PG aggregates from finely-diced human cartilage (the traditional method of 'homogenizing' the tissue prior to extraction) were often unsuccessful (Fig. 10.1(a)) (Bayliss and Ali, 1978a,b). Even when cartilage was sliced into serial 250 μm sections, in order to study the zonal variations through the depth of cartilage, very few of the purified PGs were aggregated, and yet they were capable of complexing with hyaluronan (HA) (Bayliss et al., 1983; Bayliss and Roughley, 1985) (Fig. 10.1(b)). This unusual finding was incorrectly interpreted by some investigators as evidence for the nonaggregation of PG in human articular cartilage. Although this misconception was subsequently corrected, it does serve to illustrate the care that must be taken when experimental procedures that have been successfully applied to one source of cartilage are applied to another without taking into account possible changes in macromolecular organization. This principle is not necessarily confined to different types of cartilage (nasal vs. laryngeal vs. articular), it also applies to cartilage of the same type from different species and to different ages within the same species. For example, the proportion of aggregates in a reassociated 4 M guanidine HCl extract of finely-diced mature pig or bovine articular cartilage, is far higher than that of adult human. Similarly, the aggregate content of an extract of new born or immature human articular cartilage is significantly higher than that from adult cartilage.

With hindsight it was easy to see that these variations were due to dramatic differences in the density of the collagen network. Careful powdering of human articular cartilage showed quite clearly that extraction of HA, and thus the proportion of aggregates in the PG-rich, high-density fraction of a CsCl gradient, is significantly increased (Bayliss and Ali, 1978b; Bayliss et al., 1983) (Fig. 10.1). Considerable physical disruption of human articular cartilage is therefore required before a representative extraction of HA and PG monomer is obtained. However, choosing the

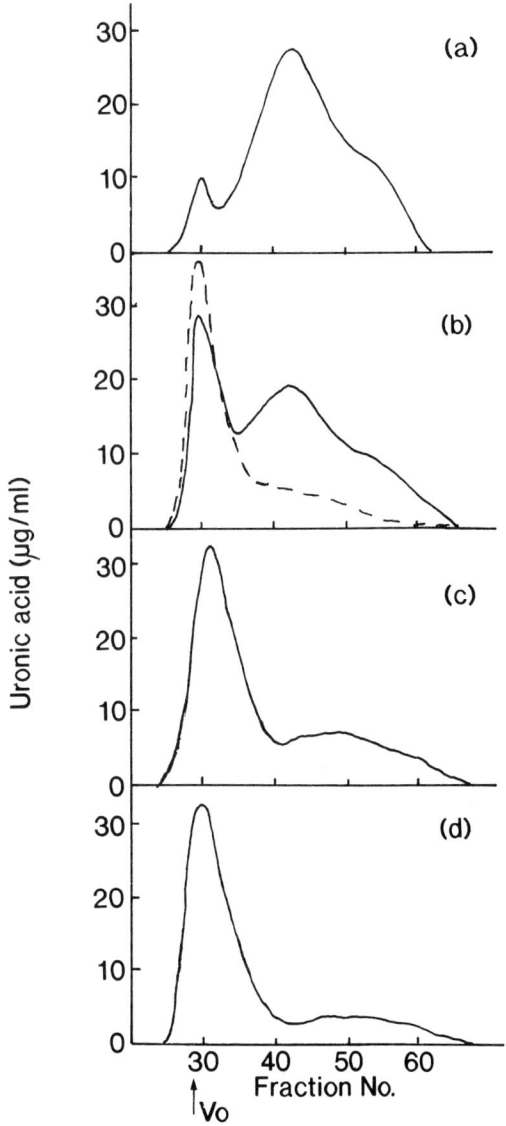

Figure 10.1 Sepharose CL-2B chromatography of proteoglycan aggregate (fraction A_1) purified from 4 M guanidine HCl extracts of adult human articular cartilage. Cartilage was (a) diced 2 mm², (b) sliced 250 μm, (c) powdered (2 g for 15 s), or (d) sectioned 20 μm, before extraction. The broken line in (b) shows the elution profile for fraction A_1 : 4% (w/w) HA.

appropriate method to effect this disruption is equally important. Although powdering of the tissue in liquid nitrogen results in an acceptable extraction of both components, it is extremely difficult to standardize the process, even when using a Spex Freezer Mill. Small changes in the amount of tissue used and the time for which it is powdered dramatically change the macromolecular structure of the final product (Bayliss and Venn, 1980). Figure 10.2 shows that, even after 15 s of powdering, extensive mechanical degradation of PG aggregate occurs.

The method that has been most successfully applied to human cartilage, and which combines efficiency of extraction with quality of product, is to 'homogenize' the tissue at 20 μm on a cryostat (Fig. 10.1(d)) (Bayliss et al., 1983; Bayliss and Roughley, 1985). It is also important to note that the way in which cartilage is treated not only determines the efficiency of extraction of individual matrix components, but where molecular heterogeneity exists (as for the PGs), it can also influence the population of macromolecules recovered. Comparison of extracts of cartilage sectioned at 20 or 250 μm showed that, in the latter case, PGs richer in keratan sulfate and of lower molecular weight were preferentially extracted (Bayliss et al., 1983). Since the rate of diffusion is proportional to the inverse of the distance squared (Chapter 59) the extraction of 20 μm thick slices is 150 times faster than from 250 μm thick slices. Thus, diffusion properties alone can explain why a larger proportion of small PGs are extracted from the thicker slices. HA extraction, however, may depend more on destruction of the collagen network, which would result in less entanglement, although diffusion of these large molecules would also be very slow in thick slices. From a teleological point of view it is noteworthy that the surface of cartilage, which is in contact with the synovial fluid and through which the PGs are therefore most likely to be lost, has also the tightest collagen network and the largest PGs.

From a practical point of view, it is of paramount importance to optimize the extraction of matrix components before a meaningful comparison of their quality and quantity in different samples of cartilage can be made (e.g. normal age-related vs. disease-related changes). In many cases this will not be achieved simply by choosing the appropriate extractant, but will also require a standardized method of fragmenting the tissue. Although cryosectioning of cartilage is tedious and does not lend itself easily to large-scale preparations, it does provide a very safe and effective means of achieving a standardized method.

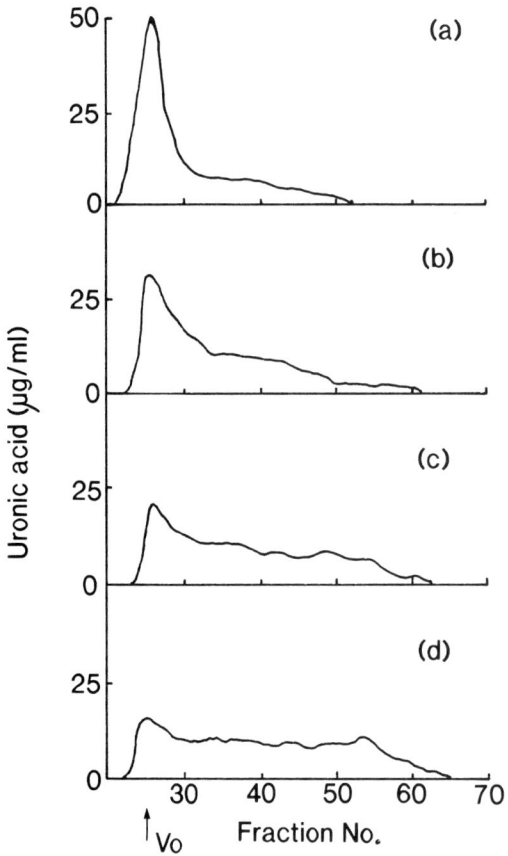

Figure 10.2 Sepharose CL-2B chromatography of proteoglycans isolated from adult human cartilage, powdered for various periods of time before extraction: (a) 2 g for 15 s; (b) 1 g for 15 s; (c) 1 g for 30 s; (d) 1 g for 60 s.

Purification

Having achieved a representative extract of all components of PG aggregate, problems can still arise during their purification if changes in composition are not allowed for. Separation of PG from soluble collagen and other noncollagenous proteins is normally carried out by equilibrium density gradient centrifugation in CsCl. The high bouyant density (low protein : carbohydrate ratio) of PG isolated from most sources of animal cartilage that are studied, enables a relatively high starting concentration of CsCl ($\varrho_0 = 1.69$ g ml^{-1}) to be used. This procedure ensures that approximately 90% of the PG is recovered in the high-density fraction of the gradient. A similar recovery is achieved for extracts of human fetal and immature cartilage, which also have a low protein : carbohydrate ratio. However, during maturation and ageing of human cartilage there is a considerable increase in the protein content of PG aggregates, reflecting extensive changes in the composition and molecular weight of the PG monomer population (Roughley and White, 1980; Bayliss, 1986). In particular, the relative proportion of the HA binding region, relatively free of carbohydrate, increases markedly. These changes reduce the bouyant density of the reformed aggregates and thus dictate the use of a lower starting CsCl concentration, $\varrho_0 = 1.5$ g ml^{-1} (Bayliss and Roughley, 1985).

The effect of different CsCl concentrations on the recovery of adult human PGs from the high-density fractions of the gradient is shown in Fig. 10.3. Not only is the proportion reduced from 90% to 50% when $\varrho_0 = 1.69$ g ml^{-1}, but the extent of aggregation in high density fractions is also decreased because the lower bouyant aggregates (containing the majority of protein-rich monomers and HA binding proteins) sediment in the middle fractions of the gradient (Fig. 10.3(c)).

extraction and purification must first be achieved before a meaningful interpretation of subsequent analytical data can be made, and that it cannot necessarily be assumed that conditions that apply to one source of cartilage are appropriate for another.

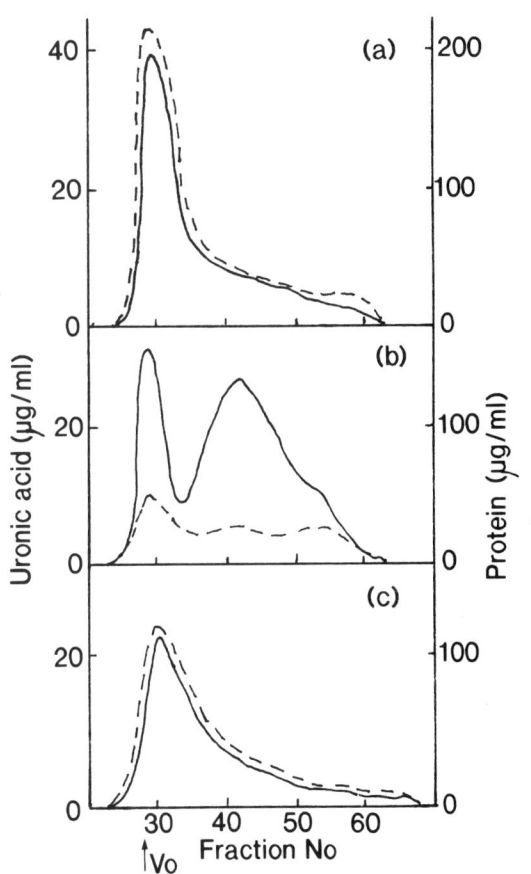

Figure 10.3 Extracts of adult human articular cartilage were subjected to CsCl density gradient centrifugation under associative conditions using a staring density of either (a) 1.5 g ml^{-1} or (b) 1.69 g ml^{-1}. The resulting high bouyant density fractions from each gradient (density > 1.54 g ml^{-1} or 1.73 g ml^{-1}, respectively) were chromatographed on Sepharose Cl-2B, as were the combined fractions from the 1.69 g ml^{-1} gradient, that had a density of 1.73–1.66 g ml^{-1} (c). The percentage of uronic acid recovered in each fraction is also shown.

CONCLUSION

Although the above examples may seem obvious to many investigators familiar with connective-tissue methodology, a survey of the current literature indicates that it is still worth reemphasizing that the best conditions of

11

Composite agarose–acrylamide electrophoresis of proteoglycans and large protein complexes

CAHIR A. McDEVITT

INTRODUCTION

Polyacrylamide gel electrophoresis remains one of the most important methods in a biochemist's repertoire of techniques for resolving proteins. The pore sizes of conventional polyacrylamide gels, which are inversely related to the concentration of acrylamide in the pre-gel monomer mixture, are not large enough to permit penetration of large proteoglycans (PGs) and protein complexes. Below 2% concentration, polyacrylamide does not form a gel. The incorporation of agarose into acrylamide solutions of less than 2%, however, results in a gel with adequate mechanical properties for electrophoresis and pore sizes large enough to allow penetration of the large PGs of cartilage (McDevitt and Muir, 1971).

PROTEOGLYCAN ELECTROPHORESIS IN AGAROSE–ACRYLAMIDE TUBE GELS

The original study undertaken in Helen Muir's laboratory (McDevitt and Muir, 1971) yielded some particularly surprising results. Firstly, in a systematic study of different gel compositions (i.e. varying agarose and acrylamide concentrations in the gel), we found that a gel composed of 1.2% polyacrylamide/0.6% agarose gave optimum separations for PGs. Roughley (1989), in a later independent study, confirmed that observation. We also noted that the quality of the gels formed and the PG separations they yielded varied with the agarose from different suppliers.

The second surprising result was that purified glycosaminoglycans and PGs that were markedly polydisperse with respect to size in gel chromatography migrated as relatively sharp bands in the composite gels. The final surprise was that cartilage PGs separated into two or more clearly-resolved bands in the gels. PG aggregates, however, did not penetrate the gels.

Three properties of PGs determine their mobility on electrophoretic gels: their size, their charge: mass ratio and, it would appear, their degree of interaction with the composite agarose polyacrylamide matrix. The technique may therefore be used to establish the number of electrophoretically distinguishable populations of PGs in a sample, i.e. the heterogeneity of a sample. A distinct advantage of the technique is that small quantities of PG (less than 1 μg) can be evaluated using toluidine blue (McDevitt and Muir, 1971) or Stains All (Jahnke and McDevitt, 1988). A limitation of the technique, compared with conventional sodium dodecyl sulfate (SDS) protein polyacrylamide electrophoresis, is that migration is not a simple function of the molecular weight of the PG. A PG may migrate fast in these gels because of a relatively large charge : mass ratio.

The composite gel method has been applied elegantly in many studies in a variety of laboratories, initially those of Roughley and Stanescu (for example see Chapter 12, also Jahnke and McDevitt, 1988; McDevitt, 1988). Curiously, the structural feature responsible for the separation of the two major bands of cartilage (and intervertebral disc) PGs remains to be established, although we do know that it resides in the glycosaminoglycan bearing portion of the molecule (Jahnke and McDevitt, 1988).

The source of the PGs influences the sharpness and number of bands obtained, presumably because of the degree of extracellular processing of the molecules. In general, PGs derived from *in vitro* chondrocyte cultures or tissue extracts of young animal cartilage (e.g. rabbits) yield sharp bands, whle those from tissue extracts of longer lived animals, such as dogs, give moderately sharp bands. Human tissues usually yield PGs that either migrate as fairly broad bands or fail to resolve into discrete populations and stain as one very diffuse band. Preliminary separation of such human PGs by density gradient centrifugation or gel chromatography, however, can yield subpopulations that migrate in the electrophoretic system as sharp, distinct bands. A study by Jahnke and McDevitt (1988) on the electrophoretic behavior of the PGs of the nucleus pulposus of the young adult disc graphically illustrates this property. The starting A1 fraction of the disc PGs, the separated aggregating and nonaggregating PG populations and chromatographic subpopulations of both the aggregating and nonaggregating pools were all evaluated by composite gel electrophoresis (Fig. 11.1). The A1 fraction (containing both aggregating and nonaggregating PGs), the aggregating (pool 1, Fig. 11.1(a)) and the nonaggregating (pool 2, Fig. 11.1(a)) all migrated as diffuse bands in the gels (Fig. 11.1(b)). Individual column fractions of a dissociative chromatographic separation of the aggregating PGs (Fig. 11.1(c)) migrated as two clearly-resolved bands in the gels (Fig. 11.1(d)). Column fractions of the nonaggregating PGs (Fig. 11.1(e)), in contrast, migrated as single bands (Fig. 11.1(f)).

SLAB GEL ELECTROPHORESIS OF PROTEOGLYCANS

Heinegard *et al.* (1985a) and Carney *et al.* (1986) have published slab gel applications of the original tube gel technique. These slab gels permit transfer onto nitrocellulose or nylon membranes and localization of specific subpopulations with anti-PG antibodies. A number of improved, unpublished modifications of the slab gel procedure are currently in use in different laboratories. The following recipe is in use in Dr Margaret Aydelotte's laboratory (Rush-Presbyterian–St Luke's Medical School, Chicago), yields good quality PG separations and is reproduced, with her permission, for the purpose of accessibility. It yields a gel that is 1.27% total acrylamide/bisacrylamide monomer and 0.64% agarose.

Recipe for slab polyacrylamide–agarose gel

Materials

One frosted- and one plain-glass plate (17.5 × 14-cm) are assembled with 1.5-mm spacers and heated to 50°C in an oven immediately prior to gel formation.

The gel buffer is 40 mM tris acetic acid, 1 mM Na_2SO_4, pH 6.8, that is left refrigerated at 4°C. The electrode chamber buffer is a 1:4 dilution of the gel buffer.

Acrylamide monomer solution is obtained by mixing acrylamide (0.912 g) with bisacrylamide (0.04 g) in 19.4 ml gel buffer and heating in an oven to 50°C.

Formation of gel

Agarose (0.48 g) in 45.0 ml gel buffer is stirred while heated to boiling. When agarose is dissolved (i.e. when solution is clear), the plates and the acrylamide mixture are removed from the 50°C oven. Ammonium persulfate (0.48 g in 10.0 ml distilled water) is added with stirring to the acrylamide mixture. TEMED (600 µm) is then quickly added to the mixture. The acrylamide mixture is then added to the agarose solution followed by 37.5 µl of Triton X-100. The mixed solution is poured into the casting apparatus with a syringe equipped with an 18 gauge needle. The combs are inserted and the apparatus placed at 4°C for 1 h. A small amount of 4 M urea in gel buffer is

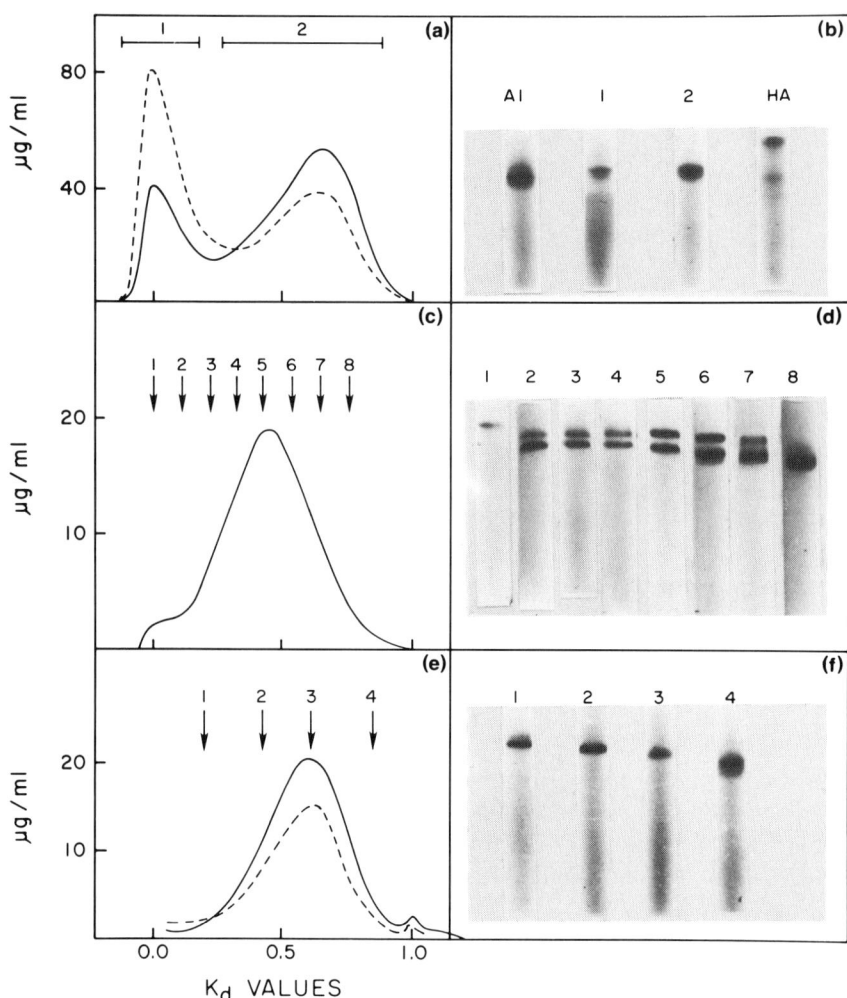

Figure 11.1 Agarose–acrylamide gel electrophoresis of human nucleus pulposus PGs. (a) Sepharose 2B gel chromatography of an A1 fraction after incubation with exogenous hyaluronic acid. The column was eluted with 0.5 M sodium acetate, pH 6.8, and fractions were pooled as indicated by the bars. (b) Agarose–acrylamide gel electrophoresis of unfractionated A1 fraction (left-hand gel), Pools 1 and 2 from (a) (center gels) and hyaluronic acid (right-hand gel). (c) Bio-Gel A-50m chromatography of aggregating PGs (Pool 1 from (a)). The column was eluted with 4 M guanidine hydrochloride/0.5 M sodium acetate, pH 5.8. (d) Selected column fractions from (c), as indicated by arrows, were analyzed by agarose–acrylamide gel electrophoresis. (e) Bio-Gel A-50m chromatography of nonaggregating PGs (Pool 2 in (a)). The column was eluted with 0.5 M sodium acetate, pH 6.8. (f) Four column fractions from (e), as indicated by arrows, were analyzed by agarose–acerylamide gel electrophoresis. (———) Uronic acid; (- - - -) protein. (Reproduced, with permission from Jahnke and McDevitt (1988).

added to the top of the gel and the apparatus is allowed to sit at 4°C overnight.

Electrophoresis

Samples (5 μl per well) that have been dissolved in equal volumes of 8 M urea and 8 M urea in 20 mM Tris, 0.5 mM Na_2SO_4, 0.2% bromophenol blue, pH 6.8, are run 60 V for 5 min and then at 160 V for 2 h.

Transblotting

Transblotting may be achieved with nitrocellulose, an electroblot buffer comprised of 25 mM Tris, 192 mM glycinine and 20% methanol, pH 8.3, and running at 0.2 A overnight or 0.5 A for 3 h at 4°C.

Double gradient polyacrylamide–agarose electrophoresis of large protein complexes

The principle of forming single concentration, large-pore electrophoretic gels with mixtures of acrylamide and agarose has now been extended to the formation of double-gradient gels for the electrophoresis of large protein complexes in the molecular weight range from 300 kDa to about 600 kDa (McDevitt, 1988). The gel consists of a polyacrylamide gradient in one direction (20% polyacrylamide at the bottom of the slab gel; 0–3% polyacrylamide at the top of the gel) and an agarose gradient in the opposite direction (0% agarose in the bottom of the gel; 0.4% agarose at the top of the gel). We employ low gelation Sea Plague agarose from the FMC Corporation in our gels. The double-gradient electrophoresis has been applied in Western Blotting in our studies of matrix adhesion proteins, type VI collagen and thrombospondin in cartilage (McDevitt *et al.*, 1988; Miller and McDevitt, 1988).

Thrombospondin migrated in the double gradient gels as a 420 kDa species under nonreduced conditions (Miller and McDevitt, 1988) in agreement with its absolute molecular weight as determined by sedimentation equilibrium analysis (Margossian *et al.*, 1981). This observation supports the validity of molecular weights determined in the 200–600 kDa portion of the gel. Under reducing conditions, the thrombospondin migrated with an apparent molecular weight of 185 kDa. The absolute molecular weight (including the carbohydrate) of thrombospondin is 138 kDa and its anomalous migration as a 185 kDa band is identical to its behavior on other gel electrophoretic systems. The development of this double-gradient system, therefore, facilitated our identification of thrombospondin in cartilage. Moreover, isotopic labeling of chondrocytes in monolayer culture and subsequent immunoprecipitation and fluorography using the double-gradient system established that the chondrocytes synthesized this protein (Miller and McDevitt, 1988).

The double-gradient system also produced a clear resolution of the four bands of the α3 chain of type VI collagen. In this study, we established that guanidine soluble type VI collagen was enriched in experimental osteoarthritic cartilage (McDevitt *et al.* 1988).

ACKNOWLEDGMENTS

I wish to thank Dr Margaret Aydelotte for permission to use her slab-gel recipe. Support from NIH grant AR39569 is acknowledged.

12

Analytical and preparative electrophoresis of proteoglycan monomers in agarose submerged gels

VICTOR STANESCU

The proteoglycan (PG) monomers of cartilage can be separated into several large and small polydisperse populations (Stanescu et al., 1977; Heinegard and Hascall, 1979; Stanescu and Sweet, 1981; Heinegard et al., 1981; Heinegard et al., 1985b; Rosenberg et al., 1985). There are several methods for separating the large PG monomer populations at the analytical level. Most of the methods are modifications of the large pore agarose–polyacrylamide gel electrophoresis first developed for protein analysis (Uriel, 1966) and then applied to nucleic acid (Peacock and Dingman, 1968) and PG chemistry (McDevitt and Muir, 1971; Stanescu et al., 1973). Later on, electrophoresis in vertical composite slab gels (Heinegard et al., 1985a; Carney et al., 1986) and in horizontal composite submerged ('submarine') gels (Stanescu and Chaminade, 1987) was used for PG monomer separation. More recently, we found that electrophoresis in simple agarose submerged gels gives monomer separations which are similar to those obtained with composite gels.

We use a Mini-gel elecrophoresis system. A Gelbond film is put into the electrophoresis chamber, sealed with agarose and 16 ml of 0.8% agarose are poured and allowed to set at room temperature for 10 min in a humidity chamber, then covered carefully with buffer (0.04 M Tris acetate, pH 6.8, 1 mM EDTA). The gel (10 cm, 7.8 cm) is kept overnight at 4°C. After removing the comb and the buffer, the slots (9 mm, 1 mm) are filled with 5–7 μl 7 M urea, 0.2 M NaCl in 0.04 M Tris acetate buffer, pH 6.8, containing 2.5–5.5 μg large PG (dry weight). Then 2 μl of 0.01% bromphenol blue 50% sucrose is added to each slot and 45 ml of electrophoresis buffer are carefully poured. Shorter slots (3 mm, 1 mm) can be also used. A 15 min premigration at 35 V is followed by migration at 48 V until the marker had migrated 3 cm (about 55 min). After staining with toluidine blue 0.2% in 0.1 N acetic acid for 15 min and destaining in acetic acid, the gels are kept in water at 4°C and dried at 37°C on the Gelbond film. For samples containing sodium dodecyl sulfate (SDS), the gel is fixed first in a solution of methanol–acetic acid–water to remove detergent and then stained. Scanning, electrophoretic transblotting and antibody stainings of fluorography can be performed if necessary.

A lot of information can be obtained using analytical electrophoresis of PG and fragments of PG combined with detection of labeled compounds or with transblotting and specific staining with antibodies. However, separation of PG monomers on a preparative or semipreparative scale is needed for more detailed studies, especially when nonlabeled PG, which have resided a long time in the tissue, are studied.

The first preparative method for the separation of the large PG monomers was based on sedimentation properties of PG and on their sensitivity to different counterions which make them more or less compact (Franzen et al., 1982). Zonal rate centrifugation with continuous monitoring at 206 nm gave two peaks with some overlap.

In our laboratory, we have developed a preparative electrophoretic method in agarose gels submerged in buffer (Stanescu and Do Pham, 1987). An 0.8% agarose slab gel (19.6 cm × 24.7 cm, 4 mm thick) is poured, as already described, in a horizontal electrophoresis system. A charge of PG monomers of 1.5–2 mg dissolved for several hours in 7 M urea, 0.2 M NaCl in 0.04 M Tris acetate, pH 6.8, is reduced and poured in a slot (3 mm × 18.7 cm) and then 2000 ml of 0.04 M Tris acetate buffer 1 mM EDTA, pH 6.8, carefully poured. The electrophoresis buffer is circulated and cooled. A premigration is performed at 20 V for 30 min. Good separations are obtained with migrations of 7 h at 70 V or 22½ h at 72 V with field inversion (10 min, 6 min). Band localization is performed by cutting three vertical slices (lateral and central), staining with toluidine blue 0.2% in 0.1 N acetic acid for 10 min and rapidly destained in 0.1 N acetic acid. From the remainder of the gel, horizontal slices corresponding to the two bands are excised. A 0.3 cm wide slice situated between the two bands is discarded. PG are obtained by a freeze–squeezing procedure with a recovery of about 60%.

An electrophoretic preparative method in 1% agarose vertical slab gel has been described (Kimura et al., 1987). The PG charge in this

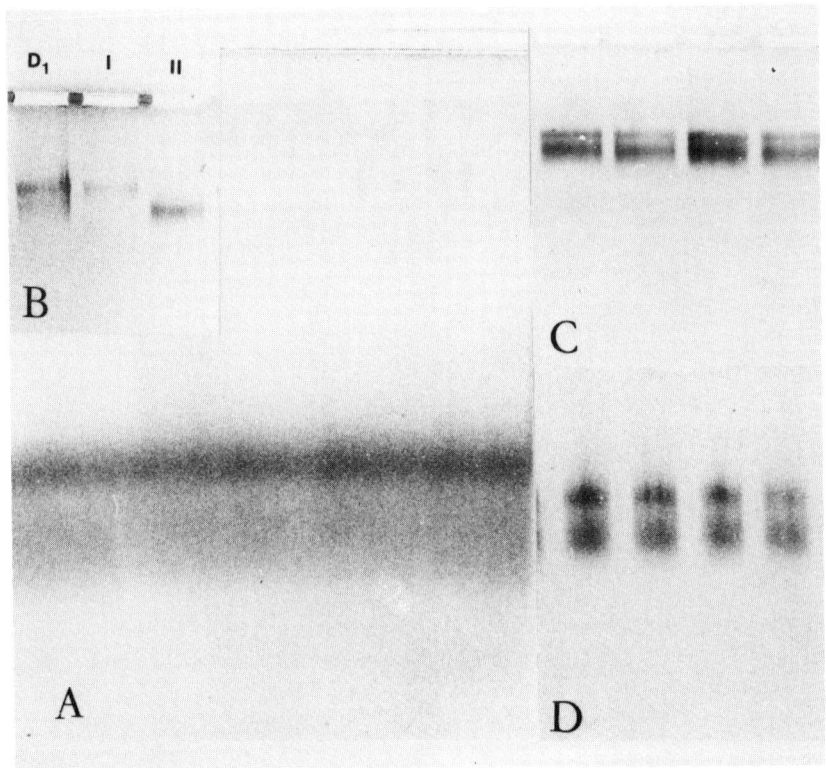

Figure 12.1 (A) Preparative separation by electrophoresis on submerged agarose gel of two aggregating PG monomers ($A_1 2B$ excl. D_1 from baboon articular cartilage). (B) Analytical electrophoresis on submerged agarose gel of the two isolated PG monomers (I and II) and of the non-separated product (D_1 from $A_1 2B$ excl.). (C) Analytical electrophoresis of PGs extracted for various areas of the cartilage of a human femoral head. PGs were purified using ion-exchange chromatography. (D) Nitrocellulose membrane with transferred PGs (D_1 baboon articular cartilage) and immunoblotting with antikeratan sulfate antibody (5-D-4, Caterson). The PGs were first separated by electrophoresis in submerged agarose gels.

method is rather small (10–20 μg per well) so its use as a preparative tool is especially indicated for the study of radiolabeled monomers.

Several points concerning the preparative electrophoresis of large PG monomers on horizontal submerged gels could be discussed. Agarose concentration depends on the monomer size. For human and baboon large monomers, we found that the best concentration is 0.8–0.9%. A highly purified agarose with low or medium electroendosmosis is recommended. Casting the agarose should follow the known rules and Gelbond films are useful for manipulating the gels. Preparation of samples should assure complete solubilization and dissociation. High concentration and overcharge are to be avoided. For purified preparations, we have found that reduction and solubilization in 7 M urea 0.04 M Tris buffer, pH 7, with gentle shaking for several hours at 4°C give satisfactory results. A good preparation of samples is important to avoid trailing. However, with some batches of agarose trailing may occur, probably due to interaction between PG and the agarose matrix. PG recovery is an important step in the technique. We cut the excised strips of gel into small pieces, add buffer and homogenize with a Polytron device operated at low speed for short periods. After freezing and thawing, followed by centrifugation, the PG of the supernatant can be concentrated and precipitated by ethanol or purified by other procedures. Pulsed-field techniques, as used in nucleic acid biochemistry, are probably worth testing. The large aggregating PG monomers of many cartilages can be separated by electrophoresis into two distinct, rather narrow bands (I and II), despite the polydispersity of each population. In some cartilages, a third aggregating population corresponding to an additional band is found (band IIB). This band (which is different from that corresponding to the small non-aggregating PG) is better separated from the second monomer band in more concentrated gels.

Our studies show that analytical and preparative electrophoresis in agarose submerged ('submarine') gels are relatively simple techniques that can be used to study PG monomers and fragments of monomers from various normal and pathological cartilages.

13

Centrifugal methodologies for studying the proteoglycans from articular cartilage

JULIO C. PITA and FRANCISCO J. MÜLLER

GENERAL CONSIDERATIONS

Centrifugation methods of purification and characterization are especially suited to the study of biological macromolecules such as cartilage proteoglycans (PG). When compared with column chromatography, ultracentrifugation represents a more gentle approach since there is no active (sometimes disruptive) interface with a stationary medium. In addition, for a detailed study of PG aggregates, centrifugal techniques are the obvious choice since these molecules on molecular sieve chromatography are excluded and cannot be resolved into the distinctive subpopulations of aggregates that have been identified in our laboratory. In this article, we will first describe the application of the three centrifugal methodologies most frequently used in PG research and then report some improvements that we have introduced in these techniques.

Equilibrium centrifugation

This method can be used for molecular-weight determination when an equilibrium is established between the centrifugal force and the opposing diffusion process. PGs, however, are difficult to analyze by this method because of their very low diffusitivity (typically 10^{-8} Ficks). However, if a significant electrolytic gradient is introduced, then an equilibrium can be established in terms of density flotation (isopycnic equilibrium). Flotation allows for the purification of PGs from proteins, free hyaluronate, etc., but not for separating aggregated from monomeric PGs since both groups float at very similar densities (A1 fraction in Fig. 13.1).

Boundary (velocity) sedimentation

This classical method is used to determine the average sedimentation coefficient, S, and/or the complete (polydisperse) distribution function, $g(S)$, of S values. The technique can distinguish all PG species, especially when centrifuged at low initial concentrations. Precision is limited, however, by the progressive dilution of the plateau and by concentration-dependent effects. In addition the presence of all components at the common plateau region disqualifies this technique for isolation of the different PG subpopulations.

Rate zonal sedimentation

Zonal sedimentation does separate the PG species from each other (very much as in chromatography

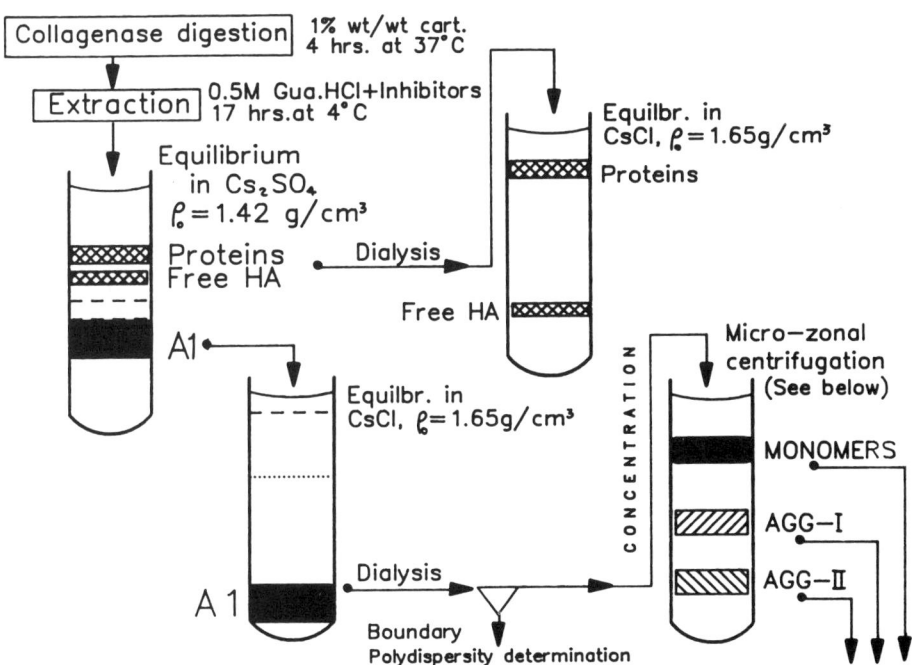

Figure 13.1 Flow diagram of sequential equilibrium and zonal centrifugation for the isolation of PG monomers and PG aggregates I and II.

or electrophoresis), but the initial layering of the macromolecules at the top of the cell introduces the danger of 'droplet sedimentation' when rectangular (or constant concentration) zones are used that contain very slowly diffusing PGs. A remedy for this situation has been to use 'triangular' or inverted PG gradients in the sample application zone. The underlying gradient required in the rest of the cell can adopt any convenient form, but it should extend also into the triangular PG zone.

SPECIFIC IMPROVEMENTS ON EARLIER TECHNIQUES

Associative extraction

Associative extraction was introduced to study the undisturbed picture of PG aggregation as it existed *in vivo*. The details of the required collagenase predigestion of the cartilage are described at the top of Fig. 13.1.

Microvolumes and transport methodology in transparent cells

It is difficult to characterize very small volumes (few microliters or even nanoliters) of PG extracts or sample solutions. The problem was solved using the transport method of centrifugation in capillary glass microcells within the preparative ultracentrifuge. This method enabled precise determinations of: average S values and molecular weights (Pita and Müller, 1972a,b); complete $g(S)$ polydisperse analysis by repeated centrifugation (Pita and Müller, 1973); and even in a single run when using slightly bigger volumes (80–500-μl) (Pita et al., 1978). To facilitate precise control over the recovery of fractions, transparent polycarbonate cells were also introduced.

Stabilizing linear gradients

Very dilute solutions (0.3–0.05-mg ml^{-1}) of PG are needed to minimize the concentration-dependent effects mentioned above. The diluted boundaries, however, are easily disturbed unless stabilized with a moderate linear electrolytic gradient across the cell as described by Pita et al. (1978).

Need of sectorial cells to avoid collision with the cell walls

Due to the radial trajectories of the sedimenting molecules, some molecules will collide with the walls of a cylindrical cell. This might introduce artifactual peaks due to accumulation on the walls. To eliminate this inconvenience, we developed and used a sectorial polycarbonate cell (Pita et al., 1983).

Use of cesium sulfate gradients

In addition to the preparative capability of the isopycnic equilibrium gradients illustrated in Fig. 13.1, Cs_2SO_4 can also be used to prepare isokinetic gradients (in cylinders) or isovolumetric gradients (in sectors) by using Noll's single mixing chamber method as described by Pita et al. (1985). These gradients prevent plateau dilution and have made possible the following zonal application.

Analytical macro- and micro-rate zonal sedimentation

The triangular zones are essential for PG zonal stability as noted above. Mathematically, however, the problem of calculating the $g(S)$ function from these types of zones is insurmountable. By using an isovolumetric Cs_2SO_4 gradient, the linearity of the equations gives a simpler $g(S)$ theory, similar to that of the rectangular zone, as proven by Müller et al. (1989b). In this way we have extended the preparative zonal methodology to analytical usage, with a precision comparable to that of boundary sedimentation.

SOME SELECTED RESULTS

Initial efforts in this laboratory concentrated on characterizing PG molecules recovered in cartilage fluids aspirated *in vivo*, using a micropuncture technique from the growth plates of rats. The results demonstrated that the PG aggregates are distributed into two distinct populations of molecules (Pita *et al.*, 1979). This bimodal distribution of the aggregates was later confirmed for PGs recovered from rat chondrosarcoma under nondissociative conditions (Faltz *et al.*, 1979). More recently, PGs were extracted associatively after collagenase predigestion of the cartilage, as described in Fig. 13.1, from articular cartilage of rabbits, dogs and humans (Manicourt *et al.*, 1986, 1988; Müller *et al.*, 1989a). The corresponding PG preparations showed remarkably similar distributions of sedimentation coefficients, as illustrated in Fig. 13.2. Again, the bimodality of the aggregates is to be noted. In the case of the human tissue, it was possible to show consistent variations across the cartilage thickness, with the fast-sedimenting aggregates being more abundant towards the middle zone of the cartilage (Müller *et al.*, 1989a).

The role of hyaluronan (HA) and link glycoproteins (LGP) in the formation and stability of the two PG aggregates was examined in a recent study of PGs from dog articular cartilage (Manicourt *et al.*, 1986, 1988). When extracted dissociatively, only monomers and one PG aggregate mode were observed. But when LGP was added to this preparation, the typical bimodality of the aggregates was reestablished. However, preliminary results seem to indicate that there is no difference between the HA molecules of the two aggregates. Rather, the difference seems to reside in the greater number of PG monomers per HA molecule in the fast, compared with the slower, sedimenting aggregate as evidenced through the chondroitin sulfate to HA ratios of each. The physiological role of aggregation bimodality is currently being explored.

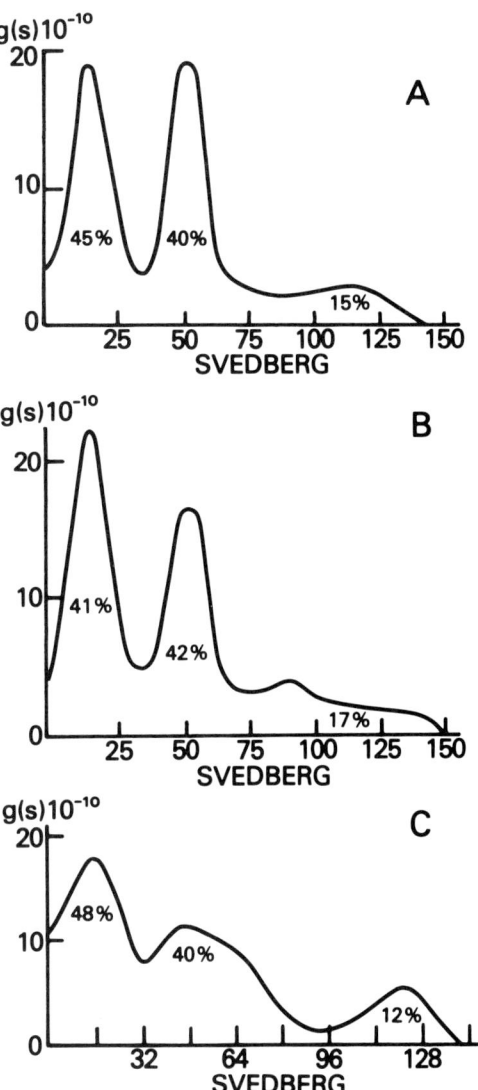

Figure 13.2 PG S value distributions in various articular cartilages: (A) rabbit; (B) canine; (C) human. The left-most peaks in all cases correspond to the PG monomers and the small peaks at the right to the faster sedimenting aggregates. (Note different horizontal scale in curve C.)

14

Microsequencing of cartilage components

M. VAN DER REST, E. DE MIGUEL, Q. NGUYEN, B. DUBLET, J.S. MORT and P.J. ROUGHLEY

INTRODUCTION

Microsequencing is usually done for one of the following objectives: (i) evidence for processing or degradation of a protein at its amino terminal end; (ii) evidence for purity or chain composition of a protein; (iii) cloning of a cDNA or genomic DNA encoding a protein of interest, using synthetic oligonucleotide probes made after backtranslation of a partial protein sequence; or (iv) identification of a protein by comparison with known sequences. The strategy for sample preparation will vary according to the objective. Objective (i) requires the isolation of the intact molecule. Objective (ii) requires the isolation of the intact native molecule or of cross-linked fragments. Objectives (iii) and (iv) are best achieved by the sequencing of internal fragments.

In our laboratory, microsequencing has been performed in the last five years on more than 700 samples, primarily proteins and peptides prepared from cartilage and other extracellular matrices. We present and discuss here our experience using this methodology.

EQUIPMENT

All the data discussed here were obtained using an ABI 470A microsequencer connected to an on-line phenylthiohydantoin– (PTH–) amino acid analyzer (ABI 120A). Standard programs for performing Edman degradation (Edman, 1956) and for the separation of PTH–amino acids were utilized as specified by the manufacturer.

PREPARATION OF THE SAMPLES

The major problems encountered in protein sequencing arise from the sample preparation: (i) insufficient amount of protein or peptide; (ii) contaminating peptides or amino acids; or (iii) blocking of the NH_2 terminus of the protein.

Some standard methods for sample preparation, such as liquid chromotography (molecular sieve, ion exchange), salt precipitation or affinity chromatography, do not usually produce samples satisfactory for microsequencing because of the frequent contamination by small peptides which copurify and remain undetected by analytical methods such as sodium dodecyl sulfate–polyacrylamide gel electrophoresis (SDS–PAGE). It takes only 5% (by weight) of a 15 amino acid contaminant to be equimolar with a 95% pure 30 kDa protein!

A final purification by high-performance liquid chromatography (HPLC) for short peptides (up to 10 kDa) (van der Rest et al., 1980; van der Rest and Fietzek, 1982) or by blotting from SDS–PAGE gels onto a polyvinylidene difluoride (PVDF) membrane for larger peptides (10–50 kDa) (Matsudaira, 1987) should eliminate these contaminants. The sequencing of larger proteins (> 50 kDa) is rarely successful: quantities tend to be overestimated (often by an order of magnitude) if a reliable protein assay, such as amino acid analysis, has not been performed; a number of proteins are naturally blocked at their amino terminal end or become blocked during purification. In addition, background can build up rapidly with long peptides due to nonspecific acid cleavage of peptide bonds during Edman degradation.

RECOMMENDED STRATEGIES

To obtain internal sequences of large matrix proteins for identification or for synthesis of oligonucleotide probes the procedure is as follows:

(i) purify the protein as much as possible by standard techniques;
(ii) cleave the protein into small fragments (trypsin, V8 protease, CNBr);
(iii) separate the fragments by HPLC (C18 large pore column, 9 mM trifluoroacetic acid as counterion);
(iv) select the largest peaks that cannot come from contaminants;
(v) Rechromatograph these peaks in a different HPLC system (heptafluorobutyric acid as counterion, for example) and collect major peaks;
(vi) determine amino acid composition of the peptides on 50% of the material and work out size, purity and quantity. If the sequence is known, a good amino acid composition will often permit the identification of the peptides (van der Rest et al., 1986); and
(vii) sequence those peptides that show the presence of interesting amino acids (e.g. methionines).

To obtain an amino terminal sequence from a large protein or fragment the procedure is as follows:

(i) purify the protein by standard techniques to the point where bands do not overlap on SDS-PAGE. Use as few steps as possible;
(ii) run your preparation on standard Laemmli gels (Laemmli, 1970). Use sucrose instead of glycerol in the same buffer;
(iii) transfer onto PVDF membranes as described by Matsudaira (1987);
(iv) stain the transfer as briefly as possible with Coomassie blue;
(v) excise the band of interest with a scalpel blade and load as such on the gas-phase sequencer;
(vi) if no sequence is obtained, recover the membrane from the sequencer, hydrolyze as such with 6 M HCl and do amino acid composition. Calculate how much protein was loaded. If quantities are sufficient (>50 pmol of protein), the amino terminus is blocked. This happens in 40–60% of cases for proteins;
(vii) it is wise to check first with a standard protein, such as myoglobin, that your electrophoresis and transfer conditions do not block the amino terminus. Some reagents of insufficient purity can be a problem; and
(viii) some proteins do not bind well to PVDF membranes. It can be useful to place two layers of membranes and stain the second one to check that no protein has gone through the membrane.

SENSITIVITY

A microbore HPLC can detect less than 1 pmol of a PTH-amino acids released from the sequencer. However, other factors limit the actual sensitivity of the procedure: (i) only 40% of the released PTH-amino acid is actually analyzed; (ii) at 92% repetitive yield, the recovery is down by 50% every 10 cycles; (iii) several amino acids (e.g. Thr, Arg, His and Ser) have recoveries between 10% and 50%; and (iv) the initial yield for most proteins is only 40–50%. For blotted proteins a 10% initial yield is frequent. For blocked proteins, it is 0%. One should, therefore, plan for 100 pmol of protein or peptide to hope to see all the identifiable residues for 20 cycles.

OTHER CONSIDERATIONS

Analysis of cysteines

Cysteines are best determined as S-β-(4-pyridylethyl) cysteine after reduction and pyridylethylation with 4-vinylpyridine (Friedman et al., 1970). The PTH derivative of this residue is indeed more stable than the PH derivative of S-carboxymethylcysteine obtained by alkylation with iodoacetamide.

Speed

A microsequencer does approximately 1 cycle h^{-1}. Polybrene coated glass filters require a 4-h precycling and it takes approximately three additional hours to see the result of the first cycle. Therefore, only one sample can be loaded per day, except in the case of PVDF membranes which do not require precycling.

EXAMPLES

Demonstration of a cross-link between type IX and type II collagen

The existence of covalent cross-links between type IX and type II cartilage collagen was demonstrated independently by Eyre *et al.* (1987a) in bovine

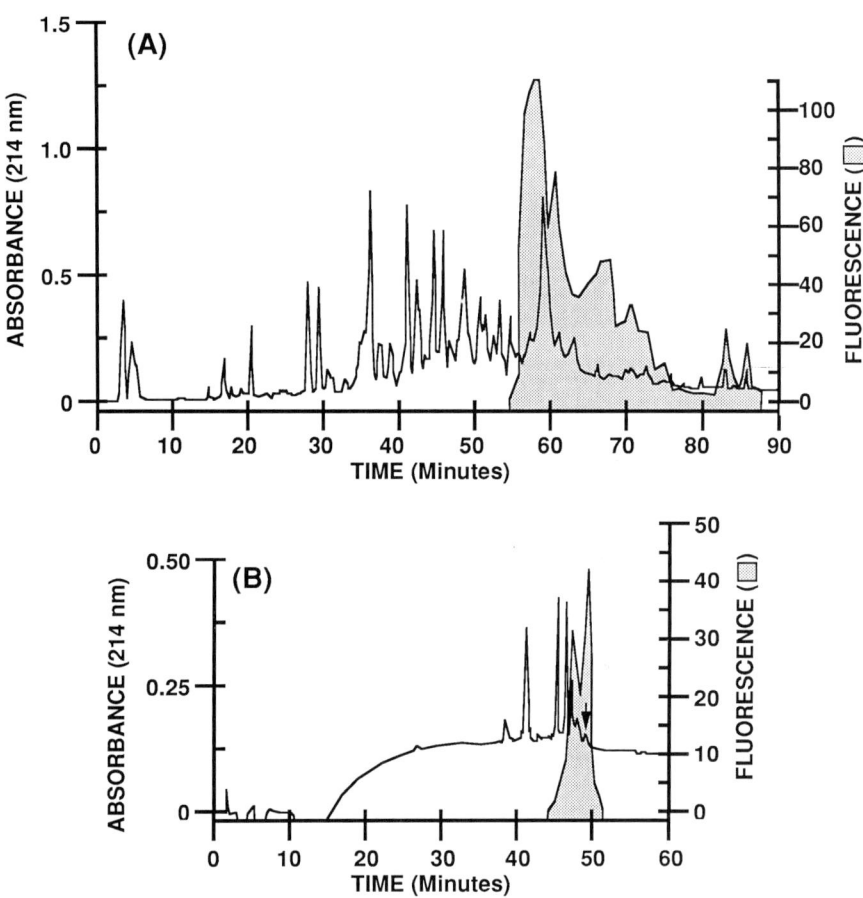

Figure 14.1 HPLC purification of the tryptic peptide containing the cross-link between $\alpha2(IX)$ and $\alpha1(II)$. The pepsin fragment C3 from chicken type IX collagen, representing the central triple helix (NC2) from the $\alpha2(IX)$ chain, was purified by standard methods (Reese *et al.*, 1982). After trypsin digestion, the resulting fragments were separated by HPLC in two steps. The chromatographies were monitored at 214 nm for the fluorescence characteristic of the pyridinium cross-link. (A) The tryptic peptides were separated by reversed phase HPLC using 9 mM trifluoroacetic acid as ion-pairing agent. (B) The fraction containing the highest fluorescence level, eluting at 59 min, was rechromatographed using 10 mM heptafluorobutyric acid as ion-pairing agent (van der Rest and Fietzek, 1982). The peak indicated by an arrow was selected for microsequencing. (Reprinted from van der Rest and Mayne (1988) with permission.)

14. MICROSEQUENCING OF CARTILAGE COMPONENTS   53

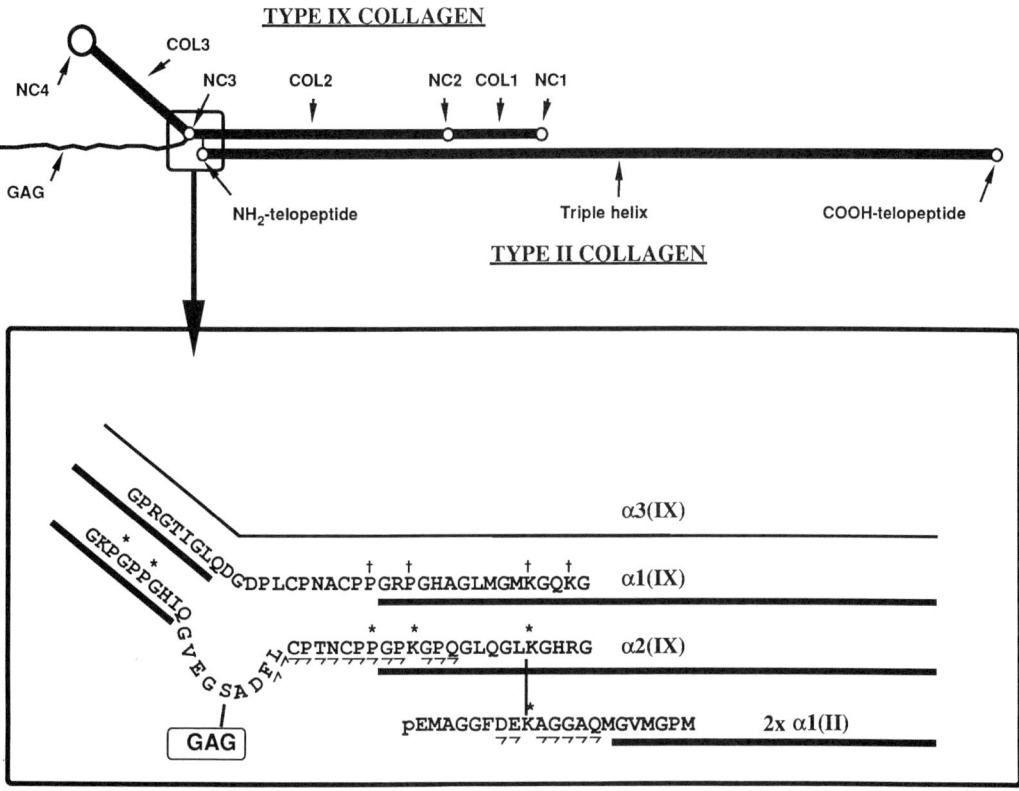

Figure 14.2 Schematic representation of the cross-link between α2(IX) and α1(II). The lower part of the figure represents the detailed arrangement of the region of the cross-link. Sequenced residues are underlined by arrows. The exact position of the cross-link in α2(IX) is indicated by analogy with the sequence of the triple-helical cross-linking sites of fibrillar collagens but could be located at the other hydroxylysine residue. The upper panel indicates schematically the position of the cross-link relative to the entire molecules. (Reprinted from van der Rest and Mayne (1988) with permission.)

cartilage and by van der Rest and Mayne (1988) in avian cartilage. In our study, we isolated a pure cross-linked peptide from a tryptic digest of a pepsin fragment from the α2(IX) in two HPLC steps (Fig. 14.1) and determined a double sequence by microsequencing. One sequence corresponded to the N-telopeptide of type II collagen, while the other, present at half the level of the type II collagen sequence, corresponded to the N-terminal end of the COL2 domain of α2(IX) (Fig. 14.2).

Study of the natural proteolysis of human link protein

Three forms of human link protein (LP) can be separated by gel elecrophoresis. With ageing, an abundance of the smallest form (LP3) is observed at the expense of the larger forms (LP1 and LP2). In an attempt to demonstrate the differences between these three forms, they were transferred onto PVDF membrane from a Laemmli gel and individually sequenced (Fig. 14.3) (Nguyen et al., 1989). LP was also treated with several different proteolytic enzymes in vitro and the resulting molecule sequenced in the same fashion (data not shown). These data, summarized below, establish that LP1 and LP2 have the identical N-terminal and probably differ only in the N-linked oligosaccharide substitution at position 6 (glycosylated residues give blank cycles) and that LP3 is 16 residues shorter at the N-terminus.

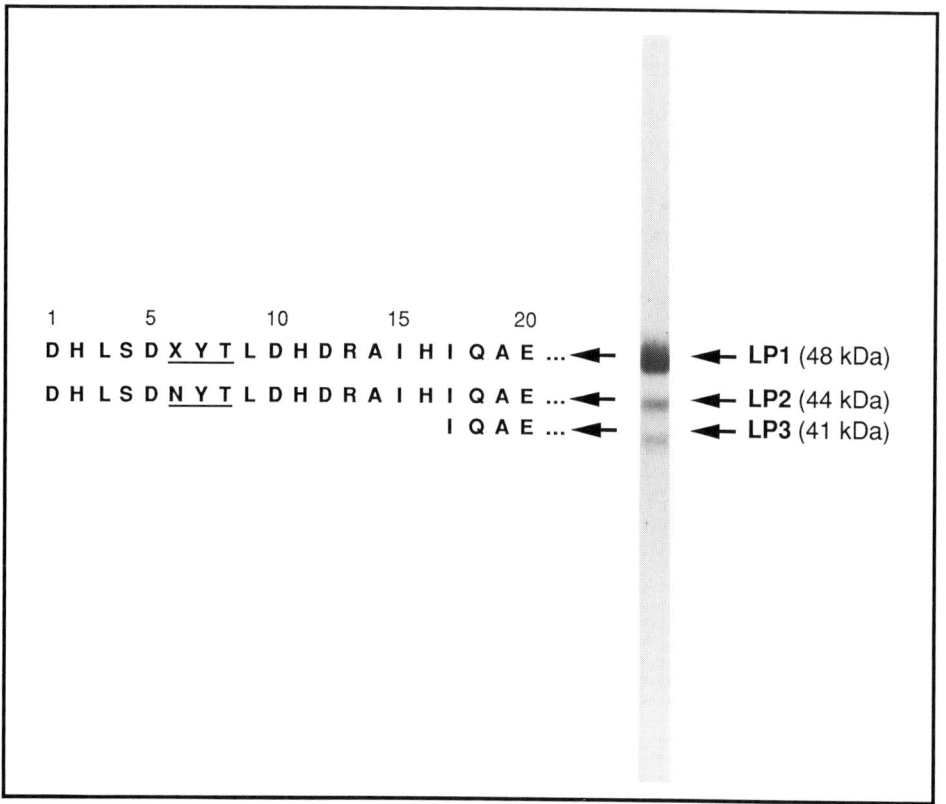

Figure 14.3 Sequence analysis of human neonatal LP. A sample of purified LPs was analyzed by SDS–PAGE, followed by electroblotting onto a PVDF membrane and stained as noted in the text. Each individual LP band was excised and submitted to microsequencing. The deduced amino acid sequences are given to the left of the figure. The X in position 6 of the LP1 sequence denotes a blank cycle, most likely due to the presence of an oligosaccharide N-linked to the asparagine residue found in that position in LP2. The consensus sequences for N-glycosylation are underlined.

Comparison with *in vitro* cleavages indicates that, in the neonatal cartilage studied, stromelysin is responsible for the generation of LP3.

The stoichiometry of type XII collagen

Type XII collagen was initially described at the nucleic acid level (Gordon *et al.*, 1987) and further characterized using a monoclonal antibody (75d7) raised against a peptide synthesized according to the cDNA sequence (Dublet *et al.*, 1989). This antibody was predicted to recognize a disulfide bonded CNBr derived peptide. The unreduced peptide was purified by affinity chromatography and the immunopurified material was shown to contain multiple bands by SDS–PAGE (Fig. 14.4). These bands were transferred onto PVDF membranes and sequenced. A unique sequence, identical to the sequence encoded in the cDNA, was obtained for all the bands, indicating that type XII collagen is a homotrimer and suggesting that the multiple bands originated from partial cleavage at the three methionines located in the carboxyl telopeptide of the predicted protein.

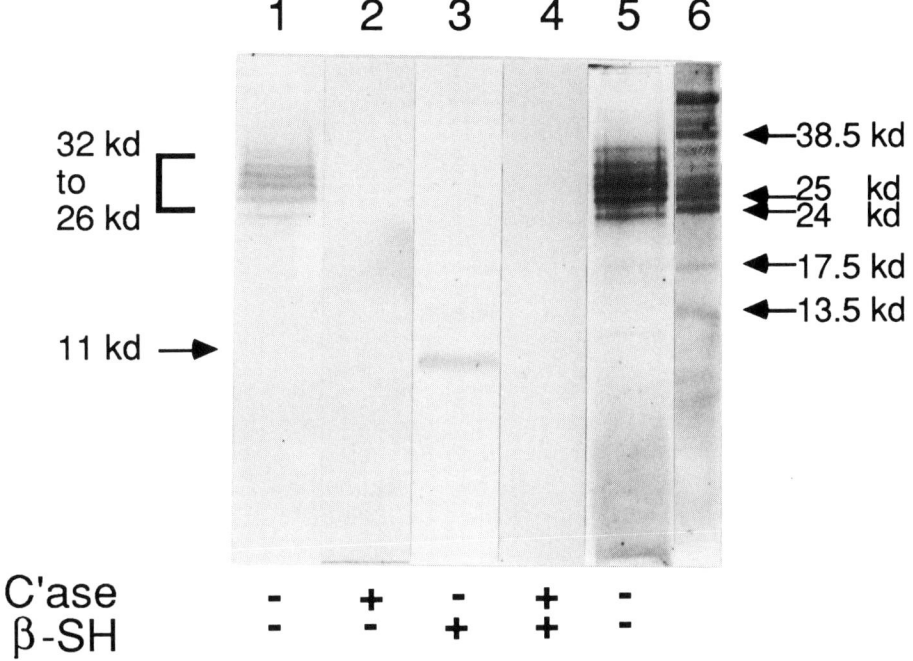

Figure 14.4 Gel electrophoresis of the CNBr derived peptide of α1(XII) containing the 75d7 epitope. Wells 1–4 were loaded with 40 μg of the CNBr collagen digest. The fractions were reduced with 1% β-mercaptoethanol (β-SH) and digested with collagenase (C'ase) as noted under the figure. After electrophoresis, lanes 1–4 were blotted and reacted with the antibody 75d7. Lane 5 corresponds to the gel electrophoresis of the unreduced affinity chromatography purified CNBr digest. Lane 6 shows type I collagen CNBr peptides used for molecular-weight determination and stained with amido-black.

ACKNOWLEDGMENTS

The work reported here was supported by the Shriners of North America, the Medical Research Council of Canada and the Arthritis Society of Canada. M.v.d.R. is a senior scholar from the Fonds de la Recherche en Santé du Québec, Q.N. is recipient of a MRC studentship award and P.J.R. is an MRC scientist.

15

Summary review

H. MUIR

Constituents of the extracellular matrix are by their very nature difficult to extract, separate and analyse because they are mostly of large molecular size, are mutually enmeshed and in many cases are strongly attached to each other either by specific covalent bonds as in the case of type II – type IX collagen or by cooperative interactions that result in very high affinities as exemplified by proteoglycan (PG) aggregates which are rather unique heteropolymers. Entrapment within the matrix is shown by the influence of collagen content on yield of extracted PGs and by the greatly increased yield when extraction is performed on finely-sectioned cartilage.

Matrix components have first to be extracted, if possible in their native form, and then separated and purified for analysis. However, conditions that are optimal for a particular constituent are not so for others and compromise is necessary. The best conditions must be chosen for each constituent in turn. The papers presented in this session address some of these difficulties, making use of recent technical developments.

In identifying the cross-links and their position in cartilage-specific collagens, all soluble constituents must first be removed, followed by specific cleavage of the residual collagens. The position of cross-links in the collagens is then indicated by microsequencing the separated collagen fragments. A similar strategy used to identify the position of disulfide bonds and specific epitopes in type XII collagen showed it to be a homotrimer. However, rigorous purity is a prerequisite of microsequencing.

Cross-linked collagens which are insoluble cannot be obtained in native form. As a compromise, a small proportion of collagen can be extracted from immature cartilage before becoming cross-linked. Fractional salt precipitation of the extracted collagens enables them to be visualized and studied in various ways in the native form. A consequence of the interlinking of molecules in the extracellular matrix is that they tend to remain *in situ* even when partially degraded, as is the case with the three native link proteins whose relationship has been shown conclusively by microsequencing.

PGs present different problems from those of the collagens. Their polyanionic nature overrides most other properties. This feature is exploited to separate them from other matrix materials, either directly or indirectly by density gradient centrifugation in the presence of appropriate counterions. Separation of individual PGs from each other is more difficult. The principal methods such as gel chromatography and gel electrophoresis depend on differences in hydrodynamic size. Mixed bed agarose/acrylamide gels offer a range of pore size for electrophoresis and has the great advantage that a variety of blotting procedures are available to identify and characterize the components. Moreover, their biosynthetic relationship may be discerned by isotopic labeling and autoradiography. The large porosity of mixed bed gels allows the migration of very large molecules of several million molecular weight. Stable agarose gels of large porosity without acrylamide have also been used. Whether separation in each type of gel depends on exactly the same properties needs to be established by comparing the migration of given proteoglycan preparations in each gel. A further sophistication is the use of double gradient mixed bed gels for separation of large protein complexes.

PG aggregates, however, are too large to penetrate even the most open-pore gels and therefore have to be characterized by physical methods such as analytical ultracentrifugation, where separation depends on size, shape and intermolecular interactions and is greatly influenced by concentration as well as ionic environment and geometry of the centrifuge cell. A proportion of native aggregates may be extracted under nondissociating conditions once the collagen has been partially degraded. Further characterization by other physical methods such as light scattering and rotary shadowing will be necessary, particularly when comparing native aggregates with dissociated–reassembled aggregates. Whether such native aggregates are representative of the total aggregate population has to be established, for example by comparing the constituent monomers and link proteins for specific epitopes on protein cores and glycosaminoglycan chains and by chemical analysis. The ultrastructural inhomogeneity of cartilage matrix and marked differences in collagen-fibre morphology add further complication to the biological significance of results. Age and anatomical site of cartilage are also extremely important factors to be taken into account.

References

Ayad, S., Evans, H.B., Weiss, J.B. and Holt, P.J.L. (1984). Type VI collagen, but not type V collagen is present in cartilage. *Collagen Rel. Res.* **4**, 165–168

Ayad, S., Kwan, A.P.L. and Grant, M.E. (1987). Partial characterization of type X collagen from bovine growth-plate cartilage. *FEBS Lett.* **220**, 181–186

Bayliss, M.T. (1986). Proteoglycan structure in normal and osteoarthrotic human cartilage. In *Articular Cartilate Biochemistry* (K. Keuttner *et al.*, eds), pp. 295–310. Raven Press, New York

Bayliss, M.T. and Ali, S.Y. (1978a). Isolation of proteoglycan from human articular cartilage. *Biochem. J.* **169**, 123–132

Bayliss, M.T. and Ali, S.Y. (1978b). Age-related changes in the composition and structure of human articular cartilate proteoglycans. *Biochem. J.* **176**, 683–693

Bayliss, M.T. and Roughley, P.J. (1985). The properties of proteoglycan prepared from human articular cartilage by using associative caesium chloride gradients of high and low starting densities. *Biochem. J.* **232**, 111–117

Bayliss, M.T. and Venn, M. (1980). Chemistry of human articular cartilage. In *Studies in Joint Disease* (A. Maroudas and E.J. Holborow, eds), pp. 2–58. Pitman Medical, London

Bayliss, M.T., Venn, M., Maroudas, A. and Ali, S.Y. (1983). Structure of proteoglycan from different layers of human articular cartilage. *Biochem. J.* **209**, 387–400

Blake, M.S., Johnstone, K.H., Russell-Jones, G.J. and Gotschlich, E.C. (1984). A rapid, sensitive method for detection of alkaline phosphatase-conjugated anti-antibody on western blots. *Anal. Biochem.* **136**, 175–179

Carney, S.L., Bayliss, M.T., Collier, J.M. and Muir, H. (1986). Electrophoresis of ^{35}S labeled proteoglycans on polyacrylamide–agarose composite gels and their visualization by fluorography. *Anal. Biochem.* **156**, 38–44

Chun, L.E., Koob, T.J. and Eyre, D.R. (1986). Sequential enzymic dissection of the proteoglycan complex from articular cartilage. *Trans. Orthop. Res. Soc.* **11**, 96

Dublet, B., Oh, S., Sugrue, S.P., Gordon, M.K., Gerecke, D.R., Olsen, B.R. and van der Rest, M. (1989). The structure of avian type XII collagen: $\alpha 1$(XII) chains contain 190 kDa non-triple-helical amino-terminal domains and form homotrimeric molecules. *J. Biol. Chem.* **264**, 13 150–13 156

Edman, P. (1956). Mechanism of the phenyl isothiocyanate degradation of peptides. *Nature* **177**, 667–668

Evans, H.B., Ayad, S., Abedin, M.Z., Hopkins, S., Morgan, K., Walton, K.W., Weiss, J.B. and Holt, P.J.L. (1983). Localization of collagen types and fibronectin in cartilage by immunofluorescence. *Ann. Rheum. Dis.* **42**, 575–581

Eyre, D.R. (1987). Collagen cross-linking amino acids. In *Methods in Enzymology* (L.W. Cunningham, ed.), pp. 115–139. Academic Press, Orlando

Eyre, D.R. and Glimcher, M.J. (1973). Isolation of crosslinked peptides from collagen of chicken bone. *Biochem. J.* **135**, 393–403

Eyre, D.R. and Wu, J.J. (1983). Collagen of fibrocartilage: a distinctive molecular phenotype in bovine meniscus. *FEBS Lett.* **158**, 265–270

Eyre, D.R., Koob, T.J. and van Ness, K.P. (1984a). Quantitation of hydroxypyridinium crosslinks in collagen by high performance liquid chromatography. *Anal. Biochem.* **137**, 380–388

Eyre, D.R., Paz, M.A. and Gallop, P.M. (1984b). Crosslinking in collagen and elastin. *Ann. Rev. Biochem.* **53**, 717–748

Eyre, D.R., Wu, J.J. and Woolley, D.E. (1984c). All three chains of $1\alpha 2\alpha 3\alpha$ collagen from hyaline cartilage resist human collagenase. *Biochem. Biophys. Res. Commun.* **118**, 724–729

Eyre, D.R., Apone, S., Wu, J.J., Ericsson, L.H. and Walsh, K.A. (1987a). Collagen type IX: evidence for covalent linkages to type II collagen in cartilage. *FEBS Lett.* **220**, 337–341

Eyre, D.R., Wu, J.J. and Apone, S. (1987b). A growing family of collagens in articular cartilage: identification of five genetically distinct types. *J. Rheumatol.* **14**, 25–27

Faltz, L.L., Reddi, A.H., Hascall, G.K., Martin, D., Pita, J.C. and Hascall, V.C. (1979). Characteristics of proteoglycans extracted from the swarm rat chondrosarcoma with associative solvents. *J. Biol. Chem.* **254**, 1375–1382

Franzen, A., Bjornsson, S. and Heinegard, D. (1982). Zonal rate centrifugation of proteoglycans in sucrose gradients. *Anal Biochem.* **120**, 38–46

Friedman, M., Krull, L.H. and Cavins, J.F. (1970). The chromatographic determination of cystine and cysteine residues on proteins as S-β-(4-pyridylethyl)-cysteine. *J. Biol. Chem.* **245**, 3868–3871

Gordon, M.K., Gerecke, D.R. and Olsen, B.R. (1987). Type XII collagen: distinct extracellular matrix component discovered by cDNA cloning. *Proc. Natl. Acad. Sci. USA* **84**, 6040–6044

Heinegard, D. and Hascall, V.C. (1979). Characteristics of the nonaggregating proteoglycans isolated from bovine nasal cartilage. *J. Biol. Chem.* **254**, 927–934

Heinegard, D., Paulsson, M., Interot, S. and Carlstrom, C. (1981). A novel low-molecular weight chondroitin sulphate proteoglycan isolated from cartilage. *Biochem. J.* **197**, 355–366

Heinegard, D., Sommarin, Y., Hedbom, E., Wieslander, J. and Larsson, B. (1985a). Assay of proteoglycan populations using agarose-polyacrylamide gel electrophoresis. *Anal. Biochem.* **151**, 41–48

Heinegard, D., Wieslander, J., Sheehan, J., Paulsson, M. and Sommarin, Y. (1985b). Separation and characterization of two populations of aggregating proteoglycans from cartilage. *Biochem. J.* **225**, 95–106

Jahnke, M.R. and McDevitt, C.A. (1988). Proteoglycans of the human intervertebral disc. Electrophoretic heterogeneity of the aggregating proteoglycans of the nucleus pulposus. *Biochem. J.* **251**, 347–356

Kimura, J.H., Shinomura, T. and Thonar, E.M.A. (1987). Biosynthesis of cartilage proteoglycan and link protein. In *Methods in Enzymology* (L.W. Cunningham, ed.), Vol. 144, pp. 391–393. Academic Press, Orlando

Klein, J. and Meyer, F. (1982). Tissue structure and macromolecular diffusion in umbilical cord. Immobilisation of endogenous hyaluronic acid. *Biochem. Biophys. Acta.* **755**, 400–411

Kwan, A.P.L., Freemont, A.J. and Grant, M.E. (1986). Immunoperoxidase localization of type X collagen in chick tibiae. *Biosci. Rep.* **6**, 155–162

Laemmli, U.K. (1970). Cleavage of structural proteins during the assembly of the head of bacteriophage T4. *Nature* **277**, 680–681

Manicourt, D.H., Pita, J.C., Pezon, C.F. and Howell, D.S. (1986). Characterization of the proteoglycans recovered under nondissociative conditions from normal articular cartilage of rabbits and dogs. *J. Biol. Chem.* **261**, 5426–5430

Manicourt, D.H., Pita, J.C., McDevitt, C.A. and Howell, D.S. (1988). Superficial and deeper layers of dog normal articular cartilage. *J. Biol. Chem.* **263**, 13 121–13 129

Margossian, S.S., Lawler, J.W. and Slayter, H.S. (1981). Physical characterization of platelet thrombospondin. *J. Biol. Chem.* **256**, 7495–7500

Maroudas, A. (1979). The physiochemical properties of articular cartilage. In *Adult Articular Cartilage* (M.A.R. Freeman, ed.), pp. 131–170. Pitman Medical, Tunbridge Wells

Matsudaira, P. (1987). Sequence from picomole quantities of protein electroblotted onto polyvinylidene difluoride membranes. *J. Biol. Chem.* **262**, 10 035–10 038

McDevitt, C.A. (1988). Proteoglycans of the intervertebral disc. In *The Biology of the Intervertebral Disc* (P. Ghosh, ed.), Vol. 1. CRC Press, Inc., Boca Raton, FL

McDevitt, C.A. and Muir, H. (1971). Gel electrophoresis of proteoglycans and glycosaminoglycans on large-pore composite polyacrylamide gels. *Anal. Biochem.* **44**, 612–622

McDevitt, C.A., Pahl, J.A., Ayad, A., Miller, R.R.,

Uratsuji, M. and Andrish, J.T. (1988). Experimental osteoarthritic articular cartilage is enriched in guanidine-soluble type VI collagen. *Biochem. Biophys. Res. Commun.* **157**, 250–255

Miller, R.R. and McDevitt, C.A. (1988). Thrombospondin is present in articular cartilage and is synthesized by articular chondrocytes. *Biochem. Biophys. Res. Commun.* **153**, 708–714

Mould, A.P., Holmes, D.F., Kadler, K.E. and Chapman, J.A. (1985). Mica sandwich technique for preparing macromolecules for rotary shadowing. *J. Ultrastruct. Res.* **91**, 66–76

Müller, F.J., Pezon, C.F. and Pita, J.C. (1989a). Macro and micro rate zonal analytical centrifugation of polydisperse and slowly diffusing sedimenting systems in isovolumetric density gradients. Application to cartilage proteoglycans. *Biochemistry* **28**, 5276–5282

Müller, F.J., Pita, J.C., Manicourt, D.H., Malinin, T.I., Schoonbeck, J.M. and Mow, V.C. (1989b). Centrifugal characterization of proteoglycans from various depth layers and weight-bearing areas of normal and abnormal human articular cartilage. *J. Orthop. Res.* **7**, 326–334

Müller-Glaser, W., Humbel, B., Glatt, M., Strauli, P., Winterhalter, D.H. and Bruckner, P. (1986). On the role of type IX collagen in the extracellular matrix of cartilage: type IX collagen is localized to intersections of collagen fibrils. *J. Cell Biol.* **102**, 1931–1939

Nguyen, Q., Murphy, G., Roughley, P.J. and Mort, J.S. (1989). Degradation of proteoglycan aggregates by a cartilage metalloproteinase. Evidence for the involvement of stromelysin in the generation of link protein heterogeneity *in situ*. *Biochem. J.* **259**, 61–67

Peacock, A.C. and Dingman, C.W. (1968). Molecular weight estimation and separation of ribonucleic acid by electrophoresis in agarose–acrylamide composite gels. *Biochemistry* **7**, 668–674.

Pita, J.C. and Müller, F.J. (1972a). Ultracentrifugal studies in capillary cells: I. Determination of sedimentation coefficients. *Anal. Biochem.* **47**, 395–407

Pita, J.C. and Müller, F.J. (1972b). Ultracentrifugal studies in capillary cells: II. Sedimentation equilibrium molecular weight determinations. *Anal. Biochem.* **47**, 408–417

Pita, J.C. and Müller, F.J. (1973). Ultracentrifugal study of polydisperse and paucidisperse biological systems using capillary microcells. *Biochemistry* **12**, 2656–2665

Pita, J.C., Müller, F.J., Oegema, T. and Hascall, V.C. (1978). Determination of sedimentation coefficient distributions for cartilage proteoglycans. *Arch. Biochem. Biophys.* **186**, 66–76

Pita, J.C., Müller, F.J., Morales, S.M. and Alarcon, E.J. (1979). Ultracentrifugal characterization of proteoglycans from rat growth cartilage. *J. Biol. Chem.* **254**, 10 313–10 320

Pita, J.C., Müller, F.J. and Pezon, C.F. (1983). A sectorial centrifuge cell for swinging bucket rotors – application to a velocity gradient centrifugation methodology. *Anal. Biochem.* **133**, 9–15

Pita, J.C., Müller, F.J. and Pezon, C.F. (1985). Boundary centrifugation in isovolumetric and isokinetic cesium sulfate density gradients: application to cartilage proteoglycans and other macromolecules. *Biochemistry* **24**, 4250–4260

Poole, C.A., Ayad, S. and Schofield, J.R. (1988). Chondrons from cartilage: 1. Immunolocalization of type VI collagen in the pericellular capsule of isolated canine tibial chondrons. *J. Cell Sci.* **90**, 635–643

Reese, C.A., Wiedemann, H., Kuhn, K. and Mayne, R. (1982). Characterization of a highly soluble collagenous molecule isolated from chicken hyaline cartilage. *Biochemistry* **21**, 826–830

Rosenberg, L.C., Choi, H.V., Tang, L.H., Johnson, T.L., Pal, S., Webber, C., Reiner, A. and Poole, A.R. (1985). Isolation of dermatan sulfate proteoglycans from mature bovine articular cartilages. *J. Biol. Chem.* **260**, 6304–6313

Roughley, P.J. (1989). Personal communication; quoted with permission

Roughley, P.J. and White, K.J. (1980). Age-related changes in the structure of the proteoglycan subunits from human articular cartilage. *J. Biol. Chem.* **255**, 217–224

Stanescu, V. and Chaminade, F. (1987). Proteoglycan electrophoresis on horizontal submerged polyacrylamide–agarose gels. *Connect. Tissue Res.* **16**, 71–77

Stanescu, V. and Do Pham, T. (1987). Preparative electrophoresis on agarose submerged gels of two aggregating proteoglycan monomers from articular cartilage. *Prep. Biochem.* **17**, 229–238

Stanescu, V. and Sweet, M.B.E. (1981). Characterization of a proteoglycan of high electrophoretic mobility. *Biochim. Biophys. Acta* **673**, 101–113

Stanescu, V., Maroteaux, P. and Sobczak, E. (1973). Gel electrophoresis of the proteoglycans of the growth and of the articular cartilage from various species. *Biomedicine* **19**, 460–463

Stanescu, V., Maroteaux, P. and Sobczak, E. (1977). Proteoglycan populations of baboon (papio) articular cartilage. *Biochem. J.* **163**, 103–109

Trueb, B., Schreier, T., Bruckner, P. and Winterhalter, K.H. (1987). Type VI collagen represents a major fraction of connective tissue collagens. *Eur. J. Biochem.* **166**, 699–703

Uriel, J. (1966). Methode d'electrophorese dans des gels d'acrylamide-agarose. *Bull. Soc. Chim. Biol.* **48**, 969–982

Vaughan, L., Mendler, M., Huber, S., Bruckner, P., Winterhalter, K.H., Irwin, M.I. and Mayne, R. (1988). D-Periodic distribution of collagen type IX along cartilage fibrils. *J. Cell Biol.* **106**, 991–997

Wu, J.J. and Eyre, D.R. (1984). Identification of hydroxypyridinium crosslinking sites in type II collagen of bovine articular cartilage. *Biochemistry* **23**, 1850–1857

van der Rest, M. and Fietzek, P.P. (1982). A comprehensive approach to the study of collagen primary structure based on high performance liquid chromatography. *Eur. J. Biochem.* **125**, 491–496

van der Rest, M. and Mayne, R. (1987). Type IX collagen. In *Structure and Function of Collagen Types* (R. Mayne and R.E. Burgeson), pp. 195–221. Academic Press, New York

van der Rest, M. and Mayne, R. (1988). Type IX collagen proteoglycan from cartilage is covalently crosslinked to type II collagen. *J. Biol. Chem.* **263**, 1615–1618

van der Rest, M., Bennett, H.P.J., Solomon, S. and Glorieux, F.H. (1980). Separation of collagen cyanogen bromide-derived peptides by reversed-phase high performance liquid chromatopgraphy. *Biochem. J.* **189**, 253–256

van der Rest, M., Rosenberg, L.C., Olsen, B.R. and Poole, A.R. (1986). Chondrocalcin is identical with the C-propeptide of type II procollagen. *Biochem. J.* **237**, 923–925

3

MORPHOLOGY OF CARTILAGE

COLLATED BY R.A. STOCKWELL

16

Overview

R.A. STOCKWELL

It is a truism that developments in techniques change our ideas about structure and function. It is of interest to explore the interplay of technique and concept in relation to the rapid progress in microscopic and biological technology over the last 30 years. Three aspects of articular cartilage structure may be considered: the articular surface; collagen fibril organization; and the chondrocytes.

THE ARTICULAR SURFACE

When transmission electron microscopy (TEM) became sufficiently established to give reliable images of biological tissues, one of the first electron micrographs of articular cartilage was of the surface of the femoral condyle (Davies et al., 1962). It showed a contour that was remarkably smooth, even where cells of the superficial zone lay immediately beneath the surface, so agreeing with opinion dating back to the eighteenth century (Hunter, 1743). Such a finding was also compatible with the well-known low-friction properties of synovial joint surfaces.

The advent of the scanning electron microscope (SEM) in the late 1960s and the use of replica techniques provided evidence (Gardner, 1972) that was at variance with the concept of smooth surfaces. After the elimination of more obvious artifacts, it became clear that the articular surfaces of the specimens examined were undulating, as observed at the microscopic level, and exhibited shallow hollows that measured 20–30 μm in diameter (Gardner and Woodward, 1969). These hollows, also seen in intact articular surfaces of opened, living joints of anesthetized animals (Gardner and McGillivray, 1971), were attributed by Clarke (1971a) to the presence of underlying superficial cell lacunae, since the hollows and the lacunae had the same frequency and diameter.

Criticism of this 'dimpled golf ball' surface appearance arose principally on account of known difficulties in avoiding shrinkage during the dehydration of unsupported tissue during preparation for scanning microscopy. Indeed, increased support by repeated impregnation of the tissue with osmium tetroxide using the thiocarbohydrazide method revealed a smooth surface by scanning microscopy (Bloebaum and Wilson, 1980). Later, however, Gardner et al. (1981) employed extremely-low-temperature techniques of SEM, below −180°C where the possibility of shrinkage due to water evaporation or sublimation was virtually eliminated. These techniques, described by Gardner et al. (Chapter 17), demonstrated not hollows but small mounds on the articular surface of nondehydrated specimens. More recent microprobe evidence (Middleton et al. 1984) shows that the mounds cover superficial cells.

Questions arise for the future. What is the state of the surface microcontour in the living, intact joint and does it vary during joint usage? Elucidation of this problem might be aided by employing imaging techniques via arthroscopy. Again, superficial cell shape and volume may respond to variations in osmotic pressure of the synovial fluid (Baumgarten et al., 1985). The chemical nature of the articular surface also requires investigation: an important topic since deposition of abnormal, electron-dense material occurs early in the onset of osteoarthrosis. This is addressed by Stanescu (Chapter 18). Lastly, too little is known about the other boundaries of articular cartilage, the osseochondral junction and the marginal transitional zone at the periphery of the articular area.

COLLAGEN FIBRIL ORGANIZATION

While there is agreement on the tangential array in the superficial zone and the radial disposition next to the calcified zone, there has been uncertainty for many years about fibril orientation in the midzone of the cartilage. Since the early findings of Benninghoff (1925), who used polarized light, it had been held that there is a radial ('arcade') fibrillar orientation in the midzone. Such a view satisfied the implicit requirements of pathology, being compatible with the vertical split lines of advanced fibrillation of the cartilage.

The radial concept was challenged by McConaill (1951) on biomechanical grounds: he proposed that the fibrils should be orientated obliquely. The early results of TEM (Davies et al., 1962; Weiss et al., 1968) provided some confirmation, suggesting a random or coiled arrangement with no evidence of a predominantly radial organization. The 'random' concept provided a structural basis for the mechanism of reversible deformation of the cartilage under static load, explained by the water-binding properties of proteoglycans (PGs) entrapped within a random fibril meshwork (Fessler, 1960). Nevertheless, scanning microscopy, particularly at low magnification, suggested that the apparently randomly orientated fibrils were organized into radial bundles or layers (Clarke, 1971b).

The radial vs. random concepts were reconciled when Broom (1984) observed the results of crack propagation on thick slices of articular cartilage under Nomarski optics. This provided the basis for a *pseudo* random but *overall* radial array, with some additional evidence for linkage molecules to maintain the high-energy three-dimensional 'chicken wire' configuration of the mesh. Broom's methods, which have served, perhaps finally, to satisfy the needs of pathology and of biomechanics, are described in Chapter 19. Future investigations must determine the mode of stabilization of the meshwork by elucidating the interactions between fibril and fibril and between fibril and PG.

THE CHONDROCYTES

The cells form 1% or less of the tissue volume, yet, since they are the only living element, they are of the greatest importance.

The low rate of respiration of articular chondrocytes, 1/20 to 1/50 of that of liver cells for example (Bywaters, 1937), and the notably poor regenerative capacity of adult cartilage, fostered the notion that these cells were effete. Early investigations with the transmission electron microscope (Davies et al., 1962; Weiss et al., 1968) demonstrated that the articular chondrocyte exhibited all the elements of fine structure found in 'more active' cells. Indeed, as biochemical research probes deeper, we realize that the chondrocyte, though specialized to create (and to be the fittest to survive in) its near anaerobic environment, is as complex and as interesting as other differentiated cells.

Improved methods of tissue preparation for electron microscopy employing high pressure/low temperature and ruthenium containing fixatives (Hunziker et al., 1983) have shown that the cell volume is not so shrunken and the contour not so 'spiky' as originally thought. These methods provide a more secure basis for applying quantitative morphometric techniques (Cruz-Orive and Hunziker, 1986) to the analysis of the fine structural organelles of chondrocytes. Hence, in small regions of tissue beyond the resolution and sensitivity of current biochemical methods, we should now be able to detect evidence of the functional response of the cells to mechanical, physicochemical and biological stimuli. Hunziker outlines the more recent morphometric techniques in Chapter 20.

Work on the microstructure of the cell lacuna (Poole et al., 1984) has led to intense interest in the 'chondron', a structure originally isolated from nasal cartilage by Szirmai (1969). Methods of extraction of chondrons, i.e. cell groups intact within their lacunae, have been greatly developed and improved so that a high yield is obtainable from articular cartilage (Poole et al., 1988a–c). The methods are described by Poole in Chapter 21. The methods provide us with an opportunity to study the cell in vitro, yet still enclosed in its natural microenvironment. This offers advantages over the use of cartilage explants or cell cultures in studying the structural and functional responses of the chondrocyte.

Despite these advances in technique and changes in concept, we still need to know, and probably always will need to know, more about articular cartilage. Thus little is known about the microstructural-molecular substratum of changes in the matrix during growth and 'degeneration' of cartilage. Shall we be able to modulate therapeutically the fibril–fibril and fibril–PG interactions that probaby occur? The physiological characteristics of the chondrocyte plasma membrane are largely unexplored. What, for example, is the nature of the mechanotransducer? Shall we ever 'induce' the cell to repair or regenerate cartilage tissue effectively?

'Much is taken, much abides'. As it was for Ulysses, so also much remains for chondrologists to seek and to find.

17

Methods for the study of cartilage by low temperature scanning electron microscopy and related techniques

D.L. GARDNER, K. OATES, D.M. LAWTON, J.G. PIDD and J.F.S. MIDDLETON

Low temperature techniques (Robards and Sleytr, 1985; Grout and Morris, 1987) have much to offer in cartilage research. An account is given of two methods that have contributed to the understanding of the fine structure of hydrated, unfixed cartilage surfaces in vitro.

The principal physical properties that enable articular hyaline cartilage to function efficiently as an interface in synovial joints, in particular its response to compressive and shear stresses, are determined by the water content. Cartilage water is chiefly retained within the domains of the hierarchies of proteoglycans (PGs) which are characteristic of this tissue. In turn, the shape and organization of these macromolecules is closely related to the water content of the cartilage. Any procedure used to study hyaline cartilage *in vitro* which changes the amount and distribution of water fundamentally alters the nature and characteristics of cartilage as a material. Fixation and dehydration, commonplace in light microscopic and ultrastructural investigations, inevitably lead to distortion, the displacement of small molecules and alterations in the properties of the very macromolecules which it is intended to study. In particular, the interrelationships of PG and collagen are likely to be disturbed.

There are, therefore, strong reasons for avoiding the movement and loss of water during the preparation of cartilage for microscopy and for minimizing the evaporation or sublimation of water during observation. To enable prolonged ultrastructural surveys of hydrated cartilage within these constraints, low-temperature methods have been developed for scanning (SEM) and for transmission (TEM) electron microscopy. The techniques aim to retain water within cartilage during SEM imaging and to circumvent the problem of water loss during TEM imaging.

COLLECTION OF TISSUE

Exposed to laboratory ambient temperatures, very small pieces of cartilage lose water quickly by evaporation. Whenever possible, the dissection of selected cartilage samples (by methods described in this volume) is conducted in a hydration chamber in an atmosphere saturated with water vapor. Within the chamber, a polystyrene bowl contains liquid nitrogen slush ($-210°C$; 63 K). Blocks of cartilage, oriented and trimmed to $c.$ $2.0 \times 1.0 \times 1.0$ mm^{-3}, are attached to aluminum stubs and frozen extremely quickly. The stubs are either expelled into the N_2 slush or slid rapidly down a cold, mirror-finished copper plate into the cryogen before transfer in liquid N_2 to a storage Dewar.

LOW TEMPERATURE SCANNING ELECTRON MICROSCOPY

At appropriate times, each cartilage block is transported to a cold pedestal in the front chamber of a scanning electron microscope (Gardner *et al.*, 1981). Here, an electrically conducting $c.$ 25-nm coat of an appropriate element (gold for morphology, aluminium for X-ray microanalysis) is applied by evaporation and the specimen advanced to the low-temperature stage in the axis of the microscope column. The design of this stage ensures mechanical and thermal stability during long periods of viewing at temperatures of $c.$ $-180°$ C (93 K). The temperatures attained during coating and imaging at accelerating voltages of 10–20 kV and beam currents of 0.1–0.4 nA have been carefully monitored (Gardner *et al.*, 1981) and evidence adduced to show that the temperature at which the sublimation of water becomes significant ($c.$ $-130°C$; 143 K) is not exceeded.

RESULTS

Normal cartilage

Images of good quality have been obtained from the bearing surfaces of the normal articular cartilages of guinea-pigs, dogs (Gardner *et al.*, 1981), mice, baboons and humans. They confirm that the articular surfaces of nonloaded cartilage *in vitro* are normally not smooth but are covered by a random array of gentle surface contours. Investigations made by X-ray microanalysis demonstrate that the elemental composition of the tissue below each feature is closely similar to that of a chondrocyte (Middleton *et al.*, 1984). The appearances of the nonloaded cartilage have been related to those of dog chondrocytes in three-dimensional culture on ceramic surfaces (Lawton *et al.*, 1989).

Abnormal cartilage

Ageing and osteoarthrotic (OA) human tibial condylar cartilages have a disorganized structure analogous to, but not identical with, that detected by conventional SEM (Fig. 17.1). After aseptic surgical division of an anterior cruciate ligament, dogs develop joint disease. Low-temperature scanning electron microscopy (LT-SEM) shows that cracking and pavementing of the articular cartilage surface begins approximately 12 weeks

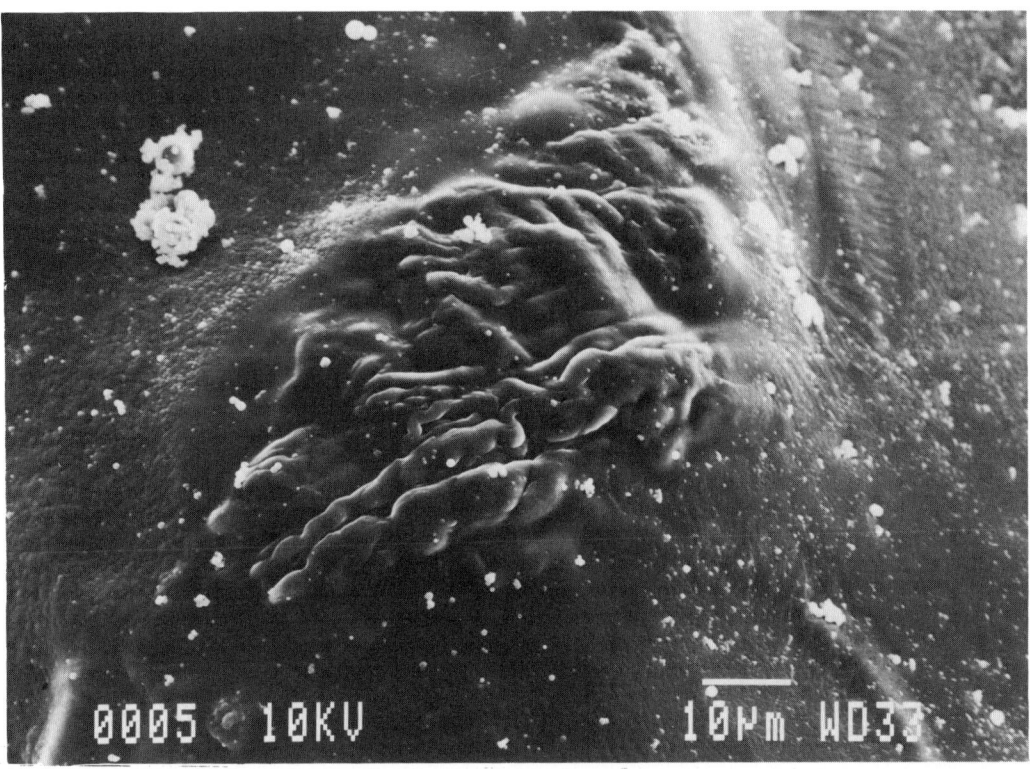

Figure 17.1 Hyaluronic acid on osteoarthrotic cartilage: human tibial condyle. Block of medial tibial condylar cartilage has been partically covered by 0.1% hyaluronic acid (MW = 1.76 kDa). Fibrillated zone is seen at the center. Note crimped collagen fiber bundles. White particles are ice. LT-SEM × 770.

after an early sequence of biochemical abnormalities (O'Connor et al., 1985). This disorganization (fibrillation) is, therefore, a relatively late manifestation of the cellular and macromolecular disorder and its origins are attributable to the continued mechanical stresses to which the increasingly abnormal extracellular matrix is subjected.

LOW-TEMPERATURE REPLICATION

Useful information concerning the structure and organization of hyaline cartilage surfaces can be gained by using LT-SEM at instrument magnifications of up to $c. \times 20\,000$, sufficient, in theory, to permit the imaging of expanded PG molecules. Beyond this magnification, images are less rewarding. A complementary low-temperature technique has, therefore, been developed to allow higher resolution TEM to be applied to the analysis of articular cartilage surfaces.

Cartilage blocks, collected as above, are transferred under liquid N_2 to a liquid N_2 cooled replication device (Gardner et al., 1983). Under vacuum, a composite layer of platinum and carbon is evaporated onto the cartilage surfaces at an angle of 45°. This application is followed by evaporation onto the block of a supporting layer of carbon which is applied from above at an angle of 90°. The thickness of the replica is $c.$ 20–25 nm. The cartilage is digested in 45% sulfuric acid for 0.5–2 h and in 75% sulfuric acid overnight. After washing, the replicas are mounted on 600 mesh copper grids and examined in a JEOL 100CX TEM at magnifications from × 1300 to × 100 000 using accelerating volatages of 80 or 100 kV.

RESULTS

Replicas of the natural, hydrated bearing surfaces of the articular cartilages of dogs (Gardner *et al.*, 1983) and of baboons (Pidd and Gardner, 1987) show two patterns of fine structure. A first amorphous surface material represents an *en face* view of the ultrastructural lamina that has been demonstrated histochemically (Orford and Gardner 1985). A second surface pattern is that of the cartilage surface revealed after the amorphous lamina has been lost (Fig. 17.2). This second structure is dominated by replicas of collagen fibers and is of sufficiently high resolution to allow their periodicity to be measured. Between the collagen fibers, gently convex contours are believed to be those of expanded PGs, not those of the cytoplasmic processes of superficial zone I chondrocytes.

DISCUSSION

The theme running through these low-temperature investigations has been the need to understand the nature and organization of the synovial fluid–articular cartilage interface, i.e. the ultrastructural, load-bearing cartilage surface (Orford and Gardner, 1985). LT-SEM and low-temperature replication (LTR) have contributed significantly to this understanding (Gardner, 1990). The methods have confirmed the presence of the non-smooth surface structure of normal,

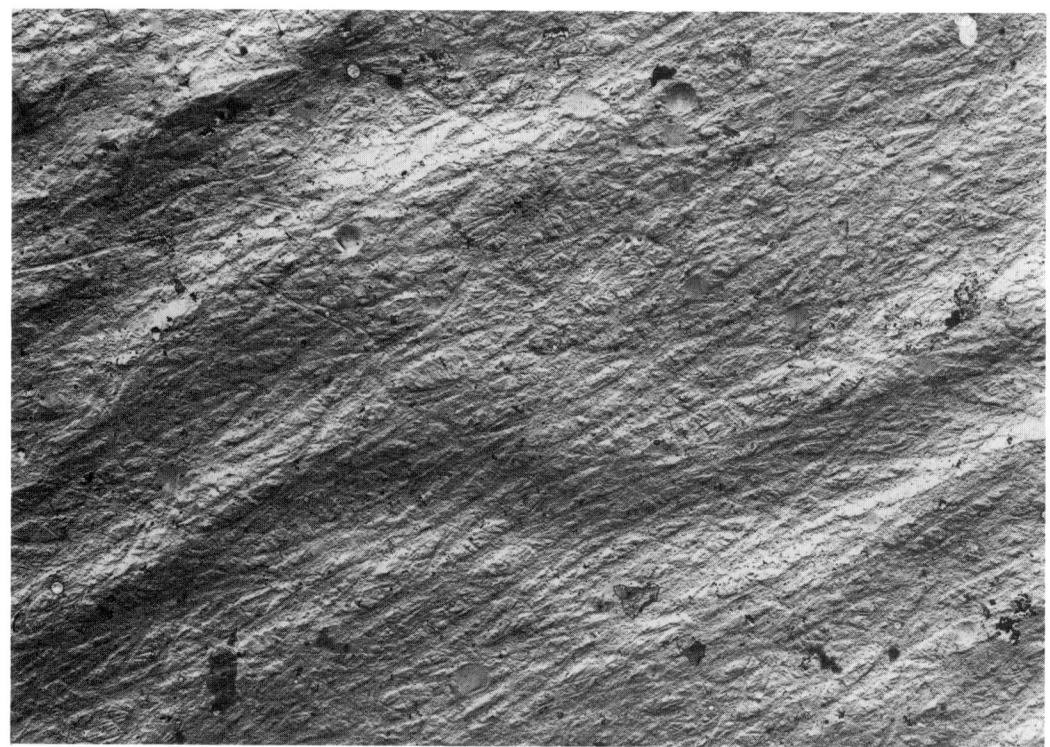

Figure 17.2 Freeze replica of nonloaded normal baboon tibial condylar cartilage surface. Replica reveals extensive fiber-rich area. Superimposed on contours are c. 5 μm ridges. Many 50–200 nm fibers lie in the plane of the surface. Occasional 400–800 nm lipid droplets are recognized. TEM × 8050.

hydrated nonloaded mammalian cartilage *in vitro* and have permitted imaging of collagen PG assemblies at the bearing surfaces. More recently, these techniques have enabled the orderly structure of hyaluronan (HA) to be seen at low temperature and have demonstrated that applied HA merges with the fibrillated surfaces of aged and OA human cartilage (Gardner *et al.*, 1989).

The *advantages* of the present methods are the ability to study hydrated, unfixed tissue in three-dimensions (LT-SEM) and at high resolution (LTR). Elemental analyses can be performed and, under circumstances not described here, indications can be obtained of the atomic composition of the tissue. The presence of individual elements and of fluorescent materials can be shown by the use of backscattered electrons and of cathodoluminescence detectors, respectively. These approaches offer the possibility of studying the localization of labeled macromolecules.

The *limitations* of these low-temperature methods are those of the cost and complexity of the equipment and of their time-consuming nature. In spite of these drawbacks, low-temperature electron microscopic methods continue to contribute to understanding cartilage fine structure.

ACKNOWLEDGMENTS

The support of the Arthritis and Rheumatism Council for Research is gratefully acknowledged.

18

Electron-microscopic study of the articular surface using cationized ferritin labeling

RITTA STANESCU

As outlined in several chapters of this book, the articular surface has a structure that differs in many respects from the rest of the cartilage. It plays a special role in joint biomechanics and cartilage nutrition (Stockwell, 1979). We have used labeling with cationized ferritin (CF) to study the charge properties of the articular surface, the morphological and chemical nature of the structures providing the charges and the alterations of the structure and charges of the surface produced by various agents and pathological conditions.

CF, a polycationic derivative of ferritin, was first prepared by Danon *et al.* (1972) for the labeling of negative charges on cell surfaces. CF is easily identifiable by electron microscopy and has a higher molecular weight than that of molecules which can penetrate normal cartilage matrix (Maroudas, 1979). We have used CF (molecular weight about 750 000, size of particles about 12 nm, pH 8.5). The labeling was performed for 30 min at room temperature with gentle shaking at a CF concentration of $0.57\,\mathrm{mg\,ml^{-1}}$ of veronal-buffered saline (VBS), pH 7.2.

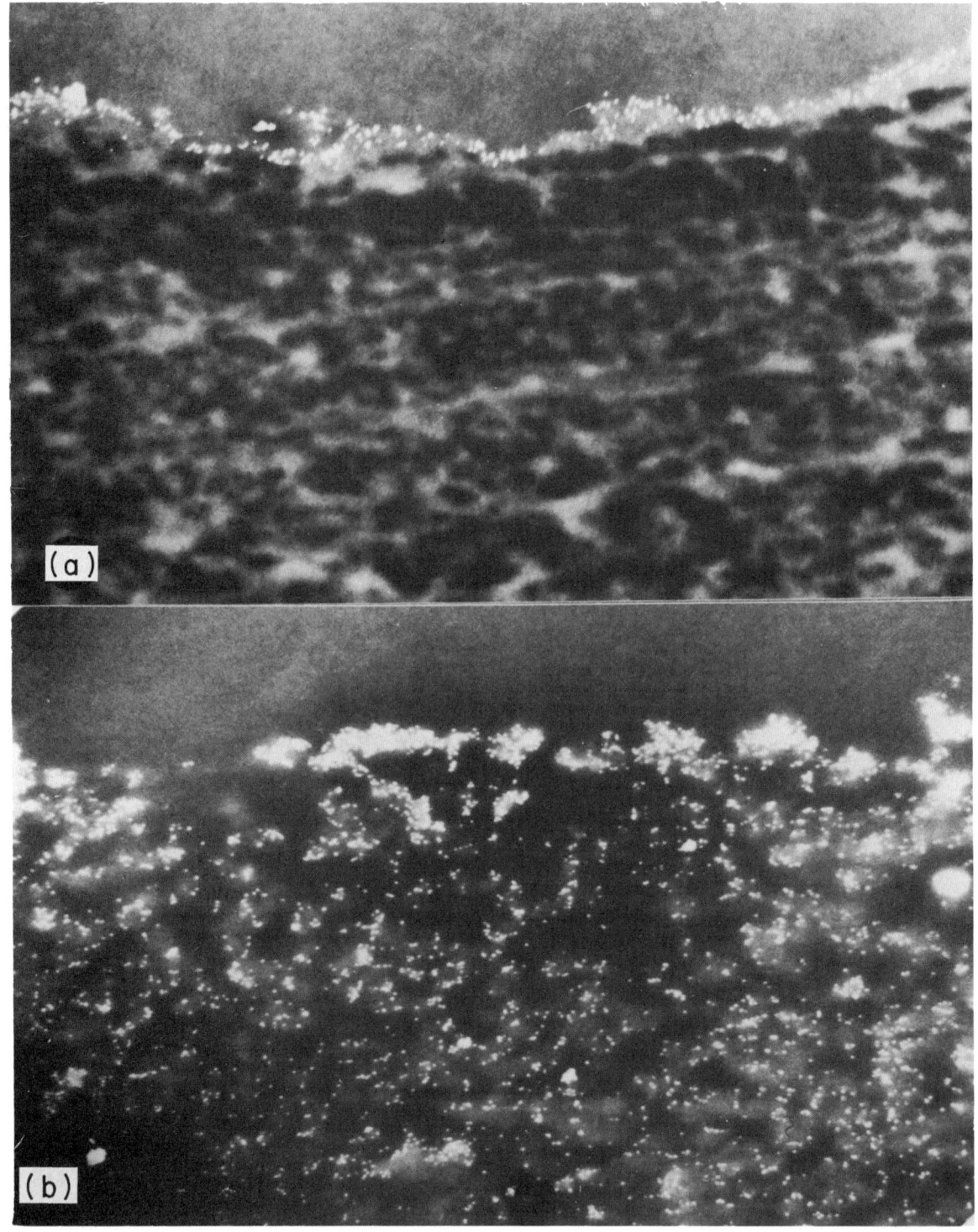

Figure 18.1 Articular surface labeled with CF, unstained sections, electron spectroscopic imaging ($\triangle E = 104$ eV). (a) Untreated surface; (b) surface digested with collagenase before labeling.

For our studies, we developed an *in vitro* model in which unfixed articular surfaces of BALB-c femoral heads were labeled with CF in various conditions and after interaction with various agents. The femoral heads were carefully removed, washed with VBS, labeled with CF, fixed, decalcified in EDTA and processed for electron microscopy as previously described (Stanescu and Leibovich, 1982). The blocks were trimmed so that transverse sections of the articular surface could be obtained. Fovea and marginal areas of the joint surface were avoided. Sections 50–60 nm thick and stained with uranyl acetate were examined with a Siemens Elmiskop 101 electron microscope, magnification 2400 and 30 000. More recently, we have used very thin unstained sections (30–35 nm) examined in an electron microscope provided with an electromagnetic prism which allows imaging with inelastically scattered electrons with a selected energy loss. CF and cartilage structure were well visualized at 140–160 eV loss.

The superficial layer of mouse femoral head contains a fine granular electron-dense material that varies in thickness or depth from 40 to 80 nm in different areas (Fig. 18.1(a)). Particles of CF were bound within this layer. The anionic sites belong to constituents of the articular surface and not to an adsorbed film or to flocculent precipitates of constituents of the synovial fluid. Washings of up to 2 h of unfixed femoral heads with water or buffers had no effect on CF labeling. The electrostatic nature of the binding was indicated by the fact that CF could be dissociated by treatment with buffers of high ionic strength. After dissociating the CF, the surface could be relabeled with CF indicating that the constituents which bind the label were not removed.

To obtain information about the morphological and chemical nature of the structure providing the anionic sites, we performed several enzymatic digestions prior to labeling (Stanescu, 1985). The material which binds CF is protein in nature. It is digested by trypsin and chymopapain, but is resistant to testicular and microbial hyaluronidase, keratanase, chondroitinase ABC and AC and neuraminidase. Thus it is unlikely that the anionic sites are on either sialyl groups of glycoproteins (e.g. lubricin, a synovial fluid glycoprotein containing sialic acid (Swann *et al.*, 1981)) the sulfate groups of chondroitin sulfate or the carboxyl groups of hyaluronan. The electron-dense material is not extracted with chloroform–methanol. Two enzymes have pronounced but different effects on the morphology and labeling pattern of the articular surface. Trypsin caused the disappearance of the electron-dense material and a partial detachment of the superficial fibrils which become labeled. Clostridial and mammalian collagenase did not remove the electron-dense material but produced discontinuities which appear to connect with the interfibrillar substance beneath the surface (Fig. 18.1(b)). The large molecules of CF penetrate deeply into a disorganized matrix with its wider separation of labeled fibers. Prior treatment with cross-linking agents protects the surface from the action of collagenase (Stanescu and Stanescu, 1988).

We have studied the action of several drugs on the articular surface using the *in vitro* model (Stanescu *et al.*, 1987a). CF labeling of human osteoarthritic femoral heads (Stanescu *et al.*, 1984) and of the articular surface in antigen-induced arthritis in the rat (Stanescu *et al.*, 1987b) showed abnormal amounts and distribution of the electron-dense material and CF penetration.

In summary, at the very surface of the articular cartilage there is a thin electron-dense layer of negatively charged protein material. This layer very probably plays a role in cartilage permeability and lubrication and undergoes early alterations in some pathologic conditions. Increased permeability of cartilage for the very large CF molecules is seen after digestion with certain enzymes and in some pathologic conditions.

19

New experimental approaches to the understanding of structure–function relationships in articular cartilage

NEIL D. BROOM

INTRODUCTION

Albert Einstein once said 'Science without religion is lame; religion without science is blind'. Perhaps it can also be said that any study of the load-bearing characteristics of articular cartilage (AC) without regard to its structure is an inadequate one, but equally so is any study of its structure or architecture without due attention to its functional implications.

It is relatively easy to study separately both the mechanical and structural characteristics of AC. However, it is my belief that by making such a separation, a potentially rich body of understanding is inevitably kept from the investigator. The reason for this is that AC, as a load-bearing material, functions over a relatively large range of deformations or strains. Most engineering materials function by virtue of their intrinsic stiffness or rigidity. Under normal service loads, there is virtually no detectable deformation. Materials such as metals, concrete, ceramics, timber, most structural plastics and certain body tissues such as bone are exploited because of their rigidity. This is an essential requirement if components are to be assembled with proper clearances in the loaded and unloaded states. We cannot build motor cars with accurately fitting doors or high-rise office blocks from floppy or compliant materials. Strength with these rigid materials is important, but nearly always subservient to stiffness. Sound engineering design always incorporates a factor of safety, thus yield strength or failure stress should never be reached under normal loading. Structurally for these rigid materials there is little difference, even at the ultrastructural level, between the loaded and unloaded state; hence it is reasonable to collect the mechanical and structural data as separate activities.

By contrast, AC, along with the wider family of soft connective tissue, is required to provide both compliancy and strength. The maintenance of sustained loading will require the cartilage to undergo considerable deformation and this in turn means large spatial or morphological rearrangement of the constituent components.

If we are to understand fully the structure–function relationships controlling the biomechanical properties of AC, these large spatial variations in the load-bearing elements must be considered, even though they will not be evident in a single histological section of the processed tissue. Rather, we must endeavor to examine the tissue directly at the highest possible resolution in a state as close as possible to its *in vivo* physiological condition while simultaneously applying mechanical loads that simulate joint function.

The aim of this chapter is to outline a number of experimental methods developed in the biomechanics laboratory in Auckland that have contributed to our present level of understanding of structure–function relationships in cartilage.

DIFFERENTIAL INTERFERENCE CONTRAST LIGHT MICROSCOPY OF THICK SECTIONS OF ARTICULAR CARTILAGE

Considerable structural information can be obtained from the examination of fully hydrated, relatively thick sections of AC (i.e. 0.1–0.2 mm as compared with 2–5-μm with conventional histology) using differential interference contrast (DIC) light microscopy. With this specialized optical method, incident light is split into two rays of a different but fixed phase relationship by one of the interferometer elements. Any phase-shifting object inserted in the path of one of these rays will produce an alteration in the interference between these two rays and hence a change in intensity corresponding to the object when they are recombined in the second interferometer element (Francon, 1961). It should be added that DIC yields a considerable improvement in image quality in relatively thick sections of AC over that achieved with ordinary bright-field or phase-contrast techniques. Sections of fully hydrated AC, 0.1–0.2 mm in thickness, can be easily and quickly prepared from full-depth scallops of tissue removed from the freshly opened joint. Excellent microscopal data can be obtained within minutes of animal death.

The thickness of section compared with the scale of size of the ultrastructural collagenous elements effectively ensures that many of the bulk tissue mechanical properties will be represented in these specimens. The opportunity is therefore available to conduct mechanical stressing experiments on AC while simultaneously observing its structural response using DIC microscopy.

TECHNIQUES FOR OBSERVING STRUCTURAL RESPONSE OF ARTICULAR CARTILAGE TO CONDITIONS APPROXIMATING PHYSIOLOGICAL COMPRESSION

The response of AC to direct compression in the surface-to-bone or radial direction can be studied

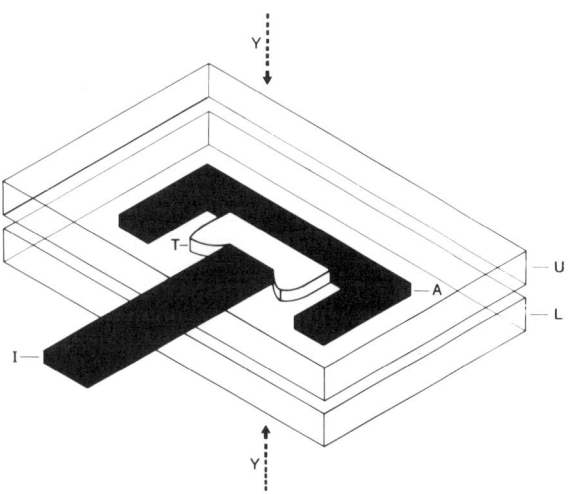

Figure 19.1 Schematic of experimental system for observing structural response of cartilage to direct compression in the radial direction. I, indentor; A, anvil-spacer; T, tissue test piece; u, upper glass surface; L, lower glass surface; Y, optical axis of interference microscope. (From Broom and Poole (1983), with permission.)

using the experimental arrangement shown in Fig. 19.1. The section of tissue incorporating the full zonal depth of structure is sandwiched between two optically flat surfaces which are separated by an amount equal to the section thickness (0.1–0.2 mm). An indentor of almost equal thickness penetrates from one side and compresses the tissue section against the rear anvil. The indentor is strain-gauged to record loads and a displacement transducer element, also attached, records displacement. Appropriate motorization provides a uniform rate of loading. Stress–strain data is recorded on an x–y plotter. The device is sufficiently miniaturized to allow insertion onto the stage of an optical microscope fitted with a DIC facility. Hydration of the tissue is maintained with saline floated into the sandwich space.

The experimental system described above provides accurate monitoring of the tissue's mechanical properties under conditions approximating plane-strain compression with simultaneous observation of the deformed structure throughout the full zonal range from the articular surface to the deep matrix. The matrix chondrocytes, as well as providing internal markers for measuring zone-related strains, can also be observed to deform under the imposed loads. In matrices that are abnormally soft, the collagen fibrils tend to aggregate into groups or bundles that are of a sufficient size for resolution with DIC optics. Again, the response of this fibrillar structure to compressive loading can be studied using the above-described technique (Broom and Poole, 1983; Broom, 1988).

INVESTIGATION OF SPECIFIC STRUCTURAL INTERACTIONS IN CARTILAGE USING MICRONOTCH/ STRESSING TECHNIQUES

The simultaneous microscopic/microcompression experiment that permits quantification of the tissue's integrated response to compressive load-bearing does not give access to the individual structural interactions within the AC matrix that this integrated response ultimately requires.

In order to investigate those specific mechanisms that provide for cohesion of the matrix within each zone, there must be some means of selectively stressing in tension the tissue in both the radial and transverse directions of a particular zonal depth. This can be achieved by preparing full-depth sections, as for the microcompression experiment discussed above, and then by cutting either a radial or transverse notch (Fig. 19.2). Under tension, the radial notch introduces a transverse tensile stress in the matrix below the notch root, whereas the transverse notch induces a radial tensile stress. By varying the initial depth of the radial notch or depth below the articular surface at which the transverse notch is cut, and by varying the orientation in which the full-depth section is taken from the original scallop of AC, it is possible to carry out an examination of the cohesive stiffness and failure strength of the various zones of the AC matrix. Furthermore, by cutting an inverted radial notch from the deep matrix up toward the articular surface, the strength properties of this layer can be investigated.

Again, all these micromechanical tests can be very effectively carried out with simultaneous DIC microscopy, so that local-strain measurements and tissue-rupture mechanisms can be studied directly with excellent structural resolution. Specifically, the rupture process can be followed as it tracks through the different zones in different directions. We find, for example, that in healthy tissue the

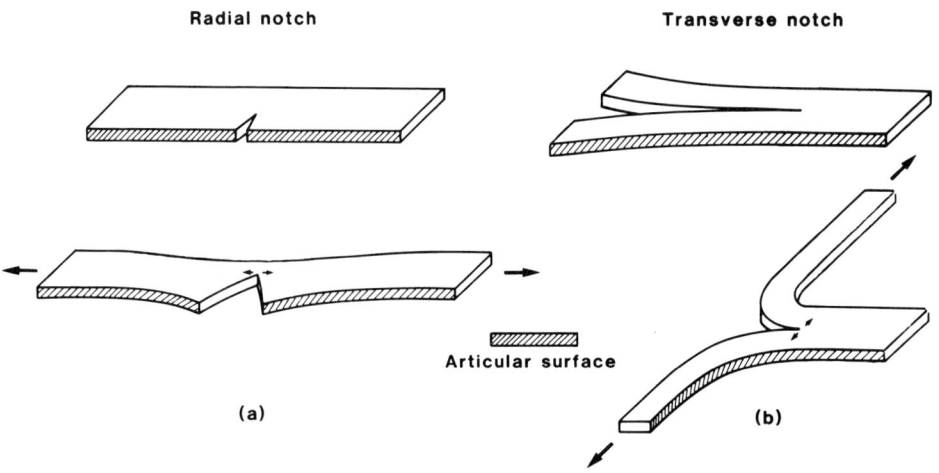

Figure 19.2 Schematic of (a) radial and (b) transverse notch geometries and their respective loading configurations. (From Broom (1984) with permission).

radial notch tracks radially downwards in a predictable manner without transverse deviation. This implies that there is a preferred radial texture of fibrils in the general matrix. Conversely, the matrix at the root of the transverse notch resists further propagation by transverse rupture; instead the matrix fails by means of a skewed radial rupture mechanism. These patterns of matrix rupture have shed considerable light on the structural principles upon which matrix cohesion is built. Whereas radial cohesion is achieved directly by the tensile strength of the collagen fibrils themselves, transverse knit is thought to involve some sort of interfibrillar link.

In degenerate matrix, the transverse notch is able to propagate transversely and this is consistent with a fundamental tensile weakening of the radially aligned collagen fibrils that are directly stressed at the transverse notch root.

It should be emphasized that the matrix deformations at the respective notch roots can involve very large strains. At the radial notch, transverse matrix extensions can be greater than 100% and the morphological rearrangements associated with such large matrix deformations can be extremely complex (Broom, 1986, 1988).

THREE-DIMENSIONAL ULTRASTRUCTURAL STUDIES USING TRANSMISSION ELECTRON MICROSCOPY STEREOSCOPY

In order to describe more accurately the spatial arrangements of the collagen fibrils in AC, the investigator must use ultrastructural techniques. Scanning electron microscopy has its own particular set of problems. Transmission electron microscopy (TEM), if carried out using conventional thin-section techniques (90–100 mm), has the disadvantage of permitting very little fibril continuity to be observed. However, in a very recent study it has been shown that a greatly enhanced picture of fibril continuity and spatial arrangement can be obtained by examining relatively thick TEM sections (0.2–0.8 μm) in stereo and at 120 KV. The application of this techique has led to the identification of a number of fibril interactions involving direct physical entwinement which are assumed to provide a mechanism for matrix cohesion in the transverse direction (Broom and Silyn-Roberts, 1989).

CONCLUSIONS

In summary, AC lends itself to a variety of novel structural/mechanical approaches that have considerably enhanced our understanding of the biomechanical principles that govern the behavior of this important tissue. The combination of the DIC/micromechanical techniques with thick-section TEM stereoscopy, and applied to the full range of matrices from normal to degenerate, offer a useful resource of research tools for those interested in the complex problem of cartilage malfunction.

ACKNOWLEDGMENT

This research has been funded by the N.Z. Medical Research Council.

20

The application of recent stereological methods in articular cartilage research

ERNST B. HUNZIKER

In articular cartilage research, morphological analyses have contributed substantially to the current state of knowledge regarding the structural organization of this tissue in the normal and pathological state. For many purposes, quantitative structural data are essential, since purely descriptive information is insufficient. A few examples of such quantitative parameters (so-called 'estimators' in stereological terms) include the proportion of tissue occupied by matrix or cells, the number of cells, the mean volume of matrix per cell, the mean cell volume or cell surface area and the cell diameters.

Such quantities cannot, however, be observed or measured in a direct, straightforward way. The morphologist's observations are made on thick or thin sections and thus represent two-dimensional projections of tissue structures. Such 'images' do not provide us directly with three-dimensional structural information, although these data are, in a statistical sense, contained within the two-dimensional sections. Stereology affords a set of methods by which three-dimensional structures may be quantitated from section analysis. For this information to be unbiased, several conditions must be fulfilled with respect to tissue sampling and sectioning (see Chapter 6).

Parameters describing quantitative structural information in tissue are called 'stereological estimators'. The most frequently determined estimators include volume, surface area and number and size of cells. The practical procedures adopted for making measurements in the two-dimensional-section plane (for example on light and electron micrographs), so-called morphometric methods (morphometry), include point or intersection counting, object counting and boundary length measurements, to name but a few examples. A frequently used estimator is the volume fraction of cells in tissue (V_V; cells/tissue). A simple approach to estimating this parameter was described in the last century by Delesse (principle of Delesse (1847)) who used the relationship:

volume fraction of cells (V_V) = area fraction (A_A)

the latter being equivalent to the number of test points of a test system hitting cell profiles divided by the number of points covering the tissue (P_p). Since this estimator is a relative value, the magnification at which the measurement is made need not be known and the arrangement of the points in the test system is irrelevant to the estimator. Moreover, plane sections need not be isotropic or uniformly random or, indeed, need the structural organization of tissue be statistically isotropic. This is also the case when estimating the number of cells, but not when determining the surface area of cells in tissue (S_V; surface (cells)/tissue). In mature articular cartilage, the structural organization of tissue is extremely anisotropic and it would be difficult or impossible to make isotropic, uniformly random sections for estimating S_V (cells) according to the relationship:

$$S_V = S \text{ (cells)} / V \text{ (tissue)} = 2 \cdot I/L$$

where I is the number of intersections between test lines and cell profile boundaries on sections and L is the total length of test lines superimposed on the tissue of interest. A novel approach to this problem, developed in recent years (Baddeley et al., 1986), permits an unbiased estimation of any type (i.e. regardless of the degree of anisotropy) of surface area from sections. The method is based on the use of 'vertical' sections and 'cycloid' test lines (systems). The basic idea is to make the test lines isotropic and uniformly random in three-dimensional space. In order to achieve this, vertical tissue sections must be cut, i.e. in a direction perpendicular to a given 'horizontal' plane. This is a plane of reference, determined by the investigator, which defines the orientation of the vertical sections. In the case of articular cartilage tissue, an intrinsic vertical direction is easily identifiable (perpendicular to the articular cartilage surface and the subchondral bone plate). All vertical sections used in a study must have a random orientation relative to the common horizontal plane. Given this condition, the cycloid test lines (Fig. 20.1) fulfil the requirement of being isotropic and uniformly random in space. With respect to test line length, this requirement is satisfied by the cycloids being proportional (in length) to the sine of any angle (between 0° and

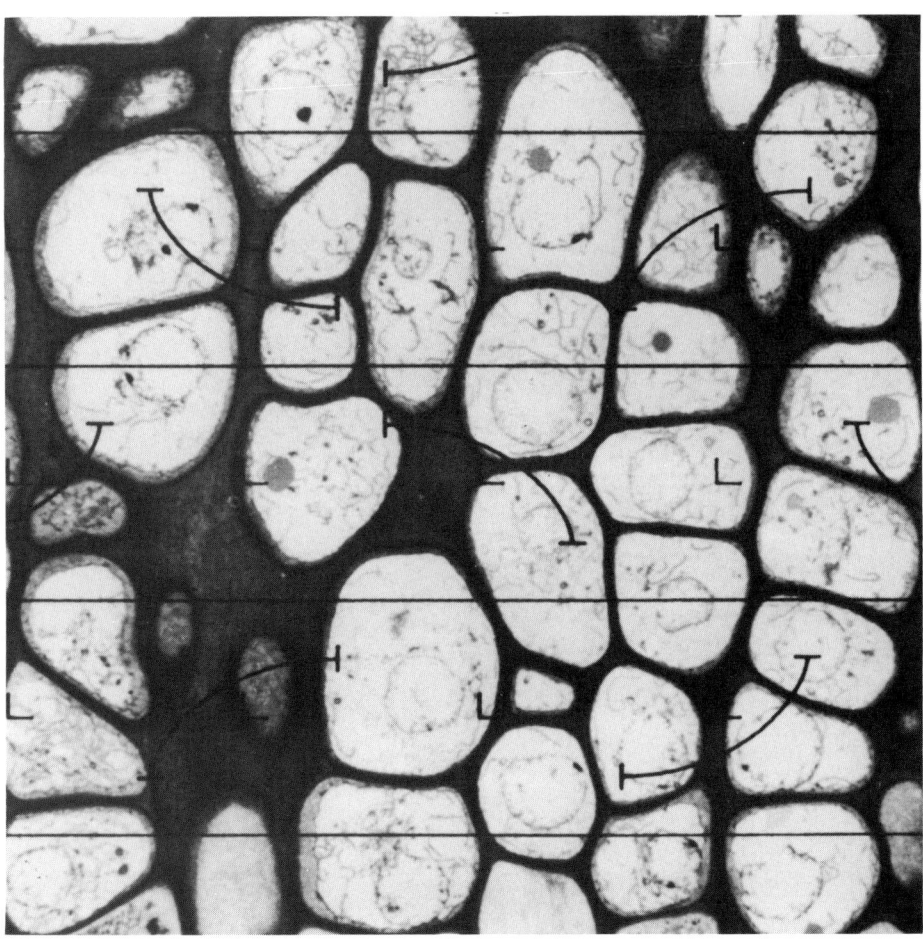

Figure 20.1 Rat growth-plate cartilage, proximal tibia. Light micrograph of hypertrophic chondrocytes on a vertical section, superimposed on which is a test system consisting of test points and test lines (cycloid arcs). The horizontal lines are used merely to follow the test arcs easily during counting (Hunziker et al. (1987) with permission of the authors and the publisher.)

90°) away from the vertical axis (Gundersen *et al.*, 1988a; Baddeley *et al.*, 1986).

The so-called disector method represents one of many novel procedures (including the nucleator, fractionator and selector) developed for estimating the number of cells in tissue (in general: particles in space, N_V), which is shape-independent and assumption free (Cruz-Orive, 1987; Gundersen *et al.*, 1988b).

A basic requirement to be fulfilled for any estimation of cell or particle number is that all cells should have a uniform (i.e. the same) probability of being sampled and counted. The disector (Sterio, 1984) is a probe by which cells are sampled in three-dimensional space with a uniform probability, irrespective of their size and shape. The probe used, i.e. the disector, thus needs to be three-dimensional and this is achieved by analyzing a section pair, S1 and S2 (Fig. 20.2). The disector volume (v(dis)) is the product of the test area (on S1 and S2) over which cell profiles are counted and the height of the disector (h, i.e. the distance between S1 and S2). An estimate of the number of cells per unit volume is determined as the number of cells present in the first section (S1), but no longer apparent in the second (S2) (ΣQ^-), divided by the disector volume, (Σv(dis)), i.e.

$$N \text{(cells)} / V \text{(tissue)} = \Sigma Q^- / \Sigma v \text{(dis)}$$

In general, one should not use sections that exceed in thickness one-quarter to one-third of the particle (cell) height. A very elegant and efficient procedure for the future is that of 'optical' disectors, which make use of confocal microscopes (Petran *et al.*, 1968; Howard *et al.*, 1985).

The mean volumes and surface areas of a cell can be efficiently estimated by using the above-presented estimators, namely, V_V, S_V and N_V. The mean cell volume ($\bar{v}_N(c)$) is thus defined as V_V/N_V and the mean cell surface ($\bar{s}_N(c)$) as S_V/N_V.

However, practical estimations of mean cell volumes (on a volume-weighted basis, $\bar{v}_V(c)$) can also be made directly, without the need to measure V_V and N_V, by using the 'point-sampling intercept'

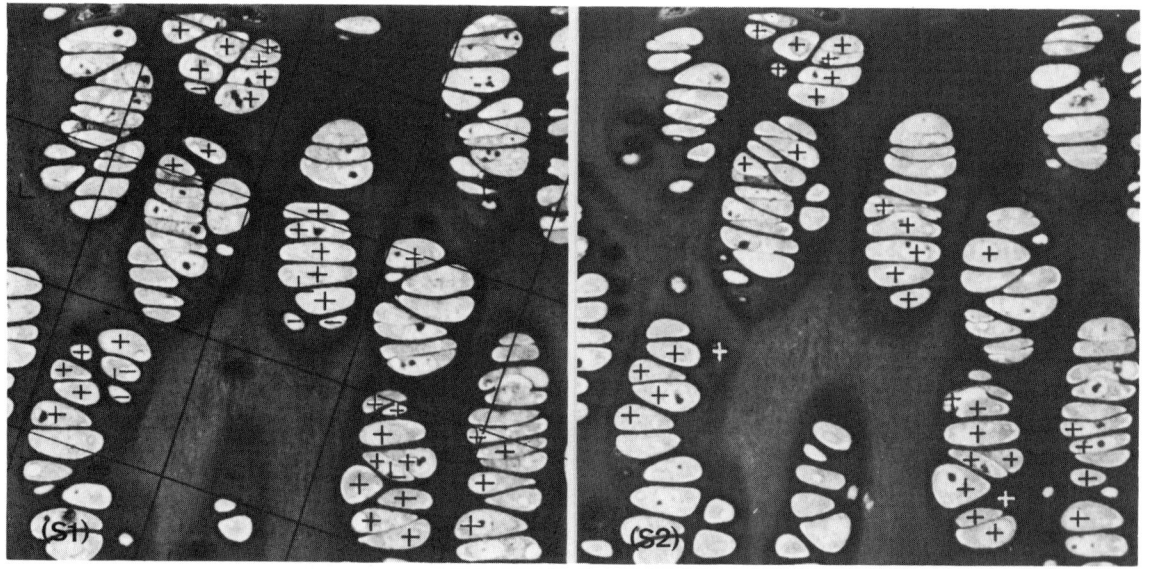

Figure 20.2 Cell counting in space using the disector method. Two sections (S1 and S2) are illustrated that were cut 4 μm apart. The number of cells present in the reference section (S1), but no longer apparent in the other (S2) (marked with a minus sign), divided by the volume of the disector, gives an estimate of the number of cells per unit reference volume. Cells that are present in both (S1 and S2) sections are marked with a plus sign. Cells are counted only in squares containing a test point. (From Hunziker *et al.* (1987) with permission of the authors and the publisher.)

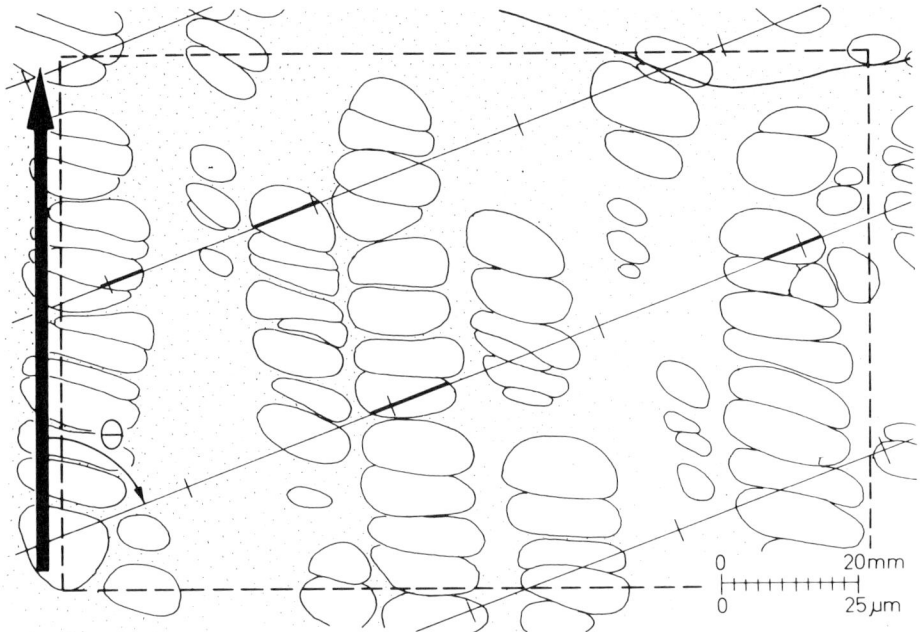

Figure 20.3 A vertical quadrant with a system of parallel lines at an angle Q with the vertical direction (black arrow). If a test point hits a cell transect, then the corresponding point-sampled intercept (thick segment in the figure) is classified using the lo-ruler at the bottom right (from Cruz-Orive and Hunziker (1986) with permission of the authors and the publisher.)

method (Cruz-Orive and Hunziker, 1986; Gundersen et al., 1988b). This method may also be particularly useful in estimating mean volumes of cells in culture. Moreover, if a confocal microscope is employed, tissue fixation, embedding and cutting can even be avoided and $\bar{v}_V(c)$ may be estimated with a very high efficiency. The procedure requires only single sections on which all profiles are sampled for measurements using a set of random points. Those points hitting cell profiles are used to measure complete linear intercepts ($lo+$) of test lines with cell profiles. The volume-weighted mean cell volume ($\bar{v}_V(c)$) is then defined as $(\pi/3) \cdot \overline{lo^3}+$ (Fig. 20.3).

The few novel stereological methods presented here, together with many others not described (Gundersen, 1986; Cruz-Orive, 1987), have provided a basis for model- and assumption-free, unbiased quantitation of tissue structural components. A number of additional methods are currently being developed for detailed quantitative characterization of individual structural elements such as single cells.

A frequent concern expressed by investigators planning a stereological study is: 'How many points, intersections, etc., need to be counted'. The answer to this is very simple: never count more than 100–150 per biological unit, i.e. per organ or animal (Gundersen et al., 1988b). On this basis, stereological studies and morphometric measurements, when performed well, become very efficient, powerful tools in structural research.

ACKNOWLEDGMENTS

This work was supported by the Swiss National Science Foundation, Grant No. 31-25723.88.

21

Chondrons extracted from articular cartilage: methods and applications

C. ANTHONY POOLE

INTRODUCTION

The chondron concept was introduced by Benninghoff (1925) to describe the functional and metabolic unit of the chondrocyte and its pericellular microenvironment in hyaline cartilages. Ultrastructural studies have subsequently shown that the chondron in adult articular cartilage consists of a chondrocyte and its pericellular matrix (Pmx) enclosed within a compacted, fibrillar capsule (Poole et al., 1984, 1987). We have now expanded on a concept introduced by Szirmai (1969) and developed new techniques to extract and isolate intact, viable chondrons from low-speed homogenates of mature articular cartilage (Poole et al., 1988a). We report here on the application of the isolated chondron model in the study of the structure, composition and function of the unique microenvironment which surrounds articular cartilage chondrocytes.

METHODS

Full-depth tibial cartilage samples were collected from mature canine, human and other mammalian joints. Small samples (1 g) were finely diced, suspended in 20 ml phosphate buffered saline (PBS) at 4°C and serially homogenized in a Polytron grinder accurately regulated at speeds of 4000–8000 rev. min^{-1} (1–10 min). The homogenate was diluted to 50 ml, gently centrifuged (100 g, 30 s) to settle larger fragments, and the flocculent supernatant collected. The sediment was washed again in PBS, gently centrifuged, the supernatants pooled and the process repeated until the sample was exhausted (6–10 times). Pooled supernatants (c. 500 ml) were filtered through a series of sterile nylon filters (pore size 1000–400 μm^2) to remove larger cartilage fragments and the filtered supernatant centrifuged at 400 g for 15–30 min. In each species examined, the loose pellet of fine flocculent material contained small cartilage 'chips', intact chondrons, capsular ghosts and collagenous debris. Chondrocyte viability was assessed using fluorescein diacetate (FDA) (Gray and Morris, 1987) and the number of viable cells in five 10 μl samples averaged to give 1–6 × 10^5 viable chondrons per preparation.

APPLICATIONS

The morphology of both fixed and viable chondrons was investigated using wet whole-mount preparations viewed by differential interference contrast (Fig. 21.1) and phase contrast microscopy (Poole et al. 1988a). A discrete Pmx, pericellular capsule (Pcp), pericellular channel (Pch) and tail (T) were readily identified by these techniques while FDA staining (Fig. 21.2) served to illustrate the unique shape of each viable chondrocyte and its relationship to the morphology of the chondron (cf Figs 21.1 and 21.2).

Histochemical and cytochemical methods have been used to map the distribution of glycosaminoglycans (GAGs), proteoglycans

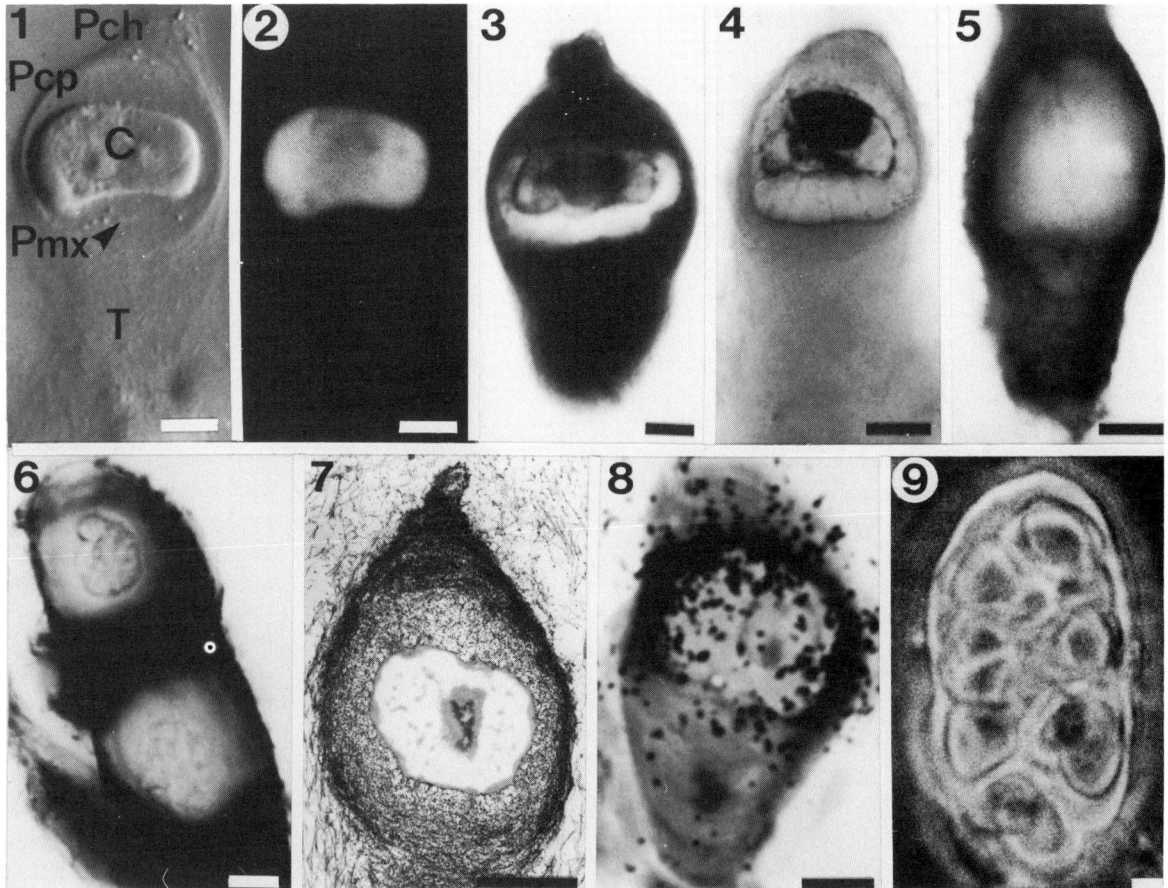

Figures 21.1–21.9 Chondrons isolated from mature canine tibial cartilage. See text for details. (1) Differential interference contrast microscopy. (2) Fluorescein diacetate viability. (3) Hematoxylin and eosin, control. (4) Hematoxylin and eosin following streptomyces hyaluronidase. (5) Distribution of antifibronectin antibody. (6) Distribution of anti C_6S antibody (MK302). (7) TEM, ruthenium red stain. (8) Autoradiographic distribution of $^{35}SO_4$. (9) Osteoarthritic chondrocyte cluster. Bar = 5 μm.

(PGs) and collagen in chondrons collected onto cellulose acetate filters (Figs 21.3 and 21.4). Samples (1 ml) of the chondron suspension were treated for 30 min to 24 h with one of the following enzymes: testicular or streptomyces hyaluronidase (Fig. 21.4), chondroitinase-ABC or -AC, keratanase and collagenase. Aliquots (100 μl) were sequentially removed from the digest, drawn onto filters, washed and fixed for 30 min. Fixatives included glutaraldehyde (with or without CPC), Karnofsky's fixative, 70% alcohol, and St Maries acid alcohol (Tuckett and Morriss-Kay, 1988).

Whole filters were stained in one of the following; hematoxylin and eosin (Fig. 21.3), toluidine blue, Safranin O, alcian blue ($MgCl_2$ CEC), PAS AB pH 1, 2.5, 4, Stains All and van Gieson. Stained filters were finally cleared in xylene, infiltrated with Eukitt and mounted under coverglass. The results indicate high concentrations of chondroitin sulphate throughout the capsule and tail, while hyaluronan appears concentrated in the Pmx.

The immunolocalization of some minor collagen species have been completed using chondron suspensions stained with fluorescein or rhodamine probes. To date, antibodies to type IX and type II collagens have been colocalized in the capsule of porcine and rat chondrosarcoma chondrons (Poole et al., 1988c), while type VI collagen was preferentially localized in the capsule and tail of canine chondrons (Poole et al., 1988b). Further experiments with filter collected chondrons treated with antifibronectin antibodies and visualized by HRP/diaminobenzidine suggests this glycoprotein also forms part of the chondron (Fig. 21.5).

Recent experiments using agarose embedded chondrons reacted with antibodies to a range of PG/GAG epitopes and visualized by HRP/4 chloro-1-naphthol have confirmed the presence of C_6S (Fig. 21.6) and keratan sulfate in the capsule. Scanning electron microscopy (SEM) studies of chondrons collected onto filters have been completed (Poole et al. 1988a) that reveal details of the fibrillar organization of the capsule. Further chondron samples (100 μl) were pelleted into loose blocks and processed for transmission electron microscopy (TEM) as described previously (Poole et al. 1984, 1987). More recently, correlative light and electron microscopy techniques (Rieder et al., 1985) have been initiated and enable selection of individual chondrons by light microscopy (LM) and correlation with structures seen by TEM. Chondrons were collected onto filters, fixed and stained with ruthenium red (Luft, 1971) or ruthenium hexamine trichloride (RHT) (Hunziker et al., 1983), infiltrated with Epon 812 or Spurrs resin and embedded flat between glass coverslips. Chondrons stained with ruthenium red (Fig. 21.7) or RHT were easily identified by LM and selected examples cut from the filter, mounted and trimmed and sectioned at 0.1–1 μm. TEM reveals an ascending gradient of particulate concentration from the plasma membrane to the outer margin of the capsule (Fig. 21.7).

In vitro experiments using both chondron suspensions and agarose gel techniques (Aydelotte and Kuettner, 1988) have been initiated and chondrons maintained up to 4 weeks in sterile culture. Autoradiographic studies have also been attempted using chondron suspensions labeled for 24 h with $^{35}SO_4$ (Fig. 21.8) or [^{3}H]-glucosamine. Labeled samples were extensively washed, gently pelleted and treated in one of two ways: (i) chondrons were mixed in agarose, spread on glass slides, fixed, air dried and dipped in Nuclear Track Emulsion; or (ii) aliquots were collected onto filters, resin embedded, sectioned at 1 μm and dipped in emulsion (Fig. 21.8). Preparations were exposed for 1–5 weeks and showed significant uptake of both labels by viable cells and a preferential sequestration of material within the microenvironment of the chondron.

Finally, studies on canine and human osteoarthritic cartilage reveal significant changes in the morphology of the chondrons isolated. These include loss of capsular organization, alteration in the histochemical profile of the chondron, the presence of dividing chondrocytes and the isolation of large chondrocyte clusters typical of osteoarthritic cartilage (Fig. 21.9).

CONCLUSIONS

Extraction of viable chondrons from articular cartilage by low-speed homogenization represents a new technique which requires further development to improve the overall yield of viable chondrons. The applications presented demonstrate that isolated chondrons can provide a valuable model to study the structure, composition and function of the chondrocyte and its unique microenvironment. The results of these studies suggest that the integrity of chondron components could have a significant effect on the fate of the chondrocyte during compression and in the genesis of degenerative joint disease.

ACKNOWLEDGMENTS

Funded by the Medical Research Council of New Zealand. The antibodies were supplied by Drs S. Ayad, B. Caterson, V. Duance, M. Gibson and T. Glant who are gratefully acknowledged.

References

Aydelotte, M.B. and Kuettner, K.E. (1988). Differences between sub-populations of cultured bovine articular chondrocytes. 1. Morphology and cartilage matrix production. *Connect. Tiss. Res.* **18**, 205–222

Baddeley, A.J., Gundersen, H.J.G. and Cruz-Orive, L.M. (1986). Estimation of surface area from vertical sections. *J. Microsc.* **142**, 259–276

Baumgarten, M., Bloebaum, R.D., Ross, S.D.K., Campbell, P. and Samiento, A. (1985). Normal human synovial fluid: osmolality and exercise-induced changes. *J. Bone Joint Surg.* **67A**, 1336–1339

Benninghoff, A. (1925). Form und Bau der Gelenkknorpel in ihren Beziehungen zur Function. II. Der Aufbau des Gelenkknorpels in seinen Beziehungen zur function. *Z. Zellforsch mikrosk Anat.* **2**, 783–862

Bloebaum, R.D. and Wilson, A.S. (1980). The morphology of the surface of articular cartilage in adult rats. *J. Anat.* **131**, 222–246

Broom, N.D. (1984). Further insights into the structural principles governing the function of articular cartilage. *J. Anat.* **139**, 275–294

Broom, N.D. (1986). Connective tissue function and malfunction: biomechanical perspective. *Pathology* **20**, 93–104

Broom, N.D. (1988). The collagenous architecture of articular cartilage: its profound influence on normal and abnormal mechanical function. In *Collagen: Chemistry, Biology and Biotechnology* (M. Nimni, ed.), pp. 243–265. CRC Press, Boca Raton, FL

Broom, N.D. and Poole, C.A.P. (1983). Articular cartilage collagen and proteoglycans: their functional interdependency. *Arth. Rheum.* **26**, 1111–1119

Broom, N.D. and Silyn-Roberts, H. (1989). The 3-dimensional knit of collagen fibrils in articular cartilage. *Connect. Tissue Res.* **23**, 261–277

Bywaters, E.G.L. (1937). The metabolism of joint tissues. *J. Pathol. Bacteriol.* **44**, 247–168

Clarke, I.C. (1971a). Human articular surface contours and related surface depression frequency studies. *Ann. Rheum. Dis.* **30**, 15–23

Clarke, I.C. (1971b). Articular cartilage: a review and scanning electron microscopy study. I. The interterritorial fibrillar architecture. *J. Bone Joint Surg.* **53B**, 732–750

Cruz-Orive, L.M. (1987). Particle number can be estimated using a disector of unknown thickness: the selector. *J. Microsc.* **145**, 121–142

Cruz-Orive, L.M. and Hunziker, E.B. (1986). Stereology for anisotropic cells: application to growth cartilage. *J. Microsc.* **143**, 47–80

Danon, D., Goldstein, L., Marikovsky, Y. and Skutelsky, E. (1972). Use of cationized verso ferritin as a label of negative charges on cell surfaces. *J. Ultrast. Res.* **38**, 500–510

Davies, D.V., Barnett, C.H., Cochrane, W. and Palfrey, A.J. (1962). Electron microscopy of articular cartilage in the young adult rabbit. *Ann. Rheum. Dis.* **21**, 11–22

Delesse, M.A. (1847). Procede mecanique pour determiner la composition des roches. *C.R. Acad. Sci. (Paris)* **25**, 544–546

Fessler, J.H. (1960). A structural function of the mucopolysaccharide in connective tissue. *Biochem. J.* **76**, 124–132

Francon, M. (1961). *Progress in Microscopy*, pp. 94–128. Pergamon Press, Oxford

Gardner, D.L. (1972). The influence of microscopic technology on knowledge of cartilage surface structure. *Ann. Rheum. Dis.* **321**, 235–258

Gardner, D.L. (1990). *Pathological Basis of the Connective Tissue Diseases*. Edward Arnold, London (in press)

Gardner, D.L. and McGillivray, D.C. (1971). Living articular cartilage is not smooth. The structure of mammalian and avian joint surfaces demonstrated in vivo by immersion incident light microscopy. *Ann. Rheum. Dis.* **30**, 3–14

Gardner, D.L. and Woodward, D. (1969). Scanning electron microscopy and replica studies of articular surfaces of guinea-pig synovial joints. *Ann. Rheum. Dis.* **28**, 379–391

Gardner, D.L., O'Connor, P. and Oates, K. (1981). Low temperature scanning electron microscopy of dog and guinea-pig hyaline articular cartilage. *J. Anat.* **132**, 267–282

Gardner, D.L., O'Connor, P., Middleton, J.F.S., Oates, K. and Orford, C.R. (1983). An investigation by transmission electron microscopy of freeze replicas of dog articular cartilage surfaces: the fibre-rich surface structure. *J. Anat.* **137**, 573–582

Gardner, D.L., Oates, K. and Simpson, R. (1989). Interaction of hyaluronic acid with osteoarthritic cartilage surfaces: a low temperature scanning electron microscope study. *J. Pathol.* **158**, 358A

Gray, D.W.R. and Morris, P.J. (1987). The use of fluorescein diacetate and ethidium bromide as a viability stain for isolated islets of langerhans. *Stain Technol.* **62**, 373–381

Grout, B.W.W. and Morris, G.J. (1987). *The Effects of Low Temperatures on Biological Systems.* Edward Arnold, London

Gundersen, H.J.G. (1986). Stereology of arbitrary particles. A review of unbiased number and size estimators and the presentation of some new ones, in memory of William R. Thompson. *J. Microsc.* **143**, 3–45

Gundersen, H.J.C., Bendtsen, T.F., Korbo, L., Marcussen, N., Moller, A., Nielsen, K., Nyengaard, J.R., Pakkenberg, B., Sorensen, F.B., Vesterby, A. and West, M.J. (1988a). Some new simple and efficient stereological methods and their use in pathological research and diagnosis. *APMIS* **96**, 379–394

Gundersen, H.J.G., Bagger, P., Bendtsen, T.F., Evans, S.M., Korbo, L., Marcussen, N., Moller, A., Nielsen, K., Nyengaard, J.R., Pakkenberg, B., Sorensen, F.B., Vesterby, A. and West, M.J. (1988b). The new stereological tools: disector, fractionator, nucleator and point sampled intercepts and their use in pathological research and diagnosis. *APMIS* **96**, 857–881

Howard, V., Reid, S., Baddeley, A. and Boyde, A. (1985). Unbiased estimation of particle density in the tandem scanning reflected light microscope. *J. Microsc.* **138**, 203–212

Hunter, W. (1743). Of the structure and diseases of articulating cartilage. *Phil. Trans. R. Soc.* **42**, 514–521

Hunziker, E.B., Herrmann, W. and Schenk, R.K. (1983). Ruthenium hexamine trichloride (RHT)-mediated interaction between plasmalemmal components and pericellular matrix proteoglycans is responsible for the preservation of chondrocytic plasma membrane in situ during cartilage fixation. *J. Histochem. Cytochem.* **31**, 717–727

Hunziker, E.B., Herrmann, W., Schenk, R.K., Mueller, M. and Moor, H. (1983). Cartilage ultrastructure after high pressure freezing, freeze substitution, and low temperature embedding. I. Chondrocyte ultrastructure — implications for the theories of mineralization and vascular invasion. *J. Cell Biol.* **98**, 267–276

Hunziker, E.B., Schenk, R.K. and Cruz-Orive, L.M. (1987). Quantitation of chondrocyte performance in growth-plate cartilage during longitudinal bone growth. *J. Bone Joint Surg.* **69A**, 162–173

Lawton, D.M., Lamaletie, M.D.J. and Gardner, D.L. (1989). Biocompatibility of hydroxyapatite ceramic: response of chondrocytes in a test system using low temperature scanning electron microscopy. *J. Dent.* **17**, 21–27

Luft, J.H. (1971). Ruthenium red and violet: chemistry, purification, methods of use for electron microscopy and mechanism of action. *Anat. Rec.* **171**, 347–368

Maroudas, A. (1979). Physico-chemical properties of articular cartilage. In *Adult Articular Cartilage*, 2nd edn (M.A.R. Freeman, ed.), pp. 215–290. Pitman Medical, Tunbridge Wells

McConaill, M.A. (1951). The movement of bones and joints. 4: The mechanical structure of articulating cartilage. *J. Bone Joint Surg.* **33B**, 251–257

Middleton, J.F.S., Oates, K., O'Connor, P., Orford, C.R. and Gardner, D.L. (1984). Demonstration by X-ray microprobe analysis of relationship between chondrocytes and tertiary surface structure of hyaline articular cartilage. *Conn. Tissue Res.* **13**, 1–8

O'Connor, P., Oates, K., Gardner, D.L., Middleton, J.F.S., Orford, C.R. and Brereton, J.D. (1985). Low temperature and conventional scanning electron microscopic observations of dog femoral condylar cartilage surface after anterior cruciate ligament division. *Ann. Rheum. Dis.* **44**, 321–327

Orford, C.R. and Gardner, D.L. (1985). Ultrastructural histochemistry of the surface lamina of normal articular cartilage. *Histochem. J.* **17**, 223–233

Petran, M., Hadravsky, M., Egger, M.D. and Galambos, R. (1968). Tandem-scanning reflected-light microscope. *J. Opt. Soc. Am.* **58**, 661–664

Pidd, J.G. and Gardner, D.L. (1987). Surface structure of baboon (*Papio anubis*) hydrated articular cartilage: study of low temperature replicas by transmission electron microscopy. *J. Med. Primat.* **16**, 301–309

Poole, C.A., Flint, M.H. and Beaumont, B.W. (1984). Morphological and functional interrelationships of articular cartilage matrices. *J. Anat.* **138**, 113–138

Poole, C.A., Flint, M.H. and Beaumont, B.W. (1987). Chondrons in cartilage: ultrastructural analysis of the pericellular microenvironment in adult human articular cartilages. *J. Orthop. Res.* **5**, 509–522

Poole, C.A., Flint, M.H. and Beaumont, B.W. (1988a). Chondrons extracted from canine tibial cartilage: preliminary report on their isolation and structure. *J. Orthop. Res.* **6**, 408–419

Poole, C.A., Ayad, S. and Schofield, J.R. (1988b). Chondrons from articular cartilage: (1) Immunolocalization of type VI collagen in the pericellular capsule of isolated canine chondrons. *J. Cell Sci.* **90**, 635–645

Poole, C.A., Wotton, S.F. and Duance, V.C. (1988c). Localization of type IX collagen in chondrons isolated from porcine articular cartilage and rat chondrosarcoma. *Histochem. J.* **20**, 567–574

Rieder, C.L., Rupp, G. and Bowser, S.S. (1985). Electron microscopy of semi-thick sections: advantages for biomedical research. *J. Elect. Microsc. Technol.* **2**, 11–28

Robards, A.W. and Sleytr, U.B. (1985). *Low Temperature Methods in Biological Electron Microscopy.* Elsevier, Amsterdam

Stanescu, R. (1985). Effects of enzymatic digestions on the negative charge of articular cartilage surfaces. *J. Rheumatol.* **12**, 833–840

Stanescu, R. and Leibovich, J.S. (1982). The negative

charge of articular cartilage surfaces. *J. Bone Joint Surg.* **64A**, 386–392

Stanescu, R. and Stanescu, V. (1988). *In vitro* protection of the articular surface by cross-linking agents. *J. Rheumatol.* **15**, 1677–1682

Stanescu, R., Stanescu, V. and Peyron, J. (1984). Labeling of articular cartilage surface with cationized ferritin: aged human normal and osteoarthritic cartilage. *J. Orthop. Res.* **2**, 151–160

Stanescu, R., Lider, O., van Eden, W., Holvshitz, J. and Cohen, J.R. (1987a). Istopathology of arthritis induced in rats by active immunization to mycobacterial antigens or by systematic transfer of T lymphocyte lines. *Arthritis Rheum.* **30**, 779–792

Stanescu, R., Peyron, J. and Stanescu, V. (1987b). Drug action on articular cartilage surface. An *in vitro* study using mouse femoral heads labeled with cationized ferritin. *Clin. Rheumatol.* **6**, 162–169

Sterio, D.C. (1984). The unbiased estimation of number and size of arbitrary particles using the disector. *J. Microsc.* **134**, 127–136

Stockwell, R.A. (1979). *Biology of Cartilage Cells*, pp. 148–163. Cambridge University Press, Cambridge

Swann, D.A., Slayter, H.S. and Silver, F.A. (1981). The molecular structure of lubricating glycoprotein-I, the boundary lubricant for articular cartilage. *J. Biol. Chem.* **256**, 5921–5925

Szirmai, J.A. (1969). Structure of cartilage. In *Aging of Connective and Skeletal Tissue* (A. Enzel and T. Larsson, eds), pp. 163–184. Nordinska Bokhandelns, Stockholm

Tuckett, F. and Morriss-Kay, G. (1988). Alcian blue staining of glycosaminoglycans in embryonic material: effect of different fixatives. *Histochem. J.* **20**, 174–182

Weiss, C., Rosenberg, L. and Helfet, A.J. (1968). An ultrastructural study of normal young adult human articular cartilage. *J. Bone Joint Surg.* **50A**, 663–674

4

CHONDROCYTE CULTURE

COLLATED BY P.D. BENYA

22

Introduction and survey of techniques for chondrocyte culture

P.D. BENYA

INTRODUCTION

Investigation of chondrocyte metabolism is essential for identifying and manipulating the pathways of normal development and pathological degeneration of cartilage. *In vivo*, chondrocytes are part of a complex joint environment or an organized developing growth plate. In both cases, chemical signals, cytokines, growth factors and physical forces emanate from surrounding tissues and cartilage itself to influence the metabolism of chondrocytes (see Section 5). The choice of *in vitro* culture as an experimental stage is predicated on reducing this complexity by removing outside stimuli and decreasing isotope and factor dilution created by the body volume. The use of cartilage slices in organ culture meet these criteria and allow investigation when original cell–surface receptors, cell–matrix, and matrix–matrix interactions remain intact (see Section 5). However, studies that require separation of cells or clonal analysis, that investigate matrix deposition, or that are negatively influenced by extensive preexisting matrix, may be performed more appropriately with released cells.

The culture of chondrocytes that have been released from their extracellular matrix is the subject of this chapter. By careful dissection of tissue and/or choice of articular surface, cartilage slices free of extraneous cell types can be obtained (Hough and Sokoloff, 1975). This is particularly facilitated by the avascular nature of cartilage. In most cases, enzymatic digestion will yield high recovery of the contained cells in a uniform suspension suitable for replicate plating, one of the major advantages of chondrocyte cell culture. However, explant outgrowths have been used, particularly with human articular cartilage (Oegema and Thompson, 1981). The enzymes used sequentially (Green, 1971; Benya *et al.*, 1978; Kuettner *et al.*, 1982) are intended to increase cartilage permeability to subsequent enzymes by degrading proteoglycans (PGs) (hyaluronidase), to degrade noncollagenous matrix molecules and unmask collagen fibers (trypsin, pronase) and to degrade the collagenous matrix (bacterial collagenase). The other proteases (clostripain, casein-degrading, etc.) present in crude collagenase preparations appear essential to the eventual release of chondrocytes from their matrix.

Released chondrocytes are ideally suited to the study of the *de novo* synthesis and deposition of extracellular matrix. High-sensitivity techniques that have capacities for only small amounts of protein or other substances can be used because large numbers of cells with minimal matrix are studied. Such cells have usually been exposed to cell-surface proteolysis by trypsin, pronase or protease in collagenase preparations during their release (for an exception see Guo et al. (1989)). Consequently, external membrane protein domains may be altered, including hormone growth factor and matrix protein receptors. Time for chondrocytes to replace these essential components should thus be provided before initiation of experimentation (Trippel et al., 1983). With this caveat, released chondrocytes may be used for short periods for the determination of receptor number and affinity using radioligand techniques (Trippel et al., 1983, 1988) because the absence of matrix removes this source of interference (Postel-Vinay et al., 1983).

The existence of chondrocyte subpopulations in both growth plate and articular cartilage provides another justification for using released cells. Although most research to date has utilized the physical separation of cartilage zones by careful dissection prior to analysis or cell release (Schmid and Conrad, 1982; Gibson et al., 1984; Aydelotte et al., 1988a; Trippel et al., 1989), the potential exists for separation of mixed populations by attachment kinetics (Sasse et al., 1984), antibody selection (Sasse et al., 1984; Zanetti et al., 1985) or other physical (Villanueva et al., 1989; O'Keefe et al., 1989) or biochemical criteria. Aydelotte et al. (Chapter 23) have emphasized the use of culture conditions that maintain the phenotypic characteristics of such separated subpopulations. Additional separation techniques would greatly facilitate our understanding of the functional differences between these cells.

Additional advantages of released chondrocytes are that cells can be cultured at high and low cell density to test for the influence of cell–cell contacts (Solursh et al., 1982; Benya and Shaffer, 1982) and cell-derived factors (Sun et al., 1986; Bruckner et al., 1989). The absence of matrix allows evaluation of defined substances (matrix molecules and analogs) for their individual effects and to identify feedback mechanisms for synthesis and/or differentiation (Nevo and Dorfman, 1972; Handley and Lowther, 1976; Solursh et al., 1980; Kato and Gospodarowicz, 1985; Guo et al., 1989; Bruckner et al., 1989).

PHENOTYPIC STABILITY

Released chondrocytes are readily modulated away from the expression of their differentiated phenotype. This must be considered in any experimental design, since such changes may be considerably greater than those caused by a test substance and the profile of receptors and associated second-messenger systems may no longer resemble that of a differentiated chondrocyte. If the experimental intent is to study the responses of normal chondrocytes to expected physiological signals and stresses, then a culture method that can maintain at least the major elements of the differentiated phenotype would be desirable (suspension culture). However, studying the process of modulation of the phenotype and investigating the mechanisms involved there and during reexpression of the phenotype will require different culture techniques (monolayer culture). Identified mechanisms may enhance our understanding of developmental and pathological processes (von der Mark, 1986; Zanetti and Solursh, 1989); and focus our attention on pathways that may serve different, but important, functions in the *in vivo* situation.

An important determinant of the chondrocyte phenotype during both development and culture is cell shape (Benya and Shaffer, 1982; von der Mark, 1986; Zanetti and Solursh, 1989). Cells in monolayer culture that are well spread and flattened will eventually stop expressing the differentiated phenotype, especially if subcultured (Mayne et al., 1976; Benya et al., 1978). In contrast, chondrocytes in liquid or agarose suspension culture or those grown in collagen gels maintain their phenotypic characteristics (see Chapters 23 and 24). The strength of the stimulus of spherical cell shape is emphasized by the fact that chondrocytes modulated by monolayer subculture can be induced to reexpress the differentiated phenotype by release and culture in the anchorage-independent environment of agarose gels where cells are entrapped with spherical shape (Benya and Shaffer, 1982).

Based on such considerations of stability of the phenotype, chondrocyte culture methods may be divided into four categories for further disccusion: (i) monolayer culture, (ii) suspension culture, (iii) composite culture, and (iv) new approaches.

MONOLAYER CULTURE

Among the principal advantages of monolayer culture are the ease of set-up, adaptability to both small and large numbers of cells and the convenience of propagation. Small numbers of cells can be cultured and expanded by passage using conventional enzymatic techniques. This is especially important in studies of genetic abnormalities and focal lesions where samples are small. However, due consideration must be given to the time-course of modulation (Benya et al., 1978) in all monolayer studies, since this represents the major disadvantage of the technique.

Replicate plates or wells can easily be established for biosynthetic and ligand-binding studies. With regard to the latter, cellular adherence and the initial absence of matrix greatly facilitate the separation of bound and free ligands under conditions of rapid-exchange kinetcs. Diffusion beneath the basal cell surface may be considerably different than that above the free cell surface and secretion may be partially polarized. These characteristics may be responsible for the release of PG aggregates into the culture medium, allowing their isolation and study under non-dissociative conditions (Fellini et al., 1981). The same characteristics may also cause the number of observed receptors to be different than the actual number.

The nature of the chondrocyte's surface attachment in monolayer culture and the fact that it is polarized and leads to formation of attachment plaques and stress fibres (Marchisio et al., 1984; Brown and Benya, 1988) may explain this method's active and/or permissive role in modulation away from the differentiated state. For example, the cell attachment protein, fibronectin, is associated with attachment plaques and the organized cytoskeleton. Fibronectin enhances the rate of modulation in monolayer culture (Pennypacker et al., 1979; West et al., 1984) while its presence in cultures of modulated chondrocytes that are spherical in agarose gels does not prevent reexpression of differentiated functions (Benya and Shaffer, 1982). Thus, the monolayer culture environment may expose regulatory pathways that could play a role in chondrogenesis (Zanetti and Solursh 1989) and, with different results, in normal homeostatic processes.

SUSPENSION CULTURE

The functional aspect of suspension culture is that cell-to-surface attachments are prevented and the cells remain spherical. This requirement has been met in stationary culture in soft agar (Horwitz and Dorfman, 1970), over agarose (Tacchetti et al., 1987; Castagnola et al., 1988) and when cells are cultured within agarose (Benya and Shaffer, 1982; Aydelotte et al., 1988a; Bruckner et al., 1989), collagen gels (Gibson et al., 1982; Yasui et al., 1982; Solursh et al., 1982; Thomas and Grant, 1988) or in viscous solutions of methylcellulose (Horton and Hassel, 1986). An example of agarose culture is presented by Aydelotte et al. in Chapter 23. Agitated or 'spinner' suspension culture also has been successful with chondrocytes (Horwitz and Dorfman, 1970; Nevo et al., 1972; Srivastava et al., 1974; Norby et al., 1977; Pacifici and Oettinger, 1985). This technique is more suitable for larger number of cells. In most cases, cellular proliferation and extracellular matrix deposition are rapid initially and then decline substantially, presumably due to matrix feedback on these processes. When experiments require rapid-exchange kinetics, diffusion may be a problem in cultures containing gels or in cultures that favor the formation of larger proliferative colonies or aggregation of cell clusters.

Aggregates without surrounding gel also allow a surface layer of flattened cells to form, which may influence the analysis of phenotype or other metabolic properties.

The matrix deposited in suspension culture is quite similar in organization to that seen *in vivo*. The presence of a surrounding gel appears to facilitate this by slowing diffusion (Aydelotte et al., 1988a; Bruckner et al., 1989). These cultures would thus be useful for studying *de novo* matrix deposition. Without a gel, the slowly depositing matrix would eventually decrease diffusion and enhance matrix deposition. The process can be accelerated by the formation of macrocell aggregates (see Chapter 24). In this case, the large dimensions (similar to the thickness of many articular cartilages) may be useful for the study of chondrolysis and associated pharmacology.

Maintenance and reexpression of the differentiated phenotype are still the major reasons for employing suspension cultures. In the former case, a good example is the use of short-term tube or multiwell plate cultures for the evaluation of growth-factor receptors and effects (Trippel et al., 1983, 1988; Ashton and Francis, 1977). Studies comparing responses and receptor number in both short-term monolayer and suspension cultures of the same chondrocyte population would help establish whether these aspects are also influenced by shape and thus may represent transducing elements for deformation-dependent effects on cartilage metabolism. Spinner cultures may be used to propagate phenotypically normal chondrocytes for the purpose of filling cartilage defects (Itay et al., 1987) (see also Chapters 26 and 76). However, such cultures are more difficult to handle and feed than anchored cells and do not divide as rapidly. Propagation in monolayer (with associated modulation) followed by shape-dependent reexpression is an alternative approach, but it is still uncertain whether all aspects of the differentiated phenotype will be regained. These two approaches have been combined by using repetitive cycles of monolayer and agarose culture to expand human chondrosarcoma chondrocytes with a stable PG phenotype (Block et al., 1989). Finally, suspension culture provides an important control for validating signaling pathways for reexpression. As monolayer cultures are stimulated to reexpress with various factors or signaling intermediates (Benya et al., 1988), it will be necessary to demonstrate that subsequent steps are shared with reexpression induced by a change in cell shape.

COMPOSITE CULTURE

Composite cultures combine cell attachment with minimal spreading to induce the chondrocyte phenotype or enhance its maintenance. Chick limb mesenchymal cells in micromass spot cultures are induced in the center of the resultant aggregate to undergo chondrogenesis, while cells on the surface and periphery maintain a mesenchymal phenotype (Ahrens et al., 1977; Zanettii and Solursh, 1989). Golowacki et al. (1983) have used different concentrations of poly(2-hydroxyethyl methacrylate) (polyHEMA) to coat culture dishes and decrease the surface contact area of chick chondrocytes. This resulted in increased cell rounding and a parallel increase in sulfate incorporation. Although cells are readily available for release and propagation, neither method has been used for the culture of large numbers of cells. In contrast, large numbers of chondrocytes have been cultured on and in porous particles of hydroxyapatite with maintenance of the collagen phenotype for periods of 8 months (Cheung, 1985). Such cells may be expanded by enzymatic release or by mixing with fresh particles; however, cells in the interior will not be available for release from this matrix. Multilayer, high-cell-density cultures on plastic (Oakes et al., 1977; Kuettner et al., 1982; Van Kampen et al., 1985) can also be considered to be composite cultures, since proliferation and matrix deposition quickly screen the majority of cells from contact or exposure with the upper and lower surfaces. This is a simple and useful approach but may not be completely effective in stabilizing the phenotype.

NEW APPROACHES

Several new approaches for stabilizing the chondrocyte phenotype during culture have been recently reported. These techniques, as well as many of those mentioned previously, have not been fully characterized but warrant further investigation. First, another composite culture method has been described by Watt and Dudhia (1988) which utilizes a gel surface composed of collagen and agarose to provide cell attachment with maintenance of spherical shape. Sparse plating density minimizes aggregation and allows for the development of small spherical colonies after longer culture. The degree of spreading can be varied by increasing the collagen content and both small and large cultures can be prepared similarly. Cells remain exposed for ready accessibility to antibodies and extraction of synthesized macromolecules. Expansion of cell populations should be similar to conventional monolayer cultures. Although initial evaluation still demonstrated a decline in type II collagen mRNA and an increase in type I mRNA, the abundance of these messages relative to one another and the effect on collagen protein expression have not yet been determined (Watt and Dudhia, 1988).

An additional suspension culture method has been described by Guo et al. (1989) which involves encapsulation of chondrocytes in alginate spheres of controllable size. Chondrocyte suspensions are injected as droplets into calcium-containing media to harden the surface of the resultant beads. The beads are cultured readily under stationary or stirred conditions and viable chondrocytes may be released by conventional enzymatic methods after dissolution of the surface by brief exposure to citrate. Considerable proliferation and matrix deposition is obtained and long-term culture is possible. A modification in the procedure allows the formation of hollow beads with different molecules (i.e. collagen, etc.) surrounding the encapsulated chondrocytes. With the alginate gel-filled beads, the PG phenotype was maintained, perhaps due to the possibility that the negatively charged alginate may serve as a PG analog. After evaluation of other phenotypic markers, this technique may prove especially useful for large-scale expansion of phenotypically normal chondrocytes.

Chondrocyte immortalization based in viral infection or transfection with selected single or multiple oncogenes (see Chapter 25) is an approach aimed at eliminating cellular senescence and perhaps stabilizing the phenotype. Such an approach has been successful with osteoblasts; two discrete cell populations have been immortalized, one with a stable osteoblast phenotype and one with a precursor phenotype which remained responsive to environmental (developmental) cues (Heath et al., 1989). Although desirable for some applications, immortalizing chondrocytes with a stable highly expressed phenotype may not be possible with present techniques. It seems unlikely that the effect of oncogene incorporation on division capacity would be sufficient also to prevent the transduction and implementation of environmental signals that lead to culture-dependent modulation. Indeed, generation of cell lines that remain responsive to physical and hormonal signals is required for use in filling cartilage defects, basic research on matrix deposition and degradation and applied pharmacology. Although many of the techniques previously described would be enhanced by such cell lines, expression of the differentiated phenotype by these cells may require the same culture conditions as normal chondrocytes.

CONCLUSION

The choice of a chondrocyte culture system should be based on careful evaluation of expected goals, expected data interpretation and the requirements of analytical methods for each experimental design. The diversity of available methods make this a difficult choice. Since our knowledge of environmental influence on chondrocytes is still considerably incomplete, it seems premature to restrict experimentation to only a few systems. Indeed, there is a need for introduction of new culture methods and further investigation and verification of those that already exist. An important part of this process will be careful description of methods in published reports and, when possible, parallel experiments made with the same cell population in different culture environments.

ACKNOWLEDGMENTS

This research was supported by a grant from the National Institutes of Health (AM-16404) and by the Cora Kaiser Foundation of Orthopaedic Hospital.

23

Subpopulations of articular chondrocytes cultured in agarose gel

MARGARET B. AYDELOTTE, BARBARA L. SCHUMACHER
and KLAUS E. KUETTNER

Studies in monolayer culture have yielded valuable information on the metabolism of chondrocytes, but a major limitation of this method stems from the phenotypic instability of chondrocytes, especially when cultured and passaged at low density. This problem can be largely overcome by keeping the chondrocytes in suspension, under conditions in which their rounded cell-shape and normal phenotype are maintained.

ADVANTAGES AND APPLICATIONS OF AGAROSE GEL CULTURES

Of the various suspension methods which have been attempted, culture within an agarose gel (Benya and Shaffer, 1982) offers some advantages over liquid medium alone (Norby et al., 1977) or culture on the surface of agarose (Watt and Dudhia, 1989). Since agarose retards diffusion of macromolecules, newly-secreted matrix components accumulate close to the cell surface to a greater extent than in liquid media. As a result, chondrocytes in agarose assemble a compact, well-organized pericellular matrix which in many respects resembles that in the tissue (Aydelotte and Kuettner, 1988). It has also been demonstrated that culture within agarose promotes a return to the normal chondrocytic phenotype after modulation in monolayer culture (Benya and Shaffer, 1982; Aulthouse et al., 1989). Thus, this agarose method is appropriate for studying anabolism and catabolism of cartilage matrix by isolated chondrocytes using quantitative biochemical methods (Benya and Shaffer, 1982; Delbrück et al, 1986; Aydelotte et al., 1988a), light and electron microscopy and histochemistry, including immunochemical methods (Delbrück et al., 1986; Raiss et al., 1987; Aydelotte and Küettner, 1988). Chondrocytes are largely immobilized in agarose and separated from surrounding cells as in cartilage, so specific cells and their associated matrix can be examined microscopically at different stages of culture and after fixation and staining. Since fibroblasts and other anchorage-dependent cells fail to grow within agarose (Horwitz and Dorman, 1970), this method allows for selection of anchorage-independent cells from a mixed population, such as that derived from chondrosarcoma tissue (Sun et al., 1986). When cells are cultured at sufficiently low density, clones can be isolated and subcultured for further analysis (Inerot et al., 1988).

An important application of the agarose culture method is in comparative metabolic studies of subpopulations of articular chondrocytes (Aydelotte et al., 1986; Aydelotte and Kuettner, 1988; Aydelotte et al., 1988a). For this purpose, any system which promotes phenotypic modulation must be avoided in favor of a method which tends to stabilize the normal phenotype. Thus, culture in monolayer at low density may foster phenotypic changes greater than the subtle interpopulation differences under investigation. It has been demonstrated that chondrocytes isolated from different depths of articular cartilage and cultured in agarose under identical environmental conditions maintain metabolic differences and show characteristics of the tissue zones from which the cells were derived (Aydelotte and Kuettner, 1988; Aydelotte *et al.*, 1988a). For example, quantitative differences in synthesis of keratan sulfate (KS) by subpopulations of cultured chondrocytes are in-keeping with concentration differences in intact articular cartilage (Fig. 23.1) (Aydelotte *et al.*, 1989).

The agarose culture method is also valuable for examining the influence on chondrocytes and their matrix of a variety of natural modulators and potential disease-modifying agents (Aydelotte *et al.*, 1986). It is encouraging that similar results can be demonstrated in different culture systems: e.g. interleukin-1 inhibits proteoglycan (PG) synthesis and stimulates chondrocyte-mediated degradation of PGs in cultures of chondrocytes in monolayer (Benton and Tyler, 1988) and in agarose gel (Aydelotte *et al.*, 1988b), as well as in cartilage explants (Tyler, 1985a,b).

TECHNICAL POINTS

Methods for the preparation and maintenance of chondrocyte cultures in agarose gel have been described previously (Benya and Shaffer, 1982; Aydelotte and Kuettner, 1988) but a few technical details should be emphasized. It is important that culture dishes be thinly, but completely, coated with agarose gel before the cell suspension in agarose is added; any gaps or loosening of this bottom layer will allow chondrocytes to attach to the dish and form a monolayer. During seeding of dishes, the cell suspension in agarose must be kept liquid at 37°C, well mixed and handled rapidly to prevent premature gelation. The final distribution of cells within the gel can be controlled partly by altering the period between seeding and chilling of the cultures. For feeding, treating or labeling cells in agarose, it is important to allow sufficient time for diffusion between the nutrient medium and the

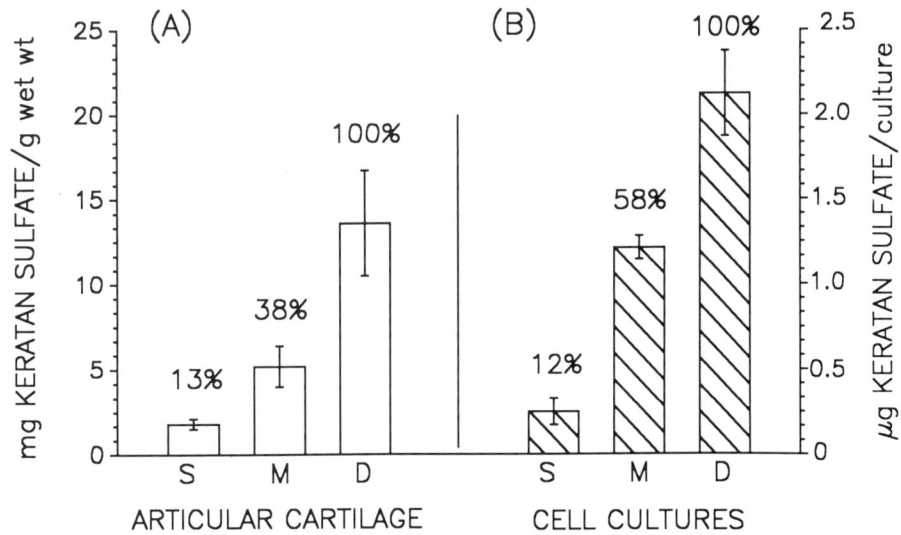

Figure 23.1 Content of KS in slices of bovine articular cartilage from different zones of the tissue according to depth (A) and also in cultures of subpopulations of chondrocytes maintained in agarose gel for 5 days (B), as determined by an ELISA-inhibition assay using the anti-KS antibody, 5-D-4, and porcine skeletal KS as the standard. Note that the content of KS in the superficial (S) zone of the tissue is only 13% of that in the deep (D) zone and that a similar difference arises when the cells are isolated and make new matrix in agarose gel culture.

gel. While subculture of cells from agarose is more difficult than from monolayer cultures, the gel can be digested with agarase and collagenase to release the chondrocytes (Schumacher and Aydelotte, unpublished observations) or the cells can be cultured in a softer agarose of ultra-low melting temperature which can be disrupted by gentle pipetting (Inerot et al., 1988). Although some biochemical studies are complicated by the necessity of separating components from the agarose, appropriate methods have been described (e.g. Benya and Shaffer, 1982; Aydelotte et al., 1988a).

COMPARISONS WITH OTHER METHODS AND LIMITATIONS OF AGAROSE GEL CULTURES

In cartilage organ cultures, normal interactions between chondrocytes and their matrix are not disturbed and a steady state of metabolism can be maintained (Handley et al., 1986). During isolation of chondrocytes for cell culture, however, some inherent artifacts arise: the digestion procedure abolishes all cell-matrix inter-relationships, removes important cell-surface molecules and disrupts the finely-regulated metabolism. In agarose, a steady state of metabolism is not regained during several weeks of culture. The freshly-isolated chondrocytes enter a phase of rapid matrix anabolism, which is nonphysiological, but which does give opportunities for studying matrix synthesis and for experimental modulation of chondrocyte metabolism. In cell culture, unlike organ culture, there is also a proliferative response of the chondrocytes which limits the comparison with conditions *in vivo*. One drawback of the organ-culture method, namely the difficulty in preparing numerous similar cultures from a nonhomogeneous tissue, is avoided for cell cultures, since many tissue slices are digested together to yield a large population of chondrocytes. Because of diffusion times and distances, the agarose method is not as suitable as monolayer cultures for kinetic experiments with very short labeling or pulse-chase times.

In summary, there are many distinct advantages, but also some limitations of the agarose method in comparison with chondrocyte culture in monolayer or organ cultures; the method of choice depends on the nature of the investigation. While more technical care and experience are necessary for the preparation of agarose than monolayer cultures, the rewards of observing the gradual accumulation of a well-structured matrix around differentiated chondrocytes grown in agarose, and the assurance that this method encourages normal phenotypic expression in chondrocytes, more than compensate for the extra effort required in the preparation and maintenance of these cultures.

ACKNOWLEDGMENTS

The authors wish to acknowledge support for this work from NIH Grant 1-P50-AR39239, and from an Arthritis Research Grant of Werk Albert, Hoechst AG, Federal Republic of Germany.

24

Three-dimensional culture model for studying human chondrocytes

C. BASSLEER, Y. HENROTIN, R. BASSLEER and P. FRANCHIMONT

INTRODUCTION

An original human chondrocyte culture model was set up (Bassleer et al., 1986). This model consists of cultivating previously dissociated human chondrocytes in three dimensions, in a liquid nutrient medium and under agitation. Under these conditions, chondrocytes form clusters, multiply and synthesize a new matrix composed of cartilage constituents. These primary cultures can be maintained for at least two months. This model is well-adapted for testing the effects of various agents on differentiated human chondrocytes.

MATERIAL AND METHODS

Chondrocyte culture

Human chondrocytes were cultivated in Dulbecco's modification of Eagle's medium (DMEM) supplemented with 10% fetal calf serum and ascorbic acid ($50\ \mu g\ ml^{-1}$). Cartilage was taken from the macroscopically normal part of human femoral heads immediately after surgery. This hyaline cartilage was cut into small fragments which were then digested by clostridial collagenase ($1\ mg\ ml^{-1}$) in carbonate–bicarbonate buffer ($CaCl_2$, 1 mM adjusted to pH 7.4) for 24 h. In this way, chondrocytes were separated from their matrix. The cellular suspension was centrifuged (1500 rpm, 5 min) and the pellet was suspended in culture medium. After six identical washings, cells were put into suspension (10^6 cells/10 ml Sovirel flask containing 2 ml of culture medium). Flasks were placed on a gyrotory shaker which was maintained at 100 rpm. The cultures were maintained at 34°C in an air atmosphere with 5% CO_2 (Bassleer et al., 1986).

Proteoglycan and type II collagen radioimmunoassays

Proteoglycan (PG) and type II collagen released into the culture medium and present inside chondrocyte clusters were assayed according to the radioimmunoassay (RIA) methods described previously (Gysen and Franchimont, 1984; Bassleer et al., 1988). Culture media were directly assayed for PG and type II collagen. Chondrocyte clusters were washed with phosphate buffered saline and homogenized by ultrasonic dissociation at 4°C (1 min, power, $200\ W\ cm^{-2}$).

Analysis of cell multiplication

After different periods of culture in the presence of the substance to be tested, chondrocyte clusters were further incubated in culture medium supplemented with the substance and [^{3}H]-methyl thymidine ($2\ \mu Ci\ ml^{-1}$, $5\ Ci\ mmol^{-1}$) during the last 24 h of the experiment. After this period of incubation, chondrocyte clusters were washed with phosphate buffered saline, incubated in a thymidine-saturated solution, washed again and ultrasonicated. Incorporated radioactivity was counted with a β counter and chondrocyte DNA content was measured according to the fluorometric method of Labarca and Paigen (1980).

RESULTS AND DISCUSSION

Human chondrocytes, after collagenase digesion, were separated and isolated from their matrix. Three-dimensional cultures allowed cells to be morphologically and biosynthetically differentiated, as demonstrated by optical, electronic and scanning microscopic observations and by histochemical and immunohistochemical methods. Cells were round in shape and situated inside a newly-synthesized matrix (Fig. 24.1) composed of type II collagen and cartilage PG (Bassleer et al., 1986, 1988).

DNA synthesis (as studied by [^{3}H]-thymidine incorporation into DNA) was more rapid at the beginning of cultivation and decreased as a function of culture duration. In general, DNA synthesis was very low in this culture model.

PG and type II collagen were assayed by specific RIA in conditioned culture medium and chondrocyte cluster extracts. While PG and type II collagen released into culture medium decreased as a function of culture duration, PG and type II collagen increased inside the clusters. This synthesis of new PG and type II collagen was accompanied by an increase in the fresh weight of the chondrocyte clusters. During the first 12 days in culture, the anabolic functions of the chondrocytes were very active; cell multiplication and synthesis of specific constituents then slowed down.

The advantages of this original human chondrocyte culture model are the following.

(i) These are primary cultures, not cell lines.
(ii) Normal or pathological human cartilage can be used.
(iii) The chondrocytes are organized spatially in three dimensions and are surrounded by the usual constituents of cartilage matrix, type II collagen and PG. These conditions are similar to those *in vivo* and different from the conditions in monolayer cultures of chondrocytes on glass or plastic.

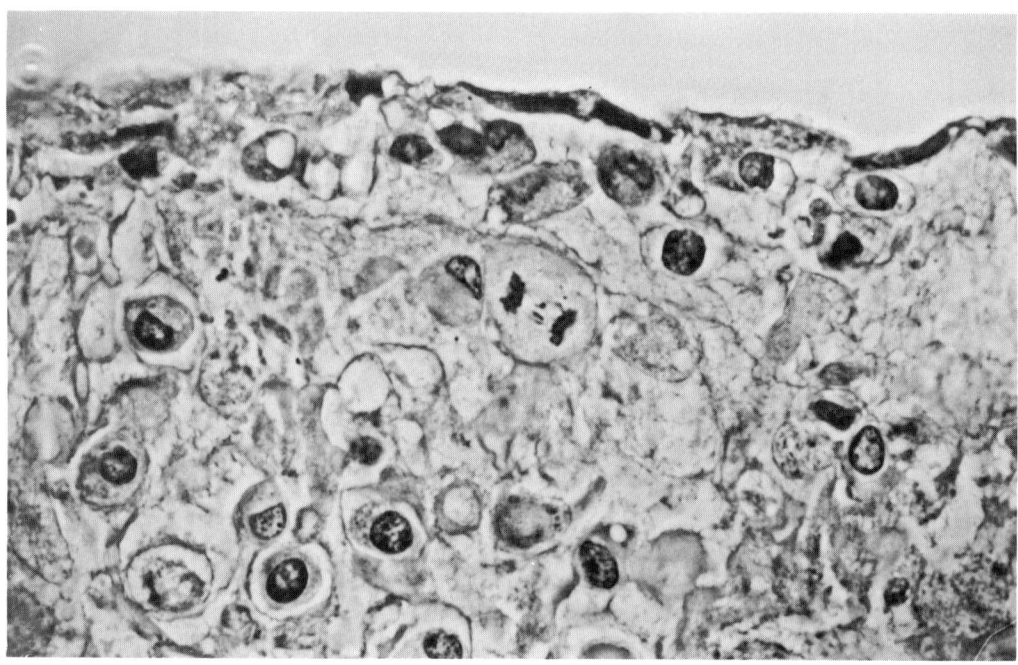

Figure 24.1 Section of a human chondrocyte cluster after 10 days in culture (×500).

(iv) The model is perfectly adapted to the analysis of the effects of various agents added to the culture medium.

The difficulties related to the use of this model are the following:

(i) human material is difficult to obtain from surgeons; and
(ii) ethical problems exist due to the use of human material.

We have used this model to test the effects of hormones, growth factors and drugs on cellular multiplication and cartilage matrix formation.

(i) Growth factors, such as EGF and IGF-1, were able to increase DNA synthesis. IGF-1 induced a dose-dependent increase in matrix component synthesis.
(ii) Calcitonin induced an increase in PG and type II collagen synthesis but had no effect on DNA synthesis (Franchimont et al., 1989).
(iii) Non-steroidal antiinflammatory drugs (NSAID), such as aspirin, decreased matrix protein synthesis by chondrocytes, while other NSAID (Tanoxicam, Naproxen, Etodolac, etc.) did not affect these anabolic parameters.
(iv) A chondroprotective agent, a peptidic–glycosaminoglycan complex (P-GAG), stimulated PG and type II collagen synthesis and increased the amount of PG inside the chondrocyte clusters.

25

Immortalization of chondrocytes in culture

SOPHIE THENET and MONIQUE ADOLPHE

INTRODUCTION

Studies using cells in culture are often hindered because of the short lifespan and/or the instability of the differentiated properties of most cell types when they are grown in culture. The generation of cell lines displaying both infinite proliferation capacity and stable phenotype would, therefore, be quite beneficial. Recombinant DNA or viruses containing oncogenes with an 'immortalizing' function have been used with various cell types to establish permanent cell lines (Evrard et al., 1986; Christian et al., 1987; Woodworth and Isom, 1987).

In the chondrocyte culture area, this approach would be particularly interesting because of the rapid modulation of the collagen phenotype that occurs following the first subculture and this results principally in the rapid decline of type II collagen synthesis and the initiation of type I, type I trimer and type III collagen synthesis (Mayne et al., 1976; Benya et al., 1978). In this regard, there are several reports of encouraging results. Gionti et al. (1985) utilized infection by the avian myelocytomatosis virus (MC29) carrying the myc oncogene to obtain immortalized quail embryo chondrocytes which still expressed type II collagen and cartilage proteoglycans (PG). More recently, the use of a recombinant retrovirus carrying the myc and raf oncogenes has permitted Horton et al. (1988) to immortalize fetal rat costal chondrocytes. These cells retained the ability to accumulate an alcian-blue-stainable matrix. However, type II collagen expression seemed to be severely reduced.

IMMORTALIZATION OF RABBIT ARTICULAR CHONDROCYTES BY SV40 EARLY GENES

Chondrocytes were obtained from articular cartilage of 1–3-month-old rabbits as described previously (Green, 1971) and plated in culture flasks in Ham's F12 medium supplemented with 10% fetal calf serum. Transfection of chondrocytes was performed on the fifth day of primary culture with the plasmid pAS containing the SV40 early function segment (expressing both large T and little t genes) without the replication origin and cloned into the EcoR1 site of pBR322 (Benoist and Chambon, 1981). This time, after initiation of culture, was chosen for transfection in order to associate as far as possible (i) cell attachment and proliferation which are required for optimum transfection efficiency using the calcium phosphate-DNA precipitation procedure (Graham and Van der Eb, 1973) and (ii) preservation of the differentiated phenotype.

SV40 DNA-transfected cells were selected by their ability to survive senscence which inevitably occurs in normal chondrocytes between passage seven and nine (Dominice et al., 1986). After nine subcultures, polygonal proliferating cells emerged from the senescent cell population and could be propagated further. After two cloning steps, clonal cell lines (Fig. 25.1(A)) were isolated and have been maintained in culture for 18 months without showing any senescence or crisis phenomenon.

Spontaneous escape from senescence by rabbit articular chondrocytes has never been reported; mock-transfected cells, which were maintained at the same time in culture, displayed no proliferation after they had reached senescence. It seems likely that SV40 early gene expression was responsible for this chondrocyte immortalization.

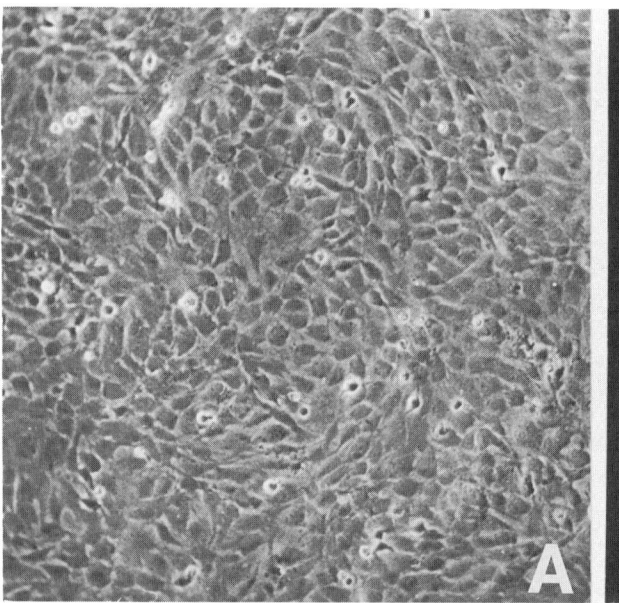 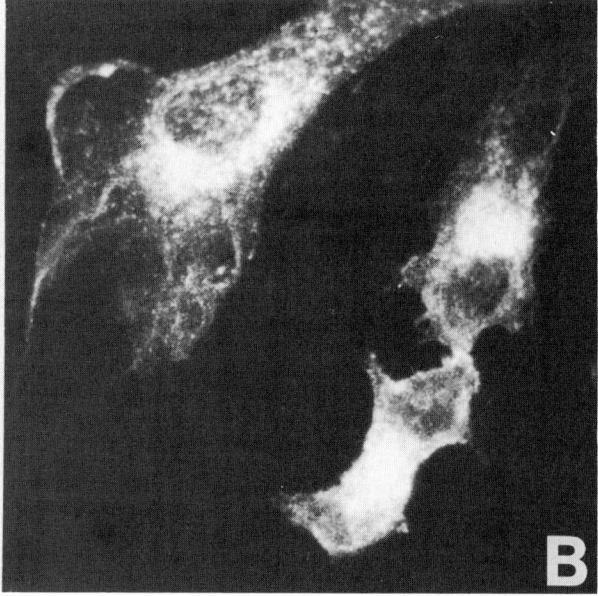

Figure 25.1 SV40 DNA-transfected chondrocytes. (a) Phase contrast photomicrograph of one clonal cell line after one year in culture (passage 80); magnification ×30. (b) Indirect immunofluorescent staining of type II collagen in one clonal cell line after 25 passages; magnification ×630.

The expression of SV40 large T-antigen was revealed by indirect immunofluorescence in all cell lines.

Growth curves of normal and SV40-transfected chondrocytes were compared and displayed similar doubling times (approximately 20 h); exponential phases were longer for the immortalized cells resulting in a two-fold higher saturation density. However, these cells retained contact inhibition properties and never developed multilayer foci. Results concerning other transformation criteria are summarized in Table 25.1. These results were sometimes difficult to interpret because normal chondrocytes share with transformed cells some unusual properties, such as growth in agar and formation of nodules when injected into nude mice. Concerning this last point, tumors provoked by immortalized chondrocytes appeared after a delay of several months and were not very aggressive; it seems, therefore, reasonable to consider that these cells are not transformed fully.

The expression of type II collagen, as assessed by immunofluorescent staining, was maintained in SV40-transfected cells (Fig. 25.1(B)), although attenuated, at least until the fortieth passage. Synthesis of alcian-blue-stainable matrix was reduced between seven and 23-fold but was still modulated by retinoic acid treatment.

Table 25.1 Summary of transformation criteria assessed for normal and SV40 DNA-transfected chondrocytes

	Normal chondrocytes	Immortalized chondrocytes
Growth in 5% or 2.5% FCS	+	++
Cloning in 5% or 2.5% FCS	−	++
Formation of multilayer foci	−	−
Colonies in agarose	+	+
Karyotype	Diploid	Hypo-tetraploid
Tumorigenicity in nude mice	±	+

In conclusion, DNA-containing SV40 early functions permitted the establishment of immortal cell lines from rabbit articular chondrocytes. Our preliminary results indicate that these cells maintained some properties of differentiated chondrocytes, but that some functions, such as PG synthesis, were disrupted.

LIMITS AND PERSPECTIVES

The main difficulty with the methods used today for immortalization is the supposed aleatory (random) focus of integration of the responsible gene into the host genome. This genomic localization is certainly very important for the properties of the resultant cell lines and its aleatory nature makes establishment of rules very difficult. For example, in contrast to the results of Horton et al. (1988), myc oncogene expression has been reported to be compatible with type II collagen synthesis in avian chondrocytes (Alema et al., 1985; Gionti et al., 1985). We may assume that this discrepancy stems from the difference in species (avian and rat), but many other reasons could explain it.

Another limitation of immortalized cells is their instability in culture. During serial subculture alterations in transformation criteria, tumorigenic properties, karyotype and differentiated properties have been reported, especially for SV40 immortalized cells (Christian et al., 1987; Neufeld et al., 1987; Woodworth and Isom, 1987).

Although immortalization of chondrocytes seems to be obtained easily by either viral infection (Gionti et al., 1985) or by using recombinant retroviruses (Horton et al., 1988), both carrying the myc oncogene, or by transfection with plasmids encoding SV40 early functions, conservation of all differentiated functions and their modulation has been imperfect. It seems that two distinct patterns of phenotypic modification were triggered in Horton's work and in ours. However, we cannot state that this difference stems from the difference between the oncogenes used.

The use of other well-known techniques could help improve these results. For example, electroporation (Shikegawa and Dower, 1988)

would be an advantageous way to transfect chondrocytes because, in contrast to the calcium phosphate procedure, this method does not require cell attachment. Therefore, chondrocytes could be transfected before being grown in culture and undergoing early modifications of their phenotype. Transgenic animals carrying an immortalizing oncogene in their germ cells (Rassoulzadegan and Cuzin, 1987) might also, in theory, permit the establishment of cell lines from differentiated chondrocytes. However, a better understanding of molecular mechanisms involved in cellular immortalization will certainly result in great improvements in this area.

Despite the actual limits, chondrocyte cell lines that remain responsive to treatments which are known to modulate the chondrocyte phenotype may be very useful tools for increasing our understanding of genetic and biochemical events involved in the process of growth, differentiation and carcinogenesis in cartilaginous tissue. Moreover, one might establish cell lines from healthy or arthritic cartilage and obtain models for pharmacological and toxicological studies. This immortalization of chondrocytes appears to be a promising approach for both fundamental research and the biotechnology and pharmacology of cartilage.

26

Culturing chondrocytes for implantation

Z. NEVO, D. ROBINSON, N. HALPERIN and S. EDELSTEIN

CELL SOURCE

Chondrocytes, the cellular elements of cartilage originate from multipotential mesenchyme cells by differentiation during embryogenesis. A typical age-related change occurring in chondrocytes early in life is a drastic reduction in the rate of cell proliferation. Therefore, it is obvious that the most common source for the isolation of actively dividing chondrocytes should be embryonic tissue.

In our screening survey of potential tissue sources of actively dividing, phenotypically stable chondrocytes, we have employed a set of three enzymatic tests. Xylosyltransferase was assayed to examine the state of differentiation and the degree of chondrogenic expression; alkaline phosphatase to evaluate the maturation of the tissue and the state of ossification; and lysozyme, to indicate the structural specificity and integrity of the cartilaginous supermolecular matrix aggregates, which are known to bind lysozyme.

A good cartilaginous tissue source is clearly one which is rich in xylosyltransferase and lysozyme, and lacks (or has a minimal content of) alkaline phosphatase. The data in Table 26.1 show that, according to our criteria, embryonic epiphyseal cartilage is the best tissue source amongst those we have tested for establishing chondrocyte cultures for implantation.

GROWTH CONDITIONS

The growth conditions for chondrocytes in cultures maintaining their phenotypic expression are

Table 26.1 Enzymatic assays of cartilaginous tissues* from four-week-old chicks compared with a reference sample of tibial and femoral epiphyses of 11-day-old chick embryos

Dietary regimen and tissue source	Xylosyltransferase (cpm ± SD/ 100 µg protein)	Alkaline phosphatase (IU ± SD/ 100 µg protein)	Lysozyme (units ± SD/ 100 µg protein)
Reference sample	13 143 ± 744	ND	350 ± 3.5
Normal epiphyses	1898 ± 82	40 ± 1.5	115 ± 1.2
Normal callus	2706 ± 161	97 ± 2.0	4 ± 0.1
Vitamin D deficient epiphyses	669 ± 39	327 ± 7.0	12 ± 0.4
Vitamin D deficient callus	3758 ± 341	79 ± 2.0	7 ± 0.1
Calcium free epiphyses	ND	53 ± 3.0	19 ± 0.6
Calcium free callus	ND	100 ± 1.0	2 ± 0.1

* The tissues were obtained from young chickens grown under three different dietary regimens: (a) a normal diet; (b) a vitamin D deficient diet since hatching, and (c) a calcium-free diet during the last (fourth) week post-hatching. Specimens of callus came from 5-day-old external callus of long bone fractures, composed largely of irritated periosteum. Xylosyltransferase was measured by following the incorporation of ^{14}C-xylose into silk peptides which replace the naturally occurring substrate, the core protein, in the assay described by Campbell et al. (1984). Alkaline phosphatase was detected spectrophotometrically by releasing p-nitrophenol from p-nitrophenylphosphate. Lysozyme was measured spectrophotometrically by the reduction of turbidity of a suspension of *Micrococcus lysodeikticus*.

One international unit (IU) of alkaline phosphatase is defined as the amount of enzyme cleaving 1 µM of p-nitrophenylphosphate per minute at the standard assay procedure. One unit of lysozyme is defined as a decrease in 0.001 units of optical density, at 450 nm, at pH 7.0 and 25°C during 3.5 h of incubation.

ND, not detected.

extensively described in Chapter 22. In addition to monolayers of initially high cell density and growth on or in hydrated gels, one should mention the growth of chondrocytes in spinner bottles (Bryan, 1968; Horwitz and Dorfman, 1970; Nevo et al., 1972; Srivastava et al., 1974; Benya and Shaffer, 1982; Pacifici and Oettinger, 1985).

The advantages of spinner growth conditions are as follows: large yields of cells are obtained; single cells and cells in small aggregates in the suspension maintain a thick differentiated matrix coat, and can be easily harvested by low-velocity centrifugation.

The nutrient medium commonly used for maintenance and growth of chondrocytes is Ham's F-12, or, less frequently, Eagle's medium, both supplemented with glutamine, antibiotics and 10% fetal calf serum. The cultures are routinely incubated at 37°C under an atmosphere enriched in CO_2 (5–10%) in air. However, old and new reports suggest that it may be advantageous to maintain chondrocytes under reduced oxygen tension (Pawelek, 1969; Nevo et al., 1972, 1988). Under conditions such as 8% O_2, 5% CO_2 in nitrogen, survival periods as actively dividing chondrocytes are lengthened and the pace of ageing is slowed down (Miller and Gay, 1979; Nevo et al., 1988).

DELIVERY SUBSTANCE

The pellets of chondrocytes harvested from the cultures to be used as cartilage-repair implants should be embedded to the desired cell concentration in a delivery substance(s). An ideal delivery substance should have several unique properties for supporting the cells and maintaining the microenvironment during storage and shipment outside the incubator at varying temperatures and in air. The viscosity of the substance should allow an even distribution of cells and the possibility of introduction through narrow-gauge arthroscopic cannulae. However, the substance should be viscous and adhesive enough to secure fixation of the cells to the implantation site. Needless to say, the substance must be biocompatible and biodegradable and offer a permissive milieu for cell proliferation and matrix production. The material must be malleable so that it can fit deep defects as well as shallow lesions of variable shape such as areas of eburnated bone in osteoarthrosis. Optimally the substance should inhibit fibroblast proliferation and prevent invasion of immune cells as well as diffusion of immunoglubulins. However, the substance must be permeable to nutrients from the synovial fluid.

Two kinds of composition were studied: (i) a fibrin based substance, and (ii), a hyaluronan (HA) based substance. The use of the fibrin based delivery substance did match several of the above-mentioned requirements, allowing the repair of defects in articular cartilage of adult chicks (Itay et al., 1987). However, the fibrin based milieu suffered from certain drawbacks. Difficulties occurred in sterilizing the fibrinogen and the resulting mixture of substances was cytotoxic to the chondrocytes; the majority of the cells lysed when cultured in it, although upon *in vivo* implantation the surviving cells did manage to proliferate. Difficulties arose in achieving an even distribution of the cells in the semisolidified mixture. Acellular islands were frequently formed. The use of a mixture containing such acellular regions for implantation clearly puts the repair process at risk. Furthermore, the viscosity of the fibrin based delivery substance is very high and could not be manipulated. This sometimes led to dislodgement of the implant as a whole. Fibrinogen is also a well-known promoter of vascular invasion and fibroblast proliferation.

The material of choice, currently under investigation in our laboratory as a delivery substance, is HA (Robinson et al., 1989, 1990). Only the high-molecular-weight (i.e. over 2 000 000 daltons) HA was found suitable. A 2% HA gel was found optimal and permissive for the growth and storage of chondrocytes *in vitro* as well as for supporting a spurt of proliferation for *in vivo* implants. HA is not antigenic. The high-molecular-weight variety stimulates chondrogenesis *in vitro* (Kujawa and Caplan, 1986; Knudson and Toole, 1987) reduces scar formation and vascular invasion (Weiss et al., 1989; Matsubara et al., 1989). This material also protects the cells both mechanically and biochemically, by reducing free-radicals which damage chondrocytes (Larsen et al., 1989). The viscosity of the chondrocyte–HA mixture can be manipulated and controlled. Sterility of HA is readily achieved. The cells thrive in the HA gel and rapidly divide while maintaining their phenotype and synthesizing new matrix. The material undergoes degradation and resorption *in vivo* within 2 weeks.

References

Ahrens, P.B., Solursh, M. and Reiter, R.S. (1977). Stage-related capacity for limb chondrogenesis in cell culture. *Dev. Biol.* **60**, 69–82

Alema, S., Tato, F. and Boettiger, D. (1985). Myc and src oncogenes have complementary effects on cell proliferation and expression of specific extracellular matrix components in definitive chondroblasts. *Mol. Cell. Biol.* **5**, 538–544

Ashton, I.K. and Francis, M.J.O. (1977). An assay for plasma somatomedin: [3H]thymidine incorporation by isolated rabbit chondrocytes. *J. Endocrinol.* **74**, 205–212

Aulthouse, A.M., Beck, M., Griffey, E., Sanford, J., Arden, K., Machado, M.A. and Horton, W.A. (1989). Expression of the human chondrocyte phenotype *in vitro*. *In Vitro Dev. Biol.* **25**, 659–668

Aydelotte, M.B. and Kuettner, K.E. (1988). Differences between sub-populations of cultured bovine articular chondrocytes. I. Morphology and cartilage matrix production. *Connect. Tiss. Res.* **18**, 205–222

Aydelotte, M.B., Schleyerbach, R., Zeck, B.J. and Kuettner, K.E. (1986). Articular chondrocytes cultured in agarose gel for study of chondrocytic chondrolysis. In *Articular Cartilage Biochemistry* (K.E. Kuettner, R. Schleyerbach and V.C. Hascall, eds), pp. 235–256. Raven Press, New York

Aydelotte, M.B., Raiss, R.X., Schleyerbach, R. and Kuettner, K.E. (1988a). Effects of interleukin-1 on metabolism of proteoglycans by cultured bovine articular chondrocytes. *Orthop. Trans.* **12**, 359

Aydelotte, M.B., Greenhill, R.R. and Kuettner, K.E. (1988b). Differences between sub-populations of cultured bovine articular chondrocytes. II. Proteoglycan metabolism. *Connect. Tiss. Res.* **18**, 223–234

Aydelotte, M.B., Thonar, E.J.-M.A., Lenz, R.E., Schumacher, B.L. and Kuettner, K.E. (1989). Differences in synthesis of keratan sulfate by sub-populations of cultured bovine articular chondrocytes. *Trans. Orthop. Res. Soc.* **14**, 83

Bassleer, C., Gysen, Ph., Foidart, J.M., Bassleer, R. and Franchimont, P. (1986). Human chondrocytes in tridimensional cultures. *In Vitro* **22**, 113–119

Bassleer, C., Gysen, Ph., Bassleer, R. and Franchimont, P. (1988). Effects of peptidic glycosaminoglycan complex on human chondrocytes cultivated in three dimensions. *Biochem. Pharmacol.* **37**, 1939–1945

Benoist, C. and Chambon, P. (1981). In vivo sequence requirements of the SV40 early promoter region. *Nature (London)* **290**, 304–310

Benton, H.P. and Tyler, J.A. (1988). Inhibition of cartilage proteoglycan synthesis by interleukin-1. *Biochem. Biophys. Res. Commun.* **154**, 421–428

Benya, P.D. and Shaffer, J.D. (1982). Dedifferentiated chondrocytes reexpress the differentiated collagen phenotype when cultured in agarose gels. *Cell* **30**, 215–224

Benya, P.D., Padilla, S. and Nimni, M.E. (1978). Independent regulation of collagen types of chondrocytes during the loss of differentiated function in culture. *Cell* **15**, 1313–1321

Benya, P.D., Brown, P.D. and Padilla, S.R. (1988). Microfilament modification by dihydrocytochalasin B causes retinoic acid-modulated chondrocytes to reexpress the differentiated collagen phenotype without a change in shape. *J. Cell Biol.* **106**, 161–170

Block, J.A., Inerot, S.E., Gitelis, S. and Kimura, J.H. (1989). Cloning and long term culture of human chondrosarcomas which produce keratan sulfate. *Orthop. Trans.* **13**, 272–273

Brown, P.D. and Benya, P.D. (1988). Alterations in chondrocyte cytoskeletal architecture during phenotypic modulation by retinoic acid and dihydrocytochalasin B—induced reexpression. *J. Cell Biol.* **106**, 171–179

Bruckner, P., Horler, I., Mendler, M., Houze, Y., Winterhalter, K.H., Eich-Bender, S.G. and Spycher, M.A. (1989). Induction and prevention of chondrocyte hypertrophy in culture. *J. Cell Biol.* **109**, 2537–2545

Bryan, J. (1968). Studies on clonal cartilage strains. I. Effect of contaminant non-cartilage cells. II. Selective effects of different growth conditions. *Exp. Cell Res.* **52**, 319–326

Campbell, P., Jacobsson, I., Benzing-Purdiel, L., Roden, L. and Fessler, J.H. (1984). Silk—a new substrate for UDP-D-xylose:Proteoglycan core protein beta-D-xylosyltransferase. *Anal. Biochem.* **137**, 505–516

Castagnola, P., Dozin, B., Moro, G. and Cancedda, R. (1988). Changes in the expression of collagen genes show two stages in chondrocyte differentiation *in vitro*. *J. Cell Biol.* **106**, 461–467

Cheung, H.S. (1985). *In vitro* cartilage formation in porous hydroxyapatite ceramic granules. *In Vitro* **21**, 353–357

Christian, B.J., Loretz, L.J., Oberley, T.D. and Reznikoff, C.A. (1987). Characterization of human uroepithelial cells immortalized *in vitro* by Simian Virus 40. *Cancer Res.* **47**, 6066–6074

Delbruck, A., Dresow, B., Gurr, E., Reale, E. and Schroder, H. (1986). *In vitro* culture of human chondrocytes from adult subjects. *Connect. Tiss. Res.* **15**, 155–172

Dominice, J., Levasseur, C., Larno, S., Ronot, X. and Adolphe, M. (1986). Age-related changes in rabbit articular chondrocytes. *Mech. Ageing Dev.* **37**, 231–240

Evrard, C., Galiana, E. and Rouget, P. (1986). Establishment of 'normal' nervous cell lines after transfer of polyoma virus and adenovirus early genes into murine brain cells. *EMBO J.* **5**, 3157–3162

Fellini, S.A., Kimura, J.H. and Hascall, V.C. (1981). Polydispersity of proteoglycans synthesized by chondrocytes from the Swarm rat chondrosarcoma. *J. Biol. Chem.* **256**, 7883–7889

Franchimont, P., Bassleer, C., Henroitin, Y. and Bassleer, R. (1989). Effects of human and salmon calcitonin on differentiated human chondrocytes cultivated in clusters. *J. Clin. Endocrinol. Metab.* **69**, 259–266

Gibson, G.J., Schor, S.L. and Grant, M.E. (1982). Effects of matrix macromolecules on chondrocyte gene expression: synthesis of a low molecular weight collagen species by cells cultured within collagen gels. *J. Cell Biol.* **93**, 767–774

Gibson, G.J., Beaumont, B.W. and Flint, M.H. (1984). Synthesis of a low molecular weight collagen by chondrocytes from the presumptive calcification region of the embryonic chick sterna: the influence of culture with collagen gels. *J. Cell Biol.* **99**, 208–216

Gionti, E., Pontarelli, G. and Cancedda, R. (1985). Avian myelocytomatosis virus immortalizes differentiated quail chondrocytes. *Proc. Natl. Acad. Sci. USA* **82**, 2756–2760

Glowacki, J., Trepman, E. and Folkman, J. (1983). Cell shape and phenotypic expression in chondrocytes. *Proc. Soc. Exp. Biol. Med.* **172**, 93–98

Graham, F.L. and Van der Eb, A.J. (1973). A new technique for the assay of infectivity of human adenovirus 5 DNA. *Virology* **52**, 456–467

Green, W.T. (1971). Behaviour of articular chondrocytes in cell culture. *Clin. Orthop. Relat. Res.* **75**, 248–260

Guo, J., Jourdian, G.W. and MacCallum, D.K. (1989). Culture and growth characteristics of chondrocytes encapsulated in alginate beads. *Connect. Tiss. Res.* **19**, 277–297

Gysen, Ph. and Franchimont, P. (1984). Radioimmunoassay of proteoglycans. *J. Immunoassay* **5**, 221–243

Handley, C.J. and Lowther, D.A. (1976). Inhibition of proteoglycan biosynthesis by hyaluronic acid in chondrocytes in cell culture. *Biochim. Biophys. Acta* **444**, 69–74

Handley, C.J., McQuillan, D.J., Campbell, M.A. and Bolis, S. (1986). Steady-state metabolism in cartilage explants. In *Articular Cartilage Biochemistry* (K.E. Kuettner, R., Schleyerbach and V.C. Hascall, eds), pp. 163–179. Raven Press, New York

Heath, J.K., Rodan, S.B., Yoon, K. and Rodan, G.A. (1989). Rat calvarial cell lines immortalized with SV-40 large T antigen: constitutive and retinoic acid-inducible expression of osteoblastic features. *Endocrinology* **124**, 3060–3068

Horton, W. and Hassel, J.R. (1986). Independence of cell shape and loss of cartilage matrix production during retinoic acid treatment of cultured chondrocytes. *Dev. Biol.* **115**, 392–397

Horton, W.E., Cleveland, J., Rapp, U., Nemuth, G., Bolander, M., Doege, K., Yamada, Y. and Massel, J.R. (1988). An established rat cell line expressing chondrocyte properties. *Exp. Cell Res.* **178**, 457–468

Horwitz, A.L. and Dorfman, A. (1970). The growth of cartilage cells in soft agar and liquid suspension. *J. Cell Biol.* **45**, 434–438.

Hough, A.J. and Sokoloff, L. (1975). Tissue sampling as a potential source of error in experimental studies of cartilage. *Connect. Tiss. Res.* **3**, 27–31

Inerot, S.E., Block, J.A., Kuettner, K.E., Kimura, J.H. and Gitelis, S. (1988). Cell cloning of human chondrosarcoma. *Trans. Orthop. Res. Soc.,* **13**, 451

Itay, S., Abramovici, A. and Nevo, Z. (1987). Use of cultured embryonal chick epiphyseal chondrocytes as grafts for defects in chick articular cartilage. *Clin. Orthop. Relat. Res.* **220**, 284–303

Kato, Y. and Gospodarowicz, D. (1985). Effect of exogenous extracellular matrices on proteoglycan synthesis by cultured rabbit costal chondrocytes. *J. Cell Biol.* **100**, 486–495

Knudson, B.B. and Toole, B.P. (1987). Hyaluronate-cell interactions during differentiation of chick embryo limb mesoderm. *Dev. Biol.* **124**, 82–90

Kuettner, K.E., Memoli, V.A., Pauli, B.U., Wrobel, N.C., Thonar, E.J.-M. and Daniel, J.C. (1982). Synthesis of cartilage matrix by mammalian chondrocytes *in vitro*. II: Maintenance of collagen and proteoglycan phenotype. *J. Cell Biol.* **93**, 751–757

Kujawa, M.J. and Caplan, A.T. (1986). Hyaluronic acid bonded to cell-culture surfaces stimulates chondrogenesis in stage 24 limb mesenchyme cell cultures. *Dev. Biol.* **114**, 504–518

Labarca, C. and Paigen, K. (1980). A simple rapid and sensitive DNA assay procedure. *Anal. Biochem.* **102**, 344–352

Larsen, N.E., Lombard, K.M. and Balasz, E.A. (1989). The effect of hyaluronan on cartilage and chondrocyte response to mechanical and biochemical perturbation. *Trans. Ortho. Res. Soc.* **14**, 151

Marchisio, P.C., Capasso, O., Nitsch, L., Cancedda, R. and Gionti, E. (1984). Cytoskeleton and adhesion patterns of cultured chick embryo chondrocytes during cell spreading and Rous Sarcoma virus transformation. *Exp. Cell Res.* **151**, 332–343

Matsubara, T., Hirata, S., Saegusa, Y. and Hirohata, K. (1989). Inhibition of vascular endothelial cell proliferation by hyaluronic acid but not by proteoglycans. *Trans. Ortho. Res. Soc.* **14**, 424

Mayne, R., Vail, M.S., Mayne, P.M. and Miller, E.J. (1976). Changes in the type of collagen synthesized as clones of chick chondrocytes grow and eventually lose division capacity. *Proc. Natl. Acad. Sci. USA* **73**, 1674–1678

Miller, E.J. and Gay, S. (1979). Chondrocytes in aging research. *Int. Rev. Cytol. Suppl.* **10**, 93–101

Neufeld, D.S., Ripley, S., Henderson, A. and Ozer, H.L. (1987). Immortalization of human fibroblasts transformed by origin defective simian virus 40. *Mol. Cell. Biol.* **7**, 2794–2802

Nevo, Z. and Dorman, A. (1972). Stimulation of chondromucoproptein synthesis in chondrocytes by extracellular chondromucoprotein. *Proc. Natl. Acad. Sci. USA* **69**, 2069–2072

Nevo, Z., Horwitz, A.L. and Dorfman, A. (1972). Synthesis of chondromucoprotein by chondrocytes in suspension culture. *Dev. Biol.* **28**, 219–228

Nevo,. Z., Beit-Or, A. and Eilam, Y. (1988). Slowing down aging of cultured embryonal chick chondrocytes by maintenance under lowered oxygen tension. *Mech. Ageing Develop.* **45**, 157–165

Norby, D.P., Malemud, C.G. and Sokoloff, L. (1977). Differences in the collagen types synthesized by lapine articular chondrocytes in spinner and monolayer culture. *Arthr. Rheum.* **20**, 709–716

Oakes, B.W., Handley, C.J., Lisner, F. and Lowther, D.A. (1977). An ultrastructural and biochemical study of high density primary cultures of embryonic chick chondrocytes. *J. Embryol. Exp. Morphol.* **38**, 239–263

Oegema, T.R. and Thompson, R.C. (1981). Characterization of a hyaluronic acid–dermatan sulfate proteoglycan complex from dedifferentiated human chondrocyte cultures. *J. Biol. Chem.* **256**, 1015–1022

O'Keefe, R.J., Crabb, I.D., Puzas, J.E. and Rosier, R.N. (1989). Countercurrent centrifugal elutriation. High-resolution method for the separation of growth-plate chondrocytes. *J. Bone Joint Surg.* **(Am) 71-A**, 607–620

Pacifici, M. and Oettinger, H.F. (1985). Stable phenotypic expression by chick chondroblasts in long-term suspension cultures as determined by proteoglycan analysis. *Exp. Cell Res.* **161**, 381–392

Pawelek, J.M. (1969). Effect of thyroxine and low oxygen tension on chondrogenic expression in cell culture. *Dev. Biol.* **19**, 52–72

Pennypacker, J.P., Hassell, J.R., Yamada, K.M. and Pratt, R.M. (1979). The influence of an adhesive cell surface protein on chondrogenic expression *in vitro*. *Exp. Cell Res.* **121**, 411–415

Postel-Vinay, M.C., Corvol, M.T., Lang, F., Fraud, F., Guyda, H. and Posner, B. (1983). Receptors for insulin-like growth factors in rabbit articular and growth plate chondrocytes in culture. *Exp. Cell Res.* **148**, 105–116

Raiss, R.X., Aydelotte, M.B., Caterson, B. and Kuettner, K.E. (1987). Immunohistochemical analysis of the extracellular matrix produced by articular chondrocytes grown in agarose with retinol and interleukin-1. *Orthop. Trans.* **11**, 392–393

Rassoulzadegan, M. and Cuzin, F. (1987). Sub-threshold neoplastic states: created in transgenic mice. *Oncogene Res.* **1**, 1–6

Robinson, D., Halperin, N. and Nevo, Z. (1989). The influence of the host's age on the fate of implants of embryonal chondrocytes into articular surfaces. *Mech. Ageing Develop.* **50**, 71–80

Robinson, D., Halperin, N. and Nevo, Z. (1990). Regenerating hyaline cartilage in articular defects of old chickens using implants of embryonal chick chondrocytes embedded in a new natural delivery substance. *Calcif. Tiss. Int.* **46**, 246–253

Sasse, J., Horwitz, A., Pacifici, M. and Holtzer, H. (1984). Separation of precursor myogenic and chondrogenic cells in early limb bud mesenchyme by a monoclonal antibody. *J. Cell Biol.* **99**, 1856–1866

Schmid, T.M. and Conrad, H.E. (1982). Metabolism of low molecular weight collagen by chondrocytes obtained from histologically distinct zones of the chick embryo tibiotarsus. *J. Biol. Chem.* **257**, 12451–12457

Shikegawa, K. and Dower, W.J. (1988). Electroporation of eukaryotes and prokaryotes: a general approach to the introduction of macromolecules into cells. *Biotechniques* **6**, 742–752

Solursh, M., Hardingham, T.E., Hascall, V.C. and Kimura, J.H. (1980). Separate effects of exogenous hyaluronic acid on proteoglycan synthesis and deposition in pericellular matrix by cultured chick embryo limb chondrocytes. *Dev. Biol.* **75**, 121–129

Solursh, M., Linsenmayer, T.F. and Jensen, K.L. (1982). Chondrogenesis from single limb mesenchyme cells. *Dev. Biol.* **94**, 259–264

Srivastava, V.M.L., Malemud, C.J. and Sokoloff, L. (1974). Chondroid expression by lapine articular chondrocytes in spinner culture following monolayer growth. *Connect. Tiss. Res.* **2**, 127–136

Sun, D., Aydelotte, M.B., Maldonado, B., Kuettner, K.E. and Kimura, J.H. (1986). Clonal analysis of the population of chondrocytes from the Swarm rat chondrosarcoma in agarose culture. *J. Orthop. Res.* **4**, 427–436

Tacchetti, C., Quarto, R., Nitsch, L., Hartmann, D.J. and Cancedda, R. (1987). *In vitro* morphogenesis of chick embryo hypertrophic cartilage. *J. Cell Biol.* **105**, 999–1006

Thomas, J.T. and Grant, M.E. (1988). Cartilage proteoglycan aggregate and fibronectin can modulate the expression of type X collagen by embryonic chick chondrocytes cultured in collagen gels. *Biosci. Rep.* **8**, 163–171

Trippel, S.B., Van Wyk, J.J., Foster, M.B. and Svoboda, M.E. (1983). Characterization of a specific somatomedin-C receptor on isolated bovine growth plate chondrocytes. *Endocrinology* **112**, 2128–2136

Trippel, S.B., Chernausek, S.D., Van Wyk, J.J., Moses, A.C. and Mankin, H.J. (1988). Demonstration of type I and type II somatomedin receptors on bovine growth plate chondrocytes. *J. Orthop. Res.* **6**, 817–826

Trippel, S.B., Corvol, M.T., Dumontier, M.F., Rappaport, R., Hung, H.H. and Mankin, H.J. (1989). Effect of somatomedin-c/insulin-like growth factor I and growth hormone on cultured growth plate and articular chondrocytes. *Pediatr. Res.* **25**, 76–82

Tyler, J.A. (1985). Chondrocyte-mediated depletion of articular cartilage proteoglycans *in vitro*. *Biochem. J.* **225**, 493–507

Tyler, J.A. (1985b). Articular cartilage cultured with catabolin (pig interleukin 1) synthesizes a decreased number of normal proteoglycan molecules. *Biochem. J.* **227**, 869–878

Van Kampen, G.P., Veldhuijzen, J.P., Kuijer, R., Van de Stadt, R.J. and Schipper, C.A. (1985). Cartilage response to mechanical force in high density chondrocyte cultures. *Arthr. Rheum.* **28**, 419–424

Villanueva, J.E., Nishimoto, S.K. and Nimni, M.E. (1989). Cells isolated from fetal rat calvaria by isopycnic separation express different collagen phenotypes. *Matrix* **9**, 40–48

von der Mark, K. (1986). Differentiation, modulation and dedifferentiation of chondrocytes. *Rheumatology* **10**, 272–315

Watt, F.M. and Dudhia, J. (1988). Prolonged expression of differentiated phenotype by chondrocytes cultured at low density on a composite substrate of collagen and agarose that restricts cell spreading. *Differentiation* **38**, 140–147

Weiss, C., Dennis, J., Suros, J.M., Delinger, J., Badia, A. and Gross, J. (1989). Sodium hylan for the prevention of post laminectomy scar formation. *Trans. Ortho. Res. Soc.* **14**, 44

West, C.M., De Weerd, H., Dowdy, K. and De La Paz, A. (1984). A specificity for cellular fibronectin in its effect on cultured chondroblasts. *Differentiation* **27**, 67–73

Woodworth, C.P. and Isom, H.C. (1987). Regulation of albumin gene expression in a series of rat hepatocyte cell lines immortalized by simian virus 40 and maintained in chemically defined medium. *Mol. Cell. Biol.* **7**, 3740–3748

Yasui, N., Ohsawa, S., Ochi, T., Nakashima, H. and Ono, K. (1982). Primary culture of chondrocytes embedded in collagen gels. *Exp. Cell Biol.* **50**, 92–100

Zanetti, N.C. and Solursh, M. (1989). Effect of cell shape on cartilage differentiation. In *Cell Shape: Determinants, Regulation, and Regulatory Role* (W.D. Stein and F. Bonner, eds), pp. 291–327. Academic Press, New York

Zanetti, M., Ratcliffe, A. and Watt, F.M. (1985). Two subpopulations of differentiated chondrocytes identified with a monoclonal antibody to keratan sulfate. *J. Cell Biol.* **101**, 53–59

Zuzuki, F. (1984). Local factors which regulate bone and cartilage growth. In "Endocrine Control of Bone and Calcium Metabolism" (eds D.V. Cohn, T. Fugita, J.T. Potts, and R.V. Talmage), pp. 78–85. Elsevier Science Publishers, B.V.

5

SHORT- AND LONG-TERM EXPLANT CULTURE OF CARTILAGE

COLLATED BY C.J. HANDLEY

27

Introduction

CHRISTOPHER J. HANDLEY, CHEE KENG NG and ANDREA J. CURTIS

Specialized resident cells (chondrocytes) from cartilage are responsible for the metabolism and maintenance of the extracellular matrix from which the tissue derives its unique mechanical properties. Chondrocytes exist *in vivo* under conditions of limiting oxygen tensions and metabolite concentrations as the result of the avascularity of cartilage. In such an environment, the nutritional and oxygen requirements of these cells are facilitated by diffusion through the extracellular matrix and further supplemented by mechanical loading and unloading of the cartilage. Energy for cellular activities is gained from substrate-level phosphorylation accompanying the conversion of glucose to lactate (Marcus, 1973). A similar manner of energy derivation also occurs in chondrocytes from tissue cultured *in vitro* under increased oxygen tensions.

Tissue culture of cartilage has a number of advantages over cell culture of isolated chondrocytes. The chondrocytes in cartilage in explant cultures maintain their differentiated state, the mitotic activity of the chondrocytes is low, the cells have not been exposed to exogenous proteolytic activity and the extracellular matrix is similar to that observed *in vivo*. However, the presence of a resilient extracellular matrix can be a disadvantage; for example, in cell receptor studies.

The purposes of this chapter are to review the current approaches used for the short- and long-term explant culture of cartilage and to introduce a series of papers dealing with specific aspects of cartilage in explant culture. These articles cover the areas of the maintenance of steady-state metabolism by articular cartilage *in vitro*, the variation in [^{35}S]sulfate incorporation into proteoglycans (PGs) by different zones of human articular cartilage in explant culture and the explant culture of intervertebral disc cartilage.

SHORT-TERM EXPLANT CULTURE OF CARTILAGE

Short-term explant culture of cartilage consists of incubating the tissue *in vitro* for periods of up to 6 h. This approach has been used by many workers mainly to incubate cartilage with radiolabeled precursors. Short-term culture can be used with cartilage immediately after it has been dissected from an animal or in conjunction with long-term explant culture where incubation of cartilage under constant, similar or optimal conditions is required.

Media used for short-term explant culture of cartilage can be simple, easily modified whenever the specific activity of metabolic precursors is required to be increased and does not require supplementation with serum or exogenous growth factors. Common media used are Dulbecco's modified Eagles medium and Ham's F-10 medium. Buffering of the medium is best achieved using CO_2/bicarbonate or organic buffers. The composition of these media can be changed so as to reduce the concentration of particular metabolites in order to optimize the specific radioactivity of the precursor used. An example of this is sulfate which is present at approximately 0.8 mM in Dulbecco's modified Eagle's medium; this value will be higher if the antibiotic streptomycin sulfate is used. If maximum incorporation of isotope is required, sulfate free medium should be considered. However, it has been shown for articular cartilage that the optimum concentration of sulfate in medium for maximal PG synthesis is approximately 0.5 mM (Robinson, 1969). Concentrations below this will result in either a lower rate of PG synthesis and/or the synthesis of under-sulfated PGs since the concentration of sulfate present in the medium will be limiting (Maroudas and Evans, 1974; Sobue et al., 1978). For experiments measuring the comparative rates of metabolism of cartilage, it is particularly important that sufficient chemical levels of the precursor are present to ascertain an unlimited supply of the radiolabeled precursor over the incubation time period.

Since the time periods used in short-term explant culture of cartilage are not more than 6 h, there is usually no need to supplement the medium with serum or exogenous factors. However, it is necessary to show experimentally that the rate of metabolism of the tissue is constant with time over the incubation period. In the case of PG synthesis by articular cartilage, it is necessary to demonstrate that the rate of incorporation of a labeled precursor, such as [^{35}S]sulfate, is constant with time over the incubation period. If the rate of synthesis decreases with time, this indicates that there is probably a decrease in the cellular pool of mRNA coding for the PG core protein which reflects changes in the rate of translation resulting from the lowering of the concentration of growth factors reaching the cells (McQuillan et al., 1986a). Alternatively, the half-life of the mRNA can be determined metabolically using inhibitors of RNA synthesis or by hybridization techniques using cDNA probes. Studies on PG synthesis by bovine articular cartilage have shown the half-life of the mRNA for the core protein to be the order of 6.3 h (McQuillan et al., 1986a).

If short-term culture of cartilage is used to determine the rate of incorporation of a radio-labeled precursor into certain macromolecules, it is necessary to maintain the culture under constant oxygen tension. The culture should, therefore, be in direct equilibrium with the gas phase. Furthermore, it is advisable to shake the incubations constantly in order to dissipate any concentration gradients resulting from the metabolic activity of the tissue.

LONG-TERM EXPLANT CULTURE OF CARTILAGE

Cartilage can be maintained in explant culture for up to 6 weeks during which time the cells remain viable. Media used for long-term culture of cartilage are similar to those previously described for short-term culture of the tissue, but are often supplemented with amino acids and metabolites (Handley and Lowther, 1976). Buffering of the medium has been achieved using CO_2/bicarbonate or organic buffers and the cultures maintained in air in open or sealed culture flasks.

Long-term cultures of cartilage have been used by many workers to study various aspects of the metabolism of the tissue. In the case of articular cartilage, long-term cultures have been used primarily to investigate aspects of PG synthesis and catabolism. To measure PG synthesis of cartilage that has been maintained in long-term culture, tissue is incubated in medium containing a suitable radiolabeled precursor (i.e. [^{35}S]sulfate). It is usual to preincubate cartilage for at least 1 h in fresh culture medium prior to labeling in order to allow the metabolism of the tissue to adjust to a situation where the supply of metabolites is not rate limiting. After preincubation, the tissue can be maintained in a common medium containing the radiolabeled precursor in short-term culture for up to 6 h. In this way cartilage can be incubated and labeled in a medium where the specific activity of the radiolabeled precursor is constant for all cultures. Where the rate of synthesis is being determined at different times within one experiment, a batch of medium containing the radiolabeled precursor should be made up and used for each determination. This will result in all the tissue in any one experiment being incubated with medium containing the radiolabeled precursor at the same specific activity. Since the time period of incubation is short, any changes in the metabolism of cartilage due to a change in the composition of medium will be minimal. After incubation, radiolabeled macromolecules can be extracted from the tissue, analyzed for radioactivity and characterized (Hascall et al., 1983a).

Measurement of PG catabolism is carried out by incubating cartilage in medium containing a radiolabeled precursor, such as [^{35}S]sulfate, for up to 6 h. The tissue is then washed to remove unincorporated radiolabeled precursor and then replaced in long-term culture in medium that can be supplemented with growth factors, cytokines and other effectors. The amount of radiolabeled macromolecules either remaining in the tissue or appearing in the medium on each day is determined (Handley and Campbell, 1987) and from the total amount of radiolabeled macromolecules present in the tissue the rate of loss of the macromolecules can be determined. Furthermore, the radiolabeled molecules remaining in the tissue during the experiment and those lost to the medium can be characterized (Campbell et al., 1984, 1989). By incubating cartilage in short-term culture in a common medium containing the radiolabeled precursor, the tissue is labeled under identical conditions.

It has been shown that the metabolism of explant cultures of articular cartilage is stimulated by the presence of serum in the culture medium. Fetal calf serum is more potent in stimulating cartilage metabolism than serum from adult animals (Hascall et al., 1983a). The active component of serum has been isolated and shown to be an insulin-like growth factor (McQuillan et al., 1986b). This has resulted in a number of workers substituting serum in long-term explant cultures of articular cartilage with recombinant or purified insulin-like growth factor-I or II, thereby giving a totally defined medium (McQuillan et al., 1986b; Luyten et al., 1988). When supplementing the medium of explant cultures with insulin-like growth factor and other peptide growth factors, it is usual to include low concentrations of serum albumin in the medium to alleviate non-specific binding of exogenous growth factors to microporous filters and culture flasks (McQuillan et al., 1986b).

Articular cartilage can be maintained in long-term culture in medium not containing added serum or growth factors. The chondrocytes respond by decreasing their biosynthetic activity which, in the case of PG metabolism, results in a lowering of this macromolecule in the extracellular matrix of the tissue. When serum or insulin-like growth factors are added to explant cultures of articular cartilage that have been maintained in medium alone, the metabolism of the chondrocytes is stimulated to levels similar to that observed in tissue maintained in culture in medium containing serum or insulin-like growth factors throughout the entire culture period. This ultimately results in the PG concentration in the extracellular matrix of the tissue returning to normal levels. The ability of chondrocytes to remain viable in tissue maintained in explant cultures in the absence of serum or added growth factors suggests that the chondrocytes are protected by the extracellular matrix.

As discussed in Chapter 28, the presence of optimal levels of serum or insulin-like growth factor in the medium of explant cultures of articular cartilage will result in the tissue attaining steady-state metabolism. In the case of PG metabolism, steady-state metabolism results in constant PG levels in the extracellular matrix as the result of the rates of synthesis and catabolism of PGs being equal. Chapter 28 describes both the practical and theoretical basis of steady-state metabolism of cartilage in explant culture.

When initially placed in culture, articular cartilage takes approximately five days to reach a constant metabolic state. This can be a steady state as discussed above or a nonsteady state where the rate of metabolism of the tissue slowly declines resulting in a loss of extracellular matrix components. Having reached such a constant metabolic state it is possible to study the mechanism, kinetics and integration of cartilage metabolism by altering the parameters of culturing conditions so that the tissue either adapts to or departs from a steady-state metabolic condition.

As pointed out above, explant cultures of articular cartilage provide an excellent model for investigating aspects of the mechanism and regulation of catabolism of the extracellular matrix of this tissue. In Chapter 29 the role of cytokines and growth factors on proteoglycan catabolism in explant cultures is discussed.

The major function of articular cartilage in synovial joints is to distribute mechanical loads over the surface of bone. This means that the cells of the tissue must exist in a constantly changing environment as the result of mechanical loading and unloading of the tissue. Chapters 30 and 31 explore the effects of mechanical loading and changes in hydration of the extracellular matrix of cartilage on the metabolism of this tissue in explant culture.

The explant culture of intervertebral disc poses a problem since this tissue will swell if conventional cartilage explant culture technology is used. Chapter 32 describes how swelling of intervertebral disc can be controlled so that this tissue can be studied in organ culture.

28

Steady-state metabolism of proteoglycans in bovine articular cartilage explants

VINCENT C. HASCALL, FRANK P. LUYTEN, ANNA H.K. PLAAS and JOHN D. SANDY

INTRODUCTION

The development of appropriate medium conditions to maintain bovine articular cartilage explants in organ culture for long time periods was initiated in Professor Dennis Lowther's laboratory in the 1970s (Sandy et al., 1980). While these initial studies suggested that explants could achieve relatively high rates of proteoglycan (PG) synthesis in basal medium over the first three days, subsequent work in the same laboratory showed that fetal calf serum was required as a medium supplement to sustain high PG synthetic rates for cultures maintained for more than four to five days (Hascall et al., 1983a). In the latter study PG catabolism in the explant cultures was also investigated, showing that the process exhibited first-order kinetics; furthermore, a half-life parameter, $t_{1/2}$, was defined as the time required in which an amount of PGs equivalent to half of those present in the matrix would be lost from the tissue. Under ideal conditions, biosynthesis replaces the PGs lost from the tissue, thereby maintaining a constant concentration of PGs in the matrix. This dynamic balance between synthesis and catabolism was referred to as *steady-state* metabolism of PGs. This concept was subsequently defined in more detail (Hascall *et al.*, 1983b). The purpose of this chapter is to discuss the criteria required for achieving a steady state experimentally and to provide an example of its use for learning more about PG metabolism in cartilage.

DEFINITION OF STEADY-STATE METABOLISM OF PROTEOGLYCANS

Steady-state metabolism of PGs in cartilage requires that the concentration of these macromolecules remain constant over the time period under consideration, usually a few weeks in the explant culture system. If the system is not in steady state, there will be a change in PG concentration with time, $d[PG]/dt$. This will be equal to the difference between the rates of synthesis and catabolism. Under many experimental conditions, the rate of synthesis will be constant, k_s, and the rate of catabolism will be first order, i.e. proportional to the concentration of PG in the matrix, $k_c \times [PG]$. This gives

$$d[PG]/dt = k_s - k_c \times [PG] \quad (28.1)$$

once steady state is achieved $d[PG]/dt = 0$, and

$$[PG]_{ss} = k_s/k_c \quad (28.2)$$

where $[PG]_{ss}$ is the PG concentration appropriate for the steady state defined by the ratio of the two rate constants.

The integral solution for equation (28.1) gives the concentration of PGs in the tissue as a function of time:

$$[PG]_t = (k_s/k_c) \times (1 - A \times e^{-(k_c \times t)})$$
$$= [PG]_{ss} \times (1 - A \times e^{-(k_c \times t)}) \quad (28.3)$$

where A, a constant of integration, can be determined from the boundary conditions of the system. At $t = 0$, the PG concentration will be the initial concentration, $[PG]_0$, and equation (28.3) becomes

$$[PG]_0 = [PG]_{ss} \times (1 - A)$$
$$A = ([PG]_{ss} - [PG]_0)/[PG]_{ss}$$

and equation (28.3) becomes

$$[PG]_t = [PG]_{ss} - ([PG]_{ss} - [PG]_0) \times e^{-(k_c \times t)} \quad (28.4)$$

CRITERIA FOR STEADY-STATE METABOLISM

Insulin-like growth factor-I (IGF-I) was found to be a major component in fetal calf serum required to sustain high levels of PG synthesis (McQuillan *et al.*, 1986b). We therefore initiated a series of experiments with IGF-I to determine if this growth factor, as the sole medium supplement, could achieve steady-state metabolism of PGs in the cartilage explant system (Luyten *et al.*, 1988). The data for three medium conditions—basal with no IGF-I, basal plus 5 ng ml^{-1} IGF-I and basal plus 20 ng ml^{-1} IGF-I—are summarized in Fig. 28.1.

The 20 ng ml^{-1} IGF-I cultures maintained steady-state conditions within experimental error throughout the experiment because the PG concentration remained constant with time (Fig. 28.1(b)). Catabolism of PGs labeled on day minus two and chased through day 26 was nearly first order from day 0 (Fig. 28.1(c)) and previous work has shown that the catabolic rates for both labeled and unlabeled PGs in these cultures are the same within experimental error (Morales *et al.*, 1984). While PG synthesis increased by 15–20% over the five weeks of the experiment, for the purposes of this analysis it will be assumed that the average synthetic rate ($k_s(20)$ in Fig. 28.1(a)) is the steady-state rate. Equations (28.2) and (28.4) can then be used to determine several parameters for the 20 ng ml^{-1} IGF-I cultures and these can then be used to predict the results for the non-steady-state basal and the 5 ng ml^{-1} IGF-I cultures.

For the 20 ng ml^{-1} IGF-I cultures, $[PG]_{ss}$ (20) = $[PG]_0 \simeq 1.9$ mg glycosaminoglycan/mg

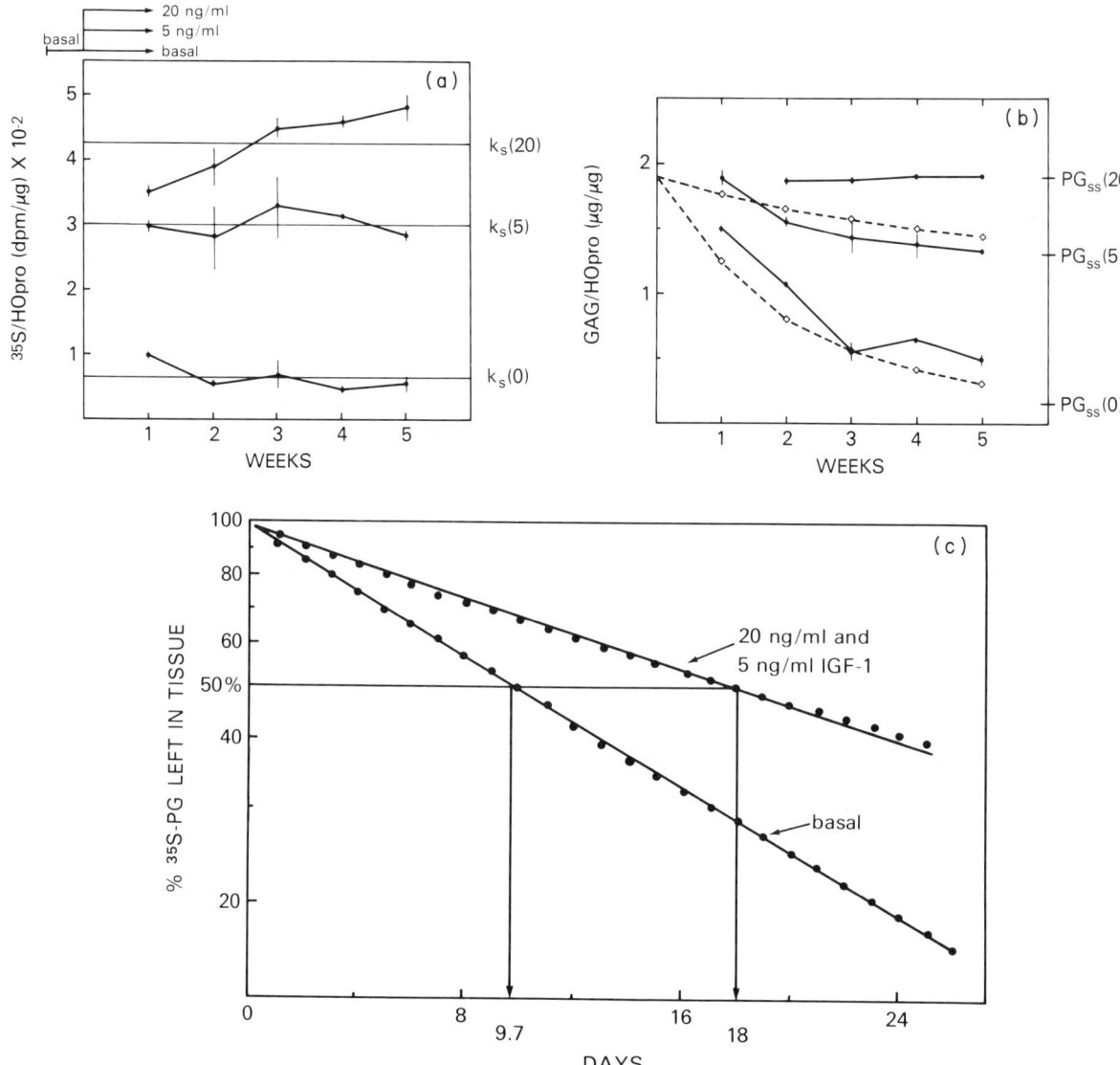

Figure 28.1 For experimental details see Luyten et al. (1988). (a) At the indicated times over 5 weeks, cultures were pulse labeled with [^{35}S]-sulfate and the amounts of activity incorporated into PGs per hydroxyproline content were determined. The bars indicate the range of duplicates for each point. The horizontal lines indicate the average values for each condition which were used to calculate the indicated k_s values as described in the text. (b) The GAG concentrations were determined by a dye-binding technique for each of the cultures described in (a) and the data are plotted as μg GAG/μg hydroxyproline with the range indicated by the bars. The dashed lines are the theoretical curves predicted from equation (28.4) as described in the text. (c) Cultures were maintained in basal, basal plus 5 ng ml^{-1} IGF-I and basal plus 20 ng ml^{-1} IGF-I for 7 days and then labeled for 6 h with [^{35}S]-sulfate (designated day minus 2). Cultures were then maintained in the same media conditions with daily changes until the end of the experiment (designated day 26). The total macromolecular [^{35}S]-activity in the cultures for each condition on day 0 was set at 100% and the data plotted as the percentage remaining in the tissue on a log scale with time. The curves for 20 ng ml^{-1} IGF-I and 5 ng ml^{-1} IGF-I were indistinguishable, yielding half-life values of c. 18 days, while that for basal medium yielded a value of c. 9.7 days.

hydroxyproline (Fig. 28.1(b)) or the equivalent of c. 2 mg PG/mg hydroxyproline. The half-life of the labeled PG is c. 18 days (Fig. 28.1(c)). For a first-order loss of labeled PGs, this defines the catabolic rate constant, $k_c(20)$:

$$[PG]_{18}/[PG]_0 = e^{-(k_c \times 18)}$$
$$k_c = 0.693/18 \simeq 0.0385 \text{ day}^{-1}$$

From equation (28.2), then:

$$k_s(20) = [PG]_{ss}(20) \times k_c(20)$$
$$= 0.0385 \times [PG]_{ss}(20)$$

The steady-state synthetic rate then is therefore, sufficient to replace c. 3.9% of the PGs day^{-1}, i.e. c. 75 µg mg^{-1} hydroxyproline. The DNA content did not change under any of the culture conditions (Luyten et al., 1988), giving a value of c. 35 µg DNA/mg hydroxyproline. Assuming c. 9 pg DNA/cell, this gives an average PG synthetic rate of c. 20 pg cell^{-1} day^{-1}. For comparison, chondrocytes from the Swarm rat chondrosarcoma synthesize c. 50 pg PG cell^{-1} day^{-1} (Kimura et al., 1981).

The parameters above can be used to calculate the changes which occur in the other culture conditions. For the 5 ng ml^{-1} IGF-I cultures, $k_s(5) = 0.70 \times k_s(20)$ (Fig. 28.1(a)) and $k_c(5) = k_c(20)$ (Fig. 28.1(c)). From equation (28.2), therefore, $[PG]_{ss}(5) = 0.70 \times [PG]_{ss}(20)$ and from equation (28.4) the PG concentration with time would be given by the dashed line for the 5 ng ml^{-1} cultures (Fig. 28.1(b)).

For basal conditions, $k_s(0) = 0.15 \times k_s(20)$ (Fig. 28.1(a)) and the half-life value of c. 9.7 days (Fig. 28.1(c)) yields a $k_c(0) = c.\ 0.0714$ day^{-1}. From equation (28.4), then, the concentration with time would be given by the dotted line for basal cultures (Fig. 28.1(b)).

As can be seen, using the kinetic parameters and the initial PG concentration in the system, the changes in PG concentration predicted agree reasonably well with those actually observed in the 5 ng ml^{-1} IGF-I and basal cultures. Furthermore, both of these culture conditions appear to be approaching the expected steady-state concentrations of PGs after five weeks of culture.

DISCUSSION

Medium conditions for attaining steady-state metabolism of PGs in bovine explants have been reported in a series of papers as described above. Briefly, tissue (25–50 mg wet wt/ml) is maintained with daily changes in a basal medium (Dulbeccos Modified Eagle's Medium containing one (Hascall et al., 1983a) or four (Morales et al., 1984) g glucose/l and organic buffers and amino acids as described by Handley and Lowther (1976)) supplemented with up to 20% fetal calf serum (Hascall et al., 1983a) or with growth factors, either IGF-I (McQuillan et al., 1986b; Luyten et al., 1988) or transforming growth factor-β (Morales and Roberts, 1988). Under these conditions, both calf (0–6 weeks) and steer (1–2 years) cartilage reach steady-state metabolism within a few days with little or no change in PG concentration from the initial, fresh-tissue level. The rapid achievement of steady-state metabolism in calf and steer tissue is consistent with their biosynthetic response to explant: steer cartilage increases PG synthetic rates to maximum levels within 1–3 days, while calf cartilage is frequently at maximum synthetic rates initially which are subsequently maintained in culture (Hascall et al., 1983a, b).

Interestingly, under the same or very similar medium conditions, cartilage tissue from mature rabbit (50–75 weeks) undergoes initial adaptation to culture in which nonsteady-state conditions prevail with rapid loss of PGs from the tissue during the first 1–4 days (Sandy et al., 1978; Sandy and Plaas, 1986). Articular cartilage from immature rabbits increased PG synthesis to a maximal level over six days while PG concentration in the tissue declined to a new steady-state level of c. 74% of the initial value. For tissue from mature rabbits, a longer time (c. 10 days) was required to attain maximal synthetic rates and a lower steady-state concentration of PGs (c. 55% of the initial value) was reached.

In summary, it appears that cartilage explants which maintain (calf) or rapidly achieve (steer) the high levels of synthesis of PGs (presumably due to high responsiveness to bovine serum IGF-I or other growth factors) required to balance the initial catabolic rates achieve a steady-state concentration close to the fresh-tissue value. Whereas in rabbit cartilage explants, the biosynthetic response is relatively slow (presumably due to low responsiveness to bovine IGF-I or other growth factors) and a marked initial catabolic phase occurs before steady-state conditions are achieved. The biphasic response of rabbit cartilage to explant culture may be related to the finding that biosynthetic and catabolic pathways in bovine cartilage explants appear to exhibit independent responses to exogenous, low concentrations of IGF-I (Luyten *et al.*, 1988). At very low concentrations (0.5–2.0 ng ml^{-1}) the synthetic rate is low but catabolism is already decreased to near minimum rates. Higher, saturating concentrations (10–20 ng ml^{-1}) are also required to increase the synthetic rates to a maximum level. The mechanisms which link the biosynthetic and catabolic responses of cartilages in this early nonsteady-state phase of culture remain to be determined.

29

Cartilage explant cultures: a model system for the analysis of matrix degradation

J. TYLER and Y. SAWYER

INTRODUCTION

Articular chondrocytes normally organize and regulate the deposition of their surrounding matrix in a highly ordered and efficient manner. In mature cartilage the synthesis and degradation of matrix molecules become balanced in a stable equilibrium. Osteoarthritis may result from a failure of the chondrocyte to maintain this balance, but little is known of the molecular basis for the mechanisms underlying degenerative disease. We describe here the use of a culture system utilizing explanted slices of cartilage to analyze *in vitro* the way in which mediators such as cytokines and growth factors influence the ability of chondrocytes to maintain a functional cartilage matrix.

METHODS

Tissue culture

Pig cartilage was excised as thin slices (approximately 12 mm × 2 mm × 0.5 mm) just from the condylar ridge of the metacarpophalangeal joints of freshly slaughtered pigs aged 5–7 months. Care was taken to exclude the underlying marrow. Macroscopically normal human cartilage was taken as full-thickness slices of similar dimensions from the surface of femoral condyles as soon as possible after their removal following femoral neck fracture. The cartilage slices were cultured in Iscove's medium supplemented with serum albumin (60 µg ml^{-1}), human transferrin

($5\ \mu g\ ml^{-1}$), soyabean lipid ($15\ \mu g\ ml^{-1}$), ascorbic acid ($50\ \mu g\ ml^{-1}$), streptomycin ($100\ \mu g\ ml^{-1}$) and penicillin 150 (units) in a humidified atmosphere of CO_2/air (1:19) at 37°C with a change of medium every 30 or 48 h. To estimate proteoglycan (PG) synthesis and degradation, six slices (each approx. 8 mg wet wt) were cultured per milliliter of medium for 72 h to allow the tissue to equilibrate and to check that the basal rates of PG release were equivalent. Cytokines of interest were added and the cultures continued for a further 72 h or longer as indicated in the legend to Fig. 29.1. To measure PG synthesis, [^{35}S]sulfate ($10\ \mu Ci\ ml^{-1}$) was added to each culture for the last 3 h. The slices were then washed in ice cold Iscove's medium and digested with papain ($25\ \mu g\ ml^{-1}$; Sigma Type III) in 50 mM sodium phosphate buffer, pH 6.5, containing 2 mM N-acetylcysteine and 2 mM EDTA at 60°C for 2 h.

Proteoglycan synthesis and degradation

PG degradation was routinely estimated as the percentage of glycosaminoglycan released into the culture medium and was determined by reaction with 1,9-dimethylmethylene blue (Farndale et al., 1986), shark chondroitin sulfate (5–50 μg) being used as standard. In some experiments done to measure proteoglycan degradation of human cartilage, the explants were prelabeled by incubation for 16 h in medium containing [^{35}S]sulfate (25–40 $\mu Ci\ mg^{-1}$; Amersham) at $10\ \mu Ci\ ml^{-1}$ and IGF ($100\ ng\ ml^{-1}$). The slices were washed well with at least four changes of warmed unlabeled medium over a period of 6 h prior to starting the experiment. [^{35}S]Glycosaminoglycans were quantitated by the amount eluting as a void-volume peak from 10 ml Sephadex G-50 columns equilibrated with 50 mM sodium acetate buffer, pH 6.0, or by precipitation with cetyl pyridinium chloride (1% in water) at room temperature as described previously (Tyler, 1985b).

Analytical procedures

Collagen was measured as hydroxyproline in neutralized acid hydrolysates of the medium and tissue (6 M HCl, 105°C, 20 h) as described by Tougaard (1973). Prostaglandin E_2 was measured by a specific radioimmunoassay (Steranti, St Albans, Herts, UK) according to the manufacturer's instructions. Tracer [^{3}H]PGE$_2$ was purchased from Amersham.

Standardization of cytokine activity *in vitro*

All cytokines and growth factors were stored as a concentrated solution at −70°C. Special grade bovine serum album ($100\ \mu g\ ml^{-1}$) was present during storage and in the medium used to dilute the samples prior to use. Human recombinant IL1α and β were from Biogen, TNFα from Genzyme and IL6 from Cambio. Natural pig IL1α and β, isolated as described by Saklatvala et al. (1985), was a generous gift. Reference cytokine and standards of known biological activity together with neutralizing antibody can be obtained on request from Dr Andy Gehring, National Institute for Biological Standards & Control (NIBSC), South Mimms, Herts, UK.

RESULTS AND DISCUSSION

Cytokines enhance matrix degradation and decrease synthesis

A dose–response curve for pig articular cartilage with recombinant human IL1α, TNFα, IL6 and native pig IL1 is shown in Fig. 29.1, based on bioassays for increased PG degradation (Fig. 29.1(b)) and decreased synthesis (Fig. 29.1(a)). When used singly IL1α is more potent by at least an order of magnitude than TNFα, but together a synergistic enhancement has been demonstrated (Saklatvala, 1986). The basal level of PG synthesis and the effects of these cytokines can also be modified by the presence of growth factors such as IGF1 (Tyler, 1989), TGFβ and FGF (Morales and Roberts, 1988; Chandraskehar and Harvey, 1988, 1989) and other cytokines such as IFNγ (Bunning and Russell, 1989). The final activity observed will, therefore, depend on the relative concentration of each factor present. The effects on PG metabolism in cultured cartilage are very similar to those found following intraarticular

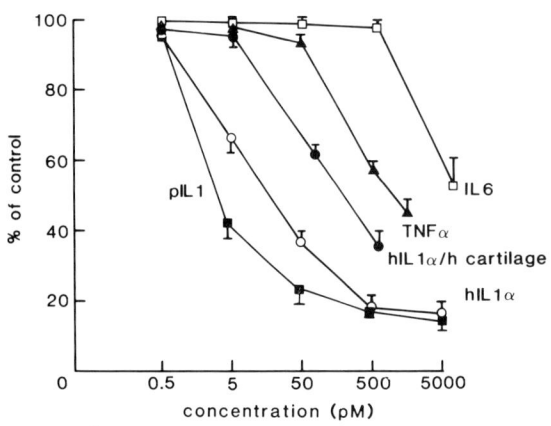

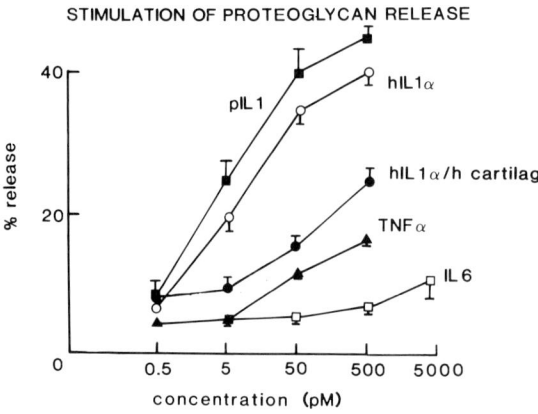

Figure 29.1 Pig articular cartilage slices were cultured for 72 h in Iscoves medium with supplements as described in the methods. The cultures contained increasing concentrations of natural pig IL1α (■), human recombinant IL1α (○), TNFα (▲) or IL6 (□). Human articular cartilage slices were cultured for 8 days with human recombinant IL1α (●). Proteoglycan synthesis was measured by incorporation of [^{35}S]-sulfate into GAG and degradation as the proportion of unlabeled PG in the medium by analysis with 1,9-dimethyl-methylene blue.

cultures have been shown to produce IL1 (Ollivierre et al., 1986; Rath et al., 1988; Shinmei et al., 1988b) which in other cell types is known to induce down regulation of IL1 receptors (Matsushima et al., 1986). Cartilage or chondrocytes cultured with IL1 also produce considerable amounts of IL6. The addition of specific neutralizing antibodies has proved useful in cartilage bioassays to determine the relative contribution of different cytokines in complex mixtures (Shinmei et al., 1988b; Guerne et al., 1989; Tyler and Richards, unpublished results).

It was not known whether IL6 could alter chondrocyte metabolism. We therefore assayed the recombinant human material in various cartilage bioassays. PG synthesis was unaffected by IL6 up to 500 pM (Fig. 29.1). A significant 50% decrease did occur at 5000 pM, although general protein synthesis was also decreased by 30% at this dose. No stimulation of PG degradation was observed and IL6 did not induce synthesis of stromelysin, PGE_2 or alter collagen synthesis (results not shown). IL6 therefore does not potentiate the biological effects of IL1 on cartilage. Significant amounts of IL6 are found in the synovial fluid of patients with rheumatoid (c. 15 ng ml^{-1}) or osteoarthritis (OA) (3–5 ng ml^{-1}) (Kishimoto et al., 1989). This cytokine can augment local antibody and corticosteroid production both in vitro and in vivo, but its main role is to stimulate hepatocytes as part of the acute phase response to trauma (Gauldie et al., 1987). This leads to a specific induction of serum proteinase inhibitors such as $\alpha 2$ macroglobulin, $\alpha 1$ proteinase inhibitor, $\alpha 1$ antichymotrypsin and anticystatin. The concentration of these inhibitors in serum can double within 8 h and also markedly increases the inhibitory capacity of synovial fluid, which indirectly provides a valuable protection mechanism against rapid cartilage degradation during inflammation. Synthesis of IL1 and IL6 can be effectively suppressed at the level of transcription by corticosteroids (Fenton et al., 1987; Gauldie, 1989). Including hydrocortisone (1 μg ml^{-1}) in cartilage cultures therefore helps to eliminate endogenous cytokine production and also has the advantage of suppressing high basal rates of PG release which are found particularly

injection of cytokines into experimental animals (Pettipher et al., 1986; van de Loo et al., 1989; Dingle et al., 1987). Even when pure recombinant proteins are added to cultures the possibility of endogenous production of cytokines by the cartilage must be considered. Some chondrocyte with bovine nasal discs; this makes the cytokine stimulated release of matrix easier to monitor.

The influence of age and species of the cartilage

There is 26% homology in the amino acid sequences of human IL1α and IL1β, and about 62% homology in the nucleotide sequences of human and murine IL1 α (Auron et al., 1984; Limedico et al., 1984). The homologous region between amino acids 150 and 186 probably contains the minimal-recognition site for the IL1 receptor. Some species specificity has been found in the cartilage resorption assay. Human recombinant IL1β acts very poorly on pig cartilage, although natural pig IL1α and β are equally effective on pig and human cartilage (Saklatvala et al., 1985) and both are more potent than human IL1α (Fig. 29.1) on pig cartilage. Despite the potent biological activity of unlabeled material on pig chondrocytes, radiolabeled iodinated human IL1α will not bind with high affinity to pig chondrocytes (Tyler and Bird, unpublished results). Even in a homologous system using pig IL1 binding to pig chondrocytes, the affinity of the IL1 receptor does not match the potency of the biological response which can often be maximal with less than 10% occupancy of the receptors (Bird and Saklatvala, 1986). The amino acid sequences of TNFα are highly conserved in different species (Marmenout et al., 1985) and no species specificity has been reported.

PG synthesis is inhibited by lower concentrations of IL1 than those required to initiate cartilage resorption (Benton and Tyler, 1988) in most systems that have been studied. It is not known whether this indicates a difference in response to the bound ligand or simply reflects the inability to monitor efficiently the onset of degradation. There is often a marked decrease in response with age which has been noted especially by those working with human explants, and very little or no increase in PG is seen in some human cartilage samples at doses of IL1 which significantly inhibit synthesis (Jubb and Saklatvala, 1985). A clear degradative response to cytokines can be demonstrated with human tissue, as shown in Fig. 29.1 (Shinmei et al., 1988a; Bunning and Russell, 1989). This was seen with less than 25% of the samples and it is not clear whether the lack of response in some cartilage is due to decreased cleavage of the core protein or the inability of degradation fragments to diffuse freely out of the more densely packed matrix. One report noted that cartilage from OA and rheumatoid arthritis patients was more sensitive to IL1 (Shinmei et al., 1988a). The assay can be optimized by slicing the cartilage thinly, increasing the time of exposure and the concentration of cytokines and by preculturing the tissue with serum or IGF1 in the presence of radiolabeled sulfate to prelabel the PG as described in the 'Methods'. Unlike pig cartilage, the newly synthesized PG in human cartilage appears to be preferentially degraded in response to IL1 (results not shown).

Characterization of degradation fragments

The degradation fragments released from cartilage cultured with IL1 have been isolated and characterized biochemically and by radio-immunoassay. A limited cleavage of the core protein occurs particularly in the G2 globular region and within the chondroitin sulfate attachment region to produce monomers with a slightly smaller average hydrodynamic size which are unable to bind to hyaluronan and, therefore, rapidly diffuse out of the matrix (Tyler, 1985a; Ratcliffe et al., 1986). PG fragments of a similar nature were isolated from unstimulated cultures and from cartilage cultured with TNF or retinoic acid, indicating that this is a general mechanism for PG turnover that is enhanced by exposure to cytokines. The large degradation fragments released remain extremely sensitive to proteolysis and can be degraded readily to small pieces by almost any freely soluble active proteinase. Freezing and thawing the culture medium will activate secreted metalloproteinases which can secondarily give rise to some very small, almost limit digest fragments of core protein. When characterizing the initial degradation products released by the explants it is, therefore, important either to include proteinase inhibitors in the culture medium or to add them before the conditioned medium is frozen prior to analysis (Tyler, 1985a, b). The fact that this does not occur within the matrix indicates that even in maximally stimulated cartilage the degradation process mediated by the chondrocyte is not rampant and indiscriminate but precise and discrete and the availability of proteolytic activity is very carefully regulated at several stages (for a review see Tyler (1990)).

Recent work with synthetic inhibitors of metalloproteinases has emphasized the importance of using explant cultures for testing potential inhibitors of matrix degradation. Concentrations of several hydroxamic derivatives that were very effective at inhibiting proteinase activity in soluble enzyme assays or on chondrocyte monolayers had no effect in the cartilage resorption assay due to poor penetration through the matrix. Concentrations of two to three orders of magnitude higher were required to show a significant decrease in PG release (DiPasquale et al., 1986; Caputo et al., 1987; Henderson and Davies, 1990).

CONCLUSIONS

The identity of mediators involved in the initiation and/or progression of some types of human OA has not yet been established, but it seems likely that the relative concentration of cytokines and growth factors at different stages may determine the rate of progress and final outcome of the disease. Cultured cartilage explants provide an efficient model system with which to investigate the mechanism of action of these factors and the way in which they influence the synthesis and degradation of matrix components. The system also provides a rapid initial method of screening large numbers of potential therapeutic agents which may modify the degradation process prior to *in vivo* testing.

30

The effect of mechanical compression on cartilage metabolism

ROBERT L.Y. SAH, YOUNG-JO KIM and ALAN J. GRODZINSKY

INTRODUCTION

Mechanical loading can significantly affect cartilage metabolism and viability, as has been observed in a variety of animal and human studies. The chondrocyte biosynthetic response *in vitro* to mechanical stimulation in cartilage explant and gel culture has been studied in an attempt to understanding the underlying transduction mechanisms (Jones *et al.*, 1982; De Witt *et al.*, 1984; Palmoski and Brandt, 1984; Bayliss *et al.*, 1986; Schneiderman *et al.*, 1986; Gray *et al.*, 1988, 1989; Urban and Bayliss, 1989; Sah *et al.*, 1989). Mechanical compression of cartilage causes hydrostatic pressure gradients to build up, which can cause fluid to exude from and redistribute within the tissue. Fluid flow also transports mobile counterions past fixed-charge groups, thereby generating streaming potentials and currents. Tissue compaction not only produces direct cell deformation and decreased matrix pore size, but also leads to increased matrix charge density (moles of fixed charge per liter interstitial fluid); this results in physicochemical changes including decreased tissue hydration, increased concentration of all mobile counterions and decreased concentration of all co-ions.

This chapter describes a system based on the explant culture of articular cartilage which we have developed in an attempt to (i) identify which of the above physical stimuli may be linked to specific changes in chondrocyte metabolic response, and (ii) distinguish between the effects of static and dynamic compression.

METHODS

Cartilage/bone cores were harvested from the femoropatellar groove of 1–2 week-old calves. After removing the top $c.$ 100 μm from the articular surface, cylindrical disks (3 mm diameter, 1 mm thick) were taken from the next 2 mm of middle-zone cartilage from the $c.$ 4–10 mm full-thickness specimen. After 2–6 days in culture (daily changes of Dulbecco's Modified Eagle's Medium (DMEM) + 10 mM N-2-hydroxyethylpiperazine-N'-2-ethanesulfonic acid (HEPES) + 10% FBS), disks swelled to $\geq$ 1.25 mm and attained relatively steady-state rates of biosynthesis (Sah et al., 1988).

Cartilage disks were then subjected either (i) to a 12 h static, radially unconfined, uniaxial compression in specially designed chambers placed within a standard incubator (control disks were free-swelling (Sah et al., 1989)) or (ii) to a 23 h sinusoidal compression (superimposed on a static compression to 1.0 mm thickness) using a dynamic compression chamber (Fig. 30.1) placed

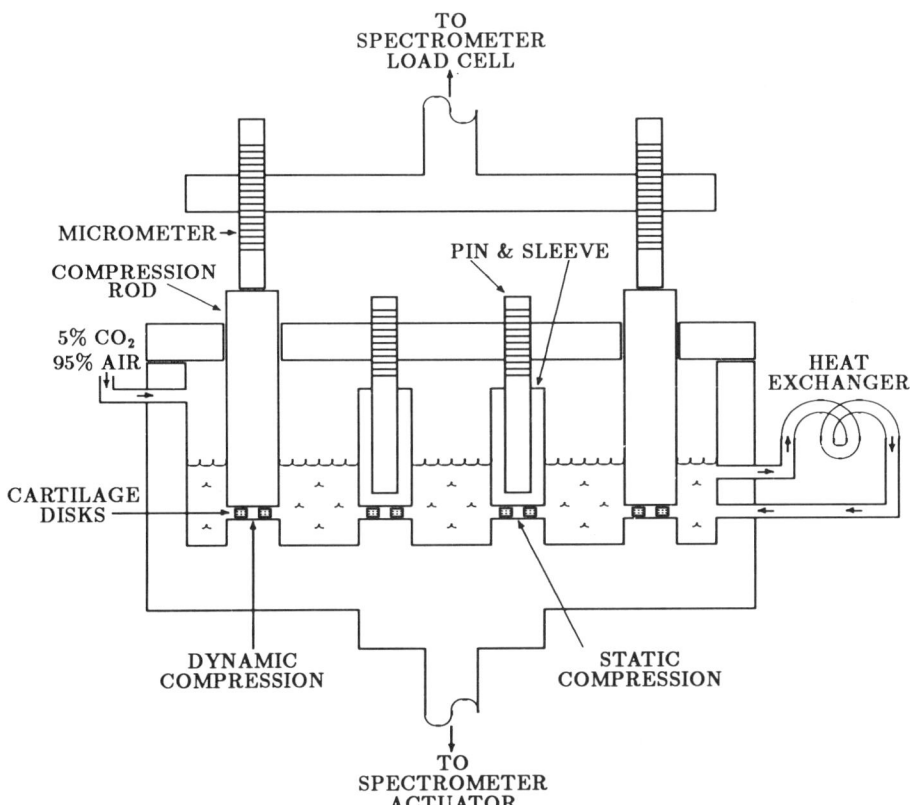

Figure 30.1 Dynamic compression chamber.

in a Dynastat mechanical spectrometer. The effect of compression on glycosaminoglycan (GAG) and protein synthesis was assessed by incorporation of [^{35}S]sulfate and L-[5-^{3}H]proline during the 12 h of static and the last 7–8 h of oscillatory compression. The design of the dynamic chamber enabled compressive load and displacement to be measured throughout the oscillatory compression/culture period; cartilage dynamic stiffness during culture was then computed as the fundamental amplitude of the load normalized to the unloaded cross-sectional area of the dynamically compressed disks and to the dynamic strain amplitude (see Sah et al. (1989) for details).

RESULTS AND DISCUSSION

Static compression caused a dose-dependent decrease in radiolabel incorporation (Sah et al., 1989). During all but the first c. 10–15 min of the 12 h static compression there is no intratissue hydrostatic pressurization, no fluid flow and, therefore, no streaming potentials. The results of these studies suggest that other physical mechanisms may inhibit biosynthesis in response to static compression, including: (i) physicochemical changes associated with compression-induced decrease in intratissue pH (Gray et al., 1988; Sah et al., 1989) and changes in hydration and other intratissue ion concentrations (Schneiderman et al., 1986; Urban and Bayliss, 1989); (ii) hindered transport of macromolecules within the matrix due to tissue compaction; and (iii) cell and cytoskeleton deformation (Benya et al., 1988; Poole et al., 1985).

The effect of 23 h of 1–2% amplitude oscillatory compression on sulfate incorporation during the last 8 h, relative to control disks statically compressed to 1 mm, is shown in Fig. 30.2(a). Such low-amplitude oscillatory compression does not significantly change cartilage-disk hydration or fixed charge density and, therefore, does not result in physicochemical changes. Therefore, this applied compression protocol selects against the mechanisms that might be associated with larger amplitude static compression, and enabled us specifically to examine the effects of dynamic compression on biosynthesis. Both sulfate and proline (not shown) incorporation were significantly stimulated (30–40%) at compression frequencies equal to or greater than 0.01 cycles^{-1} (Hz). Dynamic mechanical measurements of these same specimens during stimulation (Fig. 30.2(b)) showed stiffness to increase dramatically at $f \geq 0.01$ Hz, implying a concomitant increase in hydrostatic pressure in the central region of the cartilage disks, and in pressure gradients, fluid velocity and streaming potential near the periphery of the disks. Thus, this biosynthetic stimulation (Fig. 30.2(a)) appears unrelated to intratissue pH, but may be associated with these other dynamic fields and flows. Since the

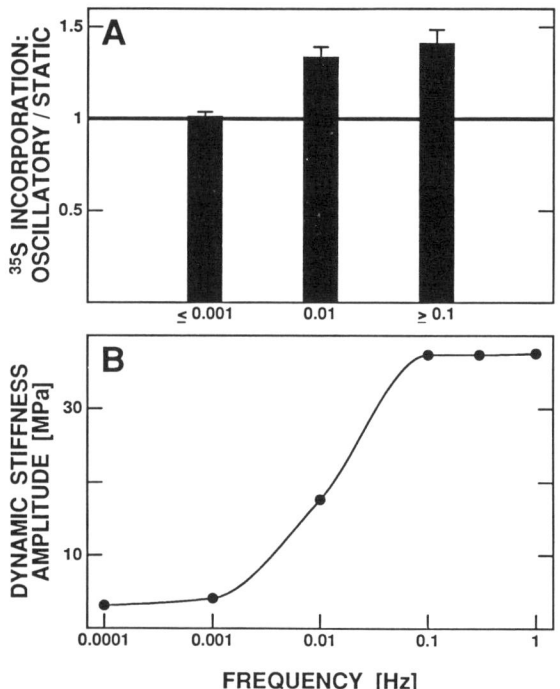

Figure 30.2 Correlation of biosynthetic response to 1–2% oscillatory compression at various frequencies with dynamic stiffness. (a) The incorporation of [^{35}S]-sulfate into cartilage disks during the last 8 h compression was normalized to that in disks held statically (mean ± SEM, $n = 12$–72). Data are compiled from Sah et al. (1989). (b) Dynamic stiffness of cartilage disks during oscillatory compression experiments. Data is from Sah et al. (1989).

intratissue profiles of hydrostatic pressure, strain, strain rate, fluid velocity and streaming potential can be estimated in radially-unconfined compression (Armstrong *et al.*, 1984; Kim, 1989), spatial variations in radiolabel incorporation within the disks may aid in distinguishing between these physical stimuli.

Several considerations arise when designing protocols to assess *in vitro* the role of putative physical mechanisms in the regulation of cartilage metabolism by mechanical loading *in vivo*. Since loading typically consists *in vivo* of a time-varying dynamic component superimposed on a time-average static component, protocols can be designed to test the effects *in vitro* of individual static and dynamic components, as we have described above. (i) It is necessary to test multiple specimens simultaneously because of the normal topographical variation in tissue composition and metabolism. (ii) For the case of sinusoidal steady-state load (displacement) components superimposed on an equilibrium static offset load (displacement), there is little difference between load control and displacement control as long as the mechanical properties of all the specimens are similar. Otherwise, to test multiple specimens dynamically with a single actuator, displacement control requires all specimens to be in parallel (as in Fig. 30.1), while load control requires all specimens to be in series. If the hypothesized mechanism to be tested is related to the magnitude of tissue hydration and charge density (and associated intratissue ion concentrations), then compressive displacement is the appropriate parameter to control. If the mechanism is related to osmotic or hydrostatic pressure, then load control may be more appropriate. (iii) Confined and unconfined tests (with or without underlying bone) each have advantages and disadvantages; while the confined test may lead to simpler mechanical analysis, the unconfined configuration may allow more rapid transport of nutrients into the explant culture (depending on the aspect ratio of the cartilage disk).

31

Effects of mechanical and osmotic pressure on the rate of glycosaminoglycan synthesis in the human adult femoral head cartilage

ALICE MAROUDAS and ROSA SCHNEIDERMAN

The matrix of cartilage, because of its strongly polyelectrolyte nature, has very different characteristics from those of other extracellular spaces. It is known now that the activity of the chondrocytes (whether anabolic or catabolic) is influenced by the conditions prevailing in the immediate surroundings of the cells. As pointed out in the previous article, these conditions are related to physicochemical factors such as matrix hydration, local changes in osmotic pressure, local concentrations of ions, and mechanical effects, resulting in direct cell deformation. It has been shown for cells from other connective tissue, e.g. bone, that mechanical stresses result in altered prostaglandin synthesis and hence in changes in other metabolic process (Rodan et al., 1975). This may also apply to articular chondrocytes. Another important phenomenon accompanying application of pressure is the loss of part of the water from the matrix (e.g. Maroudas, 1979). This might affect cell activity through a change in the concentration of the various solutes in the pericellular environment, a decrease in the diffusivity of nutrients, an increase in the proteoglycan (PG) concentration and in the osmotic pressure around the cells, or a decrease in the cell volume itself.

We have shown in our previous studies that by applying osmotically active solutions of polyethylene glycol (PEG) to cartilage the same levels of hydration could be obtained at equilibrium as with an equivalent mechanically applied stress (Maroudas, 1985). However, while in the case of osmotically active solutions being used to 'suck' water out of the cartilage matrix, the primary change in the cell's environment is a decreased hydration, in the case of unconfined mechanical compression other effects apart from water loss also come into play, such as the stretching of the tissue in one plane and an increase in the hydrostatic pressure in the matrix. The purpose of this present communication is to report the effects of changes in the water content, and hence the effective fixed-charge density (FCD), on sulfate incorporation by articular cartilage in explant culture exposed to mechanical compression or to osmotically active solutions. This will allow an assessment of whether these changes constitute one of the pathways through which mechanically applied static pressure can act on the chondrocyte.

MATERIALS AND METHODS

The procedures used have been described in detail elsewhere (Schneiderman et al., 1986; Schneiderman, 1987).

Cartilage samples

Most of the experiments were carried out using human femoral heads obtained at operations for femoral neck fractures. Full-depth plugs of cartilage, about 6 mm in diameter, were used.

Osmotic compression

The specimens were placed in small-pore dialysis sacs (spectrapor membrane No. 3, 2000 Dalton cut-off). The dialysis sacs were inserted into vials containing the radioactive medium with the osmotically active PEG solution at the chosen concentration and after initial equilibration at 4°C were incubated at 37°C for 4 h. Thereafter, the cartilage specimens were taken out of the dialysis tubing and weighed immediately. Control specimens were handled in the same manner, but the medium used did not contain PEG. Further processing included washing of the specimens to remove free [^{35}S]sulfate, measurement of FCD, determination of total water content, digestion in papain and final assessment of incorporated [^{35}S]sulfate.

Mechanical Compression

The cartilage plugs, prepared in the same way as above, were placed between two sintered pyrex discs in a Petri dish containing the radioactive medium, and compressed in an apparatus that is based on that used by Kempson for testing small cylinders of articular cartilage in uniaxial compression (Kempson, 1975). The loads used gave applied pressures equivalent to the osmotic pressures of the PEG solutions and corresponded to the lower range of physiological pressures (3–10 atm). The lateral expansion of the specimens corresponded to an increase in area of 2–10%, depending on the load used (see Chapter 68).

RESULTS

A set of typical results for the sulfate uptake, Q, of full-depth cartilage plugs versus applied pressure (mechanical and osmotic) is shown in Fig. 31.1. It can be seen that the two sets of results are very similar and that in both cases there is a steep decrease in the rate of sulfate uptake with increased pressure.

31. EFFECT OF PRESSURE ON RATE OF GLYCOSAMINOGLYCAN SYNTHESIS

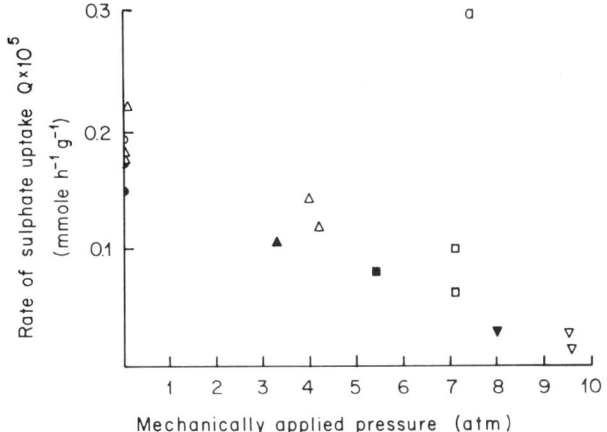

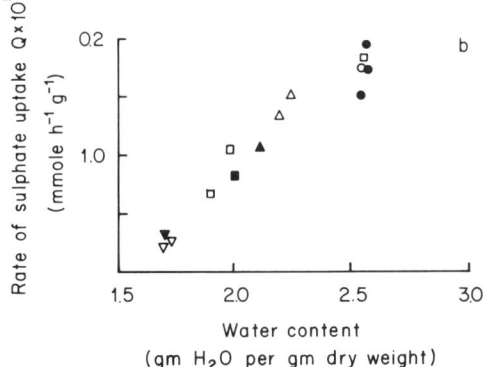

Figure 31.1 Typical variation in the rate of sulfate incorporation (Q): (a) with externally applied osmotic and mechanical pressure; (b) with hydration. (▲, ■, ●) Osmotic pressure; (△, □, ○) mechanical pressure; different symbols correspond to different pressure levels.

Since during the 37°C incubation period the cartilage generally does not achieve complete equilibrium with respect to water loss, the values of the applied pressure do not necessarily reflect the changes which these pressures would be expected to produce within the cartilage matrix at equilibrium. Thus, a better parameter to plot is the hydration at the end of the incubation period since this really does represent the conditions within the tissue (albeit the final, rather than the average, values). Figure 31.1(b) shows such a plot for the above example and Fig. 31.2(a) shows a graph of Q vs. hydration after the 37°C incubation for a large number of osmotically compressed full-depth plugs. Also in Fig. 31.2(a), the values of sulfate uptake are plotted vs. hydration for all the specimens which had been compressed mechanically. Using a t-test, we found no significant differences between either the two entire populations of results or for the values at mean water contents of 2.0 and 1.75.

However, it should be borne in mind that if specimens of different initial FCD are used, then for any given applied pressure, the equilibrium hydration is inversely related to the initial FCD. In order to overcome this complication and to attempt to normalize all our results, we calculated, wherever possible, the effective fixed-charge density corresponding to the final hydration. The effective fixed-charge density represents the actual concentration of negatively charged groups present in the extrafibrillar space at a given hydration level, and thus incorporates variations in both FCD and applied pressure (for method of calculating effective FCD, see Chapter 69). Figure 31.2(b) shows plots of Q vs. $FCD_{effective}$ for mechanically and osmotically compressed specimens; there is no statistically significant difference between the two curves. It is worth mentioning that the correlation coefficient, R, was found to be higher when Q was plotted vs. $FCD_{effective}$ than when it was plotted vs. either the applied pressure or the total hydration (Schneiderman, 1987).

It can be seen that for small losses of hydration, down to ratios of water : dry weight of approximately 2.2, and for the range of effective FCD 0.2–0.3 mEq/g H_2O, the rate of sulfate uptake is practically constant. However, as the hydration decreases from 2.2 to 1.55 and the effective FCD from 0.3 to 0.6 mEq/g H_2O, the rate of sulfate uptake decreases five-fold.

CONCLUSION

In summary, osmotic and mechanical compression seem to have much the same effect on the rate of glycosaminoglycan production by the cells. It thus appears likely that no factors other than decreased

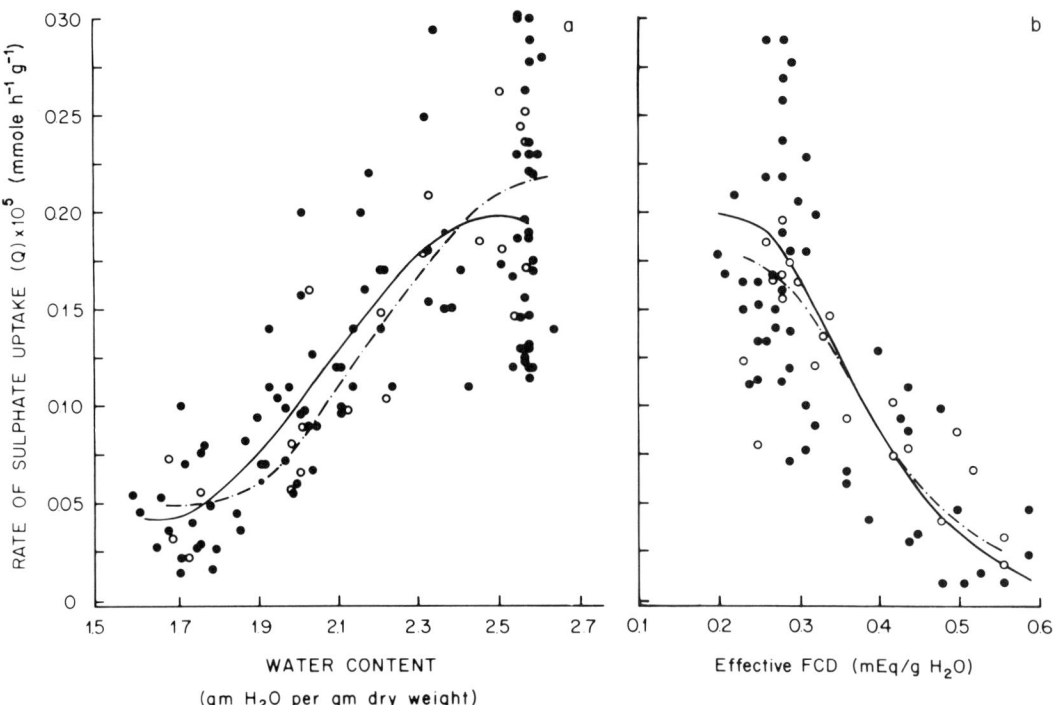

Figure 31.2 Variation in the rate of sulfate incorporation (Q) with: (a) hydration for all osmotically and mechanically compressed specimens; and (b) effective fixed charge density. (●) Osmotic compression; (○) mechanical compression.

hydration and increased PG concentration, leading to increased ionic concentrations and increased osmotic pressure around the cells, are of major importance, at least at the pressure levels used in the present investigation. Thus, the lateral expansion of the order of 2–10% which was observed to occur in the specimens undergoing mechanical compression, but not in those subjected to osmotic pressure, does not appear to have any significant effect on cell activity.

32

Explant culture of the intervertebral disc

B. JOHNSTONE

INTRODUCTION

Methods currently used for explant culture of connective-tissue samples are not suitable for intervertebral disc tissues and lead to artifactual results. When placed in aqueous solution, intervertebral discs swell considerably and matrix constituents leach out: discs can double their volume and lose more than 50% of their proteoglycans (PGs) (Pousty et al., 1975; Urban and Maroudas, 1981). These effects result in a changing pericellular environment during explant culture incubations, making it difficult to equate *in vitro* experimental findings to the *in vivo* state. Since it is difficult to quantify the effects of these changes, efforts have been made to prevent them from occurring. Studies by Urban and Maroudas (1981) introduced a method for controlling swelling, and preventing the consequent leaching, by opposing the swelling pressure of the disc with a high osmotic pressure. This can be accomplished by adding polyethylene glycol (PEG) to the bathing solution (see Chapter 69). At the appropriate PEG concentration, the osmotic pressure of the solution would be equal to the swelling pressure of the disc and the tissue would retain its postmortem hydration state. Sealing the tissue inside small-pore dialysis tubing prevents penetration of PEG and limits leaching of macromolecular material from the tissue. This method has since been adapted for use in the culture of disc slices in order to study disc cell metabolism, principally PG biosynthesis (Bayliss et al., 1986, 1988).

CULTURE METHOD

In order not to lose water from a tissue during handling in air (see Chapter 2), precautions should be taken to prevent evaporation, particularly when thin cut sections are being processed (e.g. a humidity box can be used). This was found to be extremely important for the culture of intervertebral discs. Unless the dissected disc sections were kept at high humidity, no accurate assessment of hydration changes during culture was possible. For the study of the biosynthetic rate of disc PGs, thin (c. 1 mm thick) sections were cut, weighed and enclosed in small-pore dialysis tubing sacs (c. 3500 mol. wt cut-off). The sections were then preincubated at 4°C for 1–2 h in Dulbecco's Modified Eagle's Medium (DMEM) containing 0.8 mM $MgSO_4$, 10 μCi ml^{-1} of carrier-free [^{35}S]sulfate and the appropriate concentration of PEG. This preincubation period allowed equilibration of the [^{35}S]sulfate and the medium components throughout the sections (Maroudas and Evans, 1974). Incubations proper were carried out at 37°C in a shaking water bath. After incubation, the sections were reweighed and stored frozen at −20°C. If required, sagittal sectioning was carried out before weighing and freezing. The frozen sections were then lyophilized, weighed and digested with papain. The resulting solution was eluted through Sephadex G-50 columns equilibrated in 2 M guanidine hydrochloride to separate the unincorporated [^{35}S]sulfate. The rate of incorporation was determined according to the equation described by Maroudas (1980).

DEFINING THE CULTURE CONDITIONS

Urban and Maroudas (1979) showed that the partition of sulfate throughout the disc is directly influenced by the fixed-charge density of the PGs. Furthermore, it had been shown that the rate of [^{35}S]sulfate incorporation into articular cartilage is affected by low sulfate concentrations (Maroudas and Evans, 1974; Ridgway, 1984; Schneiderman et al., 1986 also Chapter 33). In preliminary disc-culture experiments, it was established that the rate of sulfate incorporation was contingent on the inorganic sulfate concentration up to about 0.3 mM, but became independent at higher concentrations. An inorganic sulfate concentration of 0.8 mM in the medium was sufficient to have no influence on the rate of [^{35}S]sulfate incorporation within the range of accepted hydration change ($\pm 10\%$, see below).

The concentration of PEG required to control disc hydration was different for the various species from which discs were taken (Table 32.1). For a given age, rabbit and dog disc tissues were very consistent in the level of PEG required. However, it proved impossible to predict the concentration required for human discs, even for normal* discs of the same age and spinal level. The diversity in the swelling pressure of normal human discs and the even greater diversity between pathological discs made it necessary to take several serial slices from every disc studied and incubate each one in medium containing a different PEG concentration.

Slices with a postincubation hydration within $\pm 10\%$ of the in vivo value (determined from an 'unincubated' slice by drying it immediately upon excision) were used to determine the rate of sulfate incorporation. Experiments showed that a hydration change of $\pm 10\%$ had only a very small effect on the rate of [^{35}S]sulfate uptake: when serial slices of dog annulus were incubated, each in medium containing a different PEG concentration, the rate of [^{35}S]sulfate incorporation was highest in slices where the hydration remained closest to that of the unincubated control (Fig. 32.1). If the hydration change was greater than $\pm 10\%$, then the rate was reduced significantly. The effect of increased hydration was also seen in rabbit discs: adult rabbit annulus slices incubated in medium without PEG increased in hydration by 77–124% over 4 h and had rates of incorporation

Table 32.1 Polyethylene glycol concentrations selected for maintaining in vivo hydration during incubation

	% PEG selected	
	Annulus	Nucleus
Rabbit	30	35
Dog	15	20
Human		
Fetal	5	8
Young	8–12	10–12
Adult	8–15	15–20

* The definition of 'normal' used here refers to tissue taken postmortem from donors with no medical history of back problems and which was judged free of pathological signs at the time of dissection. These are by no means satisfactory criteria, but the inherent variability in adult human discs makes it very difficult to define what is normal.

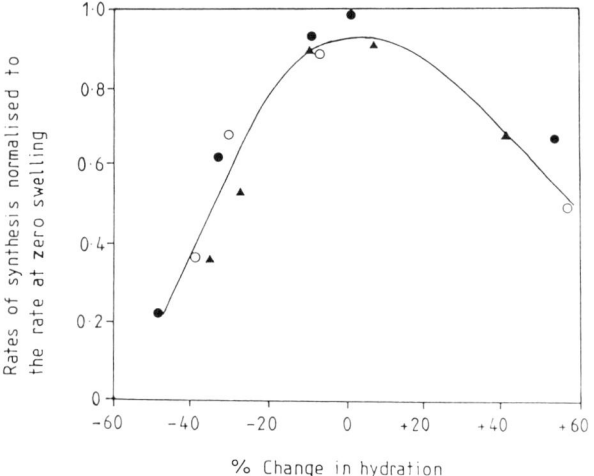

Figure 32.1 Effect of hydration on the rate of [^{35}S]-sulfate incorporation in Beagle annulus fibrosus. Serial slices were obtained from disc levels: (○) L_1–L_2; (●) L_2–L_3; (△) L_0–L_4.

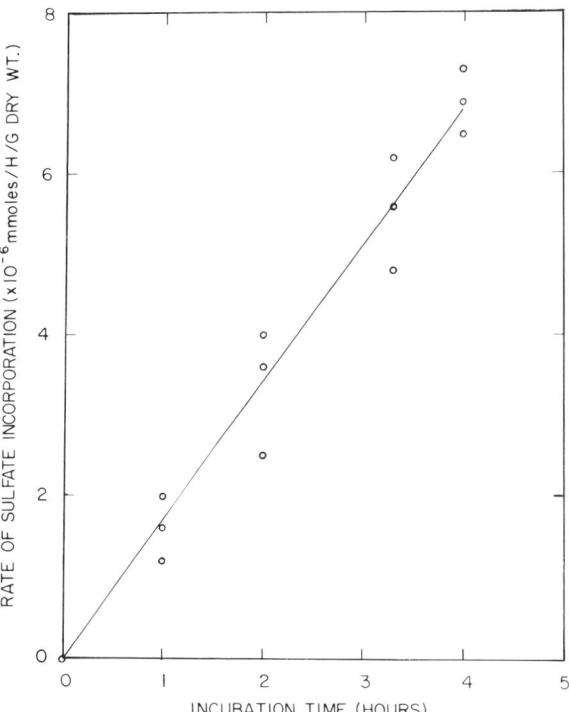

Figure 32.2 Linearity of [^{35}S]-sulfate incorporation with time in culture. Slices of adult human anterior annulus were incubated for different time periods in medium containing [^{35}S]-sulfate. All values shown are for slices where hydration was retained within ± 10% of an unincubated control.

that were 27–58% lower than slices in which hydration change was limited to within ±10%. Decreasing the hydration in human articular cartilage by the addition of PEG to the medium produced the same effect as found in the dog discs; the higher the PEG concentration, the lower the rate of [^{35}S]sulfate uptake (Bayliss et al., 1986). The results of a comparative study by Schneiderman et al. (1986) indicate that this effect is not an artifact of the PEG method since osmotic (PEG) compression reduced uptake by the same degree as mechanical compression for each amount of pressure applied (see Chapter 31).

The incorporation of [^{35}S]sulfate was linear for up to 4 h in disc slices where hydration was retained within ±10% of an unincubated control (Fig. 32.2). For all studies of the rate of PG synthesis, a 4 h incubation period was used. Slices of rabbit disc cultured under the conditions described above had rates of [^{35}S]sulfate uptake of $10–15 \times 10^{-6}$ mmol h^{-1} g dry wt^{-1} for the annulus and $20–30 \times 10^{-6}$ mmol h^{-1} g dry wt^{-1} for the nucleus. These results are similar to those determined by Maroudas (1980) using an in vivo method: $11–16 \times 10^{-6}$ mmol h^{-1} g dry wt^{-1} for the annulus and $33–37 \times 10^{-6}$ mmol h^{-1} g dry wt^{-1} for the nucleus (see Chapter 37).

APPLICATIONS OF THE METHOD

The use of the PEG method has allowed us to determine the topographical distribution of disc cell activity, both by rate determination and by the use of [^{35}S]sulfate autoradiography. The method described above was adapted to prevent swelling and PG loss during fixation of the incubated disc slices in preparation for the autoradiography (Bayliss et al., 1988). By adding a higher amount of radioactive tracer we have used the method to radiolabel newly-synthesized PGs. After extraction, the PGs were characterized using biochemical procedures: their structure and functional capabilities were compared with those of the preexisting PGs (Johnstone and Bayliss, 1988).

The problems of hydration control and matrix leaching affect other areas of study on inter-vertebral-disc tissue, such as physicochemical and histochemical measurements and biomechanical testing. The method described here has applications in all these areas.

References

Armstrong, C.G., Lai, W.M. and Mow, V.C. (1984). An analysis of the unconfined compression of articular cartilage. *J. Biomech. Eng.* **106**, 165–173

Auron, P.E., Webb, A.C. and Rossenwasser, J.J. (1984). Nucleotide sequence of human monocyte interleukin 1 precursor cDNA. *Proc. Natl. Acad. Sci. USA*, **81**, 7907–7911

Bayliss, M.T., Urban, J.P.G., Johnstone, B. and Holm, S. (1986). In vitro method for measuring synthesis rates in the intervertebral disc. *J. Orthop. Res.* **4**, 10–17

Bayliss, M.T., Johnstone, B. and O'Brien, J.P. (1988). Proteoglycan synthesis in the human intervertebral disc. Variation with age, region and pathology. *Spine* **13**, 972–981

Benton, H.P. and Tyler, J.A. (1988). Inhibition of cartilage proteoglycan synthesis by interleukin 1. *Biochim. Biophys. Res. Commun.*, **154**, 421–428

Benya, P.D., Brown, P.D. and Padilla, S.R. (1988). Microfilament modification by dihydrocytochalasin B causes retinoic acid-modulated chondrocytes to re-express the differentiated collagen phenotype without change in shape. *J. Cell. Biol.* **106**, 161–170

Bird, T.A. and Saklatvala, J. (1986). Identification of a common class of high affinity receptors for both types of porcine interleukin 1 on connective tissues. *Nature* **324**, 236–265

Bunning, R.A.D. and Russell, R.G.G. (1989). The effect of TNFα and interferon on the reabsorption of human articular cartilage and on the production of prostaglandin E and caseinase activity on human articular chondrocytes. *Arth. Rheum.* **32**, 780–784

Campbell, M.A., Handley, C.J., Hascall, V.C., Campbell, R.A. and Lowther, D.A. (1984). Turnover of proteoglycans in cultures of bovine articular cartilage. *Arch. Biochem. Biophys.* **234**, 275–281

Campbell, M.A., D'Souza, S.E. and Handley, C.J. (1989). Turnover of proteoglycans in articular cartilage cultures. Characterization of medium proteoglycans. *Biochem. J.* **259**, 21–25

Caputo, C.B., Sygowski, L.A., Wolanin, D.J., Patton, S.G., Caccese, R.G., Shaw, A. Roberts, R.A. and DiPasquale, G. (1987). Effects of synthetic metalloproteinase inhibitors on cartilage autolysis in vitro. *J. Pharmacol. E. Ther.* **240**, 460–465

Chandraskehar, S. and Harvey, A.K. (1988). TGFβ is a potent inhibitor of IL1 induced protease activity and proteoglycan degradation. *Biochem. Biophys. Res. Commun.* **157**, 1352–1359

Chandraskehar, S. and Harvey, A.K. (1989). Induction of IL1 receptors on chondrocytes by fibroblast growth factor. *J. Cell Physiol.* **138**, 236–247

DeWitt, M.T., Handley, C.J., Oakes, B.W. and Lowther, D.A. (1984). In vitro response of chondrocytes to mechanical loading: effect of short term mechanical tension. *Connect. Tissue Res.* **12**, 97–109

Dingle, J.T., King, B. and Page Thomas, P. (1987). In vivo studies of articular cartilage damage mediated by catabolin/interleukin 1. *Ann. Rheum. Dis.* **46**, 527–533

DiPasquale, G., Cacesse, R., Pasternak, R., Conaty, J., Hubbs, S. and Perry, K. (1986). Proteoglycan and collagen degrading enzymes from human IL1 stimulated chondrocytes from several species: proteoglycanase and collagenase inhibitors as potentially new disease-modifying anti arthritic agents (42416). *Proc. Sec. Exp. Biol. Med.* **183**, 262–267

Farndale, R.W., Buttle, D.J. and Barratt, A.J. (1986). Improved quantitation and discrimination of sulphated glycosaminoglycans by use of dimethylmethylene blue. *Biochim. Biophys. Acta* **883**, 173–177

Fenton, M.T., Clark, B.D., Collins, K.L., Webb, A.C. Rich, A. and Auron, P.E. (1987). Transcriptional regulation of the human prointerleukin 1β gene. *J. Immunol.* **183**, 3972–3979.

Gauldie, J. (1989). Interleukin 6. In *The Inflammatory Response in the Therapeutic Control of Inflammatory Diseases* (A.J. Lewis, N.F. Doherty and N.R. Ackerman, eds), pp. 38–46. Elsevier, Amsterdam

Gauldie, J., Richards, G., Harmish, D., Lansdrop, P. and Baumann, H. (1987). Interferon β/BSF-2 shares identity with monocyte-derived heptocyte stimulatory factor (HSF) and regulates the major acute phase protein response in liver cells. *Proc. Natl. Acad. Sci. USA*, **84**, 7251–7255

Gray, M.L., Pizzanelli, A.M., Grozinsky, A.J. and Lee, R.C. (1988). Mechanical and physiochemical determinants of chondrocyte biosynthetic response. *J. Orthop. Res.* **6**, 777–792

Gray, M.L., Pizzanelli, A.M., Lee, R.C., Grodzinsky, A.J. and Swann, D.A. (1989). Kinetics of the chondrocyte biosynthetic response to compressive load and release. *Biochim. Biophys. Acta* **991**, 415–425

Guerne, P.A., Vaughan, J.H., Carson, D.A., Terkeltaub, B. and Lotz, M. (1989). Interluekin 6 and joint tissues. *Ann. N.Y. Acad. Sci.* **557**, 558–561

Handley, C.J. and Campbell, M.A. (1987). Catabolism and turnover of proteoglycans. In *Methods in Enzymology, Structural and Contractile Proteins*, (L.E. Cunningham, ed.), Vol. 114, pp. 412–419. Academic Press, Orlando

Handley, C.J. and Lowther, D.A. (1976). Inhibition of proteoglycan biosynthesis by hyaluronic acid in chondrocytes in cell culture. *Biochim. Biophys. Acta* **444**, 69–74

Handley, C.J., McQuillan, D.J., Campbell, M.A. and Bolis, S. (1986). Steady-state metabolism in cartilage explants. In *Articular Cartilage Biochemistry*, (K.E. Kuettner, R. Schleyerbach and V.C. Hascall, eds), Chap. 14, pp. 163–179. Raven Press, New York

Hascall, V.C., Handley, C.J., McQuillan, D.J., Robinson, H.C. and Lowther, D.A. (1983a). The effect of serum on biosynthesis of proteoglycans by bovine articular cartilage in culture. *Arch. Biochem. Biophys.* **224**, 206–223

Hascall, V.C., Morales, T.I., Hascall, G.K., Handley, C.J. and McQuillan, D.J. (1983b). Biosynthesis and tunover of proteoglycans in organ cultures of bovine articular cartilage. *J. Rheum. Suppl.* **11**, 45–52

Henderson, B. and Davies, D.E. (1990). The design of inhibitors of cartilage breakdown. In *Osteoarthritis: Current Research and Prospects for Pharmacological Intervention* (R.G.G. Russell and P.A. Dieppe, eds), pp. 203–214

Johnstone, B. and Bayliss, M.T. (1988). Age-related heterogeneity of human intervertebral disc proteoglycans. *Trans. Orthop. Res.* **13**, 275

Jones, I.L., Klamfeldt, D.D.S. and Sandstrom, T. (1982). The effect of continuous mechanical pressure upon the turnover of articular cartilage proteoglycans *in vitro*. *Clin. Orthop.* **165**, 283–289

Jubb, R.W. and Saklatvala, J. (1985). Effect of pig IL1 (catabolin) on human articular chondrocytes. *Br. J. Rheumatol.* **24**, (Suppl 1), 156–157

Kempson, G.E. (1975). The effects of proteoglycan and collagen degradation on the mechanical properties of adult human articular cartilage. In *Dynamics of Connective Tissue Macromolecules*, (P.M.C. Burleigh and A.R. Poole, eds), pp. 277–307. North-Holland Publishing Company, Amsterdam

Kim, Y. (1989). Radially unconfined compression of poroelastic media with axisymmetric boundary conditions. Master's thesis, M.I.T., Cambridge, Massachusetts

Kimura, J.H., Thonar, E.J-M., Hascall, V.C., Reiner, A. and Poole, A.R. (1981). Identification of core protein, an intermediate of proteoglycan biosynthesis in cultured chondrocytes for the Swarm rat chondrosarcoma. *J. Biol. Chem.* **256**, 7890–7897

Kishimoto, T., Taga, R. and Yamazaki, K. (1989). Normal and abnormal regulation of human B cell differentiation by new cytokine BSF-2/IL6. In *Mechanisms of Lymphocyte Activation and Immune Regulation* (S. Gupta, W.E. Paul and A.S. Franci, eds), pp. 167–181. Plenum Press, New York

Lomedico, P.T., Gubler, U. and Hellman, C.P. (1984). Cloning and expression of murine IL1 in *E. coli*. *Nature* **312**, 458–462

Luyten, F.P., Hascall, V.C., Nissley, S.P., Morales, T.I. and Reddi, A.H. (1988). Insulin-like growth factors maintain steady state metabolism of proteoglycans in bovine articular cartilage explants. *Arch. Biochem. Biophys.* **267**, 416–425

Marcus, R.E. (1973). The effect of low oxygen concentration in growth, glycolysis and sulphate incorporation by articular chondrocytes in monolayer culture. *Arthr. Rheum.* **16**, 646–656

Marmenout, A., Fransen, L. and Tavernier, J. (1985). Molecular cloning and expression of human tumor necrosis factor. *Eur. J. Biochm.* **152**, 15–22

Maroudas, A. (1979). Physico-chemical properties of articular cartilage. In *Adult Articular Cartilage* (M.A.R. Freeman), pp. 215–290. Pitman Medical, London

Maroudas, A. (1980). Metabolism of cartilaginous tissue, a quantitative approach. In *Studies in Joint Diseases*, (A. Maroudas and J. Holborrow, eds), Vol. 1, pp. 59–86. Pitman Medical, London

Maroudas, A. (1985). The function of articular cartilage in terms of its structure in a healthy joint. How is it altered in the degenerative joint? Proc. 2nd Conference on Degenerative Joint Diseases. *Experta Media* 99–115

Maroudas, A. and Evans, H. (1974). Sulfate diffusion and incorporation into articular cartilage. *Biochim. Biophys. Acta* **338**, 265–279

Matsushima, K., Yadoi, J., Tagaya, Y. and Oppenheim, J.J. (1986). Down regulation of IL1 receptor expression by IL1 and fate of internalized ^{125}I labelled IL1 beta in human large granular lymphocyte cell line. *J. Immunol.* **137**, 3183–3188

McQuillan, D.J., Handley, C.J., Robinson, H.C., Ng, K. and Tzaicos, C. (1986a). The relationship of RNA synthesis to chondroitin sulphate biosynthesis in cultured bovine cartilage. *Biochem. J.* **235**, 499–505

McQuillan, D.J., Handley, C.J. and Robinson, H.C. (1986b). Control of proteoglycan biosynthesis. Futher studies on the effect of serum on cultured bovine articular cartilage. *Biochem. J.* **240**, 423–430

Morales, T.I. and Roberts, A.B. (1988). Transforming growth factor-β regulates metabolism of proteoglycans in bovine cartilage organ cultures. *J. Biol. Chem.* **263**, 12 828–12 831

Morales, T.I., Wahl, L.M. and Hascall, V.C. (1984). The effect of bacterial lipopolysaccharides on the biosynthesis and release of proteoglycans from calf articular cartilage cultures. *J. Biol. Chem.* **259**, 6720–6729

Olliviere, F., Gubler, U., Towle, C.A., Laurencin, C. and Treadwell, B.C. (1986). Expression of IL1 gene in human and bovine chondrocytes. A mechanism for autocrine control of cartilage matrix degradation. *Biochim. Biophys. Res. Commun.* **141**, 904–911

Palmoski, M.J. and Brandt, K.D. (1984). Effects of static and cyclic compressive loading on articular cartilage plugs *in vitro*. *Arthr. Rheum.* **27**, 675–681

Pettipher, E.R., Higgs, G.A. and Hendersen, B. (1986). IL1 induces leucocyte infiltration and cartilage proteoglycan degradation in the synovial fluid joint. *Proc. Natl. Acad. Sci.* **83**, 8749–8753

Poole, C.A., Flint, M.H. and Beaumont, B.W. (1985). Analysis of the morphology and function of primary cillia in connective tissues: a cellular cybernetic. *Cell Motil.* **5**, 175–193

Pousty, T., Bari-Khan, M.A. and Butler, W.F. (1975). Leaching of glycosaminoglycans from tissue by the fixatives formaline-saline and formiline-cetrimide. *Histochem. J.* **7**, 361–365

Rath, N.C., Oronsky, A.L. and Kerwar, S.S. (1988). Synthesis of IL1-like activity by normal rat chondrocytes in culture. *Clin. Immunol. Immunopathol.* **47**, 39–46

Ratcliffe, A., Tyler, J.A. and Hardingham, T.E. (1986). Articular cartilage cultured with IL1. Increased release of link protein, hyaluronate binding region and other proteoglycan fragments. *Biochem. J.* **228**, 571–580

Ridgway, G. (1984). The structure and biosynthesis of human articular cartilage proteoglycans. PhD. Thesis, University of London

Robinson, H.C. (1969). The sulfation of chondroitin sulphate in embryonic chicken cartilage. *Biochem. J.* **113**, 543–549

Rodan, G.A., Bourret, L.A., Harvey, A. and Mensi, T. (1975). Cyclic AMP and cyclic CMP mediators of the mechanical effects on bone remodelling. *Science* **189**, 467–469

Sah, R.L., Doong, J.Y.H., Kim, Y.L., Grodzinski, A.J., Plaas, A.H.K. and Sandy, J.D. (1988). Biosynthetic response of cartilage explants to mechanical and physicochemical stimuli. *Trans. Orthop. Res. Soc.* **13**, 70

Sah, R.L., Kim, Y.L., Doong, J.Y.H., Grodzinski, A.J., Plaas, A.H.K. and Sandy, J.D. (1989). Biosynthetic response of cartilage explants to dynamic compression. *J. Orthop. Res.* **7**, 619–639

Saklatvala, J., Sarsfield, S.J. and Townsend, Y. (1985). Pig IL1. Purification of two immunologically different leucocyte proteins that cause cartilage resorption, lymphocyte activation and fever. *J. Exp. Med.* **162**, 1208–1222

Saklatvala, J. (1986). Tumour necrosis factor stimulates resorption and inhibits synthesis of proteoglycan in cartilage. *Nature* **322**, 547–549

Sandy, J.D. and Plaas, A.H.K. (1986). Age related changes in the kinetics of release of proteoglycan subunits from normal cartilage explants. *Orthop. Res.* **4**, 263–272

Sandy, J.D., Brown, H.L.G. and Lowther, D.A. (1978). Degradation of proteoglycan in articular cartilage. *Biochim. Biophys. Acta* **543**, 536–544

Sandy, J.D., Brown, H.L.G. and Lowther, D.A. (1980). Control of proteoglycan sythesis. Studies on the activation of synthesis observed during culture of articular cartilages. *Biochem. J.* **188**, 119–130

Schneiderman, R. (1987). Regulation of the metabolism of weight-bearing tissues. Ph.D. thesis, Technion-Israel Institute of Technology, Haifa, Israel

Schneiderman, R. Keret, D. and Maroudas, A. (1986). Effects of mechanical and osmotic pressure on the rate of glycosaminoglycan synthesis in the human adult femoral head cartilage. An *in vitro* study. *J. Orthop. Res.* **4**, 393–408

Shinmei, M., Kikuchi, T., Masuda, K. and Shimomura, Y. (1988a). Effects of IL1 and anti inflammatory drugs on the degradation of human articular cartilage. *Drugs* **35** (Suppl. 1), 33–41

Shinmei, M., Masuda, K., Kikuchi, T. and Shimomura, Y. (1988b). Interleukin 1, tumour necrosis factor and interleukin 6 as mediators of cartilage destruction. *Sem. Arth. Rheum.* **183**, 27–32

Sobue, M., Takeuchi, J. Ito, K., Kimata, K. and Suzuki, S. (1978). Effect of environmental sulfate concentration on the synthesis of low and high sulfated chondroitin sulfates by chick embryo cells. *J. Biol. Chem.* **253**, 6190–6196

Tougaard, L. (1973). The degree of mineralization in bone tissues. The phosphorous/hydroxyproline ratio determined on small amounts of bone tissue. *Scand. J. Clin. Invest.* **32**, 351–355

Tyler, J.A. (1985a). Chondrocyte mediated depletion of articular cartilage *in vitro*. *Biochem. J.* **225**, 493–507

Tyler, J.A. (1985b). Articular cartilage cultures with catabolin (pig IL1) synthesizes a decreased number of normal proteoglycan molecules. *Biochem. J.* **227**, 869–878

Tyler, J.A. (1989). IGF 1 can decrease degradation and promaote synthesis of proteoglycan in cartilage exposed to cytokines. *Biochem. J.* **260**, 543–548

Tyler, J.A. (1990). Cartilage degradation. In *Cartilage: Molecular Aspects* (B.K. Hall and S.A. Newman, eds). Telford Press

Urban, J.P.G. and Bayliss, M.T. (1989). Regulation of proteoglycan synthesis rate in cartilage; *in vitro*: influence of extracellular ionic composition. *Biochim. Biophys. Acta* **992**, 59–65

Urban, J.P.G. and Maroudas, A. (1979). Measurement of fixed charge density and partition coefficients in the intervertebral disc. *Biochi. Biophys. Acta* **586**, 166–178

Urban, J.P.G. and Maroudas, A. (1981). Swelling of the intervertebral disc *in vitro*. *Connect. Tiss. Res.* **9**, 1–10

van de Loo, A.A.J., van Beuningen, H.M., van Lent, P.L.E.M. and van den Berg, W.B. (1989). Direct effect of murine IL1 on cartilage metabolism *in vivo*. *Agents Actions* **26**, 153–155

6

USE OF RADIOISOTOPES TO STUDY METABOLISM OF MATRIX MOLECULES

COLLATED BY V.C. HASCALL

33

Introduction

VINCENT C. HASCALL

The papers in this section explore the various ways in which radioisotopes can be used to study synthesis and catabolism of matrix macromolecules either *in vitro* or *in vivo*. For proteoglycan (PG) synthesis, radiosulfate is clearly the isotope of choice for most applications; it is relatively inexpensive, it equilibrates rapidly between extracellular and intracellular compartments, it is incorporated preferentially (usually more than 90%) into PGs as the last stage of their maturation and its specific activity in the immediate vicinity of a cell in almost all cases can be equated with the specific activity of the intracellular metabolite for sulfate transfer, phosphoadenosinephosphosulfate (PAPs). In cell or organ culture, the specific activity of the radiosulfate and its equilibration time to steady-state incorporation (usually a few minutes) can be measured directly. As discussed by Hascall *et al.* in Chapter 34, the specific activity of the radiosulfate incorporated into chondroitin sulfate or dermatan sulfate can be used to determine the specific activity of carbohydrate radioprecursors, such as [^{3}H]glucosamine, which are also incorporated into the glycosaminoglycan and oligosaccharide structures on PGs. The procedure also offers an indirect method to determine the rate of synthesis of hyaluronan which does not contain sulfate residues in its structure.

Studies *in vivo* are complicated by the difficulty in measuring specific activities of precursors, particularly as they change rapidly in single-dose experiments. Mason (Chapter 35) discusses this problem and compares the use of radiosulfate in a single-dose (pulse-chase) protocol with a controlled-infusion (steady-state label-chase) protocol to determine half-life values for PGs associated with the rat glomerular basement membrane. McAnulty and Laurent (Chapter 36) present another approach designed to circumvent the specific activity problem in studying the biosynthesis of macromolecules. In their methods, a flooding dose of unlabeled precursor is injected with the radiolabel, in this case radiolabeled proline, which essentially fixes the specific activity of the labeling precursor during the several hours of the experiment. The procedure is particularly suited to collagen synthesis because the specific activity of the hydroxyproline derived from the labeled proline can be determined and the fractional amount of collagen synthesized during the pulse period calculated directly as this amino acid is almost unique to collagen.

Maroudas (Chapter 37) deals more directly with determining the specific activity of the radiosulfate as a function of time following a single-dose injection *in vivo*, both in serum and in tissue samples taken at different times after introducing the label. Relative contributions to both synthesis and catabolism can then be evaluated directly. The assumptions inherent in this approach are assessed as is the relationship between values obtained in short-term *in vitro* labeling and values observed for the same tissue *in vivo*.

Finally, Lohmander (Chapter 38) describes how kinetic analyses of the entry of label from the precursor into different structures in mature PGs can reveal information about where synthetic steps are likely to occur during the progression of a core protein to a final PG structure. In this case, evidence is provided that xylosylation occurs as a relatively late step, possibly in an early Golgi compartment, shortly before the rest of the glycosaminoglycan chains are added.

Overall, this section presents a variety of methodological approaches which can be used to study synthesis and catabolism of matrix macromolecules with radioisotopes and provides an assessment of the underlying assumptions that need to be considered for appropriate analysis of the resulting data.

34

The use of radiolabeled glucosamine as a precursor for measuring hyaluronan synthesis

VINCENT C. HASCALL, MASAKI YANAGISHITA,
ANTONIETTA SALUSTRI and TERESA I. MORALES

INTRODUCTION

Hyaluronan (HA) is a nonsulfated glycosaminoglycan (GAG) which consists of a linear repeat sequence of the disaccharide (glucuronic acid-β-1,3-N-acetylglucosamine-β-1,4-)$_n$, where n is usually very large, 10 000 or more. HA is synthesized by a large variety of cells and its synthetic rate can vary widely depending upon the type of cell and its environment. [^{3}H]Glucosamine is widely used as a precursor for studying HA synthesis. However, the relative amount of this precursor used by the cell relative to endogenous sources for hexosamine, primarily glucose, to synthesize the metabolic precursor UDP-N-acetylglucosamine varies widely with experimental conditions. The specific activity of the glucosamine in the nucleotide sugar pool is, therefore, less than that of the glucosamine in the labeling medium, frequently by several-hundred-fold; for a given cell type, it can vary significantly depending upon changes in growth factors, hormones, nutrients, etc., in the medium. Thus, differences in the relative rates of incorporation of the isotopic precursor in two different culture conditions may not reflect the same differences in the amounts of HA being synthesized.

In this chapter we describe several experiments in which indirect methods are used to estimate metabolic parameters for HA. The methods used take advantage of the facts that: (i) [^{3}H]glucosamine is also a direct precursor for the synthesis of chondroitin/dermatan sulfate (CS/DS); and (b) radiosulfate can be used to determine the mass of this sulfated GAG synthesized during experimental protocols, thereby providing a correction for changes in specific activity of the hexosamine constituent in both HA and CS/DS.

RAT OVARIAN GRANULOSA CELLS

Rat ovarian granulosa cells synthesize DS PGs with chains consisting of a linear repeat sequence containing two predominant disaccharides (Yanagishita and Hascall, 1979, 1983):

1 (glucuronic acid-β-1,3-N-acetyl-
    -galactosamine-β-1,4-)   (c. 82%)
        |
     4-O-SO$_3$

2 (iduronic acid-α-1,3-N-acetyl-
    |
   2-O-SO$_3$
    -galactosamine-β-1,4-)   (c. 17%)
        |
     6-O-SO$_3$

After chondroitinase digestion, these disaccharides are released with the formation of 4,5-unsaturated, non-reducing terminal hexuronic acid moieties; the predominant mono-4-sulfated disaccharide unit in the chain would yield Δdi-4S (Fig. 34.1). The disaccharide digestion products can then be separated and quantitated by suitable HPLC or thin layer chromatographic procedures (Yanagishita et al., 1989).

ΔDi-4S contains one sulfate ester and one galactosamine which are metabolically labeled with [^{35}S]sulfate and [^{3}H]glucosamine, respectively. The [^{3}H]glucosamine and [^{3}H]galactosamine rapidly achieve the same specific activity by 4-epimerization at the UDP-N-acetylhexosamine level.

[^{35}S]Sulfate equilibrates rapidly with the metabolic donor for the O-sulfate esters in the DS chains, phosphoadenosinephosphosulfate (PAPS). The only other metabolic sources for sulfate, cysteine and methionine, contribute less than 2% to the sulfate pool when environmental sulfate is 100 μM or above (Yanagishita et al., 1989). Within a few minutes, therefore, the specific activity of the sulfate in PAPS is equal to that of the radiosulfate in the labeling medium (e.g. Lohmander et al., 1986).

$$\text{sa}(^{35}\text{S})_m = \text{sa}(^{35}\text{S-PAPS}) \quad (34.1)$$

Therefore, the radioactivity recovered in Δdi-4S after chondroitinase digestion provides a direct measure of the mass of disaccharide 1 synthesized during the labeling protocol for labeling times significantly longer than the equilibration time between the medium radiosulfate and the PAPS pool. Ideally, the rate of synthesis of DSPG during the labeling time will be constant, a condition which is usually the case for most experimental situations.

The situation with [^{3}H]glucosamine is different. This labeling precursor is diluted by unlabeled glucosamine derived by metabolic conversion of glucose taken up from the medium and of glucose derived from intracellular metabolic pathways. Furthermore, the equilibration time between the labeled glucosamine in the medium and that in the UDP-N-acetylhexosamine pool is longer; half-lifes to equilibration are on the order of 20–60 min (Thonar et al., 1983; Malmstrom, 1984; Lohmander et al., 1986). Thus, the ratio of specific activity of ^{3}H in the UDP-N-acetylhexosamine pool to that in the medium glucosamine will be less than 1.

In a labeling experiment with [^{35}S]sulfate, the moles of disaccharide 1 synthesized can be calculated by determining the moles of sulfate incorporated into Δdi-4S, mol(^{35}S)$_d$. This is given by the total ^{35}S radioactivity in the purified Δdi-4S, dpm(^{35}S)$_d$, divided by the specific activity of the [^{35}S]sulfate in the PAPS donor which is equal to the specific activity of the radiosulfate in the medium, sa(^{35}S)$_m$ (equation (34.1)). This value is

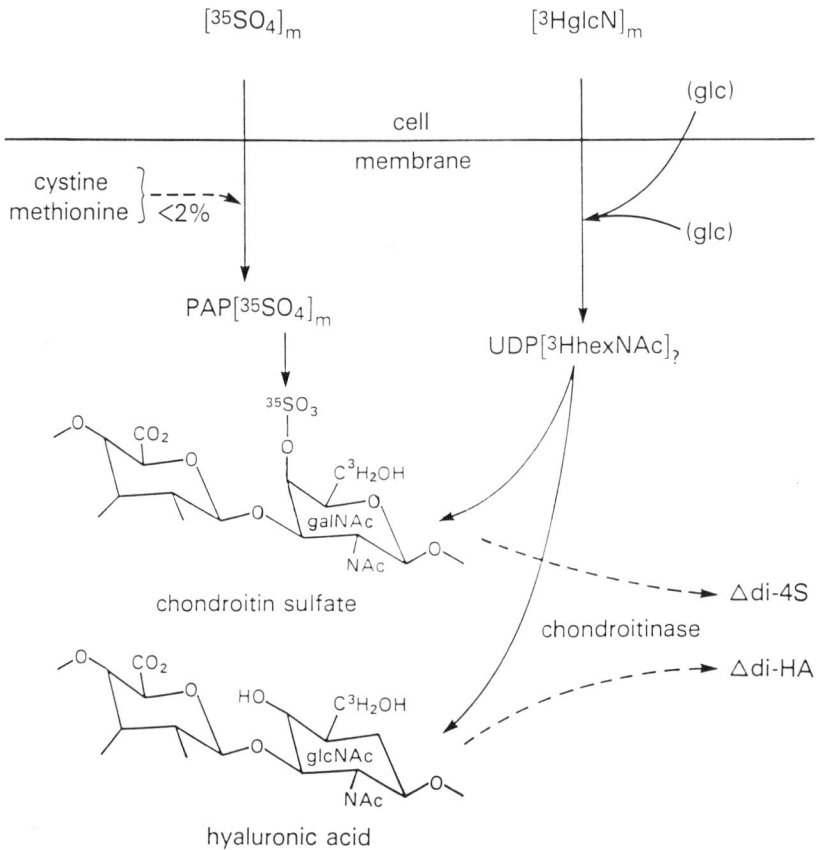

Figure 34.1 HA synthesis.

also equal to the moles of *N*-acetylgalactosamine incorporated, mol(galNAc)$_d$, because of its 1:1 stoichiometry with the sulfate moiety in the disaccharide. Therefore,

$$\text{mol}(^{35}\text{S})_d = \text{mol(galNAc)}_d = \text{dpm}(^{35}\text{S})_d/\text{sa}(^{35}\text{S})_m \quad (34.2)$$

For a double-labeling experiment with [^{3}H]-glucosamine as well as [^{35}S]sulfate, the specific activity of the *N*-acetylgalactosamine in disaccharide **1** synthesized during the labeling protocol, sa(^{3}H-galNac)$_d$, will be the total ^{3}H radioactivity in the purified Δdi-4S, dpm(^{3}H)$_d$, divided by the moles of *N*-acetylgalactosamine in the disaccharide, mol(galNAc)$_d$.

$$\text{sa}(^3\text{H-galNAc})_d = \text{dpm}(^3\text{H})_d/\text{mol(galNAc)}_d \quad (34.3)$$

which, from equation (34.2) gives

$$\begin{aligned}\text{sa}(^3\text{H-galNAc})_d &= [\text{dpm}(^3\text{H})_d/\text{dpm}(^{35}\text{S})_d] \times \text{sa}(^{35}\text{S})_m \quad (34.4)\\ &= A \times \text{sa}(^{35}\text{S})_m\end{aligned}$$

where A is the ratio of dpm, ^{3}H/^{35}S, in Δdi-4S. The dilution, D, between the specific activity of [^{3}H]glucosamine in the medium, sa(^{3}H)$_m$, and that of the [^{3}H]galactosamine in Δdi-4S, sa(^{3}H-galNAc)$_d$, is then given by their ratio, which from equation (34.4) gives

$$D = \text{sa}(^3\text{H-galNAc})_d/\text{sa}(^3\text{H})_m$$
$$= [A \times \text{sa}(^{35}\text{S})_m]/\text{sa}(^3\text{H})_m \quad (34.5)$$
$$D = A \times B$$

where B is the ratio of the specific activities, ^{35}S/^{3}H of the labeling precursors in the medium. D is defined as the dilution factor.

Table 34.1 summarizes the results of an experiment in which identical cultures of granulosa cells were labeled for 20 h in media with equal dpm and constant specific activity of [^{3}H]glucosamine in combination with equal dpm but different specific activities of [^{35}S]sulfate. Table 34.2 summarizes the results of the reciprocal experiment in which the media contained equal dpm and constant specific activity of [^{35}S] sulfate in combination with equal dpm but different specific activities of [^{3}H]glucosamine. Δdi-4S was purified from each culture and the parameters calculated from the equations above (see Tables 34.1 and 34.2).

Table 34.1 Effect of environmental sulfate concentration on incorporation of [^{35}S]sulfate into Δdi-4S

[SO$_4$]$_m$ (μM)	sa(^{35}S)$_m$ (mCi mmol^{-1})	sa(^{35}S)$_d$ (mCi mmol^{-1})	D sa(^{35}S)$_m$/sa(^{35}S)$_d$
80	125	123	1.02
130	77	92	0.84
180	56	61	0.92
280	36	39	0.92
880	11	11*	1.00*

* The specific activity of ^{35}S in Δdi-4S, sa(^{35}S)$_d$, for the highest sulfate concentration, 880 μM, was assumed to be equal to the specific activity of the sulfate in the medium, sa(^{35}S)$_m$ for the reasons discussed in the text and the dilution factor, D, calculated from the ratio of specific activity of the sulfate in the medium to that in the disaccharide for the other sulfate concentrations. The concentration of glucosamine in the medium was 3 μM and the specific activity of the glucosamine in the medium, sa(^{3}H)$_m$ was 29.5 Ci mmol^{-1}. D for the ^{3}H was constant, c. 1/780, for all the cultures (Table 34.2).

Table 34.2 Effect of environmental glucosamine on incorporation of ^{3}H from [^{3}H]glucosamine into Δdi-4S*

[glcNAc]$_m$ (μM)	sa(^{3}H)$_m$ (mCi mmol^{-1})	A	B	D†
3	29.5	3.45	0.37 × 10^{-3}	1/780
13	6.8	3.36	1.62 × 10^{-3}	1/180
100	0.90	3.00	12.2 × 10^{-3}	1/27
300	0.29	2.72	37.9 × 10^{-3}	1/9.7
1000	0.088	2.36	125 × 10^{-3}	1/3.4

* The sulfate concentration was 880 μM and the specific activity of the sulfate in the medium, sa(^{35}S)$_m$, was 11 mCi mmol^{-1} for all cultures.
† $D = AB$, see equation (34.5).

In the first experiment, the dilution factor for the hexosamine, D, did not change because the dpm of [^{3}H]galNAc in Δdi-4S was the same for all cultures. For the reasons discussed above, the specific activity of ^{35}S in the disaccharide was assumed to be the same as that of ^{35}S in the medium for the culture with the highest concentration of sulfate in the medium and D was calculated from the data for all the other cultures as indicated in Table 34.1. The specific activity of ^{35}S in Δdi-4S decreased in proportion to the decrease in the specific activity of the [^{35}S]sulfate in the medium, as reflected by the nearly constant value of $D \simeq 1$. This is the result expected for a classic isotope dilution experiment and confirms the assumption that the specific activity of the sulfate in the medium is equivalent to that in PAPS (equation (34.5)).

In the second experiment, the dpm of ^{35}S in Δdi-4S was constant for all cultures, as expected. However, the dpm of ^{3}H in the disaccharide, as reflected by the labeling ratio, A, did not decrease to nearly the same extent as for the specific activity of the [^{3}H]glucosamine in the medium, sa(^{3}H)$_m$, as reflected by the large increase in B which is inversely proportional to sa(^{3}H)$_m$ (equation (34.5)). The labeling ratio only decreased by c. 1/3 while sa(^{3}H)$_m$ decreased by more than 300-fold. At the highest specific activity of the precursors, D was c. 1/780, while at the lowest specific activity D was

c. 1/3.4. This indicates that only 1 out of c. 780 (or 1 out of c. 3.4) of the galactosamines recovered in Δdi-4S was derived from the [^{3}H]glucosamine in cultures with the highest (or lowest) sa(^{3}H)$_m$.

MOUSE CUMULUS CELL–OOCYTE COMPLEX MUCIFICATION

The procedure described above was used to study HA synthesis by mouse cumulus cell–oocyte complexes (COCs) induced to mucify *in vitro* with follicle-stimulating hormone (FSH) or with dibutyryl cyclic AMP (Bt$_2$cAMP) (Salustri et al., 1989). Increases in HA synthesis and its deposition in the extracellular matrix of the cumulus cells surrounding the oocyte correlate with COC expansion during mucification. Stimulation with optimal concentrations of Bt$_2$cAMP consistently gave higher dpm of ^{3}H in Δdi-HA, the disaccharide derived from HA after chondroitinase digestion, than did FSH (Table 34.3). However, when the specific activities of ^{3}H in Δdi-4S derived from the DSPG synthesized by the COCs were determined as described above, the value for Δdi-4S from the FSH-treated cultures was only c. 56% of that obtained with Bt$_2$cAMP. Thus, when a correction was made for the specific activity differences, the amount of HA synthesized in the FSH treated cultures was increased (Table 34.3). This analysis assumes that the specific activity of the UDP-N-acetylglucosamine used for synthesis of HA is the same as that of the UDP-N-acetylgalactosamine used for synthesis of the DSPG in the same cells. This is likely to be the case since cytoplasmic nucleotide sugars would be the common source for both synthetic systems even though that for the DSPG is in the Golgi compartment (Lohmander et al., 1986), while that for HA appears to be associated with a cytoplasmic compartment near the cell surface (Prehm, 1984).

HYALURONAN METABOLISM IN ARTICULAR CARTILAGE EXPLANTS

HA forms the backbone structure for the CS/keratan sulfate (KS)PG aggregates in cartilage (Hascall, 1988). Chondrocytes in articular cartilage regulate both synthesis and catabolism of the CS/KSPGs and aspects of these metabolic processes have been studied extensively in explant cultures of young bovine articular cartilage (Hascall et al., 1983). PG parameters in this model system can be studied conveniently with [^{35}S]sulfate as a metabolic precursor because almost all of the incorporated activity resides in the PGs. Double-labeling experiments with [^{35}S]sulfate and [^{3}H]glucosamine were done with cultures maintaining steady-state metabolism of PGs throughout the 23 days of the experiment (Hascall et al., 1983) to compare metabolic parameters for HA with those of the PGs (Morales

Table 34.3 Effects of FSH and Bt$_2$cAMP on synthesis of HA in mouse COCs*

Treatment	^{3}H-Δdi-HA (cpm COC^{-1})	sa(^{3}H-glcNAc)$_d$ (μCi nmol^{-1})	net HA synthesis (pmol glcNAc/COC)
Basal	100	0.16	0.56
FSH	610 (6.1)	0.10	5.54 (9.9)
Bt$_2$cAMP	720 (7.2)	0.18	3.64 (6.5)

* COCs were isolated and cultured for 18 h as described by Salustri et al. (1989) in medium alone (basal) or with 1 μg FSH ml^{-1} (FSH) or with 2 mM Bt$_2$cAMP (Bt$_2$cAMP). For each treatment, the specific activity of the glucosamine in Δdi-HA was determined from that for galactosamine in Δdi-4S as described in the text and this value used to calculate the net amount of glucosamine incorporated in HA during the labeling period. The values in parentheses are the ratios for treated to basal cultures.

and Hascall, 1988). The chemical ratio of HA to CS in the tissue was constant (range 1.4–1.8) and equivalent to their ^{3}H labeling ratio (range 1.1–1.6) for cultures labeled for 6 h on days 8, 18 and 23. This ratio is approximately the value expected for CS/KSPG aggregates.

The equivalence of the chemical and ^{3}H labeling ratios in steady-state conditions indicates that the catabolic half-lifes for HA and CS in the tissue must be the same. Furthermore, if most of the HA is in aggregates, the catabolic mechanism would involve coordinate removal of both the HA backbone and the CS/KSPG monomers in aggregates. This was tested directly in pulse-chase experiments. Cultures were labeled for 20 h on experimental day 0, washed and then chased for 2 or 20 days with daily replacement of medium. Native PG aggregates, i.e. ones which were not exposed to dissociative solvents, in which many CS/KSPG monomers are bound to individual HA molecules, were isolated by a protocol including: digestion of 30 μm sections of the tissue with purified collagenase; extraction with an associative solvent; and centrifugation in both zonal and isopycnic density gradients. The final preparations represented c. 35% of the total PG in the original tissue. The net amount of ^{3}H in both HA and CS decreased to c. 50% from day 2 to day 20, as did the net amount of ^{35}S in CS. The loss of both isotopes from CS yielded the same value for the half-life of the CS/KSPG in aggregates, c. 18 days, and also validates the use of the ^{3}H label for monitoring catabolism of HA. The result confirms that HA in native aggregates is catabolized with the same half-life as the bound monomers.

As with the studies on COC mucification described above, HA metabolic parameters in the cartilage explant model were determined by comparison with the metabolic properties of a sulfated PG synthesized by the same cells.

35

Assessment of turnover of proteoglycans *in vivo*

ROGER M. MASON

INTRODUCTION

There are two advantages in measuring proteoglycan (PG) synthesis and turnover *in vivo* rather than *in vitro*. Firstly, the tissue remains intact during the course of the experiment and is subject to all the normal physiological factors which may influence the metabolism of PGs within it. This may be important in studies on cartilage or intervertebral disc. These tissues are difficult to remove for *in vitro* studies without causing them mechanical damage and are liable to swell when placed in tissue culture media. Furthermore, chondrocytes in these tissues are responsive to a variety of physiological stimuli, including hormones, cytokines and dynamic pressure changes, which are difficult to reproduce precisely *in vitro*. Secondly, animal models of disease can be used in *in vivo* experiments to investigate whether PG metabolism undergoes changes in specific tissues. For example, we showed that intervertebral disc PGs in normal, 30-day-old, male CBA mice turn over with rates that follow first-order kinetics and with metabolic half-lives ($t_{1/2}$) of 12.5, 10.5 and 10.7 days in the cervical, thoracic and lumbar discs, respectively (Venn and Mason,

1983). Similar turnover rates were found in the intervertebral discs of ky/ky mice of the same age and sex (Venn and Mason, 1986). In contrast, PG synthesis was elevated in discs at the cervicothoracic junction, where disc degeneration occurs in these animals (Mason and Palfrey, 1984).

METHODS

There are two approaches: (i) pulse-labeling followed by a chase period; and (ii) steady-state labeling followed by a chase period. The former approach has been used most frequently but the second method, which is currently under development in our laboratory, may have a number of advantages. In both methods, the animal is given a dose of [^{35}S]sulfate to label PGs, followed by a dose of nonradioactive sulfate to chase out and dilute out any remaining unincorporated [^{35}S]sulfate. Animals are sacrificed at various periods thereafter and tissues analyzed for [^{35}S]PGs and [^{35}S]glycosaminoglycans (GAGs) (Venn and Mason, 1983; Beavan et al., 1989).

Pulse-chase

Sodium [^{35}S]sulfate is the precursor of choice to label PGs synthesized in vivo. It diffuses readily into the blood from subcutaneous or intraperitoneal injection sites and is taken up rapidly by cells. Plasma radioactivity reaches a maximum of about 7×10^7 ^{35}S-dpm ml^{-1} 40 min after an intraperitoneal injection of 1.8 mCi sodium [^{35}S]sulfate into a 180 g rat and decreases to half this value within about 3.0–3.5 h. The plasma sulfate concentration in rats of this size is 0.33–0.60 mM (mean 0.43 ± 0.1 SD) and is of the same order as found in many tissue-culture media (e.g. DMEM 0.8 mM).

In experiments to measure the turnover of [^{35}S]PGs in intervertebral discs of 30-day-old mice (Venn and Mason 1983), the pulse period was 3 h following an intraperitoneal injection of 20 mCi Na$_2$[^{35}S]O$_4$ (5 mCi/μg sulfur, carrier free)/kg body weight. After 3 h, an intraperitoneal injection of 1 mg Na$_2$SO$_4$ in 0.5 ml of saline was given as a chase. During the labeling period, about 2×10^4 [^{35}S]dpm were incorporated into PGs/μg DNA in intervertebral discs from all spinal regions. Mice were sacrificed between 1 and 45 days after the chase and the radioactivity remaining at each stage was assessed. It is essential that all extraction and purification procedures for [^{35}S]PGs give quantitative recoveries and they should be checked for this. It is important to recognize that procedures such as extraction with 4.0 M guanidine hydrochloride will probably extract a progressively smaller proportion of the total [^{35}S]PGs remaining in either cartilage or intervertebral discs with increasing chase times (Venn and Mason, 1983). Experimental protocols should include tissue digests with papain to establish the total [^{35}S]GAG content and provide a baseline for assessing recoveries. With care, reproducibility between animals is good (e.g. Table II in Beavan et al., 1989) and experiments can be carried out with three or four animals per time point. However, for statistical analyses it may be necessary to use larger numbers (e.g. Figure 1 in Venn and Mason, 1986).

We have refined the basic pulse-chase protocol to measure the turnover of rat glomerular [^{35}S]PGs (Beavan et al., 1989). The pulse-labeling period was 7 h with sodium [^{35}S]sulfate given in two intraperionteal injections at 3.5 h intervals. At various times after the chase (1 mg Na$_2$SO$_4$/ml, 2 ml/100 g body wt), rats were anesthetized and the kidneys perfused with a 0.01% solution of cetylpyridinium chloride to precipitate PGs in the tissue prior to isolation of glomeruli from the renal cortex (Beavan et al., 1988). This yields recoveries of glomerular [^{35}S]PGs two to three times greater than recoveries from 'unfixed' glomeruli. The cetylpyridinium can be dissociated from the GAGs later in high ionic strength salt solutions. Perfusion-fixation is unlikely to have a role in experiments done in vivo involving cartilage since it is avascular and its matrix macromolecules are relatively insoluble at physiological ionic strength. However, such fixation may be required to optimize recoveries in experiments involving other connective tissues. In the analysis of the turnover of glomerular [^{35}S]PGs, quantiative autoradiography and specific immunoprecipitation procedures were used in addition to more standard biochemical analyses to identify particular populations of PGs. In principle, similar methods could be applied to *in vivo* experiments involving cartilage PGs.

Steady-state label-chase

Pulse-labeling has several disadvantages. Firstly, the labeling period, by necessity, is relatively short. Thus macromolecules which are synthesized at a low level and turn over at a slow rate may not be labeled sufficiently to detect them. Nevertheless, they may be quantitatively and physiologically important in the tissue. Secondly, the continuously changing level of the blood ^{35}S radioactivity during a pulse-labeling protocol makes it difficult to calculate the mean specific activity of the blood sulfate over the period of interest (see Chapter 37). However, if the blood ^{35}S specific radioactivity can be kept constant and the labeling period prolonged, it may be assumed that the intracellular 3'-phosphoadenosine-5'-phosphosulphate (PAPS) pool (the sulfate donor in GAG chain synthesis) will reach the same specific activity. The molar amounts of sulfate present in ^{35}S-labeled PGs can then be calculated from the radioactivity and expressed per nanogram of tissue DNA. This is a more absolute indicator to follow the turnover of PGs in *in vivo* experiments than are ^{35}S radioactivity levels. Apart from compensating for the fact that blood sulfate concentration varies between animals within a normal range (see above), this approach also allows comparisons to be made between normal animals and animals with disorders which may alter blood sulfate concentration. For example, rats with alloxan-induced diabetes have reduced blood sulfate concentrations (Spiro, 1987).

We have developed a steady-state *in vivo* labeling procedure using a constant infusion of sodium [^{35}S]sulfate from an Alzet mini-osmotic pump implanted subcutaneously in the rat's neck scruff. The pump chamber (volume 200 μl) is filled with sodium [^{35}S]sulfate (15 mCi ml^{-1}) which is released at a constant rate (1 μl h^{-1}) after implantation. Blood radioactivity reaches a maximum level within 12 h of implantation. It decreases during the next 12 h to about 50% of the maximum level and thereafter remains almost constant over the next five days. Typical blood ^{35}S-radioactivity levels during this phase are 8 to 10×10^5 dpm ml^{-1} for 180 g rats. Serum sulfate concentration is readily measured with a microassay based on the precipitation of [^{133}Ba]SO$_4$ (Cole *et al.*, 1979) and thus the ^{35}S-specific activity during the labeling period can be found.

Modified chase conditions are required to minimize the biosynthetic reutilization of [^{35}S]sulfate released by catabolism of tissue components during the chase period. At the end of the labelling period, the rat is anesthetized, given an intraperitoneal injection of unlabeled sodium sulfate (1 mg ml^{-1}, 1 ml/100 g body wt) and the ^{35}S-minipump removed and replaced by another delivering 100 mM Na$_2$SO$_4$ (1 μl h^{-1}). Measurements of the serum sulfate concentration 3 h after this procedure show that it is the same as prechase levels but the ^{35}S-specific activity is reduced by about 40%. Twenty-four hours after initiating the chase, specific activity is only 15% of initial values and remains at this level over the next 100 h.

Using the steady-state label-chase protocol and the *in vivo* perfusion-fixation procedure, initial experiments have shown that the glomerular PGs turn over at rates similar to those found in pulse-label experiments. In principle, the steady-state label-chase procedure could be used to measure the turnover of PGs in cartilaginous tissues of small laboratory animals such as rats and mice. Used in conjunction with other techniques, such as quantitative autoradiography, immunoprecipitation and agarose-gel electrophoresis, it may provide a powerful tool for exploring this aspect of cartilage matrix biology and pathology.

36

In vivo measurement of collagen metabolism in cartilage and bone

R.J. McANULTY and G.J. LAURENT

INTRODUCTION

Collagens of various types represent the major structural elements of connective tissues. Bone consists predominantly of type I collagen, whereas in cartilage type II is the major component with small amounts of type VI, IX, X and XI. Arthritic diseases are associated with erosion of joint, cartilage and bone. This is likely to be due at least partly to the failure of chondrocytes to maintain a balance between synthesis and degradation of matrix components, including collagens. Altered collagen deposition can result from changes in either synthesis, degradation or both synthesis and degradation. It is therefore important to understand the changes in these processes during disease. The uncertainties arising from studies of chondrocytes in culture, due to the difficulties involved in maintaining phenotype with respect to collagen production (Nimni, 1983), make the study of these processes *in vivo* particularly important.

METHODS FOR MEASURING COLLAGEN TURNOVER *IN VIVO*

The pioneering studies of collagen turnover *in vivo* were based on the uptake of radiolabeled amino acids into protein, followed by subsequent extraction of tissue collagens and measurement of the radioactive-protein decay curves over long periods of time (Neuberger *et al.*, 1951; Neuberger and Slack, 1953; Gerber and Altman, 1960; Kao *et al.*, 1961; Popenoe and Van Slyke, 1962). These studies suggested extremely slow rates of turnover for collagen and led to the belief that collagen was almost inert. The subsequent realization that measurements of protein turnover obtained from decay studies may be severely underestimated due to reutilization of the labelled amino acid resulted in renewed interest in measuring rates of collagen turnover. Two approaches have evolved which overcome the problems associated with precursor reutilization.

Studies employing the decay approach have been developed with the use of nonreutilizable isotopes such as $^{18}O_2$ (Jackson and Heininger, 1974, 1975; Molnar *et al.*, 1986). This isotope is incorporated into collagen during the posttranslational hydroxylation of proline. Since hydroxyproline is not incorporated directly into proteins, it cannot be reutilized when the labeled collagen molecules are degraded. Estimates obtained from studies where reutilizable tritiated or deuterated amino acids were administered simultaneously with $^{18}O_2$ demonstrated that turnover rates may be underestimated by as much as 50% when reutilizable isotopes are used (Jackson and Heininger, 1975; Molnar *et al.*, 1986). The disadvantage of this type of approach is that expensive, specialized equipment is required both for the administration of the isotope and its subsequent measurement in proteins. Furthermore, many animals have to be used over long periods of time, sometimes several-hundred days, to obtain a single rate. The method is, therefore, unsuitable for assessing short-term changes in collagen metabolism. However, the advantage of this method is that accurate estimates are obtainable for the rate of collagen degradation, which may be important when studying the degenerative changes in collagen which occur in joint diseases such as osteoarthritis (OA) and rheumatoid arthritis.

The second approach has been developed with the aim of limiting the effect of isotope reutilization. Collagen synthesis, rather than degradation, is estimated by measuring the rate of incorporation of a radiolabeled precursor into collagen over short periods of time (several hours). Early studies employing this approach involved continuous infusions of radiolabeled proline to obtain constant, specific radioactivity of the free amino acid (Laurent et al., 1978; Robins, 1979; Palmer et al., 1980). More recently, the methods have been simplified by administering a single injection of the radiolabeled amino acid with a large 'flooding' dose of unlabeled amino acid (Laurent, 1982; McAnulty and Laurent, 1987). With the flooding-dose approach, the free amino acid specific activity rises rapidly to a plateau level which is maintained for a variable length of time. This time will depend on the size of the flooding dose and on the rate of amino acid metabolism. Since metabolism tends to be more rapid in smaller animals (McAnulty and Laurent, 1987), the dose may need to be adjusted in different species to maintain a plateau precursor-pool specific activity for sufficient time for estimates of collagen synthesis to be made. Measurements of the specific radioactivities of tissue hydroxyproline and of proline in the precursor pool for protein synthesis, together with the time over which incorporation of isotope is measured, allow estimation of a fractional rate of collagen synthesis using the formula given below.

$$\text{Fractional rate of collagen synthesis (\% day}^{-1}) = \frac{\text{Tissue hydroxyproline specific activity (dpm}\,\mu\text{mol}^{-1})}{\text{Precursor-pool specific activity (dpm}\,\mu\text{mol}^{-1}) \times \text{time (days)}} \times \frac{100}{1}$$

The main difficulty with this type of approach is to determine the appropriate precursor-pool specific activity. The most accurate estimates are likely to come from measurements of prolyl tRNA-specific activities (Kelley et al., 1984) or of the specific activity of proline or hydroxyproline in procollagen (Robins, 1979; Palmer et al., 1980; Laurent, 1982; Kelley et al., 1984). However, these are present in very small amounts and their specific activity can only be measured where large tissue samples are available. This problem largely has been overcome by the single injection of a 'flooding' dose of unlabeled proline with the radiolabeled proline, with the aim of eliminating pools of amino acid with widely varying specific activities (Laurent, 1982; McAnulty and Laurent, 1987). Laurent (1982) showed that the specific activity of proline in type I procollagen of rabbit skin was between that of the free proline in plasma and skin, suggesting that rates estimated using the specific activity of these pools represent minimum and maximum rates, respectively. The difference between specific activities of these pools was such that use of either would not result in large errors in the estimated rates. The precursor specific activity rose to plateau levels within 15 min, making errors in the calculation of protein synthesis rates over a period of 180 min, using the plateau precursor specific activity, insignificant. The advantages of this approach are that a rate of collagen synthesis can be obtained for each animal and can be measured over short periods of time, thus allowing assessment of short-term changes in collagen synthesis. In addition, no specialized equipment, other than a β scintillation counter, is required. Collagen degradation can also be deduced from the difference between synthesis and the fractional rate of change of the collagen pool (Laurent and McAnulty, 1983) although this does involve quite large cumulative errors. Estimates of degradation obtained in this way give useful information on collagen kinetics. However, a major assumption is that all collagens are equally susceptible to degradation. It is known that this is not the case and recently synthesized collagens are more susceptible to degradation than those with mature cross-links. Ideally, studies should give information on the various collagen pools, but current techniques are still inadequate and new approaches are required.

Table 36.1 Rates of collagen synthesis in cartilage and bone of rabbits*

Animal	Hydroxyproline (μmol g^{-1})	(dpm g^{-1})	Specific (dpm μmol^{-1})	Collagen synthesis rate (% day^{-1})
Cartilage				
1	60	31 300	520	4.2
2	110	38 500	350	2.6
3	90	28 100	310	2.2
4	150	46 100	310	2.3
Bone				
1	150	54 000	360	3.0
2	160	116 200	730	5.4
3	150	74 800	500	3.6
4	130	86 400	660	4.8
5	120	114 200	950	7.0

* Rabbits weighing 2051 ± 27 g aged approximately 3 months were injected intravenously with L-[5-^{3}H]proline (400 μCi/kg body wt) together with a large dose of unlabeled proline (800 mg/kg body wt). Animals were killed 180 min after injection and samples of blood, rib and sternal cartilage removed for analysis. The specific activity was determined for proline in plasma and tissue-free pools. Hydroxyproline specific activities were obtained for trichloroacetic acid insoluble protein and estimates of fractional rates of collagen synthesis determined as described previously (Laurent, 1982; Laurent et al., 1982).

COLLAGEN SYNTHESIS IN CARTILAGE AND BONE

Neither of the approaches discussed has been used previously to estimate rates of collagen synthesis in cartilage or bone. Here we give rates for these tissues, obtained in young New Zealand White rabbits, using measurements of incorporation of radiolabeled proline into collagen as hydroxyproline after injection with a flooding dose of unlabeled proline (Table 36.1). The mean specific activity of free proline in plasma (107 000 ± 900 dpm μmol^{-1}) was close to that in the tissue-free pool for bone (94 300 ± 8100 dpm μmol^{-1}). Cartilage samples (approximately 50 mg) were too small to obtain accurate measurements of the free-proline specific activity. Since free-proline specific activities in plasma and bone were similar and close to that of the injected solution (125 700 dpm μmol^{-1}) it may be assumed that pools of amino acids with widely varying specific activities have been eliminated. Therefore, synthesis rates have been calculated using the plasma free-proline specific activity as an estimate of the precursor for protein synthesis. Mean rates for cartilage and bone were 2.8 ± 0.5 and 4.7 ± 0.7% day^{-1}, respectively. These rates are similar to those reported previously for collagen in heart, skin and skeletal muscle of rabbits of similar age, but slower than observed in lung (Laurent, 1982).

37

Determination of the rate of glycosaminoglycan synthesis *in vivo* using radioactive sulfate as tracer: comparison with *in vitro* results

ALICE MAROUDAS

INTRODUCTION

Measurements of the rate of proteoglycan (PG) synthesis and catabolism in cartilaginous tissues are of considerable basic interest because of their relevance to questions of tissue renewal and repair under various physiological and pathological conditions. Hence, large numbers of experiments *in vitro* and *in vivo* have been done in the past but few have been designed to yield quantitative results. However, it is possible using tracer techniques to obtain quantitative values for the rates of glycosaminoglycan (GAG) synthesis, both *in vivo* and *in vitro*. Clearly, for certain purposes experiments *in vivo* are necessary. However, most tests for assessing the effects of individual factors on GAG metabolism and thus separating the variables involved are best carried out *in vitro*, particularly since this is the only way in which human cartilage can be studied. In recent years, 'long-term' culture systems have been developed for *in vitro* studies (e.g. Hascall *et al.*, 1983); most researchers employ serum or growth factors as additives (e.g. see Chapter 28), but some prefer to use serum-free media (e.g. Bayliss *et al.*, 1989).

In view of the above considerations, we feel it is important to know how the rates of synthesis and catabolism obtained *in vitro* under different conditions compare with the values obtained *in vivo* for the same species, the same age and the same tissue location. In what follows, a short description is given of the method we have used *in vivo* to study quantitatively the overall rate of GAG synthesis and catabolism in cartilage and in the disc (Maroudas, 1975, 1980; Urban *et al.*, 1978). The comparison with some results *in vitro* is also given.

METHOD FOR DETERMINING THE RATE OF SULFATE INCORPORATION *IN VIVO* AFTER A PULSE INJECTION OF RADIOACTIVE TRACER

The principle of the method for determining the rate of sulfate tracer incorporation is as follows. The radioactive tracer is introduced into the animal in the blood stream, and thence into the joint cavity, or directly into the joint cavity and diffuses into the aqueous phase of the tissue matrix where it is taken up by the cells and used in the synthesis of the GAG. It is known that the equilibration time for [^{35}S]sulfate between the extracellular fluid and the intracellular metabolic donor, PAPS, is very short and that the specific activity of ^{35}S in the PAPS can be taken as equal to that of [^{35}S]sulfate in the extracellular fluid (see Chapter 34). The latter observation indicates that there is virtually no reutilization of ^{35}S originating from the degradation of freshly made GAG compared with the direct supply of free tracer from the external solution.

THEORY

The tissue area under consideration will be assumed to be of uniform composition. Let the concentration of sulfate present in GAG be $\bar{G}$ mol/g tissue and that of *free* sulfate present in the extracellular water be $\bar{M}$ mol/g tissue. Because in the adult the tissue composition remains constant, i.e. in steady state, free sulfate must be converted into incorporated sulfate in GAG at the same rate as the latter is catabolized. Let this rate be Q moles per hour per gram of tissue, i.e.

$$\text{Free } SO_4^{2-} \xrightarrow{Q} \text{Incorporated } SO_4^{2-}$$

$$\xrightarrow{Q} \text{Out of the system}$$

If tracer [^{35}S]sulfate is introduced into the system as a pulse at time t_0 and the concentration of free tracer is $\bar{m}(t)$ and that of incorporated tracer $\bar{g}(t)$ at any time thereafter, then a mass balance of the tracer in GAG at time t gives

$$\frac{d\bar{g}}{dt} = Q\frac{\bar{m}}{\bar{M}} - Q\frac{\bar{g}}{\bar{G}} \tag{37.1}$$

Integrating between t_0 and time t_1 gives

$$Q = \frac{\int_0^{\bar{g}(t_1)} d\bar{g}}{\int_{t_0}^{t_1} (\bar{m}/\bar{M} - \bar{g}/\bar{G}) \, dt} \tag{37.2a}$$

where $\bar{m}/\bar{M}$ is the specific activity of free tracer at time t and $\bar{g}/\bar{G}$ is the specific activity of incorporated tracer at time t in the tissue. Instead of integrating between the limits t_0 and t_1 and 0 and $\bar{g}(t_1)$, it is possible to use any other limits, such as t_1, t_2, $\bar{g}(t_1)$ and $\bar{g}(t_2)$. It should be noted that the initial few minutes usually give unreliable results, so it is better to start with, for example, $t > 30$ min.

During the incorporation period, the specific activity of incorporated tracer is several orders of magnitude lower than that of free tracer. Hence the term $\bar{g}/\bar{G}$ becomes negligible compared with $\bar{m}/\bar{M}$ and equation (37.2a) can be rewritten as

$$Q = \frac{\int_0^{\bar{g}(t_1)} d\bar{g}}{\int_{t_0}^{t_1} (\bar{m}/\bar{M}) \, dt} \tag{37.2b}$$

Unfortunately, $\bar{M}$, the steady-state concentration of free sulfate, is not easily measurable in tissues as it is small compared with that of GAG sulfate. However, it can easily be estimated from equilibrium partition studies *in vitro* (Maroudas and Evans, 1974). Thus, if there is no consumption of the sulfate (as, for example, at 4°C), we have the relation

$$\bar{M} = KM \tag{37.3}$$

where K is the molar partition coefficient and M is the concentration of sulfate in the external equilibrating solution (*in vivo* synovial fluid and, indirectly, plasma, for example). If the solute is being consumed, then $\bar{M} < KM$. However, the error thus introduced is small—approximately 1% for adult cartilages—if the GAG turnover is not very fast.

For rabbit and dog sera, the values of M are c. 0.7 and c. 0.75 mM, respectively, and the corresponding values of K are c. 0.45 and c. 0.36 (Maroudas, 1975).

In the experiment in which a pulse of tracer is introduced into the blood stream or into the joint cavity, the radioactivity due to free [^{35}S]sulfate first rises steeply and then gradually decays with time as the tracer diffuses away. As time progresses, the local concentration of tracer in the joint tissues (i.e. $\bar{m}(t)$) will also rise and decrease. Obviously, it is not possible to measure $\bar{m}$ as a function of time for one given animal since $\bar{m}(t)$ can only be obtained after the joint has been dissected. However, if experiments are carried out on a number of carefully matched animals for different periods of time, the variation in $\bar{m}(t)$ with time can be established and the integration according to equation (37.2b) carried out graphically. (The term $\bar{g}(t)/\bar{G}$ in equation (37.2a) is usually negligible compared with the term $\bar{m}(t)/\bar{M}$ and can, therefore, be disregarded; that is, at early times very little of the newly labeled PG has entered the catabolic pool.)

EXPERIMENTAL PROTOCOL

Animals are given a dose of [^{35}S]sulfate, either into the blood stream or into the joint cavity, and are sacrificed at various periods thereafter—usually 15 min to 12 h for measuring rates of synthesis of GAG. Blood samples usually are taken just prior to sacrifice to check the radioactivity in plasma and compare it with that in the tissue. It is essential to excise the joint or spine as rapidly as possible and plunge it into liquid nitrogen to stop movement of free tracer. The cartilage or disc (or any other tissue) is then sliced whilst kept frozen; the free [^{35}S]sulfate is desorbed from each slice and quantified and the residual slice digested in papain for determination of the tracer in GAG. The detailed protocols have been described previously (e.g. Maroudas, 1975; Urban *et al.*, 1978; Gershuni *et al.*, in preparation). An alternative procedure to determine both free and incorporated [^{35}S]sulfate is to use a G50 column, thus avoiding the desorption step.

If one also wishes to determine the rates of PG degradation, groups of animals can be kept over long periods of time (months or years, depending on age) and sacrificed at regular time intervals until the tracer reaches suitably low values. Note that in this case it is $\bar{m}(t)$ which can be disregarded and $\bar{g}(t)$ dominates (see equation (37.2a)). Due to safety problems associated with radioactivity, this method clearly can be applied only to small animals. It has been used for guinea-pigs by Lohmander (Lohmander *et al.*, 1973) and for rabbits by Maroudas (1980) and Maroudas *et al.* (unpublished data).

SOME EXAMPLES

If the cartilage is very thin (e.g. rabbit articular cartilage), the [^{35}S]sulfate in the tissue is practically in equilibrium with synovial fluid and plasma throughout the experiment. The illustration in Fig. 37.1 is for rabbit articular cartilage and the patten of the decay of free radioactivity from cartilage follows the semilogarithmic pattern observed in blood (Richmond and Hastings, 1960). If the specific activity is plotted vs. time, its mean value up to time t can be estimated from the area under the curve; Q can then be calculated from equation (37.2b) as illustrated numerically.

However, in larger animals, such as labrador dogs, another factor needs to be considered. In such cases, the intervertebral disc is large (about 5 mm thick) and only at the surface is it in tracer equilibrium with the plasma. Thus, the rate of transport of tracer into the tissue must also be taken into account and the disc cannot be treated as one well-mixed compartment (Urban *et al.*, 1978).

Because the change in free tracer with time will be different for different positions in the tissue, the counts of incorporated tracer will vary correspondingly throughout the tissue, even if the *incorporation rate* itself *does not* vary with location. Therefore, to obtain Q at any site, the variation in free-tracer concentration with time at that site needs to be known as well as the total counts due to incorporated tracer. Figure 37.2 shows the variation in radioactivity due to free and incorporated tracer in two areas of a dog's disc as a function of time. It should be noted that the topographical differences in the radioactivity of free sulfate are due to a combination of two effects, *viz.* differences in the values of the equilibrium partition of the sulfate ion as well as in the rates of transport mentioned above. For instance, the molar partition coefficients for the sulfate ion vary from 0.55 in the outer annulus to 0.3 in the nucleus of a dog's disc.

Another example of our method is given by a recent study (Gershuni *et al.*, in preparation) to determine the effect of continuous passive motion (CPM) on the rate of synthesis of GAG in rabbit menisci and ligaments. In this study, knee joints were injected immediately after sacrifice with [^{35}S]sulfate and one knee was exercised for a given period of time up to 8 h. The menisci and anterior cruciate ligaments were removed immediately after treatment and then analyzed for free and incorporated radioisotope concentration. The *free*-tracer content of the menisci and ligaments was *substantially* lower and the incorporated

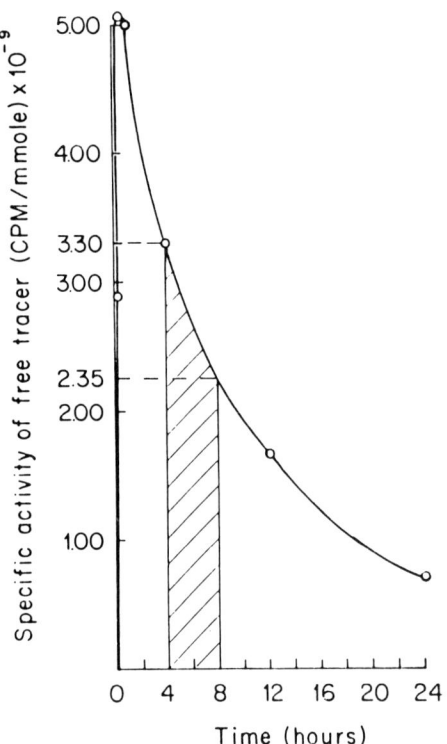

Figure 37.1 Typical variation in specific activity of free tracer, $^{35}SO_4^{2-}$, in rabbit articular cartilage, with time after intravenous injection. Example of calculation of mean specific activity of tracer and of rate of sulfate incorporation into GAG. Mean specific activity of free sulfate between 4 and 8 h =

$$\frac{\text{shaded area}}{4} = 2.82 \times 10^9$$

hence:

$$\int_{t=4}^{t=8} \frac{\bar{m}}{\bar{M}} \, dt = \text{shaded area} = 4 \times 2.82 \times 10^9$$

The mean increase in incorporated radioactivity over the same period (i.e. from 4 to 8 h) was

$$\int_{t=4}^{t=8} d\bar{g} = 1.46 \times 10^5 \text{ cpm g}^{-1}$$

Hence, rate of sulfate incorporation per hour per gram of cartilage, Q, (see equation (37.2b)) will be given by:

$$Q = \frac{\int_{t=4}^{t=8} d\bar{g}}{\int_{t=4}^{t=8} \frac{\bar{m}}{\bar{M}} \, dt} = \frac{1.46 \times 10^5}{4 \times 2.82 \times 10^9}$$

$$= 1.3 \times 10^{-5}$$

Since the GAG sulfate content of rabbit cartilage is approximately 0.09 mmol g^{-1}, it follows that the turnover time, T, will be given by

$$T = \frac{0.09}{24 \times 1.3 \times 10^{-5}} = 288 \text{ days}$$

---

tracer content *somewhat* lower in the menisci and ligaments subjected to CPM. However, when the respective free-tracer concentrations were taken into account, the *actual* rates of sulfate incorporation were significantly *higher* in the tissues subjected to CPM. Thus CPM facilitates transport of free sulfate from the knee while at the same time stimulating the rate of GAG synthesis in the meniscus and anterior cruciate ligament. The conclusions could not have been reached if the specific activities of both free and incorporated tracer had not been measured.

The procedure described above, whilst relatively straightforward, is clearly time-consuming. In the case of small animals, the method using a constant infusion of tracer (see Chapter 35) has definite advantages. It should be borne in mind, however, that in many types of investigations larger animals have to be used because their cartilaginous tissues mimic better the characteristics of human tissues and are more suitable for certain studies, e.g. those involving topographical variations. Due to the practical problems associated with keeping animals with a high content of radioactivity over longer periods of time the infusion method cannot be employed in these cases.

COMPARISON OF *IN VIVO* AND *IN VITRO* VALUES

Our procedures for short-term culture *in vitro* have been described previously (Maroudas and Evans, 1974; Maroudas, 1980). The comparison between the *in vivo* and *in vitro* values for articular cartilage is given in Table 37.1 and it is clear that the correspondence is very close. Moreover, the depth profiles obtained *in vivo* for canine cartilage exhibited the same shape as the *in vitro* ones with lowest sulfate uptake in the superficial zone

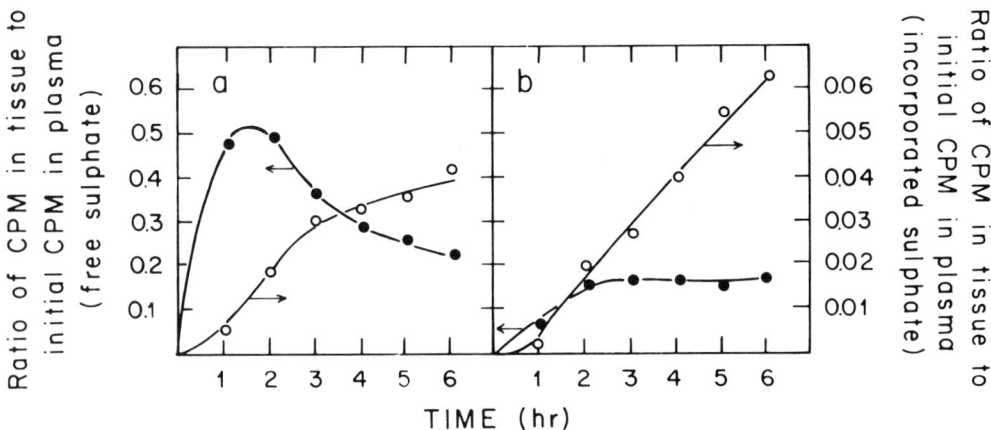

Figure 37.2 Variation of free and incorporated tracer sulfate with time after intravenous injection of tracer in areas of a dog's disc. (a) The outer annulus; (b) the nucleus. (●) Free sulfate; (○) incorporated sulfate.

Table 37.1 Sulfate incorporation into articular cartilages: comparison between *in vitro* and *in vivo* results

Animal	Conditions of test	Rate of sulfate uptake per mass of tissue ($\times 10^5$ mmol h^{-1} g^{-1})	PG sulfate per mass of wet cartilage (mmol g^{-1})	Approximate mean life of sulfated PGs (days)
Young rabbit (4 weeks)	*in vivo*	18	0.075	16
Young rabbit (3–5 months)	*in vivo*	2.4	0.055	90
	in vitro	1.7	0.055	130
Adult rabbit (2½ years)	*in vivo*	1.2	0.09	310
	in vitro	1.1	0.09	340
Adult dog (greyhound)	*in vivo*	1.3	0.085	280
	in vitro	1.2		300

(Maroudas, unpublished data). Autoradiographic data reported in the literature (Mankin and Lippiello, 1969; Meachim, 1963) also show that in the rabbit *in vivo* the surface zone incorporates less radioactivity than do deeper zones. It thus seems that the general patterns of variation in sulfate uptake by articular cartilage in minimal medium and in short-term culture reflect those prevailing *in vivo*. Similarly, close agreement has been obtained between results *in vivo* for the disc and those observed *in vitro* in short-term serum-free culture provided the disc was kept under the same hydration as *in vivo* (Bayliss *et al.*, 1986, 1988).

It should be noted, however, that recent work by Hascall (Hascall *et al.*, 1983) as well as by other groups, including our own (Maroudas, *et al.*, 1988), has shown that in long-term culture, in the presence of added serum or growth factors, sulfate uptake shows a considerable increase (two- to four-fold) as compared with the initial value in medium alone. Moreover, we found that the depth profile itself shows a dramatic change after about two days in culture, with the surface zone incorporating much more sulfate than before and at least as much as the other zones (Maroudas et al., 1988 also Chapter 4). It is not clear at present how the conditions in such experiments correspond to those normally prevailing in vivo, particularly with regard to the availability to chondrocytes in vivo of the various factors present in serum. The finding that the depth profiles of sulfate uptake obtained in short-term culture agree with those seen in vivo, together with the fact that a considerable length of time is required for the profile, as well as the level, to alter in culture in the presence of serum would indicate, in our view, that it is the short-term culture which gives results reflecting more closely the situation in vivo.

38

Biosynthesis of cartilage proteoglycan: an analysis of posttranslational events by different in vitro labeling protocols

L. STEFAN LOHMANDER

INTRODUCTION

Chondroitin sulfate (CS) chain synthesis on the proteoglycan (PG) core protein precursor is initiated when xylose is transferred from UDP-xylose by xylosyltransferase onto appropriate serines in the peptide chain of the PG precursor. The intracellular location of this step has been debated. Schwartz and coworkers (Geetha-Habib et al., 1984; Rodén et al., 1985; Campbell and Schwartz, 1988) immunolocalized xylosyltransferase in the rough endoplasmic reticulum and proposed that xylosylation occurs in this intracellular compartment, perhaps on the nascent core protein precursor. However, Hirschberg and coworkers (Nuwayhid et al., 1986) showed that most of the antiport activity for UDP-xylose and essentially all the endogenous acceptor activity resided in vesicles derived from the Golgi complex of hepatocytes, a result consistent with xylosyl transfer occurring mainly in the Golgi complex. We have addressed this conflicting evidence by the use of two different protocols of in vitro labeling with radioactive precursors using the Swarm rat chondrosarcoma as a model system (Thonar et al., 1983; Kimura et al., 1984; Lohmander et al., 1986; Lohmander and Kimura, 1986; Lohmander et al., 1989).

The core protein of the completed large PG from the Swarm rat chondrosarcoma is a peptide chain of 2105 amino acids which contains 279 serines and 198 threonines (Doege et al., 1986). This protein is substituted with: (i) about 100 CS chains in glycosidic linkage to serines; (ii) about 130 O-linked oligosaccharides attached via N-acetylgalactosamine in glycosidic linkage to serines and threonines; (iii) up to eight N-linked oligosaccharides attached to asparagine (Lohmander et al., 1980); and (iv) about seven monophosphates attached to serines (Oegema et al., 1984). The biosynthesis of this large macromolecule requires an extensive series of posttranslational modifications of the core protein. For CS, the chain synthesis is initiated by adding xylose to appropriate serines. Subsequent chain completion involves adding the remaining residues of the linkage region and the repeating disaccharide backbone of the glycosaminoglycan.

CONTINUOUS LABELING UNDER STEADY-STATE CONDITIONS AND ANALYSIS OF COMPLETED PG

The intracellular half-life of the core protein precursor of the Swarm rat chondrosarcoma PG is about 50 min (Kimura et al., 1981; Mitchell and Hardingham, 1981; Shinomura et al., 1986) and at least 70% of this time is spent in the rough endoplasmic reticulum (Fellini et al., 1984; Kimura et al., 1984). These parameters were arrived at partly through the use of continuous labeling protocols with radioactive precursors to determine the kinetics of incorporation of precursor into the completed PG.

In continuous labeling experiments, there will always be time delays in the entry of label into the finished macromolecule associated with the equilibration of the labeled precursor in the culture medium with the intracellular precursor compartments. After this delay, incorporation kinetics into the completed macromolecules under study will become linear with time. In the case of labeling of the core protein of the completed PG, an initial delay will be caused by the time required for equilibrium of, for example, [^{3}H]-serine in the culture medium with intracellular seryl-tRNA pools and nascent polypeptides on polyribosomes. A measurable further delay will be caused before the label enters PG molecules, since they require extensive posttranslational processing before completion. The delay caused by this considerable posttranslational modification can be estimated by comparing the time lag until linear incorporation of the precursor into total protein and PG respectively. Simplified kinetic equations previously used for the kinetic analysis of DNA and polysaccharide synthesis (Rubinow and Yen, 1972; Thonar et al., 1983) may be used to describe the entry of label into the completed molecules and to calculate the time delays caused by the different posttranslational processing steps (Kimura et al., 1984). After linear incorporation is obtained, the slopes of the linear labeling curves may be used further to calculate the relative rates of synthesis of the different pools of molecules or of different components of the same molecule (Kimura et al., 1984; Lohmander et al., 1986). In addition, if the specific activity of the precursor pool is known, the absolute amount and number of labeled macromolecules synthesized per labeling period may be calculated (Lohmander and Kimura, 1986).

The principles described for kinetic analysis of continuous labeling protocols and the fact that the chondrosarcoma PG core protein precursor has a measurable intracellular half-life were used to determine the timing of the addition of the linkage sugars of the CS chain to the core protein precursor (Lohmander et al., 1986). In these experiments, [1-^{3}H]glucose was used as a labeling precursor in the culture medium in the presence of high levels of unlabeled glucose (4.5 g l^{-1}) in order to ensure the presence of a precursor pool with constant specific activity for the duration of the labeling period.

The chondrosarcoma cells were labeled in vitro for periods of 0.5 to 8 h and the completed labeled PG molecules extracted and purified by density gradient ultracentrifugation and ion-exchange chromatography. After a short equilibration lag period, the total incorporation of radioactivity into PG was linear up to 5 h. The linkage region of CS to the PG core protein was isolated by treatment of the PG with alkaline borohydride, followed by ethanol precipitation of the β-eliminated CS chains. After digestion with chondroitinase-AC, the linkage region consisting of xylitol–galactose–galactose-unsaturated uronic acid residue was separated from the unsaturated repeating disaccharides produced by the action of the enzyme through gel permeation chromatography. The linkage region was then hydrolyzed in trifluoroacetic acid and the labeled monosaccharides separated by HPLC (Lohmander, 1986).

The kinetics of incorporation of label from [1-^{3}H]glucose into xylitol and galactose of the CS linkage region are shown in Fig. 38.1. In each case, after a lag period, incorporation of radioactivity became linear through 5 h. The points through 5 h

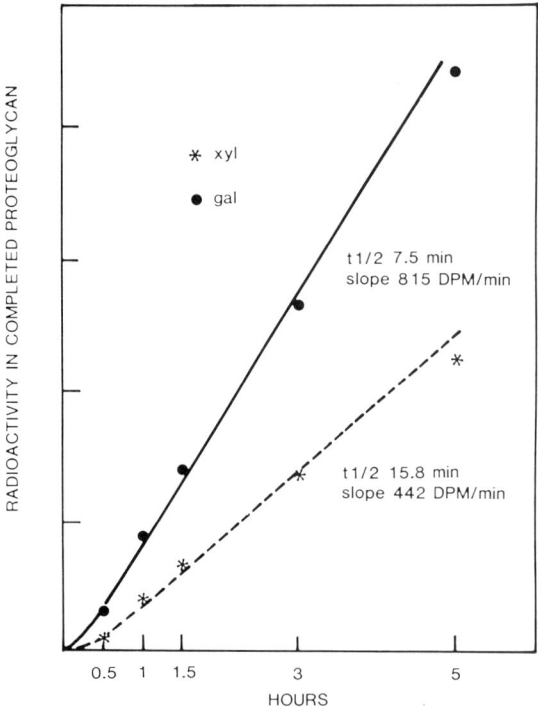

Figure 38.1 Kinetics of incorporation of label from [1-³H]glucose into xylitol and galactose of the CS linkage region.

were fit to first-order rate equations (Kimura *et al.*, 1984) and the final slope values and the $t_{1/2}$ values until linear incorporation estimated. The $t_{1/2}$ values thus calculated were 7.5 min for galactose and 15.8 min for xylitol. The UDP-nucleotide sugar precursor pools for galactose and xylose are both derived metabolically from UDP-glucose and will have identical specific activities at equilibrium. Assuming that these nucleotide precursor pools are small and turn over rapidly, it is likely that the differences in their half-lives to constant specific activity will likewise be small. If they are identical, then the differences in $t_{1/2}$ to linear incorporation for [³H]galactose and [³H]xylose, obtained by kinetic analysis, would indicate that xylosyl transfer to the appropriate serine residues would precede addition of the galactose residues by about 8 min, or the difference in half-life to linear incorporation for the two sugars. The 2 : 1 labeling ratio of galactose to xylitol is close to the theoretical and provides support for the validity of the rate equations used. The half-life to equilibrium labeling for glucuronic acid, a part of the backbone of CS, was about 6 min, or about the same as for galactose. This indicates that the addition of the linkage galactose residues occurs at almost the same time as the chain elongation of CS occurs. The significantly longer half-life to linear xylose labeling, on the other hand, suggests that the xylose residues may be added about 8 min earlier to the core protein precursor than the rest of the chain. Since the intracellular half-life of the core protein precursor in the chondrosarcoma cells is about 50 min, these data strongly suggest that the addition of xylose is not completed to any significant extent while the polypeptide is still nascent or shortly after release in the rough endoplasmic reticulum. Our interpretation of the labeling kinetics after continuous labeling and analysis of the completed PG is thus consistent with the suggestion that xylosyl transfer to PG core protein is mainly a Golgi-related event (Nuwayhid *et al.*, 1986).

PULSE LABELING AND ANALYSIS OF PROTEOGLYCAN CORE PROTEIN PRECURSOR

Another approach in order to address the same problem is to isolate the intracellular PG core protein precursor and then directly analyze its degree of substitution of serine residues with xylose. Initial experiments showed, however, that the amount of radioactive label possible to incorporate *in vitro* into CS linkage sugars of the PG precursor was insufficient for further analysis. We therefore chose to analyze the degree of substitution of the precursor by utilizing the sensitivity of O-glycosidically substituted serine residues to treatment with alkali (Anderson *et al.*, 1967). In the prescence of borohydride, the β-eliminated dehydroalanine residues will be converted to alanine residues, while unsubstituted serines are insensitive to this treatment (Lohmander *et al.*, 1989). The degree of substitution for the intracellular PG precursor may thus be directly compared with that for the completed PG of the same cultures.

The rat chondrosarcoma chondrocytes were pulse-labeled *in vitro* with L-[3-^{3}H]serine. Intracellular PG core protein precursor was purified from cell lysates by immunoprecipitation with polyclonal antibodies against the hyaluronic acid-binding region, followed by sodium dodecyl sulfate (SDS)–polyacrylamide gel electrophoresis (PAGE). The core protein precursor was eluted from the gels and then treated with alkaline borohydride as explained above in order to convert O-substituted serines to alanines. Radioactively labeled serine and alanine were then separated by high performance liquid chromatography (HPLC) and quantified and the results compared with those obtained for the completed PG from the same cultures. In the completed PG about 55% of the serine residues were substituted with xylose or N-acetylgalactosamine, while the corresponding value for the intracellular precursor was less than 5% (Fig. 38.2) (Lohmander *et al.*, 1989).

If all the serines in the precursor that are destined to carry CS chains in the completed PG were xylosylated at translation, about 35% of the serines would be alkali-labile (279 serine residues total, 100 CS chains), while only less than 5% are. If xylosylation occurs in a distinct compartment during a short time period, our results suggest that no more than about 1/7 of the total core protein molecules would be xylosylated. With an intracellular half-life of about 50 min for the precursor in the chondrosarcoma cells, xylosyl transfer would occur about 43 min after

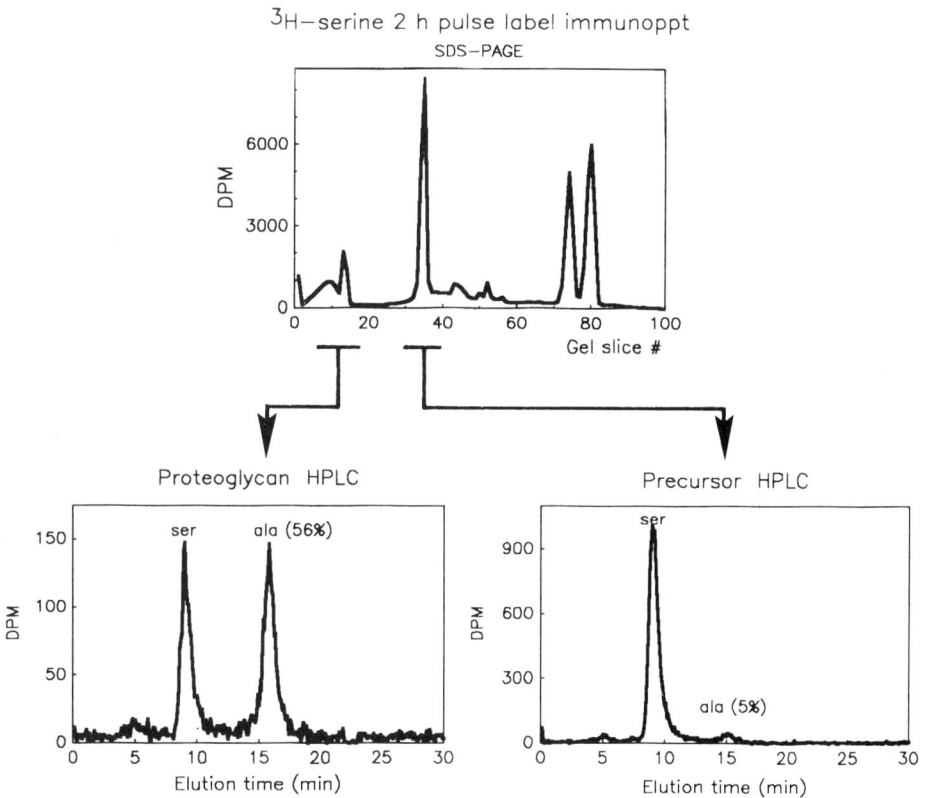

Figure 38.2 Substitution of serine residues with xylose or N-acetylgalactosamine.

translation and no more than about 7 min before the addition of the rest of the CS chain and completion of the molecule.

These results indicate, in agreement with our kinetic data described above, that the major part of the xylosyl transfer to the chondrosarcoma PG precursor must take place late in the processing sequence. This provides further support that the PG precursor resides mainly in a pre-Golgi compartment and that most of the xylosyl transfer to the core protein occurs in a Golgi compartment.

CONCLUSIONS

Two different *in vitro* labeling protocols were used to study the timing and intracellular location of the addition of the CS linkage sugars to the chondrosarcoma PG core protein precursor. Both protocols led to same conclusion: the major part of the xylosyl transfer to the chondrosarcoma PG precursor must take place late in the post-translational processing sequence and occurs mainly in a Golgi compartment.

ACKNOWLEDGMENTS

Supported by the Swedish Medical Research Council, the King Gustaf V 80th Birthday Fund, the Lundberg Foundation, the Axison Johnson Foundation, the Österlund Foundation and the Medical Faculty of Lund University.

References

Anderson, Bray, B., Lieberman, R. and Meyer, K. (1967). Structure of human skeletal keratosulfate—the linkage region. *J. Biol. Chem.* **242**, 3373–3380

Bayliss, M.T., Urban, J.P.G., Johnstone, B. and Holm, S. (1986). *In vitro* method for measuring synthesis rates in the intervertebral disc. *J. Orthop. Res.* **4**, 10–17

Bayliss, M.T., Johnstone, B. and O'Brien, J.P. (1988). Proteoglycan synthesis in the human intervertebral disc. Variation with age, region and pathology, Vol. 13. *Spine* **9**, 972–981

Bayliss, M.T., Vilim, V., Hardingham, T.E. and Muir, H. (1989). *Trans. 35th Annual Meeting*, p. 329, Orthopics Research Society, Las Vegas

Beavan, L.A., Davies, M. and Mason, R.M. (1988). Renal glomerular proteoglycans. An investigation of their synthesis *in vivo* using a technique for fixation *in situ*. *Biochem. J.* **251**, 411–418

Beavan, L.A., Davies, M., Couchman, J.R., Williams, M.A. and Mason, R.M. (1989). *In vivo* turnover of the basement membrane and other heparan sulfate proteoglycans of rat glomerulus. *Arch. Biochem. Biophys.* **269**, 576–585

Campbell, S.C. and Schwartz, N.B. (1988). Kinetics of intracellular processing of chondroitin sulfate proteoglycan core protein and other matrix proteins. *J. Cell. Biol.* **106**, 2191–2202

Cole, D.E.C., Mohyuddin, F. and Scriver, C.R. (1979). A microassay for analysis of serum sulfate. *Anal. Biochem.* **100**, 339–342

Doege, K., Fernandez, P., Hassell, J.R., Sasaki, M. and Yamada, Y. (1986). Partial cDNA sequence encoding a globular domain at the C terminus of the rat cartilage proteoglycan. *J. Biol. Chem.* **261**, 8108–8111

Fellini, S.A., Hascall, V.C. and Kimura, J.H. (1984). Localization of proteoglycan core protein in subcellular fractions isolated from rat chondrosarcoma. *J. Biol. Chem.* **259**, 4634–4641

Geetha-Habib, M., Campbell, S.C. and Schwartz, N.B. (1984). Subcellular localization of the synthesis and glycosylation of chondroitin sulfate proteoglycan core protein. *J. Biol. Chem.* **259**, 7300–7310

Gerber, G. and Altman, K.I. (1960). Studies on the metabolism of tissue proteins. 1. Turnover of collagen labeled with proline-U-C^{14} in young rats. *J. Biol. Chem.* **235**, 2653–2656

Gershuni, D.H., Maroudas, A., Hargens, A.R., Skyhar, M.J., Danzig, L., Schneiderman, R. and Barg, F. The effect of continuous passive motion on the transport and metabolism of ^{35}S sulfate in the knee menisci and anterior cruciate ligaments, in prep.

Hascall, V.C. (1988). Proteoglycans: the chondroitin sulfate/keratan sulfate proteoglycan of cartilage. *ISI Atlas Sci. Biochem.* **1**, 189–198

Hascall, V.C., Handley, C.J., McQuillan, D.J., Hascall, G.K., Robinson, H.C. and Lowther, D.A. (1983). Effect of serum on biosynthesis of proteoglycans by bovine articular cartilage in culture. *Arch. Biochem. Biophys.* **224**, 206–223

Hascall, V.C., Morales, T.I., Hascall, G.K., Handley, C.J. and McQuillan, D.J. (1983). Biosynthesis and turnover of proteoglycans in organ culture of bovine articular culture. *J. Rheum.* **10**, 45–52

Jackson, S.H. and Heininger, J.A. (1974). A study of collagen reutilization using an $^{18}O_2$ labeling technique. *Clin. Chim. Acta* **51**, 163–171

Jackson, S.H. and Heininger, J.A. (1975). Proline recycling during collagen metabolism as determined by concurrent $^{18}O_2$ and ^{3}H-labeling. *Biochim. Biophys. Acta* **381**, 359–367

Kao, K.T., Hilker, D.M. and McGavack, T.H. (1961). Connective tissue. V. Comparison of synthesis and turnover of collagen and elastin in tissues of rat at several ages. *Proc. Soc. Biol. Med.* **106**, 335–338

Kelley, J., Stirewalt, W.S. and Chrin, L. (1984). Protein synthesis in rat lung. Measurements *in vivo* based on leucyl-tRNA and rapidly turning-over procollagen I. *Biochem. J.* **222**, 77–83

Kimura, J.H., Thonar, E.J.-M.A., Hascall, V.C., Reiner, A. and Poole, A.R. (1981). Identification of core protein, an intermediate in proteoglycan biosynthesis in cultured chondrocytes from the Swarm rat chondrosarcoma. *J. Biol. Chem.* **256**, 7890–7897

Kimura, J.H., Lohmander, L.S. and Hascall, V.C. (1984). Studies on the biosynthesis of cartilage proteoglycan in a model system of cultured chondrocytes from the Swarm rat chondrosarcoma. *J. Cell Biochem.* **26**, 261–278

Laurent, G.J. (1982). Rates of collagen synthesis in the lung, skin and muscle obtained *in vivo* by a simplified method using [^{3}H] proline. *Biochem. J.* **206**, 535–544

Laurent, G.J. and McAnulty, R.J. (1983). Protein metabolism during bleomycin-induced pulmonary fibrosis in rabbits. *Am. Rev. Respir. Dis.* **128**, 82–88

Laurent, G.J., Sparrow, M.P., Bates, P.C. and Millward, D.J. (1978). Turnover of muscle protein in the fowl. Collagen content and turnover in cardiac and skeletal muscles of the adult fowl and changes during stretch-induced growth. *Biochem. J.* **176**, 419–427

Laurent, G.J., McAnulty, R.J. and Oliver, M.H. (1982). Anomalous tritium loss in the measurement of tissue hydroxy-[5-^{3}H]-proline specific activity following chloramine T oxidation. *Anal. Biochem.* **123**, 223–228

Lohmander, L.S. (1986). Analysis by high-performance liquid chromatography of radioactively labeled components of proteoglycans. *Anal. Biochem.* **154**, 75–84

Lohmander, L.S. and Kimura, J.H. (1986). Biosynthesis of cartilage proteoglycan. In *Articular Cartilage Biochemistry* (K.E. Kuettner, R. Schleyerbach and V.C. Hascall, eds). Raven Press, New York, pp. 93–110

Lohmander, L.S., Antonopoulos, C.A. and Friberg, U. (1973). Chemical and metabolic heterogeneity of chondroitin sulfate and keratan sulfate in guinea pig cartilage and nucleus pulposus. *Biochim. Biophys. Acta* **304**, 2130

Lohmander, L.S., DeLuca, S., Nilsson, B., Hascall, V.C., Caputo, C., Kimura, J.H. and Heinegard, D.H. (1980). Oligosaccharides on proteoglycans from the Swarm rat chondrosarcoma. *J. Biol. Chem.* **255**, 6084–6091

Lohmander, L.S., Hascall, V.C., Yanagishita, M., Kuettner, K.E. and Kimura, J.H. (1986). Post translational events in proteoglycan synthesis: kinetics of synthesis of chondroitin sulfate and oligosaccharides on the core protein. *Arch. Biochem. Biophys.* **250**, 211–227

Lohmander, L.S., Shinomura, T., Kimura, J.H. and Hascall, V.C. (1989). Xylosyl transfer to the core protein precursor of the rat chondrosarcoma proteoglycan. *J. Biol. Chem.* **264**, 18 775–18 780

Malmstrom, A. (1984). Equilibration of [^{3}H]-glucosamine and [^{35}S]sulfate with intracellular pools of UDP-N-acetylhexosamine and 3'-phosphoadenosine-5'-phosphosulfate (PAPS) in cultured fibroblasts. *Arch. Biochem. Biophys.* **235**, 692–698

Mankin, H.J. and Lipiello, L. (1969). The turnover of adult rabbit articular cartilage. *J. Bone Joint Surg.* **51A**, 1591–1600

Maroudas, A. (1975). Glycosaminoglycan turnover in articular cartilage. *Phil. Trans. R. Soc. London B* **271**, 293–313

Maroudas, A. (1980). Metabolism of cartilaginous tissue: A quantitative approach. In *Studies in Joint Diseases* (A. Maroudas, E.J. Holborow and T. Wells, eds), pp. 59–86. Pitman, London

Maroudas, A. and Evans, H. (1974). A study of ionic equilibria in cartilage. *Conn. Tiss. Res.* **1**, 69–79

Maroudas, A., Chiriqui, C. and Weinberg, P. (1988). The stimulation of proteoglycan synthesis in cartilage by serum: variation with depth and influence of cyclic compression. *Trans. 34th Ann. Meeting Orthop. Res. Soc.*, Atlanta, Orthopaedic Research Society

Mason, R.M. and Palfrey, A.J. (1984). Intervertebral disc degeneration in adult mice with hereditary kyphoscoliosis. *J. Orthop. Res.* **2**, 333–338

McAnulty, R.J. and Laurent, G.J. (1987). Collagen synthesis and degradation *in vivo*. Evidence for rapid rates of collagen turnover with extensive degradation of newly synthesized collagen in tissues of the adult rat. *Collagen Rel. Res.* **7**, 93–104

Meachim, G. (1963). The effect of scarification on articular cartilage in the rabbit. *J. Bone Joint Surg.* **45B**, 150–161

Mitchell, D. and Hardingham, T. (1981). The effects of cycloheximide on the biosynthesis and secretion of proteoglycans by chondrocytes in culture. *Biochem. J.* **196**, 521–529

Molnar, J.A., Alpert, N., Burke, J.F. and Young, V.R. (1986). Synthesis and degradation rates of collagens *in vivo* in whole skin of rats, studied with $^{18}O_2$ labeling. *Biochem. J.* **240**, 431–435

Morales, T.I. and Hascall, V.C. (1988). Correlated metabolism of proteolgycans and hyaluronic acid in bovine articular cartilage explants. *J. Biol. Chem.* **263**, 3632–3638

Neuberger, A. and Slack, H.G.B. (1953). The metabolism of collagen from liver, bone, skin and tendon in the normal rat. *Biochem. J.* **53**, 47–52

Neuberger, A., Perrone, J.C. and Slack, H.G.B. (1951). The relative metabolic inertia of tendon collagen in the rat. *Biochem. J.* **49**, 199–204

Nimni, M.E. (1983). Collagen: structure, function and metabolism in normal and fibrotic tissues. *Sem. Arthr. Rheum.* **13**, 1–86

Nuwayhid, N., Glaser, J.H., Johnson, J.C., Conrad, H.E., Hauser, S.C. and Hirschberg, C. (1986). Xylosylation and glucuronysylation reactions in rat liver Golgi apparatus and endoplasmic reticulum. *J. Biol. Chem.* **261**, 12 936–12 941

Oegema, T.R., Kraft, E.L., Jourdian, G.W. and Van Valen, T.R. (1984). Phosphorylation of chondroitin sulfate in proteoglycans from the Swarm rat chondrosarcoma. *J. Biol. Chem.* **259**, 1720–1726

Palmer, R.M., Robins, S.P. and Lobley, G.E. (1980). Measurement of the synthesis rates of collagens and total protein in rabbit muscle. *Biochem. J.* **192**, 631–636

Popenoe, E.A. and Van Slyke, D.D. (1962). The formation of collagen hydroxylysine. *J. Biol. Chem.* **237**, 3491–3494

Prehm, P. (1984). Hyaluronate is synthesized at plasma membranes. *Biochem. J.* **220**, 597–600

Richmond, J.E. and Hastings, A.B. (1960). Distribution of sulfate in blood and between cerebrospinal fluid and plasma *in vivo*. *Am. J. Physiol.* **199**, 814–820

Robins, S.P. (1979). Metabolism of rabbit skin collagen: differences in the apparent turnover of type I and type III collagen precursors determined by constant intravenous infusion of labelled amino acids. *Biochem. J.* **181**, 75–82

Roden, L., Koerner, T., Olson, C. and Schwartz, N.B. (1985). Mechanisms of chain initiation in the biosynthesis of connective tissue polysaccharides. *Fed. Proc.* **44**, 373–380

Rubinow, S.I. and Yen, A. (1972). Quantitation of some DNA precursor data. *Nature New Biol.* **239**, 73–74

Salustri, A., Yanagishita, M. and Hascall, V.C. (1989). Synthesis and accumulation of hyaluronic acid and proteoglycans in the mouse cumulus cell-oocyte complex during FSH-induced mucification. *J. Biol. Chem.* **264**, 13 840–13 847

Shinomura, T., Kuettner, K.E., Madsen, L. and Kimura, J.H. (1986). Quantitative immunoprecipitation of proteoglycan core protein and fibronectin from cultures of Swarm rat chondrosarcoma. *Trans. Orthop. Res. Soc.* **11**, 443

Spiro, M.J. (1987). Sulfate metabolism in the alloxandiabetic rat: relationship of altered sulfate pools to proteoglycan sulfation in heart and other tissues. *Diabetologia* **30**, 259–267

Thonar, E.J.-M.A., Lohmander, L.S., Kimura, J.H., Fellini, S.A., Yanagishita, M. and Hascall, V.C. (1983). Biosynthesis of *O*-linked oligosaccharides on proteoglycans by chondrocytes from the Swarm rat chondrosarcoma. *J. Biol. Chem.* **258**, 11 564–11 570

Urban, J.P.G., Holm, S. and Maroudas, A. (1978). Diffusion of small solutes into the intervertebral disc: an *in vivo* study. *Biorheology* **15**, 203–223

Venn, G. and Mason, R.M. (1983). Biosynthesis and metabolism *in vivo* of intervertebral disc proteoglycans in the mouse. *Biochem. J.* **215**, 217–225

Venn, G. and Mason, R.M. (1986). Changes in mouse intervertebral disc proteoglycan synthesis with age. *Biochem. J.* **234**, 475–479

Yanagishita, M. and Hascall, V.C. (1979). Biosynthesis of proteoglycans by rat granulosa cells cultured *in vitro*. *J. Biol. Chem.* **254**, 12 355–12 364

Yanagishita, M. and Hascall, V.C. (1983). Characterization of low buoyant density dermatan sulfate proteoglycans synthesized by rat ovarian granulosa cells in culture. *J. Biol. Chem.* **258**, 12 847–12 856

Yanagishita, M., Salustri, A. and Hascall, V.C. (1989). Determination of the specific activity of hexosamine precursors by analysis of double labeled disaccharides from chondroitinase digestion of chondroitin/dermatan sulfate. *Methods Enzymol.* **1179**, 435–455

7

Immunochemical methods in cartilage research

COLLATED BY T. HARDINGHAM

39

Introduction

TIM HARDINGHAM

The sensitivity and specificity of antibodies has been exploited in many different ways in investigations of cartilage. Chapter 40 provides a range of examples from studies on proteoglycans (PGs) that illustrate the strengths and some of the weaknesses of different techniques. These include assay and localization methods with polyclonal and monoclonal antibodies with specificity for either protein or carbohydrate epitopes. The strategy and techniques involved in raising monoclonal antibodies (mAbs) are presented by Bruce Caterson and coworkers (Chapter 41). Their studies with PGs show how pretreatment of antigens, such as reduction/alkylation or removal of carbohydrate chains, can be used to select for mAbs to particular types of epitope, or for epitopes on defined regions of the molecule. The sensitivity of detection of antigens by immunoblotting is demonstrated with PGs resolved on acrylamide/agarose composite gels and transferred to nylon membranes.

The preparation of polyclonal antibodies to different collagens and the advantages they offer over mAbs is described by Daniel Hartmann (Chapter 42). This involves important criteria for establishing specificity for collagen type and the extent of species cross-reactivity and possible contamination with antibodies to other native or denatured collagens.

The major interest in detecting cartilage-derived components in body fluids as a measure of cartilage damage in joint disease has resulted in several immunoassay methods for different cartilage components being tested for this purpose. The value of an ELISA method for determining keratan sulfate (KS) epitopes has been explored in a number of clinical and experimental disease studies and Eugene Thonar and coworkers (Chapter 43) describe the details of this method, emphasizing a number of experimental conditions for optimizing it to provide a reliable and reproducible assay. The determination of KS (and other carbohydrate epitopes) presents some problems, particularly as the antigens may contain multiple epitopes on multiple-chain structures. This causes the antigens to behave differently in different assay methods and Tony Ratcliffe and coworkers (Chapter 44) contrast the results using different mAbs to keratan sulfate in different techniques.

The section is rounded off with a discussion by Tibor Glant (Chapter 45) of the production of PG-specific T-lymphocyte clones. This approach may help in understanding more about joint pathology and the possible role of cartilage derived autoantigens in its development. The identification of antigenic sequences capable of T-cell stimulation may lead to new approaches for controlling chronic joint disease.

40

Immunochemical methods and their use in characterizing cartilage proteoglycans

TIM HARDINGHAM

The development of techniques using antibodies has enabled great advances to be made in the study of cartilage and its components. The exquisite structural specificity with which antibodies can recognize and bind to antigens and the sensitivity and fidelity of the detection methods they permit have opened up new areas of study that could not have been envisaged without them.

The complex structure of cartilage proteoglycan (PG) has presented many problems in the structural interpretation of experimental results showing heterogeneous composition and polydisperse size (Muir and Hardingham, 1975). The multidomain structure of the protein core and different attached chondroitin sulfate (CS) and keratan sulfate (KS) chains have been shown to present a range of distinctive antigenic structures and antibodies to both protein and carbohydrate epitopes and have been used extensively in PG research to help unravel their structural details (Baker et al., 1982; Caterson et al., 1985, 1986; Poole, 1986; Fosang and Hardingham, 1989). Techniques for exploiting antibodies have also advanced dramatically since the 1970s, when most detection and discrimination were based on immunodiffusion and the generation of precipitation lines of Ouchterlony plates. Immunochemical methods currently offer a range of powerful techniques for identifying and quantifying different cartilage components.

POLYCLONAL AND MONOCLONAL ANTIBODIES

PGs and other cartilage components present no special problems for the preparation of polyclonal or monoclonal antibodies by the application of the appropriate techniques of immunization (Furthmayr, 1982). In general, cartilage PGs have not been found to be strongly antigenic. The titers obtained in antisera have frequently been low and have required repetitive boosting by the injection of the antigen to obtain reasonable responses. Nevertheless, the antisera obtained have been successfully exploited in a broad range of applications and any failure to achieve high titers has not seriously handicapped their usefulness.

The specificity of a polyclonal antiserum is critically dependent on the purity of the antigen initially used for the immunization. Here biochemical criteria for purity, such as the appearance of a single band on a stained SDS-PAGE analysis, may not be good enough to ensure the absence of small amounts of other antigenic proteins. It is therefore important that the antisera are tested not only against the primary antigen, but also against a range of likely contaminants. In the case of cartilage components, this would be the complete mixture of proteins in a cartilage extract. The components could be tested, after separation by sodium dodecyl sulfate – polyacrylamide gel (SDS-PAGE), by immunoblotting with the antiserum after transfer to nitrocellulose (De Blas and Cherwinski, 1983). Activities against proteins other than the primary antigen would then be identified. The presence of contaminating antibodies in an antiserum may be of major importance for some techniques. For immunolocalization in a tissue section with an antiserum, the presence of a weak response to components other than the main antigen could lead to erroneous results and completely negate the use of the antiserum by this method. If this problem exists, then affinity purification and isolation of the antibodies from the antiserum, such that they no longer show response to other components, would be essential before using them for tissue localization. However, in some other techniques such as radioimmunoassay (RIA), the specificity of the method resides in the purity of the radiolabeled antigen used in the assay rather than in the specificity of the antiserum. The presence of antibodies in the antiserum to other unrelated antigens will not affect the precipitation of the radiolabeled antigen and provided that the radiolabel is principally (> 95%) in the main antigen, the use of the system for competitively detecting unlabeled antigen is then highly specific and usually very sensitive.

The preparation of monoclonal antibodies does not require rigorously purified antigen for the initial immunization of mice (or rats) and has been pursued with crude mixtures of tissue components for some purposes (Zanetti et al., 1985). However, at the screening and selection stage, purified antigen is required. This is usually carried out by enzyme-linked immunosorbent assay (ELISA) technique with antigen coated to the wells of plastic plates. Here, the final selection stage at which hybridomas producing antibodies to specific antigens are identified would require testing with antigens of the highest purity. There are some clear advantages offered by monoclonal antibodies amongst which the large, unlimited supply possible in their production is very important. The selection of a single epitope may also be an important aspect of experimental design and may assist greatly in the interpretation of results. Polyclonal antisera may offer advantages over a single monoclonal antibody in some situations. The general level of detection of a protein antigen may be enhanced by having many antibodies to different epitopes on the protein. This was apparent when the binding of a monoclonal antibody (1-C-6) (Caterson et al., 1985, 1986) to a single epitope on a full size PG was found to be insufficient to cause its precipitation when mixed with *Staphylococcus aureus*, whereas the same PG was precipitated by a polyclonal antiserum (anti G1) under the same conditions (Ratcliffe and Hardingham, unpublished results). This appeared to be mainly a physical problem as the binding of the same monoclonal to the epitope on a much smaller fragment of PG was able to precipitate it.

Although the antibodies within an antiserum are rarely characterized by the number and type of epitopes they interact with or their affinity of interaction, they may in practice work well and provide very useful research tools. Likewise, with monoclonal antibodies, the proof of their value lies in how well they work in practice and experience currently suggests no easy way of predicting this. The application of antibodies and the use obtained from them are thus entirely dependent on their validation in different experimental systems in comparison with appropriate controls.

RADIOIMMUNOASSAYS FOR PROTEOGLYCAN BINDING REGION (G1 DOMAIN) AND LINK PROTEIN

Polyclonal antisera were raised in rabbits following their immunization with purified binding region (G1 domain) or link protein prepared from pig laryngeal cartilage PG (Ratcliffe and Hardingham, 1983). The antisera were shown to be able to immunoprecipitate ^{125}I-labeled G1 or ^{125}I-link proteins when tested using *Staph. aureus* which precipitates all the immunoglobulins. Rabbit antibodies bind well to the protein A on the cell wall of the formaldehyde and heat-treated *Staph. aureus* and extremely short incubation (c. 15 min at room temperature) with mixing is sufficient to bind all antibodies and antibody–antigen complexes. Several mouse monoclonals IgG or IgM, although generally reported to be poor in binding to protein A, have been found to bind effectively to the *Staph. aureus* without using a second antibody (B. Caterson, personal communication). Competitive radioimmunoassay (RIAs) were established with dilutions of the antisera giving approximately 50% of maximum antigen binding (about 1 in 500 for link protein and 1 in 100 for G1). These produced assays sensitive down to 2 ng of link protein and 10 ng of G1. The cross-specificity was tested with the antiserum and showed that purified link protein contained 1.7% contamination with G1 which could be removed by immunoabsorption and purified G1 contained only 0.4% link protein (Ratcliffe and Hardingham, 1983). The antisera did not show any significant titer against the contaminating antigen and did not localize it on an immunoblot.

In applying the RIAs to link protein and G1 in preparations of PG aggregates, it was immediately found that link protein and, to a lesser extent, G1 were not freely accessible to the antibodies when part of the aggregate, and this was in spite of the presence of the detergents nonidet and deoxycholate (Ratcliffe and Hardingham, 1983). In order to overcome this problem, it was found necessary to devise a method to ensure dissociation of the PG–link protein–hyaluronan interaction before assaying. The most efficient way devised was by heating the samples for 15 min at 80°C in incubation buffer containing 0.025% SDS. This concentration of SDS was sufficient to promote disaggregation and yet did not interfere with the subsequent assay. Low concentrations of SDS have previously been shown to be well tolerated in RIAs and to help suppress nonspecific binding (Dimitriadis, 1979). Where analysis is thus being carried out on crude mixtures in tissue extracts or body fluids and there is the possibility of association or insolubility amongst the components present, brief heating in dilute SDS may be useful in fully solubilizing samples and making antigens which are more efficiently detected. Whereas antibodies appear to tolerate low concentration of SDS well, some are interfered with by deoxycholate. In general, it was found that omitting deoxycholate from RIA or ELISA procedures (but retaining nonidet p-40) resulted in modest increases in antibody titers without any increase in nonspecific binding (Dunham, Fosang and Hardingham, unpublished results).

A study of low-molecular-weight PGs isolated from porcine and human cartilage used a polyclonal antiserum to show evidence of their partial structural identity (Sampaio et al., 1988). The antiserum (rabbit) was raised against the purified small PG (CS-PG II) from porcine cartilage. The antiserum, in addition to recognizing the porcine PG, also recognized the corresponding PG from human cartilage but with lower titer (Fig. 40.1(a)). The antiserum thus contained fewer antibodies that recognized the human PG. In an RIA established with the antiserum, the human PG was able to inhibit antibody binding to the porcine PG, but the inhibition was only partial showing that they shared some, but not all, antigenic sites (Fig. 40.1(b)). However, if antibody binding to human PG was tested in an RIA, both human and porcine PG were equally competitive and both showed full inhibition (Fig. 40.1(b)). The epitopes recognized by the antibodies on the human PG were thus completely shared with the porcine PG, but the antiserum contained additional antibodies that recognized epitopes only present on the porcine PG. The detection of common protein epitopes on two proteins is good evidence for their close structural relationship. However, the failure to detect any shared epitopes is, on its own, no evidence for a lack of structural relationship.

When the antisera to aggregating PG G1 domain and link protein were originally prepared, the close structural relationship between the antigens was unknown. It has now been shown that they have homologous protein structures with considerable similarity in amino acid sequences, although there are no continuous sequences of more than a few amino acids that are identical (Perkins et al., 1989). The fact that the antiserum

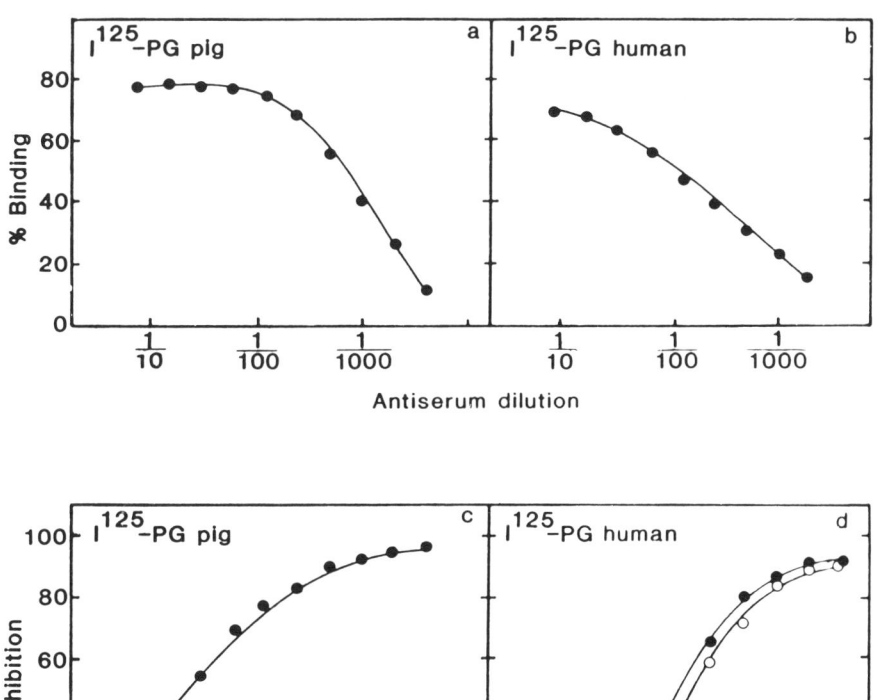

Figure 40.1 Titration of a rabbit antiserum raised against porcine CS/DS-PG II and its use in a RIA for porcine and human CS/DS PG II (from Sampaio et al., 1988). A rabbit polyclonal antiserum raised against the small pig CS-PG II was tested for its ability to precipitate (a) ^{125}I-labeled porcine cartilage CS-PG II, and (b) ^{125}I-labeled human cartilage DS-PG II. RIAs with this antiserum at (c) 1 in 1000 dilution with ^{125}I-labeled porcine CS-PG II, and (d) 1 in 350 dilution with ^{125}I-labeled human DS-PG II were used to determine separately the extent of competition with porcine CS-PG II (●) and human DS-PG II (○). The results showed the antiserum to have a weaker titer against the human DS-PG II (b) than against the primary antigen porcine CS-PG II (a). The subsequent RIA showed the human DS-PG II to be only partially competitive with antibodies recognizing the ^{125}I-porcine CS-PG II (c), but both antigens showed similar and complete competition with antibodies recognizing the ^{125}I-human DS-PG II (d).

raised against G1 does not contain significant antibodies that recognize link protein and *vice versa*, shows that their major antigenic determinants are different, although the structures are homologous. Examination of the species specificity of the antibodies showed that link proteins from human, cow, rat or dog cartilage were all well-recognized by the antibodies raised against pig link protein in a rabbit (Ratcliffe and Hardingham, 1983). Comparison of the amino acid sequences of many species of link protein show them to be highly conserved structures

(Perkins et al., 1989) which would explain their common antigenic identity. The species cross-reaction for the antibodies to G1 was weaker than for link protein. The antiserum raised against pig G1 domain showed a declining ability to react with PG preparations from cow (89%), dog (78%), rat (37%), human (22%) or rabbit cartilage (15%). Few species of G1 domain have been completely sequenced, but this may reflect a rather less-conserved structure than with link protein.

ANTIBODIES TO NATIVE OR DENATURED PROTEIN STRUCTURES

Globular proteins such as G1 domain have a complex structure that is greatly altered by unfolding on denaturation by detergents together with the reduction of intramolecular disulfide bridges. Experiments with the antiserum to PG G1 domain showed that it contained antibodies to both native and denatured epitopes (Fig. 40.2; Ratcliffe and Hardingham unpublished results). In the RIA, it was shown that antibodies binding to ^{125}I-labeled native G1 domain were completely inhibited by native PG monomer, but not inhibited at the same concentrations by reduced and alkylated G1 domain (Fig. 40.1(a)). The preparation of reduced and alkylated G1 domain therefore contained few of the epitopes recognized on the native G1. However, the same antiserum also showed a titer against ^{125}I-labeled, reduced and alkylated G1 domain and, therefore, contained antibodies to the reduced and alkylated protein. However, their binding was very poorly inhibited by the native G1 preparation (Fig. 40.2(b)). The native and reduced and alkylated preparations thus both contained antigenic determinants but contained few in common. It also showed that, although immunization was with the native G1 preparation, antibodies to both the native and unfolded protein were produced in the subsequent immune response of the animal. The presence of antibodies to both types of structure has important implications for the application of the antiserum. In localization techniques on immunoblots or in tissue sections, both native and denatured proteins or fragments of proteins may be detected, whereas a competitive RIA with an ^{125}I-labeled native antigen would specifically

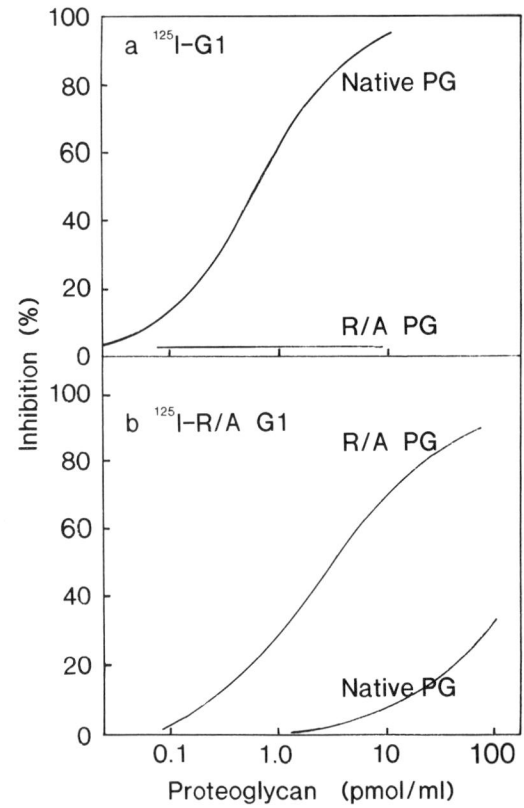

Figure 40.2 Evidence for antibodies with different specificities to native and denatured protein epitopes in a rabbit antiserum to cartilage PG G1 domain (binding region) (Ratcliffe and Hardingham, unpublished results). A rabbit polyclonal antiserum raised against cartilage PG G1 domain (pig) was able to precipitate purified ^{125}I-labeled G1 domain before or after reduction and alkylation of disulphide bonds. RIAs were established with (a) ^{125}I-labeled native G1 or (b) ^{125}I-labeled R/A PG and competition of native PG and R/A PG were compared. (a) The R/A PGs showed no detectible competition with antibodies recognizing native G1 domain. (b) The native PG also showed very weak competition with antibodies recognizing the denatured R/A C1 domain. The results show that the epitopes on native and denatured G1 recognized by the antiserum were different and that it contained some antibodies that were specific for the native structure and others that were specific for the denatured structure.

detect only native antigen and any unfolded or denatured antigen would not compete. The range of epitopes detected can therefore be selected for by the technique in which they are used. This may also give rise to apparently conflicting results where, for example, proteolytic fragments detected by immunoblotting may go undetected in an immunoassay using the same antiserum.

The situation is clearly much simpler for a monoclonal antibody that recognizes a single protein epitope. The epitope may be part of a native protein structure, or it may only be detected after reduction and alkylation. If the epitope of a globular protein is buried in the native protein and only available after reduction of disulfide bonds and unfolding of the protein, it may be efficiently detected following reduction with dithiothreitol in denaturing solvent (4 M guanidine HCl) and alkylation with iodoacetate. However, conditions for reduction may be less ideal in samples absorbed on nitrocellulose or within tissue sections and thus under these conditions detection may be far from quantitative. Monoclonal antibodies to buried protein epitopes may thus have limited use for tissue localization of antigens.

MONOCLONAL ANTIBODIES TO CARBOHYDRATE EPITOPES, KERATAN SULFATE AND CHONDROITIN SULFATE

Carbohydrate epitopes do not have 'native' and 'denatured' states to be discriminated between and they also show a range of other properties that are different from protein epitopes. There is a large number of CS and KS chains on the cartilage PG and a single PG may thus contain several copies of an epitope. The antigen may thus be multivalent and, as immunoglobulins are bivalent in IgG or decavalent in IgM, this can lead to an increase in the apparent affinity of the antibody for the antigen (Caterson *et al.*, 1989a; Poole *et al.*, 1989). A single glycosaminoglycan (GAG) chain such as KS may also contain a chain sequence providing more than one epitope site.

The presence of several copies of an epitope on a single antigen may provide an advantage in some applications involving immunoprecipitation or immunolocalization, but can create considerable problems in devising quantitative assays of the epitope. This is well-illustrated with KS (Caterson *et al.*, 1989a; Poole *et al.*, 1989). Several monoclonal antibodies have been described which, although not all identical, appear to recognize oversulfated sequences of KS that contain two sulfate groups per disaccharide (Mehmet *et al.*, 1985). These sequences are not present in all KS chains and are enriched in those of greatest length and highest charge density (Oeben *et al.*, 1987; Caterson *et al.*, 1989a). The content of this epitope thus varies in KS from different tissue sources and with different animals and at different ages. The assay of the epitope does not therefore provide an assay of the number or mass of KS chains. An assay for KS epitope was developed using an RIA procedure with chondroitinase ABC-digested PG as the radiolabeled antigen (Zanetti *et al.*, 1985). A sensitive inhibition curve was obtained with PG (with or without chondroitinase digestion), but the competitiveness decreased if the PG was proteolytically digested to give fragments containing fewer KS chains. Single KS chains were only 1% as competitive as intact PG. This showed that a polyvalent epitope (a PG with many KS chains) was a much better inhibitor of antibody binding to a polyvalent antigen than a monovalent antigen. However, in an assay procedure developed using ELISA technique (Thonar *et al.*, 1985) in which the antigen is absorbed to the surface of the plate, there appeared to be much less difference in competition between multichains and single-chain antigens. The assays developed using KS monoclonals can, therefore, provide quantitative measures of KS only when certain criteria are fulfilled and the content of epitope in the KS chains remains constant (see Chapters 43 and 44).

Monoclonal antibodies directed against CS were originally developed using chondroitinase ABC-digested PG as the antigen. Antibodies were identified that were specific for 4- sulfated, 6-sulfated or non-sulfated disaccharides at the ends of the chains (Caterson *et al.*, 1985). Other antibodies have now been prepared that do not require chondroitinase digestion for the creation of the epitope but recognize sulfated epitopes that form particular structures within chain sequences (Yamagata et al., 1987). These antibodies are of great interest as the distribution of epitopes amongst CS chains from different sources is quite varied and preliminary results show that the expression of epitopes may change during tissue development and in pathology (Caterson et al., 1989b; Hardingham et al., 1989). This has provided evidence that the structure of the chain is controlled by the cells during synthesis and is modulated during cellular responses to environmental or regulatory factors. The antibodies provide a sensitive means for detecting these changes and enable the structural details and their biological significance to be studied.

LOCALIZATION IN TISSUE SECTIONS

Antibodies have been used extensively to reveal by light microscopy and immunofluorescence the distribution of PG antigens in tissue sections. The technique is extremely informative for identifying the presence of antigen in relation to other morphological features such as collagen fibers, basement membranes and cell surfaces. However, it is not a quantitative technique as the extent of penetration of the antibody into the section and the extent to which the antigen is lost during preparation of sections are usually unknown factors. In particular, with soluble components such as PGs, the loss during fixing, sectioning and staining may be high and methods need to be tested to minimize it.

Localization by electron microscopy requires more specialist techniques but has the potential for reflecting the quantitative distribution of antigens. By using antibodies to PG G1 domain, the distribution of PG in sections of articular cartilage was determined in superficial, middle and deep zones and in pericellular and intercellular regions (Ratcliffe et al., 1984) (Fig. 40.3). The results compare well with the analysis of the tissue content of the same zones determined after extraction. The technique used involved a low-temperature embedding resin (Lowicryl K4M) which preserves protein structure by avoiding the excessive heating involved in the polymerization of most embedding resins. Localization was then carried out on the surface of ultrathin sections cut after embedding. The antibodies localize the epitope at the section surface which avoids the problem of variable penetration and the antibodies are then detected with colloidal gold particles which have been coated with protein A. The distribution of gold particles on the surface of a section (number per unit area) is therefore proportional to the concentration of PG found within the section. The technique was also used to investigate intracellular pathways of PG synthesis (Ratcliffe et al., 1985) and by using gold particles of two different and distinct sizes, it was possible to localize both protein core and CS epitopes within the same section. Using this technique, it was possible to show that the medial *trans* Golgi rather than *cis* Golgi was the site for CS chain synthesis on PG protein core. It was also shown that both PG and link protein were found within the same intracellular Golgi compartments (Ratcliffe et al., 1987).

MOLECULAR IMAGING BY ELECTRON MICROSCOPY

Electron microscopy of PGs has been particularly useful in establishing the structural features of PGs. Originally, this was done by contrasting the GAG chains with cytochrome C as developed for visualizing DNA (Rosenberg et al., 1975; Buckwalter and Rosenberg, 1982). More recently, the technique has been extended by using rotary shadowing or negative staining to visualize the globular protein domains (Wiedemann et al., 1984; Paulsson et al., 1987; Mörgelin et al., 1988). As PGs present large expanded structures by electron microscopy, there are clear opportunities for identifying the sites of epitopes within the molecular structure by localizing antibodies bound to the spread molecules. This has been achieved by using antibodies to binding region and KS (Sheehan et al., 1987). The technique used protein A–gold for antibody localization and was

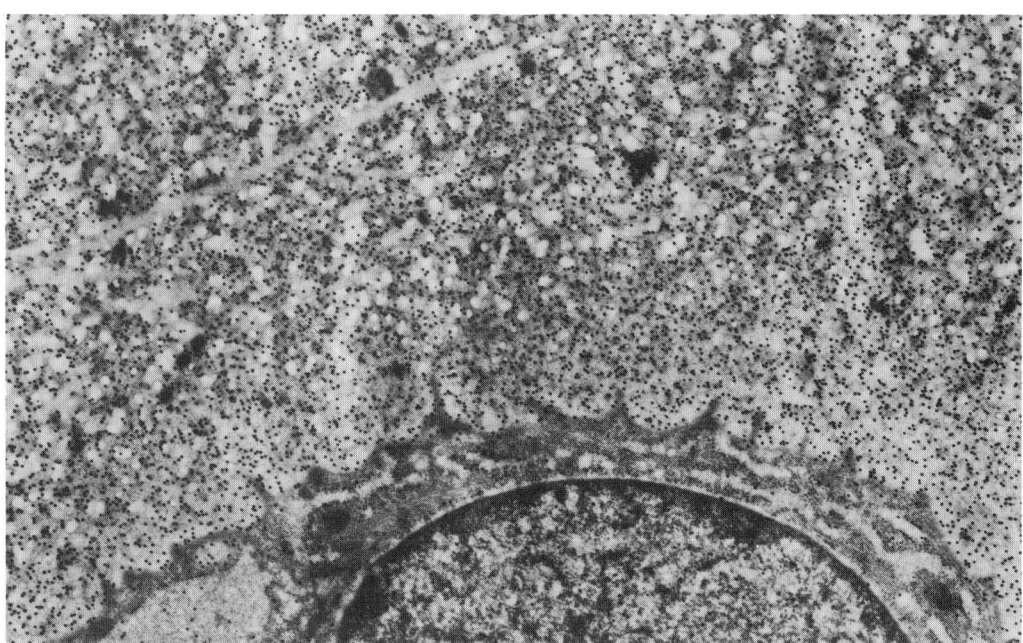

Figure 40.3 Immunogold localization of PG in articular cartilage (Ratcliffe et al., 1984). Porcine articular cartilage was embedded in low-temperature Lowicryl K4M resin and polyclonal rabbit anti-PG G1 domain was used on ultrathin sections following chondroitinase ABC-digestion to localize PGs with protein A–gold (15 nm diameter). A vertical section in the mid zone of porcine articular cartilage close to a chondrocyte is shown. The density of PG localization is higher in the pericellular region compared with the intercellular region. Collagen appears as largely unstained fibers in longitudinal or cross-section in the matrix and PGs localized in the space between the fibers.

designed to avoid the problem of heavy background staining obtained when antibody and protein A–gold were applied directly to molecules already spread on the electron-microscope. The technique was also compatible with using simple antisera rather that purified antibodies. The PG preparation was incubated with the antiserum (anti-G1 domain) and then the PG and attached antibodies were separated by gel chromatography from unbound antibodies and other proteins. The PG–antibody complex was then incubated with protein A–gold and the PG–antibody–protein A–gold complex formed was likewise separated from unbound protein A–gold by gel chromatography. The diluted solution of the complex was then spread on the electron-microscope grid and the molecules were contrasted with benzylalkylammonium chloride. With anti-G1 antibodies, there was strong localization of gold particles at one end of the PG structure which corresponded with the known N-terminal location of the G1 domain. With anti-KS monoclonal antibodies, there was also localization toward one end of the PG which appeared to correspond to the KS-rich region of PG. In some molecules with one KS monoclonal antibody (5-D-4), there was a different distribution of antibody as it bound more extensively along the protein core and caused the GAG chains to be extended rather than collapsed, as they are usually visualized with benzylalkylammonium chloride. This may reflect some different structural arrangement of KS chains in some molecules or possibly the presence of larger concentrations of KS epitope in the KS attached to some PGs.

SUMMARY

Antibodies can provide useful reagents for a broad range of applications for detecting, identifying, locating and quantifying PGs and other cartilage components. They have become part of the essential techniques of research on cartilage and with careful validation they can provide a most valuable insight into the molecular and cellular processes that characterize the tissue.

ACKNOWLEDGMENT

This work was carried out with the support of the Arthritis and Rheumatism Council (UK).

41

Methods for production and characterization of monoclonal antibodies against connective-tissue proteoglycans

BRUCE CATERSON, TONY CALABRO, TERRY BLANKENSHIP-PARIS, MARK ADAMS, RICHARD PEARCE and ANDREW MALCOLM

Over the past ten years the primary objectives of research in our laboratory have been directed towards the production and characterization of monoclonal antibodies against connective-tissue proteoglycans (PGs). Our goals here have been to produce monoclonal antibodies that recognize epitopes on different structural and functional domains of connective-tissue PGs. To achieve these goals we have utilized a wide variety of different methodological approaches and experimental strategies; a summary of some of the conclusions made from these studies is the subject of this chapter.

PGs are in general extremely large and inherently heterogeneous macromolecules that present several problems in monoclonal antibody production and characterization. PG heterogeneity is derived from several sources which include the occurrence of different classes of glycosaminoglycan (GAG) and also N- and O-linked oligosaccharide substitutions present on either common or different polypeptide backbones. Furthermore, connective tissues are usually composed of several different classes (families) of PG, their isolation and purification for antibody production and screening usually involving many laborious and time-consuming steps.

METHODS FOR PRODUCING MONOCLONAL ANTIBODIES AGAINST PROTEOGLYCANS

In general, it is best to begin monoclonal antibody production with the most purified sample, as this minimizes the chances of wasting valuable time and reagents in the identification of monoclonal antibodies directed against minor contaminants. However, if it is difficult or impractical to prepare large quantities of 'pure' antigen for immunization purposes, one can also use partially purified sample as the immunizing antigen and utilize small amounts of the 'highly purified antigen' in selective screening procedures once putative hybridomas have been initially identified.

Mice and rats are generally the animals used as a source of activated β-lymphocytes for cell fusion and hybridoma production. Rats are often preferred if mouse-derived material is used as antigen for immunization. In this laboratory we have successfully used Balb-C mice for the production of almost all our monoclonal antibodies against PG structures. Retrospective analysis of their epitope specificity has indicated that many of these antibodies recognize epitopes (both protein and carbohydrate) in structures that have been highly conserved in nature and are common to PGs from a wide variety of animal species. This phenomenon may result from our use of a short-term hyperimmunization protocol and the draining of lymph nodes rather than the spleen as the source of activated β-lymphocytes (see Caterson et al., 1985). This protocol does not necessarily lead to production of a high frequency of IgG producing hybridomas, our analyses to date indicating that approximately two-thirds (22/34) of those tested are of the IgM subclass and all but two of these expressed κ rather than λ immunoglobulin light chains.

The strategies employed in our laboratory also involve various forms of enzymatic and chemical modification of PG antigens (Calabro, 1987; Caterson et al., 1985, 1986, 1987a, b) to facilitate the production of monoclonal antibodies to different domains present in cartilage PG monomer, (Fig. 41.1). Treatment of PGs with enzymes such as chondroitinase or mammalian hyaluronidase removes chondroitin sulfate (CS) GAG chains from the PG leaving short oligosaccharide stubs containing the CS linkage region and some nonreducing terminal disaccharides that are characteristic of the various different sulfate isomer forms of CS (Caterson et al., 1985). When chondroitinase-treated PGs are used as immunogens, we have observed that we generate with high frequency monoclonal antibodies that are directed against the terminal unsaturated disaccharide unit with a δ-4,5-unsaturated hexuronate group at the nonreducing

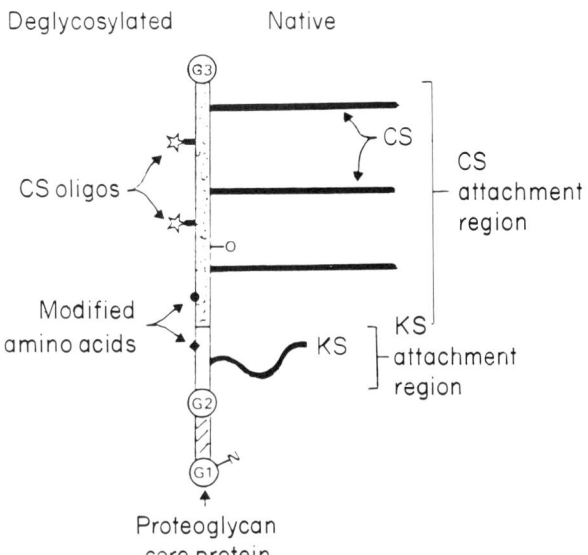

Figure 41.1 Schematic representations of the antigenic structures on 'native' and 'deglycosylated' cartilage PG monomer. CS-oligos indicate oligosaccharide 'stubs' that remain attached to the protein core after chondroitinase digestion of the CS chains of the PG monomer. Antibodies to the protein polypeptide of the CS and KS attachment regions of the PG, (◆) and (●) denote modified amino acids in the PG core protein that result from β-elimination of O-linked glycosaminoglycans and oligosaccharides. O- and N- depict O- and N-linked oligosaccharides, respectively. G1, G2 and G3 indicate the three disulfide bonds containing globular domains of the PG monomer. (G1 contains the HA binding region of the PG.) Antibodies to these domains were produced after reduction and alkylation of the disulfide bonds. Over-sulfated domains of the native CS and KS GAGs are also antigenic if untreated PG is used as immunogen.

terminal of these oligosaccharide stubs. From these studies we have now identified several hybridomas (Caterson et al., 1985, 1987, a,b) that are specific for the three most common sulfate isomers of CS (i.e. 4-, 6- and non-sulfated CS). In general, these antibodies require samples to be pretreated with chondroitinase in order to generate the unsaturated nonreducing terminal hexuronic acid moiety that is required for antibody recognition. These antibodies are being used in a wide variety of immunohistochemical and immunochemical studies to identify specifically connective-tissue PGs that contain these different CS isomers (see Caterson et al., 1985, 1986, 1987b).

We have also generated monoclonal antibodies to native (unmodified) GAG chains of connective-tissue PGS. It has been our experience (Caterson et al., 1983, 1986, 1987b, 1989a) that keratan sulfate (KS) structures are particularly immunogenic to mice and, therefore, one always finds several hybridomas producing antibodies against a wide variety of different epitopes that are often present in over-sulfated domains of the KS glycosaminoglycan (Mehmet et al., 1986). Removal of the KS by enzymatic or chemical procedures reduces the chance of getting unduly large numbers of hybridomas producing antibodies against this PG substructure.

In recent studies (Sorrell et al., 1988; Mahmoodian, 1988), we have also identified five hybridomas that produce monoclonal antibodies against epitopes in 'native' CS GAGs. Preliminary analysis of their specificity has indicated that these antibodies also recognize over-sulfated or uncommon disaccharide domains of the CS GAG similar to that reported by others (Yamagata, 1987). These uncommon CS domains (epitopes) seem to be differentially expressed during normal growth and development (Sorrell et al., 1988; Mahmoodian, 1988).

In order to generate monoclonal antibodies against protein epitopes on the core protein of cartilage PGs we have used chemical-modification procedures to introduce 'foreign' amino acids into different protein structural domains of the proteoglycan (see Fig. 41.1). Reduction and alkylation of disulfide bonds in the PG has facilitated the production of several monoclonal antibodies recognizing epitopes in the G1, G2 and G3 domains of the PG. In addition, alkali elimination of O-linked GAGs in the presence of reducing agents such as sodium sulfite (Caterson et al., 1983; Knight and Robinson, 1984) has resulted in the identification of several monoclonal antibodies that recognize protein domains adjacent to the sites of KS, CS and O-linked oligosaccharide attachment to the PG protein core. The studies described above have produced a bank of monoclonal antibodies that recognize epitopes present in many of GAG substructures (KS and CS) and the substructural protein

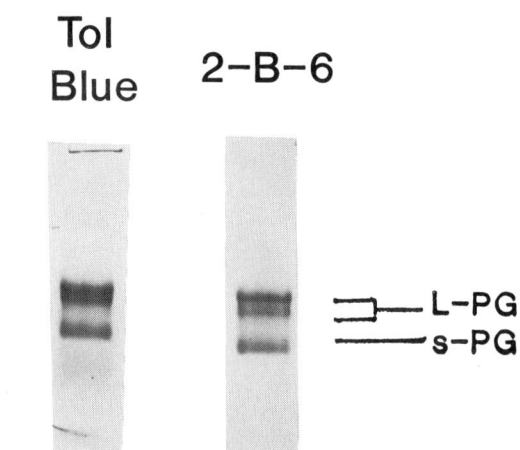

Figure 41.2 Biochemical and immunochemical analysis of PG subpopulations separated by composite agarose–polyacrylamide gel electrophoresis. Guinea-pig articular cartilage (10 mg wet wt) was extracted at 4°C in 4 M guanidine HCl (1 ml) containing proteinase inhibitors. The extract was dialyzed against distilled water overnight at 4°C, lyophilized and dissolved in electrophoresis buffer (8 M urea, 0.25 mM Na_2SO_4, 40 mM (tris)-acetate, pH 6.8). Replicate samples (5–10 μl) containing 0.1–5.0 μg PG were then subjected to composite gel electrophoresis (Carney et al., 1986). The PG bands were identified by staining with toluidine blue on the track loaded with c. 2.5 μg PG and were immunolocalized with monoclonal antibody 2-B-6 on the track loaded with c. 0.1 μg PG. This antibody recognized 4-sulfated CS oligosaccharides attached to the PG core proteins after chondroitinase ABC-digestion. The results identify two populations of 'large' PG (L-PG) and one of 'small' PGs (S-PG). Both procedures specifically stain the PGs without detecting other macromolecules present in the 4 M guanidine HCl extract. The immunolocalization method is ideal for multiple analyses with a wide variety of monoclonal antibodies of different specificity, thus providing a comprehensive biochemical/immunochemical analysis of the PG subpopulations.

domains of cartilage PGs (see Fig. 41.1). Because many of these structures occur in other families of PG some of the monoclonal antibodies can also be used biochemically to characterize PGs from a wide variety of connective tissues and animal species.

BIOCHEMICAL ANALYSIS OF PROTEOGLYCAN SUBPOPULATIONS USING MONOCLONAL ANTIBODIES AND AGAROSE—ACRYLAMIDE GEL ELECTROPHORESIS

In collaborative studies (West Virginia University and The University of British Columbia) (Caterson *et al.*, 1987a,b), we combined the techniques of composite agarose–polyacrylamide gel electrophoresis (Carney *et al.*, 1986) and 'Western Blot' immunolocalization to facilitate the detailed analysis of different PG subpopulations found in extracts of connective tissues. An example of this procedure is shown in Fig. 41.2 with PGs from guinea-pig articular cartilage.

Using this procedure, different PG subpopulations ('small' and 'large' PG) can be electrophoretically separated from one another and the use of cationic dyes or monoclonal antibodies allows one to identify specifically the PGs within the complex milieu of molecules present in the tissue extracts. In this method, the use of monoclonal antibodies for immunolocation has several advantages over the use of cationic dyes such as toluidine Blue or Alcian Blue: detection with monoclonal antibodies is 10–50 times more sensitive; the use of several different monoclonal antibodies allows for the detection of subtle biochemical differences in both protein and carbohydrate components present on the different PG subpopulations; and protein epitopes can be detected with the monoclonal antibodies, whereas cationic dyes only react the polyanionic GAG chains. This procedure is particularly useful in studies involving small animal species where only limited tissue is available for study. Extracts from as little as 15 mg wet wt cartilage can be used to perform 25–30 different immunolocation analyses using different monoclonal antibodies, thus providing a comprehensive biochemical analysis of different PG subpopulations separated by this electrophoretic method. Using this procedure we have been able to detect PG subpopulations containing differences in the presence or absence of various globular domains (G1, G2 or G3), their substitution with different GAGs (CS or KS) and also variability in the occurrence of subtle carbohydrate structures within these GAG side chains. These methods have provided a sensitive means of assaying a large number of PGs in a relatively short time and are particularly useful for studying the affects of factors that perturb PG metabolism.

ACKNOWLEDGMENT

This work was supported by N.I.H. grants AR32666 and AR38726.

42

Characterization and use of polyclonal antibodies to collagen

D.J. HARTMANN

Polyclonal antibodies to collagen have been used extensively for histological, biological and clinical studies on connective tissue (Furthmayr and Timpl, 1976; Michaeli, 1977; Timpl and Risteli, 1982; Timpl, 1984; Gay and Fine, 1987; Risteli and Risteli, 1989). The preparation of specific polyclonal antibodies to collagens is still difficult, since many closely related proteins are present in the extracellular matrix and thus specific antigens cannot be purified easily. Collagen antibodies that have been raised using classical immunization procedures have some distinctive features: (i) a low titer due to the weak immunogenicity of collagens (except for types IV and VI); (ii) an affinity, measured by their equilibrium constant, that is within the range 10^9–10^{11} l mol^{-1} and determines the potential sensitivity of quantitative assays; and (iii) specificity with regard to type of collagen, animal species and conformation. With regard to the first criterion, the antibody must recognize only one type of collagen and not other types or other connective-tissue proteins; purification by affinity chromatography is often required. Collagen antibodies are not usually considered as species specific since they can stain tissues of different species, however, in competitive radioimmunoassays (RIAs) or inhibition in solid-phase RIAs or enzyme-linked immunosorbent assays (ELISAs), the major antibody population preferentially recognizes the species of collagen against which it was raised, and not others. For example, Fig. 42.1 shows that neither bovine nor mouse type II collagen can displace the binding of labeled human type II collagen with its antibody, but bovine (or mouse) type II collagen can displace the binding of labeled

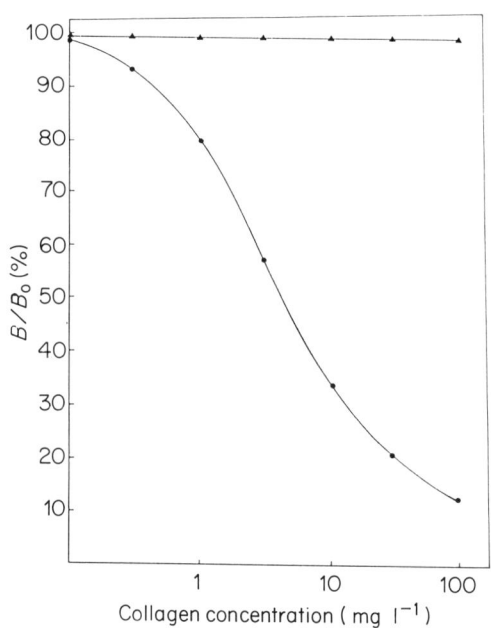

Figure 42.1 RIA for human type II collagen with ^{125}I-labeled human type II collagen and anti-human type II collagen antibody. The inhibitors used were human (●) and mouse of bovine (▲) type II collagens.

bovine (or mouse) type II collagen with the antibody to human type II collagen. In our experience, polyclonal antibodies to interstitial collagens are very sensitive to conformation even when the major antigenic sites are located at the ends of the molecule, as shown for type II collagen by rotary shadowing (Fig. 42.2). This specificity to conformation can be seen by RIA in liquid phase:

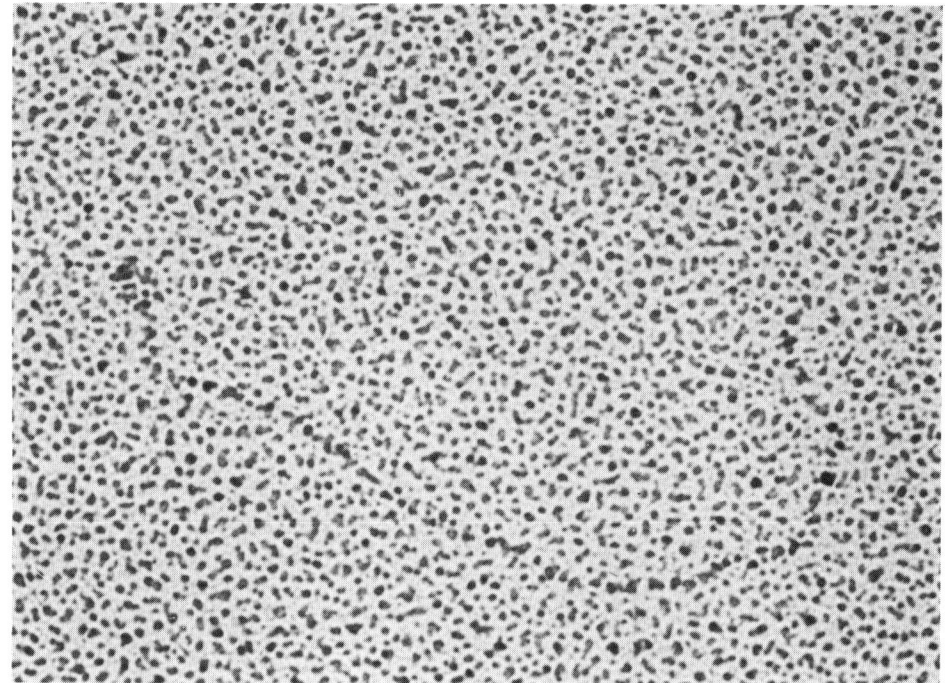

Figure 42.2 Electron-microscopic visualization of the terminal determinant detected by a polyclonal antibody on human type II collagen using the rotary shadowing technique. (Courtesy of Annie Barge.)

denatured type II collagen is recognized at least 100-fold less than native type II collagen by the anti-type II. This fact may be of great importance when western blotting is the only technique used to characterize antibodies, particularly when assessing specificity. With this technique, the antigens are denatured, and, therefore, only minor populations are involved.

The major use of these antibodies besides immunostaining is for quantifying collagens in biological fluids or cell-culture media. Such quantitative determinations comprise two main problems. First, there is no international reference standard (expressed on a molar basis) that allows comparison of the results of different laboratories. Second, the measured molecule must be as similar as possible to the molecule that was used to raise the antibody. For instance, antibodies directed against acid-soluble molecules and against pepsinized molecules do not give the same responses in cell-culture media. The detection of bovine and human type II and type III collagens in culture media of bovine chondrocytes and human fibroblasts is increased after pepsin treatment since our antibodies are directed against pepsinized molecules.

Moreover, in biological fluids, the distribution of the collagen antigenic forms is often heterogeneous; for instance, the antigenicity of serum type I collagen is separated by gel filtration into two fractions of completely different molecular weights and these fractions do not have the same affinity for the antibody (Hartmann *et al.*, in preparation).

Despite the development of monoclonal antibodies to different collagen types, polyclonal antibodies remain useful for many studies, particularly for quantitative immunoassays, as monoclonal antibodies often have low affinity constants and weak bindings of radiolabeled collagen (5–30%) due to the microheterogeneity of collagen preparations (Timpl, 1984).

43

Measurement of antigenic keratan sulfate by an enzyme-linked immunosorbent assay

EUGENE J.M.A. THONAR, MARY ELLEN LENZ, BRIAN MALDONADO, LORI OTTEN, TIBOR GLANT and KLAUS E. KUETTNER

The enzyme-linked immunosorbent assay (ELISA) offers some advantages over radio-immunoassays (RIA) for the quantification of antigenic molecules. The color reaction can be measured using an inexpensive apparatus, all reagents are stable over long periods of time and multiwell microtiter plates allow large number of assays to be performed in a semiautomated fashion (Kemmeny and Challacombe, 1988). Competitive indirect ELISAs have been developed to measure the concentration in solution of different constituents of the cartilage matrix, i.e. hyaluronan binding region (Thonar et al., 1982), link protein (Thonar et al., 1982), keratan sulfate (KS) (Thonar et al., 1985, 1986; Williams et al., 1988), and lysozyme (Thonar et al., 1988a), etc.

In developing a competitive indirect ELISA, it is necessary to examine important technical aspects in order to optimize the conditions and to determine whether the assay can provide an accurate measure of the concentration of the antigen present. Theoretical and practical aspects of ELISAs are thoroughly described in a recent book by Kemmeny and Challacombe (1988) which provides useful information for the novice and expert alike. This report focused on some technical aspects which were taken into consideration in optimizing the ELISA for the quantification of keratan sulfate (KS). The ELISA we have developed is shown in Fig. 43.1. The conditions were optimized to give as accurate a representation of the amount of KS epitope present as possible. Although many anti-KS antibodies are available, we have only used two of these [1/20/5-D-4 (a generous gift from Dr Bruce Caterson, University of West Virginia) and ET-4-A-4] in all the studies performed thus far. Unless indicated otherwise, all observations described in this chapter were made using one of these two antibodies which recognize a similar, if not identical, domain of over-sulfated disaccharides (Mehmet et al., 1986; Thonar et al., 1986) which has recently been shown to be present near the non-reducing end (Stuhlsatz et al., 1989) of the longest KS chains. These two antibodies have a very high affinity for long KS chains but do not recognize KS chains of shorter length (Maldonado et al., 1988). In the ELISA, the antibodies form as stable complexes with intact proteoglycan (PG) molecules containing many KS chains as with single long KS chains and recognize equally well KS chains in the KS-rich and the chondroitin sulfate (CS)-rich regions of the PG molecule (Maldonado et al., 1988). The ELISA is sensitive (50% inhibition is obtained at approximately 5 ng pig costal cartilage KS/ml) and yields very reproducible results from day to day (standard deviation < 4%) (Thonar et al., 1988b).

Because KS chain length may vary with age and cartilage of origin (Stuhlsatz et al., 1989), the amount of epitope detected in the ELISA does not necessarily provide an absolute measure of the amount of KS present. For example, the ratio of antigenic/nonantigenic KS is higher in the aggregating PGs of bovine articular cartilage than in those of bovine nasal cartilage of the same age.

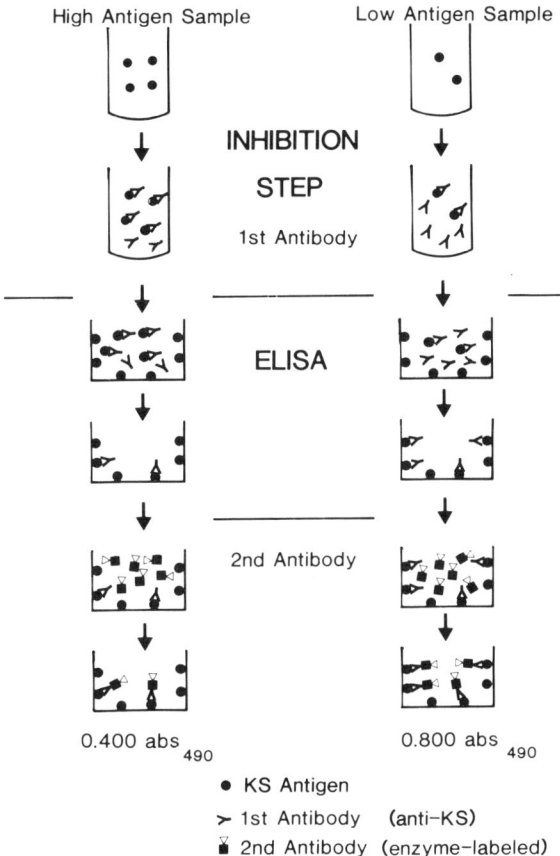

Figure 43.1 Competitive indirect ELISA for the quantification of KS. The KS antigen to be quantified competes with coated KS antigen for binding to the anti-KS antibody. The concentration of KS antigen present in unknowns is calculated by comparing the absorbance value in each case to values generated from known concentrations of costal cartilage KS antigen treated in an identical fashion and run in parallel.

Since the KS chains in bovine articular cartilage do not show significant age-related differences in length, it is not surprising that there are no age-related differences in the ratio of antigenic/nonantigenic KS in this tissue. On the other hand, the ratio shows a several-fold increase with age in human articular cartilage aggregating PGs, the KS chains of which show a marked age-related increase in length (Glant and Thonar, unpublished observations; also see Chapters 53 and 54). In all the studies which have made use of the KS ELISA, we have used the same preparation of highly purified skeletal KS from pig costal cartilage as a standard (a kind gift from Drs M.B. Mathews and A.L. Horwitz, The University of Chicago, Chicago, IL). Consequently, all concentrations of serum KS reported in those studies reflect equivalents of this international standard of KS.

A number of observations help illustrate how important the selection of the anti-KS antibody is in obtaining a meaningful interpretation of the amount of epitope present. First, some antibodies, such as the MZ15 (a generous gift from The Kennedy Institute, London) (Zanetti et al., 1985) and our HAC-232 or HFPG-529 anti-KS antibodies, show a marked preference in this ELISA for KS-bearing molecules containing many KS chains, i.e. they bind with low affinity in solution to single chains of KS (half inhibition > 1000 ng pig costal cartilage KS/ml). Thus, it is not possible to use these antibodies in the ELISA to quantify the amount of KS epitope present. In contrast, other antibodies bind with high affinity to single chains of KS. For example, 50% inhibition of binding of the 1/20/5-D-4 or ET-4-A-4 anti-KS antibodies to the bovine nasal PG coated to the plate can be achieved by preincubating the antibody with single chains of pig costal cartilage KS at 5–10 ng ml^{-1} (Thonar et al., 1985, 1986). Second, some anti-KS antibodies (MK-202 or MK-172) find corneal KS is richer in epitope than purified KS from pig costal cartilage. When other antibodies (HAC-655 or 1/20/5-D-4) are used in the ELISA, the converse is true. Third, some antibodies (EFG-11, MK-202) recognize KS in fetal PGs well, while others do not (HAC-655 or HAC-232). These observations suggest that the amount of KS epitope detected depends, at least in part, on the anti-KS antibody used and that the relative concentration of epitope in some KS preparations is higher than in others. One should be able to take advantage of differences in the specificity or affinity of two or more anti-KS antibodies to differentiate between different types of KS-bearing molecules.

Changes in the pH of the solution in which the antigen and anti-KS antibody are incubated (inhibition step) may have a profound effect on the shape of the inhibition curve. For example, at pH 7.0, KS-bearing molecules in rabbit serum or plasma do not inhibit binding of the 1/20/5-D-4 anti-KS antibody to the coated antigen by more than 60%. This problem can be remedied by lowering the pH of the phosphate buffered saline (PBS) in the incubation mixture of pH 5.3 (Williams et al., 1988). ELISAs performed at the lower pH yield for both standards and unknowns steeper inhibition curves, therefore increasing the ability to discriminate between concentrations of antigen that are not markedly different. The lower pH also helps in reducing the background. For these reasons, we now use PBS at pH 5.3 in our analyses of serum KS (Williams et al., 1988). It should be noted that although PBS does not buffer well at this pH, this seldom creates a problem because of the high sensitivity of the ELISA, the samples to be assayed are usually diluted at least 20 times in PBS buffer prior to analysis.

We have observed that changes in the concentration of some of the interactants, i.e. coated antigen and first antibody, may create problems with the quantification process. For example, at much lower concentrations of the ET-4-A-4 antibody, the complex formed between antibody and single KS chains dissociates more rapidly than the complex antibody–cartilage PG.

Other observations worth noting include the following. First, the KS standard is very stable when dissolved in water containing 1% bovine serum albumin +0.05% Tween 20 and stored at −80°C. Serum or plasma stored at −80°C for 3 years similarly shows no loss in content of KS epitope. Second, repeated freezing and thawing of samples produces no significant loss in antigenicity. Third, the use of some salts which appear to complex with the epitope should also be avoided. For example, sodium borate at concentrations as low as 35 mM totally inhibits antibody binding to the KS epitope (Maldonado and Thonar, unpublished observations). Fourth, the presence of guanidinium chloride and/or some detergents (e.g. deoxycholic acid) may reduce or abolish antigen–antibody binding in the ELISA.

The time required to perform the analysis can be reduced to 60 min (Maldonado and Thonar, unpublished observations). In this modified rapid ELISA-inhibition assay, the inhibition step can be shortened to 1 min and the sequential incubations of the inhibition mixture and peroxidase-labeled second antibody to a few minutes. It is, however, necessary to increase the concentrations of the first and second antibody 3–4 times. Importantly, the shapes of the inhibition curves and the sensitivity are not markedly different from those obtained using the longer method.

In summary, the ELISA for the quantification of KS epitope is an extremely useful tool which can be developed in the laboratory at relatively little cost. Like other immunoassays, investigators should exercise caution in using it to obtain an absolute measure of the antigenic KS present. Accurate quantification can, however, be achieved by rigorous characterization of all factors which influence recognition of the antigen by the antibody in this ELISA.

ACKNOWLEDGMENTS

This work was supported in part by The William Noble Lane Foundation, grants AG-04736 and 1-P50-AR-39239 from The National Institutes of Health and by the National Council of Research Foundation (OTKA), Hungary.

44

Quantitation of keratan sulfate epitope in bovine and human cartilage proteoglycans: comparison of immunoassay procedures and anti-keratan sulfate antibodies

M.J. SEIBEL, R. JELSMA, F. SAED-NEJAD and A. RATCLIFFE

INTRODUCTION

The majority of keratan sulfate (KS) in the body is present in the proteoglycans (PG) of cartilage and intervertebral disc (Muir and Hardingham, 1975), and it has been suggested that KS may have some specificity for cartilage (Thonar et al., 1985). Quantitative analysis of KS in body fluids is therefore regarded as having a certain potential in monitoring articular cartilage catabolism (Thonar et al., 1985; Hascall and Glant, 1987). Quantitation of KS in synovial fluid and serum is presently achieved by immunoassay procedures such as radioimmunoassays (RIA) and enzyme-linked immunosorbent assays (ELISA), using monoclonal antibodies to KS (Caterson et al., 1983; Zanetti et al., 1985). However, recent studies of these techniques have shown the quantitation of KS epitope to be strongly influenced by factors such as the monoclonal antibody used and the structural presentation of the antigen (i.e. KS chain length, degree of sulfation, number of KS chains attached to a protein core) (Mehmet et al., 1986; Poole et al., 1989; Caterson et al., 1989; Seibel et al., 1989).

In this study we have determined the influence of antibody, structure and presentation of antigen, and type of immunoassay, on the quantitation of KS epitope using (i) purified PG preparations from bovine nasal and human articular cartilage and (ii) body fluids (synovial fluids and sera).

MATERIAL AND METHODS

PG monomer (AlDl fraction) was prepared from both bovine nasal and human articular cartilage. This was digested with chondroitinase ABC (0.1 U mg^{-1}, 4 h, 37°C), to yield a KS-bearing PG core protein preparation devoid of chondroitin sulfate (PG-core). Smaller KS-bearing peptides were further prepared by (i) digestion of the PG-core preparation with trypsin (1 μg mg protein, 4 h, 37°C), followed by purification on a diethylaminoethyl-Sephacel (DEAE-Sephacel) column (KS peptide 1), and (ii) digestion of KS peptide 1 with papain (0.5 μg mg protein, 16 h, 60°C), followed by heat inactivation (100°C, 30 min) of the enzyme (KS peptide 2).

The monoclonal anti-KS antibodies investigated were: 1/20/5-D-4, 5/29/2-D-3 and 4/8/1-B-4 (provided by Dr B. Caterson, Morgantown, WV), 1110-S-12.1 (provided by Ciba-Geigy Ltd, Basel, Switzerland), ET-4-A-4 (provided by Dr E. Thonar, Chicago, Il) and MZ15 (provided by The Kennedy Institute, London, UK). KS epitope was determined using an RIA with ^{125}I-labeled PG core, and an ELISA as described previously (Thonar et al., 1985; Ratcliffe et al., 1988). Determinations were done in duplicate, using AlDl as standard. Total sulfated glycosaminoglycan (S-GAG) concentrations were determined using the 1,9-dimethylmethylene blue dye binding assay (Ratcliffe et al., 1988).

Gel filtration chromatography was performed on a column (1.0 × 120 cm) of Sepharose CL-6B eluted with 2 M guanidine HCl. Fractions were analyzed for S-GAG and apparent KS epitope content. Affinity chromatography was performed using a CNBr activated Sepharose 4B column containing covalently bound antibody MZ15. Samples were applied in PBS, and bound antigen was eluted using 0.1 M (tris)HCl, pH 2.8.

Synovial fluids and sera were randomly chosen from a pool of samples from healthy individuals and patients with a variety of inflammatory and degenerative joint disorders. Differences in KS epitope concentration between paired samples were analyzed using either Wilcoxon's paired sample test (synovial fluids) or the paired sample t-test (sera). Correlations were tested using Spearman's rank correlation coefficient (r_s).

RESULTS

Gel filtration and affinity chromatography of proteoglycan fragments

The PG preparations of human articular cartilage were applied to Sepharose CL-6B chromatography, and the fractions were analyzed for S-GAG and KS epitope content. PG core eluted at the V_o of the column (Fig. 44.1(a)). When KS peptide 1 was applied, S-GAG analysis showed it to elute as two distinct peaks, both included in the column (Fig. 44.1(b)). However, ELISA and RIA analysis for KS epitope, using the antibodies 12.1, 5-D-4 and MZ15, consistently revealed KS epitope to be present only in the high M_r fragments, eluting in the first peak (Fig. 44.1(b)). When human KS peptide 2 was applied to the column it eluted as a single peak close to the

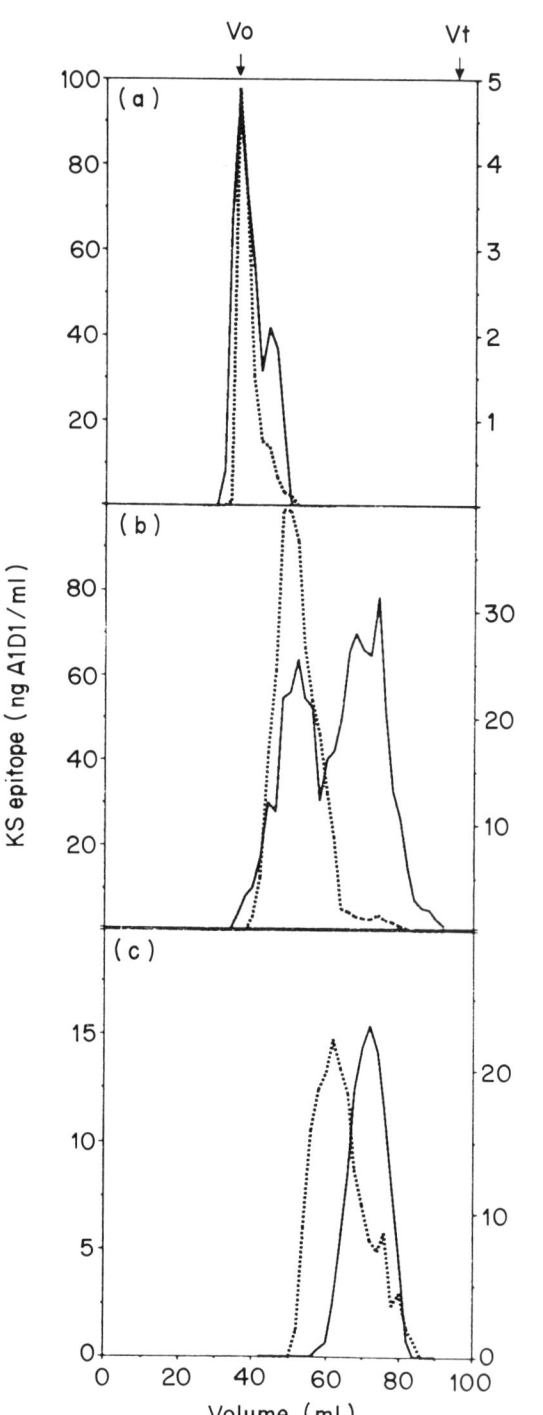

Figure 44.1 Gel filtration chromatography of human PG core (a), KS peptide 1 (b) and KS peptide 2 (c). Samples were chromatographed on a Sepharose CL 6B column in 2 M guanidine HCl. Column fractions were analyzed for S-GAG (———) and for KS epitope (····) determined by ELISA using antibody 5-D-4. Similar results were observed using the RIA and using antibodies 12.1 and MZ15.

position of the second peak of KS peptide 1, with KS epitope being detected preferentially in the higher M_r fractions (Fig. 44.1(c)). Similar results were obtained when analyzing PG fragments of bovine origin (data not shown).

Bovine KS peptide 2 was applied to a CNBr activated Sepharose 4B column containing antibody MZ15. Unbound and bound fractions were analyzed for total S-GAG and KS epitope using MZ15 in both the RIA and ELISA. The ratio of KS epitope to S-GAG was 10- to 15-fold higher in the bound fraction compared with the starting material, indicating that a small proportion (approximately 10%) of KS chains contain the majority of the epitope as recognized by antibody MZ15.

Inhibitory capacity of proteoglycan fragments

The lower limits of KS epitope detectability (defined as the amount of inhibitor resulting in 20% inhibition of antibody binding) varied according to the type of immunoassay and the antibody used. For one antibody, the ELISA generally had a lower detection limit than the RIA. Within one assay, the lower detection limits of KS epitope varied as a function of the antibody used and greatest detectability was always achieved with antibodies 12.1 and 4A4. The lower detection limit for bovine monomer using antibody 12.1 was 20 ng AlDl/ml in the ELISA, and 200 ng AlDl/ml in the RIA. In contrast, antibody MZ15 required 1000 ng ml^{-1} for detection in both the RIA and the ELISA. Between antibodies, variability of detection limits was greater in the ELISA than in the RIA.

In order to compare the inhibitory capacity of purified KS-bearing PG fragments, the amount of inhibitor (in terms of KS content) required for 50% inhibition of antibody binding was determined. In both the RIA and the ELISA, KS-bearing PG fragments of human and bovine origin consistently showed a gradual loss of inhibitory capacity with a reduction in size (number of KS chains per core) of the fragments analyzed (Fig. 44.2). The difference between the inhibitory capacity of the PG core and the significantly smaller preparation of KS peptide 2 ranged from a minimum of 1.7-fold to a maximum of 58-fold using bovine PG fragments and from 3.2-fold to 88-fold using human articular cartilage PG fragments (Table 44.1). Thus, the amount of apparent epitope in a given KS preparation may be dependent on the type of assay and the antibody, even though the same standard may be used.

Analysis of human synovial fluid and sera
(see Chapter 80)

The concentration of KS epitope was determined in human synovial fluids ($n = 15$) and sera ($n = 15$) using the antibodies 12.1, 5-D-4 and MZ15 in both immunoassays. Apparent KS epitope concentrations in synovial fluids, as determined by either RIA or ELISA using all the antibodies, showed no significant difference ($p > 0.05$).

In contrast, determinations of apparent KS epitope concentration in sera using one antibody, by RIA and ELISA, were significantly different ($p < 0.001$) and did not correlate between assays ($p > 0.05$). RIA determination of concentration in sera did show significant differences between antibodies ($p < 0.001$), although the results still showed good correlations. ELISA determinations of KS epitope revealed that concentrations of apparent KS epitope were found to be significantly different between all antibodies tested and results obtained with antibody MZ15 did not correlate with those obtained with either antibody 12.1 or 5-D-4.

Table 44.1 Loss of inhibitory capacity with reduction of antigen size. (Values represent the ratio of the inhibitory capacity of KS peptide 2 and of PG core; for details see text)

	Human articular cartilage		Bovine nasal cartilage	
	ELISA	RIA	ELISA	RIA
12.1	3.2	4.7	1.7	5.9
4-A-4	4.2	7.7	1.8	7.3
2-D-3	3.6	5.1	2.7	4.8
5-D-4	4.2	10.1	5.3	4.3
1-B-4	88.4	26.4	50.4	40.5
MZ15	24.4	47.8	7.8	58.8

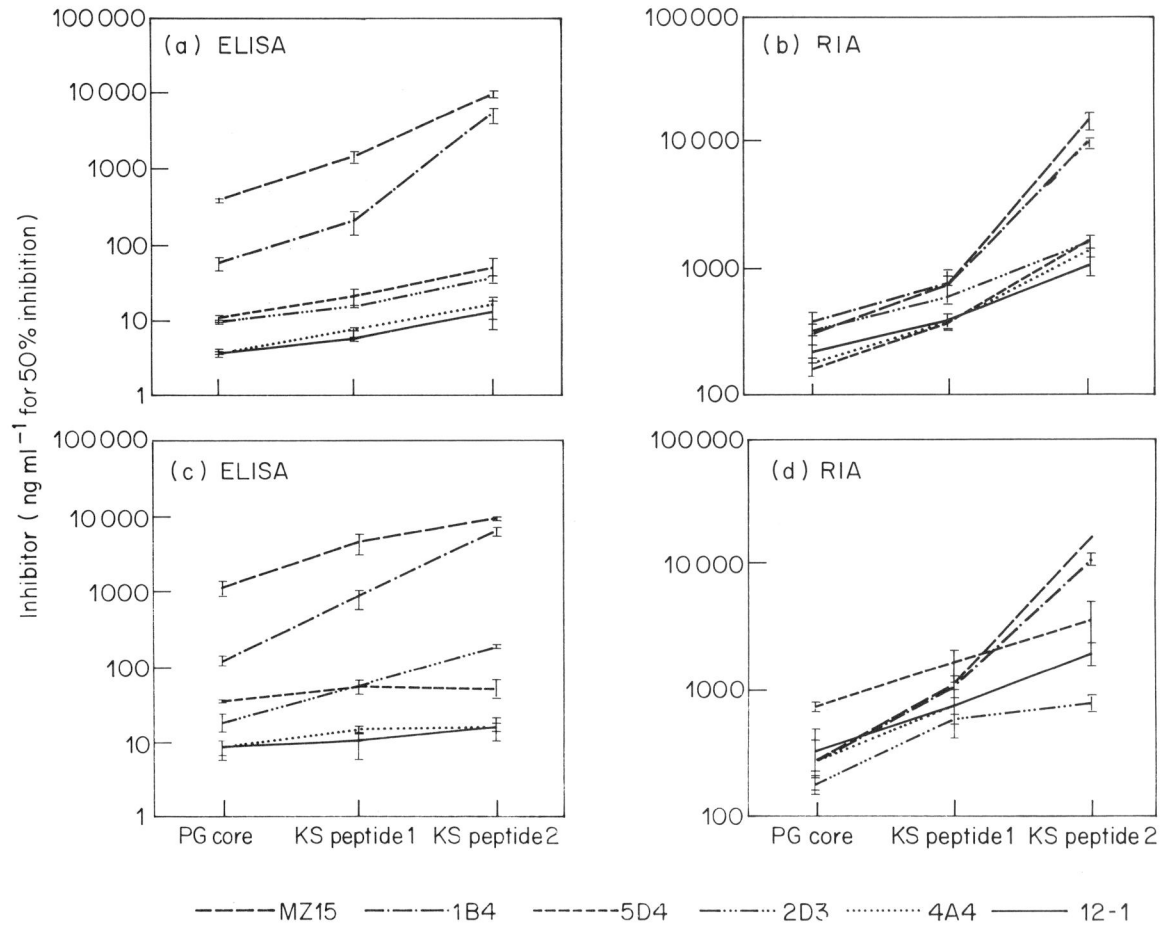

Figure 44.2 Inhibitory capacity of PG fragments isolated from human articular cartilage (a, b) and from bovine nasal cartilage (c, d). The amount of inhibitor (in terms of KS content) required for 50% inhibition of antibody binding was determined. Values represent the mean ± SD of three independant experiments.

DISCUSSION

Recent studies have shown skeletal KS to be heterogeneous in structure (Thornton *et al.*, 1989). In the present study, gel filtration chromatography has shown a heterogeneous distribution of the epitope within the KS chains, the epitope being detected only in the larger chains. It was also shown that the majority of the KS epitope was present only on a minority of KS chains. The immunochemical detection of KS epitope in skeletal KS is therefore a determination of a proportion of the KS chains and is not a measure of the total KS population. The size distribution of the KS chains could have a major influence on the level of epitope in a KS population.

Quantitation of apparent KS epitope in both the RIA and ELISA was shown to be dependent on (i) the antibody and (ii) the presentation of the antigen used. In both immunoassays, and for all antibodies investigated, there was a significant loss of inhibitory capacity with a decrease in size of the KS-containing PG fragments. The magnitude of this effect varied depending on the immunoassay and the antibody used; it was highest in the ELISA using antibody 1-B-4 and human PG fragments and lowest also in the ELISA using antibody 12.1 and bovine PG fragments. In most cases, the loss of inhibitory capacity with decrease in size appeared to be more pronounced in the RIA than in the ELISA. The dependence of quantitation on fragment size, i.e. number of KS chains attached to a protein core, is due in part to the bivalency of the antibodies (Caterson *et al.*, 1989a,b; Poole *et al.*, 1989). Differences between the antibodies are likely to be due to subtle differences in specificity and affinity.

Analysis of synovial fluids with different antibodies and assays, using PG monomer as standard, showed no significant variation in apparent KS epitope concentrations. This observation is consistent with the majority of the epitope in these samples being present as high-molecular-weight fragments of PG of similar size to the PG used as standard. In contrast, quantitation of KS epitope in the sera, using PG monomer as standard, was strongly dependent on the antibody and assay used. This is consistent with the KS epitope in serum being located on PG fragments of lower molecular weight than the PG monomer standard and the PG fragments in the synovial fluid.

It is clear that when RIA or ELISA is used, the quantitation of KS epitope is dependent on several factors and there is, therefore, potential for misinterpretation of data. This may be reduced by the appropriate preparation of the samples and the use of appropriate standards. The results indicate that particular care should be taken when comparing quantitative evaluations samples of unknown content, particularly if they may contain different PG structures. However, the appropriate use of quantitation of KS epitope in biological samples is an important technique. The possibility of a change in the expression of KS epitope with age and pathology offers potential in the detection and understanding of events in PG synthesis and turnover in development and disease.

ACKNOWLEDGMENTS

MJS was supported by a grant from the Deutscher Akademischer Austauschdienst, Bonn, FRG.

45

Antigen-specific T-lymphocyte clones as a new tool in proteoglycan research

TIBOR T. GLANT

Cartilage is one of the few immunologically privileged tissues in the body in that it is essentially avascular and, therefore, not subjected to close 'internal' immunological surveillance. Only when this tissue is degraded do antigenic cells and matrix components become exposed, released and, subsequently, recognized by the immune system. Many of the antibodies (either polyclonals or monoclonals) raised against cartilage proteoglycans (PG) react with the carbohydrate moiety of the PG. These carbohydrate components, however, do not appear capable of participating in any autoimmune process. The key involvement of T-lymphocytes in the pathological mechanism of human rheumatic diseases and experimental arthritis, induced by cartilage PGs or type II collagen, makes it important to isolate these cells and to identify the amino acid sequence of core protein fragment(s) that are critical for interaction with T-cell receptors. In general, the interaction of antigen with a T-cell receptor requires a short peptide (12–15 amino acid) sequence within which only one or two amino acids are responsible for the immune response (Schwartz, 1982; Finnegan et al., 1986; Strominger, 1989). Antigen-specific T-cell clones, once they are isolated, can simply be recultured and/or assayed for proliferation and, in addition, can be used to produce a variety of lymphokines which are additional factors in the progression of joint inflammation. In our laboratory, studies on protein-related epitopes on the core protein of human articular cartilage PGs recognized by monoclonal antibodies (Glant et al., 1986a,b) and by T-cells (Mikecz et al., 1988a,b) are performed in parallel to identify immunodominant regions of cartilage PGs, which may trigger or maintain autoimmune reactions in humans and animals (Glant et al., 1980; Mikecz et al., 1987). In this chapter basic methodology (Von Boehmer and Haas, 1985; Fathman and Engleman, 1986; Cantor, 1986) used for isolating PG-specific T-lymphocytes and hybridomas is described and complementary remarks on technical difficulties are given.

GENERAL GUIDELINES FOR ESTABLISHING ANTIGEN-SPECIFIC T-CELL LINES

Methods used to obtain cloned T-cells depend on the presence of antigen processed for presentation to T-lymphocytes by antigen-presenting cells (APC) and growth factors (Schwartz, 1982). Lymphocytes are usually collected after initial sensitization with antigen *in vivo* and placed in culture with the appropriate antigen (Fig. 45.1). These cultured lymphocytes are then exposed repetitively and alternatively to T-cell growth factor (interleukin 2, **IL-2**) and stimulating antigen, which is processed by Ia-positive antigen-presenting cells before cloning (Fig. 45.1).

Antigen

Core proteins of cartilage PGs in native, nondegraded form are 'weak' immunogens. This is because (i) their immunodominant regions are highly protected (hidden) by the negatively charged glycosaminoglycan side chains (Loewi and Muir, 1965; Sandson et al., 1966; Brandt et al., 1973; Glant et al., 1975); (ii) repetitive core protein structures are identical in different species (Dorfman et al., 1980; Kresina and Malemud, 1986; Glant et al., 1986a,b; Oldberg et al., 1987); and (iii) they express phylogenetically stabilized protein domains (Stevens et al., 1984; Doege et al., 1986, 1987; Sai et al., 1986, Neame et al., 1987; Perkins et al., 1989) which are not recognized by the immune system. Thus, manipulations on the molecular structure (reduction and alkylation, depletion of chondroitin sulfate (**CS**) side chains which leads to conformational change of core protein, proteolytic cleavages, etc.) may increase the immunogenicity of PGs in terms of both humoral and cellular immunity.

Lymphocytes

Lymphocytes from a variety of tissue sources, such as peripheral blood, lymph node, thoracic duct, spleen, tonsil, etc., can be used, although the use of a population enriched for the specificity to the given antigen (e.g. lymphocytes from the regional lymphoid organs or from tissues of the inflamed joint) offers a better opportunity for establishing a successful primer culture. Human lymphocytes should be tested first for sensitization with the given antigen in microassays (12 h incorporation of 1μCi of [^{3}H]thymidine measured on day five in the presence of antigen). In addition, setting up of analogous microcultures in parallel with the bulk stimulations is highly recommended, since the rate of antigen stimulation detected by incorporation of [^{3}H]thymidine gives useful results during the whole procedure. If the stimulatory effect with the given antigen leads to less than a doubling of [^{3}H]thymidine incorporation in the primer culture

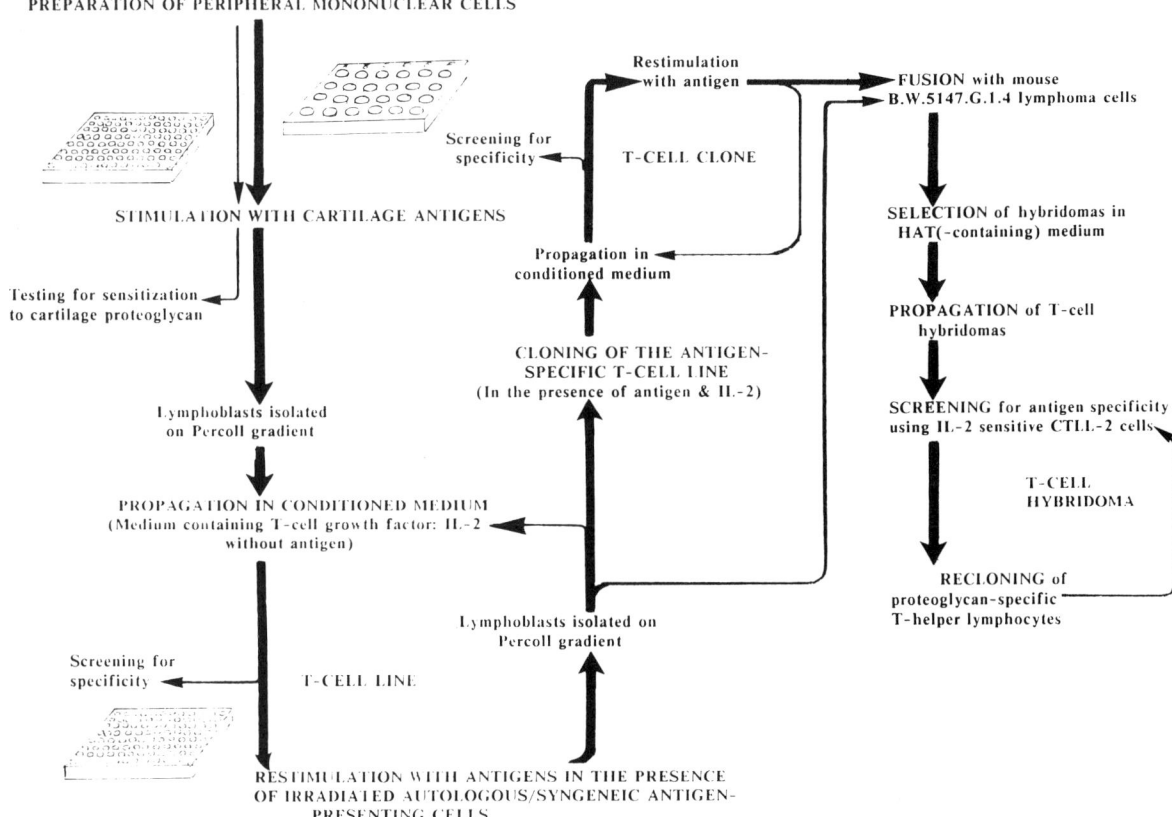

Figure 45.1 Isolation and propagation of T-lymphocyte cell lines, clones and T-cell hybridomas.

in the presence of antigen, the chance of getting a stable clone is very low. If this happens, which is not uncommon using PGs (or collagen type II) for stimulation of human lymphocytes, an enrichment of T-cells either by removing Ig$^+$ B-cells on a plastic surface coated with antiimmunoglobulin specific for the species (Mage, 1984), or by separation of T-lymphocytes on a T-cell recovery column, may help to solve the problem.

Antigen-presenting cells

Antigen-presentating cells (APC) (cells of the mononuclear phagocyte system) must be obtained from autologous (human) or syngeneic (e.g. mouse) sources to avoid a mixed lymphocyte reaction and irradiated with 4000–6000 rad to inhibit their *in vitro* proliferation. Mononuclear cells (monocytes/macrophages) for antigen presentation are prepared from peripheral blood (human) or spleen (mouse) on Ficoll-Hypaque gradient centrifugation. Monocytes may also be enriched by adherence to plastic or glass Petri dishes at 37°C for 1 h and harvested by pipetting with Ca^{2+}-free medium containing 0.1% EDTA.

Growth factors

In practice, partially purified or crude conditioned medium derived from either mitogen-stimulated (e.g. concanavalin A, 5 μg ml^{-1}, 5–8 × 10^6 cells ml^{-1}, 24–36 h stimulation at 37°C) rat or mouse spleen cells or mixed lymphocyte cultures (Fathman and Engleman, 1986) may be used as growth factor. In addition, there are murine and human lymphoma cell lines (e.g. EL4, HuT78, HuT102 and MLA144) which spontaneously or after exposure to T-cell mitogens or phorbol esters produce a significant amount of IL-2. Human or rat IL-2 support the growth of murine T-cells, but the reverse is not the case; therefore, human IL-2 (either purified or recombinant) is required for propagation of human T-cells.

CULTURE CONDITION AND CLONING OF PROTEOGLYCAN-SPECIFIC T-LYMPHOCYTE LINES

The long-term culture of lymphocytes requires the use of *complete medium* (recommended Dulbecco's Modified Eagle's Medium (DMEM) with 4.5 g glucose/l) supplemented with 2 mM l-glutamine, 1 mM sodium pyruvate, 0.1 mM nonessential amino acids, 20 mM Hepes, 0.5 μM 2-mercaptoethanol, antibiotics (either $100\,\mu g\,ml^{-1}$ gentamicin or 100 μg streptomycin and 100 units ml^{-1} penicillin) and 10% heat-inactivated (autologous or fetal bovine) serum. This standard medium may then be supplemented further with antigens ($50\,\mu g\,ml^{-1}$ of proteoglycan protein) and/or IL-2 (100 unit ml^{-1}). Primer cell cultures ($3–5 \times 10^6$ mononuclear cells ml^{-1}) are recommended to establish without excess antigen presenting cells. On day 7–8 of primer culture, viable human T-cells are recovered on Ficoll-Hypaque (Davidson and Parish, 1975) or an enriched lymphoblast population may be harvested from the 1.055/1.060 g ml^{-1} density interface of a discontinuous Percoll gradient (Mikecz et al., 1988a). These cells are cultured at 1×10^6 cell ml^{-1} in complete medium with 5% autologous human serum and 100 unit/ml IL-2 without antigen for a 5-day period to propagate human T-cells. Restimulation ($2–3 \times 10^5$ responder cells ml^{-1}) with antigen (for 7–8 days) in the presence of irradiated autologous peripheral mononuclear cells ($2–3 \times 10^{-6}\,ml^{-1}$) and resting phase (5–6 days) should be repeated several times before cloning (Fig. 45.1). In a murine system, these alternative steps may be combined in 12–14 day cycles, i.e. cells may be simply left in the presence of residual antigen, since the large number of antigen-sensitive T-cells produces a sufficient amount of IL-2.

Cloning

Cells of T-cell lines may be cloned either in soft agar ($0.3–5 \times 10^5$ responder cells ml^{-1}) or by limiting dilution (average is 0.3 cell/200 μl/well) in the presence of antigen, IL-2 and antigen presenting filler cells (Fathman and Engelman, 1986; Mikecz et al., 1988a) at the concentrations described above. Cloned cells can be assayed on day 7–14 after propagation (Fig. 45.1) by taking aliquots from each clone (2×10^4 cells) and restimulating them in the presence of appropriate antigen processed by irradiated autologous (human) or syngeneic (mouse) APC ($3–5 \times 10^5$ cells) in 200 μl of complete medium. Cells should be harvested at 48–72 h prior to the addition of 1 μCi of [^{3}H]thymidine for 12 h.

The major problems in the cloning of PG-specific human T-cells are: (i) an inability to immunize humans with these antigens; (ii) limited availability of cells from lymphoid organs or synovial tissue for primer culture; (iii) difficulties in obtaining antigen-presenting cells from the same individual in 10–12 day intervals for several months; and (iv) the limited lifetime of human T-cells *in vitro*.

Proteoglycan-specific murine T-cell hybridomas

An alternative source of homogeneous population of T-cells, which has the advantage of continuous growth with 'unlimited' lifetime in the absence of exogenous growth promoters and antigen, is the T-cell hybridoma. Unfortunately, we do not have stable fusion partner cell lines for human systems (Taussig, 1985; Fathman and Engelman, 1986), thus only murine T-cell hybridomas are discussed here. T-lymphocytes (1×10^8) with defined epitope specificity can be fused with BW 5147.G.1.4 mouse lymphoma cells ($2–3 \times 10^7$ by the method developed originally for monoclonal antibody technology (Köhler and Milstein, 1975). This BW 5147.G.1.4 mouse lymphoma has a deficiency in the enzyme hypoxanthine–guanine–phosphoribosyl–transferase, making it and the fused cells unable to grow in hypoxanthine, aminopterin- and thymidine- containing (HAT) medium. Likewise, for the generation of B-cell hybridomas, the presence of filler cells is also important. The use of spleen mononuclear cells, however, assures a faster growth of hybridomas then peritoneal macrophages. A convenient method for identifying antigen-specific T-cell hybridomas is to expose them to PG presented by syngeneic antigen presenting cells and, thereafter, to measure the production of IL-2 content in the supernatants using an IL-2 dependent T-cell line (CTLL) (Gillis and Smith, 1977) in a 24 h bioassay (Robb, 1985). This proliferation is generally measured by [^{3}H]thymidine uptake or the viability test. However, it is extremely important to use parallel cultures with or without antigen because there is a high risk of isolating T-cell hybridomas from BALB/c mice, which are able to produce IL-2 even in the absence of soluble PG as antigen (Buzás and Mikecz, unpublished observations). On the other hand, the proliferation and viability of CTLL cells can often be affected by reagents (salts, azaserine, aminopterin, etc.). Thus, the supernatants of hybrids should be subjected to the same serial dilution as the IL-2 standard in order to avoid false reactions. Selected cell lines should be cloned 2–3 times and stored under nitrogen. Their doubling time is about the same as for B-cell hybridomas (8–18 h). T-cell hybridomas can be used for *in vitro* studies to determine epitope specificity of T-cell receptors using either core protein fragments of PGs or analogous synthetic peptides and for *in vivo* experiments to test their arthritogenic potential in susceptible animals.

References

Baker, J.R., Caterson, B. and Christner, J.E. (1982). Immunological characterization of cartilage proteoglycans. *Methods Enzyol.* **83**, 216–235

Brandt, K.D., Tsiganos, C.P. and Muir, H. (1973). Immunological relationships between proteoglycans of different hydrodynamic size from articular cartilage of foetal and mature pigs. *Biochim. Biophys. Acta* **320**, 453–468

Buckwalter, J. and Rosenberg, L. (1982). Direct evidence for the variable length of the chondroitin sulfate-rich region of the proteoglycan subunit core protein. *J. Biol. Chem.* **257**, 9830–9839

Calabro, T. (1987). Monoclonal antibodies directed against proteoglycan core protein. Ph.D. Thesis, West Virginia University

Cantor, H. (1986). Overview: T cell clones. In *Cellular Immunology, Handbook of Experimental Immunology* (D.M. Weir, ed), Vol. II, pp. 75. 1–75.7. Blackwell Scientific, Oxford.

Carney, S.L., Bayliss, M.T., Collier, J.M. and Muir, H. (1986). Electrophoresis of ^{35}S-labelled proteoglycans on polyacrylamide–agarose composite gels and their visualization by fluorography. *Anal. Biochem.* **156**, 38–44

Caterson, B., Christner, J.E. and Baker, J.R. (1983). Identification of a monoclonal antibody that specifically recognizes corneal and skeletal keratan sulfate. *J. Biol. Chem.* **258**, 8848–8854

Caterson, B., Christner, J.E., Baker, J.R. and Couchman, J.R. (1985). Production and characterization of monoclonal antibodies directed against connective tissue proteoglycans. *Fed. Proc.* **44**, 386–393

Caterson, B., Calabro, T., Donohue, P.J. and Jahnke, M.R. (1986). Monoclonal antibodies against cartilage proteoglycans and link protein. In *Articular Cartilage Biochemistry* (K. Kuettner, R. Schleyerbach, and V. Hascall, eds), pp. 59–73. Raven Press, New York

Caterson, B., Adams, M.E., Calabro, T. and Pearce, R.H. (1987a). Agarose/acrylamide gel electrophoresis and monoclonal antibody immunolocation as a means of characterizing proteoglycan subpopulations. *Orthop. Res. Soc. Trans. (USA).* **12**, 60

Caterson, B., Calabro, T. and Hampton, A. (1987b). Monoclonal antibodies as probes for elucidating proteoglycan structure. In *Biology of the Extracellular Matrix: A Series, 'Biology of Proteoglycans'* (T. Wight and R. Mecham, eds), pp. 1–26. Academic Press, New York

Caterson, B., Brooks, K., Sattsangi, S., Ratcliffe, A., Hardingham, T.E. and Muir, H. (1989a). Factors affecting the determination of keratan sulfate using monoclonal antibodies in immunoassay procedures. In *Keratan Sulfate* (H. Greiling and J.E. Scott, eds), pp. 199–204. Biochemical Society, London

Caterson, B., Mahmoodian, F., Sorrell, J.M., Bayliss, M.T., Hardingham, T.E. and Muir, H. (1989b). Monoclonal antibodies that recognize novel chondroitin sulfate structures that are specifically expressed during development and in disease. *Orthop. Res. Soc. Trans. (USA)*, **14**, 12

Davidson, W. and Parish, C.R. (1975). A procedure for removing red cells and dead cells from lymphoid cell suspension. *J. Immunol. Methods* **7**, 291–300

De Blas, A.L. and Cherwinski, H.M. (1983). Detection of antigens on nitrocellulose paper immunoblots with monoclonal antibodies. *Anal. Biochem.* **133**, 214–219

Dimitriadis, G.J. (1979). Effect of detergents on antibody–antigen interaction. *Anal. Biochem.* **98**, 445–451

Doege, K., Fernandez, P., Hassell, J.R., Sasaki, M. and Yamada, Y. (1986). Partial cDNA sequence encoding a globular domain at the C terminus of the rat cartilage proteoglycan. *J. Biol. Chem.* **261**, 8108–8111

Doege, K., Sasaki, M., Horigan, E., Hassell, J.R. and Yamada, Y. (1987). Complete primary structure of the rat cartilage proteoglycan core protein deducted from cDNA clones. *J. Biol. Chem.* **262**, 17 757–17 767

Dorman, A., Hall, T., Ho, P.-L. and Fitch, F. (1980). Clonal antibodies for core protein of chondroitin sulfate proteoglycan. *Proc. Natl. Acad. Sci. USA* **77**, 3971–3973

Fathman, C.G. and Engleman, E.G. (1986). T cell lines and hybrids in mouse and man. In *Cellular Immunology. Handbook of Experimental Immunology* (D.M. Weir, ed), Vol. II, pp. 69.1–69.12. Blackwell Scientific, Oxford

Finnegan, A., Smith, M.A., Smith, J.A., Berzofsky, J., Sachs, D.H. and Hodes, R.J. (1986). The T cell repertoire for recognition of a phylogenetically distant protein antigen. *J. Exp. Med.* **163**, 897–910

Fosang, A.J. and Hardingham, T.E. (1989). Isolation of N-terminal globular protein domains from cartilage proteoglycans. *Biochem. J.* **261**, 801–809

Furthmayr, H. (1982). *Immunochemistry of the Extracellular Matrix*, Vol. I, pp. 143–178. CRC Press Boca Raton, Florida

Furthmayr, H. and Timpl, R. (1976). Immunochemistry of collagens and procollagens. *Int. Rev. Connect. Tiss. Res.* **7**, 61–99

Gay, S. and Fine, J.D. (1987). Characterization and isolation of poly- and mono-clonal antibodies against collagen for use in immunohistochemistry. *Methods Enzymol.* **145**, 148–167

Gillis, S. and Smith, K.A. (1977). Long-term culture of tumor-specific cytotoxic T cells. *Nature* **268**, 154–156

Glant, T., Hadhazy, Cs. and Csernyansky, H. (1975). Species-common antigen of connective tissues. *Acta Biol. Acad. Sci. Hung.* **26**, 197–208

Glant, T., Csongor, J. and Szucs, T. (1980). Immunopathologic role of proteoglycan antigens in rheumatoid joint diseases. *Scand. J. Immunol.* **11**, 247–252

Glant, T., Mikecz, K. and Poole, A.R. (1986a). Monoclonal antibodies to protein-related epitopes of human articular cartilage proteoglycans. *Biochem. J.* **234**, 31–41

Glant, T., Mikecz, K., Roughley, P.J., Buzas, E. and Poole, A.R. (1986b). Age-related changes in protein related epitopes of human articular cartilage proteoglycans. *Biochem. J.* **236**, 71–75

Hardingham, T.E., Caterson, C., Bayliss, M.T., Carney, S.L., Ratcliffe, A. and Muir, H. (1989). Appearance of novel chondroitin sulfate structures in the articular cartilage from experimental canine osteoarthritis joints. *Orthop. Res. Soc. Trans. (USA)* **14**, 505

Hascall, V.C. and Glant, T. (1987). Proteoglycan epitopes as potential markers of normal and pathologic cartilage metabolism. *Arthr. Rheum.* **30**, 586–588

Kemmeny, D.M. and Challacombe, S.J. (1988). *ELISA and Other Solid Phase Immunoassays*. Wiley, New York

Knight, K.R. and Robinson, H.C. (1984). The structure of the linkage region of the bovine nasal cartilage proteoglycan after β-elimination and sulfite addition. *Conn. Tiss. Res.* **12**, 119–131

Köhler, G. and Milstein, C. (1975). Continuous cultures of fused cells secreting antibody of predefined specificity. *Nature* **256**, 495–497

Kresina, T.F. and Malemud, C.J. (1986). Murine monoclonal antibodies recognizing rabbit proteoglycans. *Collagen Rel. Res.* **6**, 15–39

Loewi, G. and Muir, H. (1965). The antigenicity of chondromucoprotein. *Immunology* **9**, 119–127

Mage, M.G. (1984). Separation of lymphocytes on antibody-coated plates. *Methods Enzymol.* **108**, 118–124

Mahmoodian, F. (1988). Biochemical characterization of embryonic chick bone marrow proteoglycans. Masters Thesis, West Virginia University

Maldonado, B., Kuettner, K.E. and Thonar, E.J.-M.A. (1988). Characterization of antigenic keratan sulfate in the KS-rich and CS-rich regions of cartilage proteoglycans. *Orthop. Res. Soc. Trans.(USA).* **13**, 11

Mehmet, H., Scudder, P., Tang, P.W., Hounsell, E.F., Caterson, B. and Feizi, T. (1985). The antigenic determinants recognized by three monoclonal antibodies to keratan sulfate involve sulfated hepta- or larger oligosaccharides of the poly(N-acetyllactosamine) series. *Eur. J. Biochem.* **157**, 385–391

Michaeli, D. (1977). Immunochemistry of collagen. In *Immunochemistry of Proteins* (M.Z. Atassi, ed.), Vol. I, pp. 371–399. Plenum, New York

Mikecz, K., Glant, T. and Poole, A.R. (1987). Immunity to cartilage proteoglycans in BALB/c mice with progressive polyarthritis and ankylosing spondylitis induced by injection of human cartilage proteoglycan. *Arthr. Rheum.* **30**, 306–318

Mikecz, K., Glant, T., Baron, M. and Poole, A.R. (1988a). Isolation of proteoglycan specific T cells from patients with ankylosing spondylitis. *Cell Immunol.* **112**, 55–63

Mikecz, K., Glant, T., Buzas, E. and Poole, A.R. (1988b). Cartilage proteoglycans as potential autoantigens in humans and experimental animals. *Agent Actions* **23**, 63–66

Mörgelin, M., Paulsson, M., Hardingham, T.E., Heinegard, D. and Engel, J. (1988). Cartilage proteoglycans: assembly with hyaluronate and link protein as studied by electron microscopy. *Biochem. J.* **253**, 175–185

Muir, H. and Hardingham, T. (1975). Structure of proteoglycans. ser. I. *MTP Int. Rev. Sci. Biochem.* **5**, 153–220

Neame, P.J., Christner, J.E. and Baker, J.R. (1987). Cartilage proteoglycan aggregates. The link protein and proteoglycan amino-terminal globular domains have similar structures. *J. Biol. Chem.* **262**, 17 768–17 778

Oeben, M., Keller, R., Stuhlsatz, H.W. and Greiling, H. (1987). Constant and variable domains of different disaccharide structure in corneal keratan sulfate chains. *Biochem. J.* **248**, 85–93

Oldberg, A., Antonsson, P. and Heinegard, D. (1987). The partial amino acid sequence of bovine cartilage proteoglycan deduced from a cDNA clone, contains numerous Ser-Gly sequences arranged in homologous repeats. *Biochem. J.* **243**, 255–259

Paulsson, M., Mörgelin, M., Wiedemann, H., Beardmore-Gray, M., Dunham, D., Hardingham, T.E. Heinegård, D., Timpl, R. and Engel, J. (1987). Extended and globular protein domains in cartilage proteoglycans. *Biochem. J.* **245**, 763–772

Perkins, S.J., Nealis, A.D., Dudhia, J. and Hardingham, T.E. (1989). Immunoglobulin fold and tandem repeat structures in proteoglycan N-terminal domains and link protein. *J. Mol. Biol.* **206**, 737–753

Poole, A.R. (1986). Proteoglycans in health and disease structures and functions. *Biochem. J.* **236**, 1–14

Poole, A.R., Webber, C., Reiner, A. and Roughley, P.J. (1989). Studies of the monoclonal antibody to skeletal keratan sulfate; importance of antibody valancy. *Biochem. J.* **260**, 849–856

Ratcliffe, A. and Hardingham, T.E. (1983). Cartilage proteoglycan binding region and link protein. Radioimmunoassays and the detection of masked determinants in aggregates. *Biochem. J.* **213**, 371–378

Ratcliffe, A., Fryer, P. and Hardingham, T.E. (1984). The distribution of aggregating proteoglycan in articular cartilage. Comparison of quantitative immunoelectron microscopy with radioimmunoassay and biochemical analysis. *J. Histochem. Cytochem.* **32**, 193–201

Ratcliffe, A., Fryer, P. and Hardingham, T.E. (1985). Proteoglycan biosynthesis in chondrocytes: protein A-gold localization of proteoglycan, chondroitin sulfate and link protein within Golgi sub-compartments. *J. Cell Biol.* **101**, 2355–2365

Ratcliffe, A., Hughes, C., Fryer, P.R., Saed-Nejad, F. and Hardingham, T.E. (1987). Immunochemical studies on the synthesis and secretion of link protein and aggregating proteoglycan by chondrocytes. *Collagen Rel. Res.,* **7**, 409–421

Ratcliffe, A., Doherty, M., Maini, R.N. and Hardingham, T.E. (1988). Increased levels of proteoglycan components in the synovial fluids of patients with acute, but not chronic joint disease. *Ann. Rheum. Dis.* **47**, 826–832

Risteli, L. and Risteli, J. (1989). Noninvasive methods for detection of organ fibrosis. In *Focus on Connective Tissue in Health and Disease* (M. Rojkind, ed), pp. 1–114. CRC Press, Boca Raton, Florida

Robb, R.J. (1985). Human interleukin 2. *Methods Enzymol.* **116**, 493–525

Rosenberg, L., Hellmann, W. and Kleinschmidt, A. (1975). Electron microscopic studies of proteoglycan aggregates from bovine articular cartilage. *J. Biol. Chem.* **250**, 1877–1883

Sai, S., Tanaka, T., Kosher, R.A. and Tanzer, M.L. (1986). Cloning and sequence analysis of a partial cDNA for chicken cartilage proteoglycan core protein. *Proc. Natl. Acad. Sci. USA* **83**, 5081–5085

Sampaio, L. de O., Bayliss, M.T., Hardingham, T.E. and Muir, H. (1988). Dermatan sulfate proteoglycan from human articular cartilage: variation in its content with age and its structural comparison with a small chondroitin sulfate proteoglycan from pig laryngeal cartilage. *Biochem. J.* **254**, 757–764

Sandson, J., Rosenberg, L. and White, D. (1966). The antigenic determinants of the protein polysaccharides of cartilage. *J. Exp. Med.* **123**, 817–828

Schwartz, R.H. (1982). The cloning of T lymphocytes. *Immunol. Today* **3**, 43–46

Seibel, M.J., Towbin, H., Braun, D.G., Kiefer, B., Mueller, W. and Paulsson, M. (1989). Serum keratan sulfate in rheumatoid arthritis and different subsets of osteoarthritis. In *Keratan Sulfate Chemistry, Biochemistry, Biology and Chemical Pathology* (H. Greiling and J.E. Scott, eds). Biochemical Society, London

Sheehan, J.K., Ratcliffe, A., Oates, K. and Hardingham, T.E. (1987). The detection of substrates within proteoglycan molecules: electron-microscopic immuno-localization with the use of Protein A-gold. *Biochem. J.* **247**, 267–276

Sorrell, J.M., Lintala, A.M., Mahmoodian, F. and Caterson, B. (1988). Indirect immunocytochemical localization of chondroitin sulfate proteoglycans in lymphopoietic and granulopoietic compartments of the developing bursae of fabricus. *J. Immunol.* **140**, 4263–4270

Stevens, J.W., Oike, Y., Handley, C., Hascall, V.C., Hampton, A. and Caterson, B. (1984). Characteristics of the core protein of the aggregating proteoglycan from the Swarm rat chondrosarcoma. *J. Cell Biochem.* **26**, 247–259

Strominger, J.L. (1989). The T cell receptor and class Ib MHC-related proteins: enigmatic molecules of immune recognition. *Cell* **57**, 895–898

Stuhlsatz, H.W., Keller, R., Becker, G., Oeben, M., Lennartz, L., Fischer, D.C. and Greiling, H. (1989). Structure of keratan sulfate proteoglycans: core proteins, linkage regions, carhobydrates chains. In *Keratan Sulfate, Chemistry, Biology, Chemical Pathology* (H. Greiling and J.E. Scott, eds), pp. 1–15. The Biochemical Society, London

Taussig, M.J. (1985). In *T Cell Hybridomas* (M.J. Taussig, ed.). CRC Press, Boca Raton, Fl.

Thonar, E.J.-M.A., Kimura, J.H., Hascall, V.C. and Poole, A.R. (1982). Enzyme-linked immunosorbant assay analyses of the hyaluronate binding region and the link protein of proteoglycan aggregates. *J. Biol. Chem.* **257**, 14 173–14 180

Thonar, E.J.-M.A., Lenz, M.E., Klintworth, G.K., Caterson, B., Pachman, L.M., Glickman, P., Katz, R., Huff, J. and Kuettner, K.E. (1985). Quantification of keratan sulfate in blood as a marker of cartilage catabolism. *Arthr. Rheum.* **28**, 1367–1376

Thonar, E.J.-M.A., Meyer, R.F., Dennis, R.F., Lenz, M.E., Maldonado, B., Hassell, J.R., Hewitt, A.T., Stark, W.J., Stock, E.L., Kuettner, K.E. and Klintworth, C.K. (1986). Absence of normal keratan sulfate in the blood of patients with macular corneal dystrophy. *Am. J. Opthalmol.* **102**, 561–569.

Thonar, E.J.-M.A., Feist, S.D., Fassbender, K., Lenz, M.E., Matijevitch, B.L. and Kuettner, K.E. (1988a). Quantification of hen egg white lysozyme in cartilage by an enzyme-linked immunosorbent assay. *Conn. Tiss. Res.* **17**, 181–198

Thonar, E.J.-M.A., Pachman, L.M., Lenz, M.F., Hayford, J., Lynch, P. and Kuettner, K.E. (1988b). Age related changes in the concentration of serum keratan sulfate in children. *J. Clin. Chem. Clin. Biochem.* **26**, 57–63

Thornton, D.J., Morris, H.G., Cockin, G.H., Huckerby, T.N., Nieduszynski, I.A., Carlstedt, I., Hardingham, T.E. and Ratcliffe, A. (1989). Structural and immunological studies of keratan sulfates from mature bovine articular cartilage. *Biochem. J.* **260**, 277–282

Timpl. R. (1982). Antibodies to collagens and procollagens. Methods Enzymol. **82**, 472–498

Timpl, R. (1984). Immunology of the collagens. In *Extracellular Matrix Biochemistry* (K.A. Piez and A.H. Reddi, eds), pp. 159–190, Elsevier, New York

Timpl, R. and Riseli, L. (1982). Radioimmunoassays in studies of connective tissue proteins. In *Immunochemistry of the Extracellular Matrix* (H. Furthmayr, ed.), pp. 199–235. CRC Press, Boca Raton, Florida

Von Boehmer, H. and Haas, W. (1985). Cytolytic T cell clones and hybridomas. In *T Cell Clones. Research Monographs in Immunology* (H. Von Boehmer and W. Haas, eds). Vol. 8. Elsevier, Amsterdam.

Wiedemann, H., Paulsson, M., Timpl, R., Engel, J. and Heinegard, D. (1984). Domain structure of cartilage proteoglycan visualized by rotary shadowing of intact and fragmented molecules. *Biochem. J.* **224**, 331–333

Williams, J.M., Downey, C. and Thonar, E.J.-M.A. (1988). Increase in levels of serum keratan sulfate following cartilage proteoglycan degradation in the rabbit knee joint. *Arthr. Rheum.* **31**, 557–560

Yamagata, M., Kimata, K., Oike, Y., Tani, K., Maeda, N., Yoshida, K., Shimomura, Y., Yoneda, M. and Suzuki, S. (1987). A monoclonal antibody that specifically recognized a glucuronic acid 2-sulfate containing determinant in intact chondroitin sulfate chain. *J. Biol. Chem.* **262**, 4146–4152

Zanetti, M., Ratcliffe, A. and Watt, F.M. (1985). Two subpopulations of differentiated chondrocytes identified with a monoclonal antibody to keratan sulfate. *J. Cell. Biol.* **101**, 53–59

8

RECOMBINANT DNA AND CARTILAGE MATRIX

COLLATED BY M.L. TANZER

46

Overview

MARVIN L. TANZER

The application of contemporary molecular biologic approaches to the study of cartilage matrix has proceeded apace with similar areas of research. Initially, progress was made in the study of type II collagen of cartilage, soon followed by other components, e.g. link proteins, cartilage matrix protein, chondroitin sulfate (CS) proteoglycans (PGs) and other collagen types. The full impact of this approach has not yet been reached, although considerable information has already accrued.

The power of recombinant DNA techniques potentially allows many different aspects of cartilage biology to be explored. Inroads have already been made in some areas while others are just beginning to be developed. A full perspective of future directions would include:

(i) deduction of protein structures;
(ii) determination of corresponding genomic structures;
(iii) understanding genomic expression and regulation;
(iv) analyzing protein folding and domain specificity;
(v) revealing previously unknown proteins;
(vi) deciphering cell lineages and pattern formation;
(vii) detecting and correcting genetic defects; and
(viii) producing novel proteins and diagnostic reagents.

All these directions have been explored, to varying degrees, in other aspects of contemporary biology and should be amenable to use in the study of cartilage matrix. Clearly, the power of the techniques will allow answers to long-standing problems in cartilage matrix biology. Tailoring of the general recombinant DNA methods to the particular idiosyncracies of cartilage has become an important issue. For example, during the recent Bat-Sheva Workshop on methods used in cartilage research, a prominent topic of discussion was the lack of adequate methods for isolating or for quantitating mRNA species in adult cartilage. Indeed, much of the cloning success and mRNA assays to date have been accomplished using embryonic or tumor cartilages which have very different properties from normal adult cartilage. Similar considerations apply to using *in situ* hybridization protocols on such material. Hopefully, the progress which has been made using embryonic and tumor samples will be readily applicable to normal, mature cartilages. It would seem that a systematic approach, employing internal standards and other controls, may provide the solution to the technical problems.

To date, recombinant DNA approaches have provided information concerning deduced protein structures and the corresponding gene structures of various matrix components of cartilage, including collagens, CS PGs, link proteins and cartilage matrix protein. Some insight into genomic expression and regulation has also been obtained. Precise elucidation of genetic defects is just beginning to appear, as illustrated by nanomelia in chickens and spondyloepiphyseal dysplasia in humans. Some insight into the lectin activity of the COOH terminal domain of the large CS PG of cartilage, which had been predicted by structure comparisons, has been forthcoming. The approach using transgenic animals (Hogan and Lyons, 1988; Jaenisch, 1988; Westphal, 1989) may be the most powerful means of determining structure–function relationships.

The papers in this section provide a sample of some of the applications of recombinant DNA technology to the study of cartilage. The structural studies made by Hardingham *et al.* (Chapter 47) provide a comprehensive picture of the large aggregating PG of cartilage which has served as the prototype PG for many years. The deduced amino acid sequences have revealed new putative domains of the molecule and have detected fascinating homologous sequences upon comparison with link protein and with noncartilaginous proteins. The power of 'reverse genetics' is illustrated by Michel van der Rest in Chapter 48 where he describes the initial detection of type XII coliagen at the nucleic acid level, followed by its elucidation and characterization at the protein level. His description vividly shows how the interactions of molecular biologists, immunologists and protein chemists rapidly yielded detailed information about a previously unknown collagen molecule. Keating and Pritzker (Chapter 49) demonstrate how contemporary *in situ* hybridization clearly localizes the mRNA for lysozyme over the cytoplasm of chondrocytes, resolving a long-standing dilemma concerning the origin of this enzyme in cartilage. Horton and Chandrasekhar (Chapter 50) provide an analysis of approaches for studying the regulation of chondrocyte gene expression. Their overview describes strategies for introducing DNA containing reporter genes into cells and measuring the level of expression of such genes. They demonstrate that studies of regulatory molecules such as growth factors may be readily performed and forecast the next level of regulation, that of identifying regulatory genomic sequences which bind specific proteins, as well as characterizing such intrinsic proteins themselves. Jiminez (Chapter 51) outlines a strategy to determine if some individuals with familial osteoarthritis may harbour mutations in the Type II collagen gene. His approach includes RFLP screening, PCR amplification, and transfection of the human Type II collagen gene into mouse fibroblasts for ultimate expression of the protein. Potentially, this scheme may yield new insights into a subset of the osteoarthritis population.

The appearance of multiple 'cookbooks' which provide recipes for all aspects of recombinant DNA approaches (see Bibliography below) has allowed many laboratories to become proficient in such methods. In addition, the availability of continuing education courses, including laboratory exercises, has provided investigators with opportunities to develop their skills. Thus, the prospects for using recombinant DNA methods to explore the biology of cartilage are very bright and only require the concerted efforts of interested investigators.

ACKNOWLEDGMENT

Supported in part by NIH grants AR 12683 and AR 17720.

BIBLIOGRAPHY

Ausubel, F.M., Brent, R., Kingston, R.E., Moore, D.D., Seidman, J.G., Smith, J.A. and Struhl, K. (1988). *Current Protocols in Molecular Biology.* Wiley-Interscience, New York

Berger, S.L. and Kimmel, A.R. (1987). *Guide to Molecular Cloning Techniques.* Academic Press, New York

Davies, K.E. (1988). *Genome Analysis: A Practical Approach*. IRL Press, Oxford

Glover, D.M. (1985–1987). *DNA Cloning: A Practical Approach*. Vols I–III. IRL Press, Oxford

Marcus-Sekura, C.J. (1988). Techniques for using antisense oligodeoxy-ribonucleotides to study gene expression (review). *Anal. Biochem.* **172**, 289–295

Pardue, M.L. (1985). *In situ* hybridization. In *Nucleic Acid Hybridization: A Practical Approach* (B.D. Hames and S.J. Higgins, eds), pp. 179–202. IRL Press, Oxford

Sambrook, J., Fritsch, E.F. and Maniatis, T. (1989). *Molecular Cloning: A Laboratory Manual* 2nd edn. Cold Spring Harbor, New York

Wu, R., Grossman, L. and Moldave, K. (1989). *Recombinant DNA Methodology*. Academic Press, New York

47

Domain structure and sequence homologies in cartilage proteoglycan

TIM HARDINGHAM, JAYESH DUDHIA and AMANDA J. FOSANG

The most abundant proteoglycan (PG) in cartilage is a high-molecular-weight aggregating species bearing chondroitin sulfate (CS) and keratan sulfate (KS) side chains on a large protein core (M_r = 225 kDa (Hardingham *et al.*, 1986). Rotary shadowing techniques (Paulsson *et al.*, 1987) and DNA sequences (Doege *et al.*, 1987) have shown this PG to be a multidomain structure that consists of three globular (G1, G2 and G3) and two extended regions (Fig. 47.1).

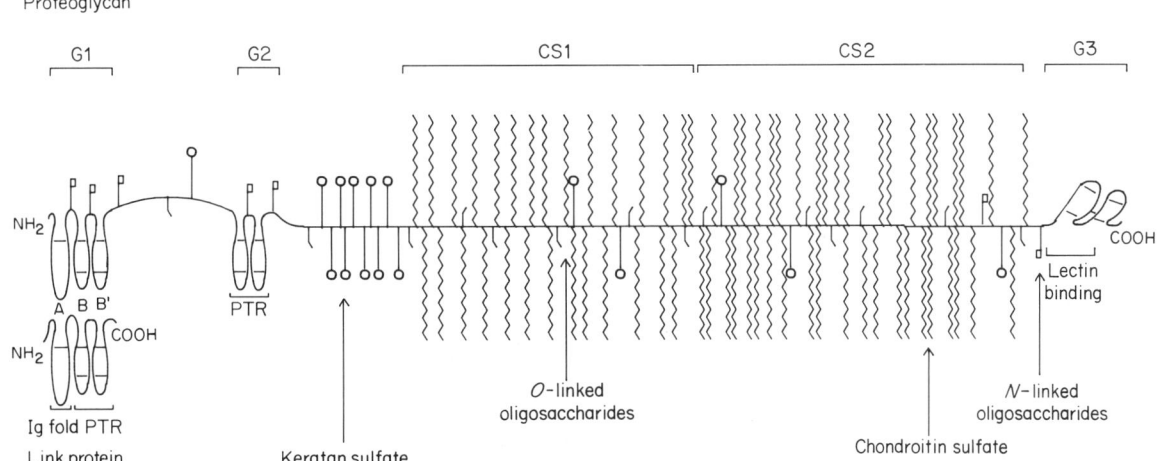

Figure 47.1 Schematic representation of cartilage PG and link protein structure. The domain structures of cartilage PG and link protein are shown including; Ig fold, immunoglobulin variable region fold, PTR, and CS1 and CS2 attachment region sequences. Disulfide bonds are marked with dashed lines. The polypeptide chains are drawn approximately to scale. (Reproduced with permission from the Biochemical Society.)

The aggregation properties are due to interactions involving the G1 globular domain lying at the NH$_2$ terminal. This disulfide bonded G1 domain is composed of two structural motifs, an Ig fold and a tandem repeat, which have also been identified in link protein from its DNA sequences from pig and human cartilage (Perkins et al., 1989), rat chondrosarcoma (Rhodes et al., 1988) and chick sternal cartilage (Deak et al., 1986). These two structural motifs together constitute the whole of link protein (M_r = 39-kD) as a disulfide-bonded looped structure. One motif (loop A, Fig. 47.1) at the NH$_2$ terminal of G1 and link protein is a 90-residue sequence that shows homology with an immunoglobulin-variable-region fold (Ig fold) and, although the homology is not high, secondary structure predictions (Perkins et al., 1989) show significant identity with the Ig fold in the number and position of β-sheet sequences. The second motif is a tandem repeat structure that contains two homologous loops (B and B', Fig. 47.1), each of 99 amino acid residues lying adjacent to the Ig fold and toward the carboxy terminal. This PG tandem repeat (PTR) is also found in a second globular domain (G2) in the PG protein core, where it is separated by a short extended segment from G1. The sequences of the PTR B loops of PG and link protein taken together for all four species determined show a homology of about 48%, while that of the B1 loops is 35%. For link protein alone, comparison amongst different species shows the amino acid sequence homology between these two loops to be almost 60%.

The G1 domain has been shown to bind specifically to hyaluronan (HA) (Ratcliffe and Hardingham, 1983). Evidence from immunochemical data using antibodies raised specifically to G1 and G2 domains (Fosang and Hardingham, 1989) clearly suggests that, while G1 can interact with link protein and HA, G2 does not possess this functional property. The G2 domain also does not appear to bind to collagen or other matrix proteins and its precise functional role in PG organization remains obscure.

The third globular domain (G3) is located at the carboxy terminal of PG and has a sequence quite different from G1 and G2 domains. G3 contains 10 cysteine residues and exhibits 90% homology between chicken (Sai et al., 1986), rat (Doege et al., 1987), bovine (Oldberg et al., 1987), and human and pig (Dudhia and Hardingham, 1989) sequences. Although highly conserved, the function of G3 remains unclear. A part of G3 containing six cysteine residues has sequence homology with verterbate hepatic lectins specific to terminal galactosyl or N-acetylglucosaminyl residues. A carboxy terminal G3-like domain found in a PG from human fibroblasts (Krusius and Ruoslahti, 1986) is related in sequence to the G3 domain of the chondrocyte PG. It contains the lectin-like portion and ten cysteine residues whose spacing is completely conserved between these two PGs expressed by different cell types. The human chondrocyte PG G3 domain is less homologous (68% homology) with that of the human fibroblast than it is with the G3 domains of chondrocytes from other species (> 90% homology).

Adjoining the G2 and G3 domains is an extended region that contains two parts both rich in hydroxy amino acids and containing many Ser–Gly sequences but with different sequence patterns. From the available partial sequences for an M_r = 50 kD region (region CS2, Fig. 47.1) for human, rat and bovine PG, it contains 65% of common sequence, although within it a 150-residue portion low in Ser–Gly sequences immediately adjacent to G3 is less than 50% conserved. The total number of Ser–Gly dipeptides varies between species, being 24 in rat, 35 in bovine and 28 in human, of which 18 are maintained in common positions in all three species. The Ser–Gly dipeptides are found as a series of ten amino acid repeats and could serve as substitution points for bearing CS chains. This region is less well-conserved than the globular G3 domain and suggests that the precise pattern and numbers of Ser–Gly dipeptides is not critical to its function in bearing large numbers of CS chains.

A general feature of the Ser–Gly dipeptide-containing repeats is the presence of adjacent acidic amino acid residues. This arrangement has been postulated (Bourdon et al., 1987) to stimulate in vivo glycosylation in synthetic Ser–Gly containing peptides. The two extended regions of the core protein thus provide large numbers of substitution sites for glycosaminoglycan attachment and the density of CS chains found on each extension is reflected by the respective numbers of the Ser–Gly containing repeats. Hence the extended sequence (CS2) adjacent to G3 contains CS chains that are arranged in clusters, while in the CS1 regions they are evenly distributed. The CS attachment region thus appears to have arisen from the amplification of genes for two different Ser–Gly rich sequences.

The multidomain structure of PG and the conservation of domain structure between species and their relationship with domains of other proteins implies that the gene for this protein has arisen from exon movement from a number of gene families. The PTR loops (B and B') share significant homology to a human lymphocyte homing receptor Hermes (cell adhesion molecule) (Stamenkovic et al., 1989; Goldstein et al., 1989), while the lectin-like region in G3 is related to a sequence found in a mouse lymphocyte homing receptor (Lasky et al., 1989). The human Hermes molecule has only one copy of the PTR motif located at the NH_2 terminal and its homology to the B loops of link protein and PG is approximately 35% and to the B' loops about 25%. The PTRs of these three proteins may thus share a common ancestral gene. The presence of an Ig fold at the N-terminal also classes the PG (and link protein) as members of the immunoglobulin superfamily (Williams and Barclay, 1988) in which there are many examples of proteins involved in recognition and adhesion. Amongst the different gene sequences that make up the PG protein core, there are thus strong relationships with several prominent families of cell surface proteins that each provide elements of the globular protein structures that flank the heavily glycosylated CS attachment region. The PG thus provides a further example of the interesting close relationships that exist amongst proteins at the cell surface and secreted components of the extracellular matrix.

The value of determining the sequence structure of PGs from cDNA cloning as an aid to developing a clearer understanding of the function of its different domains is best illustrated by considering the close structural relationship that is present between link protein and G1 domain.

Immunochemical evidence had shown that the G1 domain of PG was unrelated to link protein (Ratcliffe and Hardingham, 1983) and it was only when some sequences were determined, initially from peptide analysis and later by cDNA cloning, that their structural relationship was revealed (Naeme et al., 1987; Doege et al., 1986, 1987). Both proteins contained related Ig fold and PTR motifs. The application of secondary-structure-prediction analysis to the Ig fold of link protein and G1 domain and their comparison with Ig folds of known crystal structure enabled a characteristic β-sheet pattern to be identified (Perkins et al., 1989). This showed that, not only was there some homology within the sequences, but that they were also likely to form comparable three-dimensional protein structures and that this part of the sequence of link protein and G1 is a largely independent structural domain.

Some experimental evidence has shown that the N-terminal region of link protein (containing the Ig fold) was involved in binding to the PG G1 domain, whereas the C-terminal region (containing the PTR) was involved in binding to HA (Périn et al., 1987). This would be supported by the ability of Ig folds in other proteins to participate in protein–protein interactions. It would also imply that the Ig folds in link protein and G1 domain have evolved to bind selectively to each other. If the sequences of the Ig folds of link protein and G1 domain are compared, the regions of greatest divergence are those corresponding to the hypervariable loops in the immunoglobulin V region (Perkins et al., 1989). In immunoglobulins, these loops provide the sites for determining the specificity of antigen recognition and it is possible that in link protein and G1 domain they specify the interactions between each other.

The C-terminal region of link protein and G1 domain is also likely to form an independent structural domain as a closely homologous PTR is the only component of the G2 domain which, by rotary shadowing electron microscopy, is clearly globular (Paulsson et al., 1987). As indicated above, the PTR is likely to be responsible for binding to HA and it is interesting to consider why it contains two homologous loops. Both link protein and G1 domains show specificity in binding to an HA chain sequence of nine or ten sugar residues (Hardingham, 1981). In an extended form, this implies quite a large binding site — over 4-nm long. It is possible that each loop of the PTR provides half this site by binding to HA down to two disaccharide units. Other proteins that bind to HA are known which show specificity for hyaluronate down to two disaccharide units but none have yet been sequenced (Evered and Whelan, 1989). It will be interesting to see if any of these proteins contain sequences with homology to a single PTR loop. The lymphocyte homing receptor (Hermes antigen) was shown to contain a sequence with low homology to a single PTR loop (Stamekovic et al., 1989; Goldstein et al., 1989). This molecule is involved in cellular recognition and the PTR loop may provide it with some lectin properties.

The comparison of sequences and the structural predictions derived from them can thus lead to the creation of hypotheses concerning the functions of protein structures. These can be tested by determining the properties of isolated protein substructures (Fosang and Hardingham, 1989) and by experiments on specifically modified proteins prepared from the expression of new cDNA constructs in which selected sequences have been deleted or changed.

48

From the gene to the protein: the discovery of type XII collagen

MICHEL VAN DER REST

INTRODUCTION

The repetitive structure of the collagen triple helix, made of Gly–Xaa–Yaa repeats with Xaa being frequently a prolyl residue and Yaa a hydroxyprolyl residue, is reflected at the nucleic acid level by highly repetitive coding sequences of the type $(GGNCCNCCN)_n$. The resulting nucleic acid sequence similarities among all collagenous sequences have permitted the use of a probe for a given collagen chain for the identification of clones encoding other collagen chains in cDNA or genomic DNA libraries. Furthermore, part of this sequence corresponds to the cleavage site of the restriction enzyme Sau961 (G↓GNCC) and sequences encoding collagen triple helical domains are, therefore, fragmented by this enzyme into a number of small fragments, all of nine or a multiple of nine base pairs, giving rise to a characteristic ladder by gel electrophoresis.

Most of the presently available collagen probes have been isolated by searches in cDNA libraries from appropriate tissues with a probe for another collagen type and subsequent identification of the encoded chain by comparison with protein sequence data for purified collagen chains. Type XII collagen, however, was initially discovered by Gordon et al. (1987) in a search at the nucleic acid level for an analogue of type IX collagen in matrices containing type I collagen as the major fibrillar collagen without prior knowledge of the structure or even of the existence of the protein. I will briefly summarize here the strategies that have been used at the nucleic acid and protein levels to discover and characterize this molecule.

INITIAL cDNA CLONING

The strategy developed by Gordon et al. (1987) was based on the assumption that a tendon analog of type IX collagen would have a relatively small molecular weight like the type IX chains (van der Rest and Mayne, 1988), i.e. less than 100 kDa. Such collagenase-sensitive chains did indeed show up in cell-free translations of mRNA isolated from embryonic chick tendons. Poly(A)$^+$ RNA was enriched by size-fractionation in messages coding for chains of this size and used to create a cDNA library. 1000 minipreparative isolations of DNA were analyzed by electrophoresis and 77 plasmids with inserts >500 base pairs were digested with the restriction enzyme Sau96I. Ten clones produced the ladder characteristic of collagen cDNAs and the plasmid pMG377, which did not hybridize to type I probes, was further analyzed. The insert contained an open reading frame of 351 base pairs. The conceptual translation product clearly was similar to the COL1 domain of type IX collagen chains, particularly α1(IX), with sequence similarities of 42.7% at the amino acid level and 46.5% at the nucleic acid level. Particularly striking were the conservations of the two cysteinyl residues at the carboxy terminal end of COL1 and of the two imperfections of the triple helix found in this domain. The polypeptide partially encoded in pMG377 has been called the α1(XII) collagen chain. Since pMG377 was a very partial clone, no conclusion could be drawn regarding the size and overall structure of the encoded collagen.

CHARACTERIZATION OF THE PROTEIN

Pepsin fragments

The sequence similarity between the α1(XII) chain and the type IX chains led us to postulate that short disulfide bonded collagenous fragments similar to the type IX LMW and HMW fragments should be produced by pepsin digestion of type XII containing tissues. An initial purification was performed from the leg tendons of 50-dozen 17-day-old chick embryos since pMG377 had been isolated from a cDNA library from this tissue. The collagens were fractionated by a standard NaCl precipitation in 0.5 M acetic acid and disulfide bonded collagenous fragments (10 and 16 kDa, after reduction) were isolated from the 2 M precipitate. These fragments represented only a small proportion of the collagen present in tissues (< 0.5%). The purified fragments were digested with trypsin and the resulting peptides were separated by high performance liquid chromatography (HPLC) and submitted to sequential Edman degradation. Most sequences precisely matched the sequence of the protein encoded in pMG377 (Dublet and van der Rest, 1987) and, in recently isolated extended cDNAs (Gordon et al., 1989), demonstrating that type XII collagen is a genuine component of the extracellular matrix. However, some peptides gave triple helical sequences that do not correspond to cDNA sequences, suggesting the presence of additional chains similar to type XII and type IX collagens.

Immunochemical studies

A 12 amino acid long sequence from the carboxy terminal non-triple helical end of the protein encoded in pMG377 was chosen by Sugrue et al. (1989) to synthesize a peptide that was used to raise a monoclonal antibody (75d7) after coupling to hemocyanin. As this sequence was predicted to be comprised in a 99 amino acid long CNBr derived peptide that included part of the triple helical COL1 domain and two cysteines, the specificity of this antibody was demonstrated by showing by immunoblotting that it reacted with a disulfide bonded and collagenase sensitive peptide of 10 kDa after reduction. This specificity was further demonstrated by the purification of an unreduced CNBr derived peptide by affinity chromatography on an antibody column. This peptide was shown to have a unique amino terminal amino acid sequence, identical to the one predicted from the sequence of pMG377. These data established that the α1(XII) collagen chain forms a homotrimeric molecule $(\alpha1(XII))_3$ (Dublet *et al.*, 1989).

The 75d7 antibody was used to show that type XII collagen is localized in dense connective tissues containing type I collagen as the major collagen type, such as tendons, ligaments, perichondrium and periosteum (Sugrue *et al.*, 1989).

Characterization of the intact molecule

The 75d7 antibody was also used to study the intact form of the molecule and its processing. By immunoblotting, intact type XII collagen was shown to be much larger than type IX collagen with an apparent molecular weight of 220 kDa for the reduced chain. Additional higher molecular weight bands were also stained by the antibody. The exact nature of these higher molecular weight compounds has not been established yet. Intact type XII collagen was then purified from a 1 M NaCl extract of leg tendons from 17-day-old chick embryos (Dublet *et al.*, 1989). Dot immunoblots, done with the 75d7 antibody, were used to monitor the various purification steps since the relative abundance of type XII collagen was too low in the extract to detect the molecule in Coomassie-blue-stained polyacrylamide gels. Type XII collagen is very difficult to concentrate from the extract since it could be redissolved after precipitation only after heat denaturation in the presence of 0.1% sodium dodecyl sulfate and, therefore, only partially renatured molecules were initially purified. It was later discovered that native molecules could be partially purified and concentrated by affinity chromatography onto a Concanavalin A-Sepharose column and by Sephacryl S-500 chromatography. Contrary to

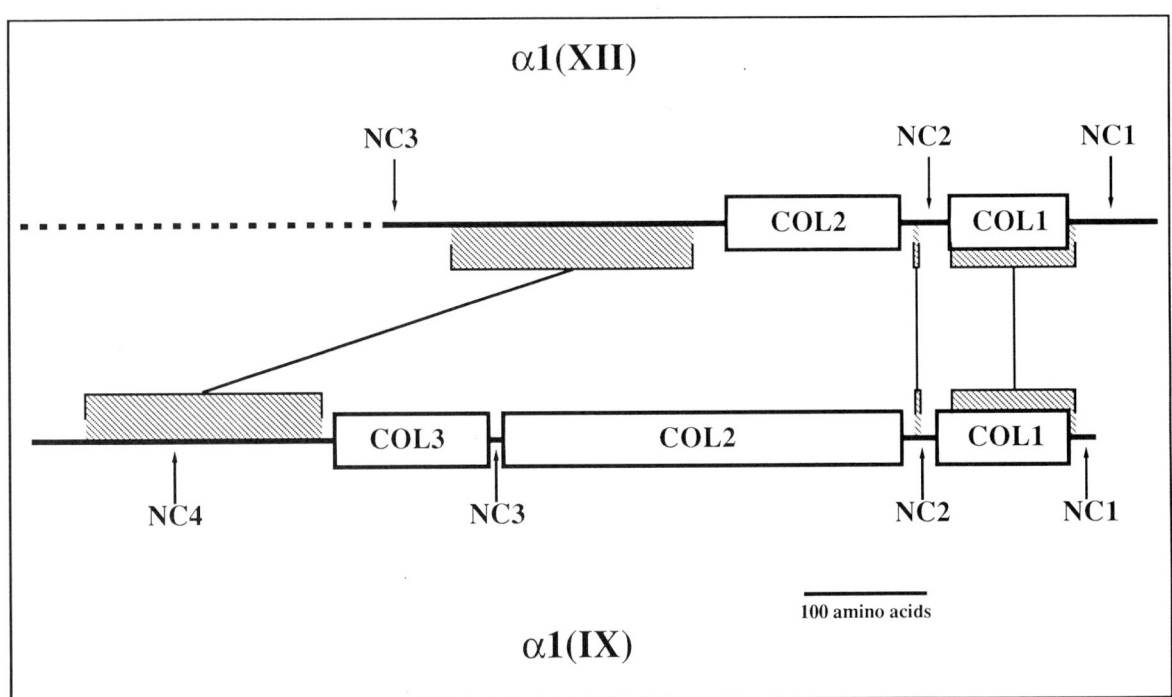

Figure 48.1 Linear comparison of the domain structure in $\alpha1(XII)$ and $\alpha1(IX)$ collagen chains. The triple-helical (COL) domains are represented in boxes while the non-triple-helical (NC) domains are represented by solid lines. The structures are derived from cDNA sequences. Regions of sequence similarities are shaded. The full sequence and the exact size of the NC3 domain of $\alpha1(XII)$ are not known. Protein analysis predicts that this domain should be almost eight times larger than the NC4 domain of $\alpha1(IX)$.

type IX collagen, type XII collagen is not a proteoglycan although its affinity for concanavalin A indicates that it is a glycoprotein.

The purified molecules were studied by rotary shadowing electron microscopy (Dublet et al., 1989). Native molecules showed a characteristic cross structure with a large central globule, a thin 75 nm collagenase sensitive tail, often kinked near its center and three 65 nm collagenase resistant fingers. Partially renatured molecules had a 'lollipop' appearance showing only the collagenous tail and a larger globule. This structure is in complete agreement with the extended cDNA data that recently have been obtained (Gordon et al., 1989) and show that type XII collagen contains only two triple-helical domains (COL1 and COL2) and a large non-triple-helical domain (NC3) at its amino-end. Homology with type IX collagen is restricted to the COL1 domains and to a segment of the NC3 domain which is homologous to part of the NC4 domain of $\alpha 1$(IX).

DISCUSSION

The discovery and the characterization of type XII collagen were based on a triangle of interactions among molecular biologists, protein chemists and immunocytochemists. None of the approaches, alone or used separately, would have led to such a rapid unraveling of the many facets of this fascinating molecule.

The initial identification by nucleic acid analysis has led, however, to specific problems that have not been fully resolved yet. For example, the size and the tissue concentration of the molecule could not be predicted from the initial cloning experiment. In fact, the size of type XII collagen turned out to be much larger than anticipated. Since the initial cell-free translation experiment demonstrated the existence of collagenase sensitive translation products of a size similar to the type IX collagen chains (Gordon et al., 1987), one might expect that other and probably closer analogs of type IX collagen are still to be discovered. Along the same line, the size of the intact type XII molecule has been demonstrated by immunoblotting to be 220 kDa per chain. It is quite

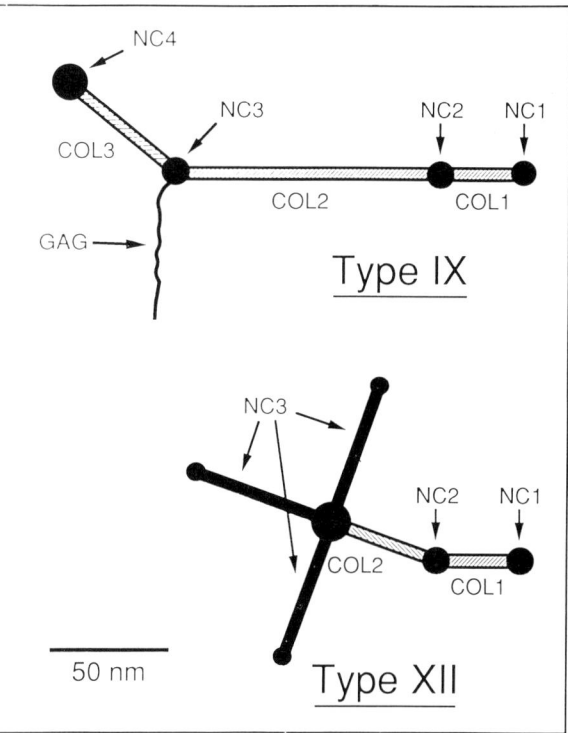

Figure 48.2 Comparison of the structures of type IX and XII collagens. The molecular organization of types IX and XII collagens are represented schematically according to the structures revealed by rotary shadowing electron microscopy. Triple-helical (COL) domains are represented by shaded boxes and non-triple-helical (NC) domains are represented in black.

possible, however, that type XII collagen is only one among a larger number of molecules sharing structural homologies with type IX collagen and that the present preparations of intact molecules are heterogeneous. Recent data from our laboratory do actually demonstrate the existence of another member in this family of molecules, type XIV collagen (Dublet and van der Rest, manuscript in preparation).

Type IX and type XII collagens only present limited homologies (Fig. 48.1). It is likely, however, that the homologous regions play similar functions. The short carboxy terminal triple-helical domain (COL1) is of particular interest.

The model that was derived for the type IX-type II interaction (van der Rest and Mayne 1988) suggests that this domain is in alignment with the gap region of the fibril. Since this domain is homologous to type IX in type XII and probably type XIV collagens, we speculate that it may serve as a site of interaction with the fibril, probably in the gap region (Fig. 48.2).

49

The source of lysozyme in chick embryo cartilage

SARAH J. KEATING and KENNETH P.H. PRITZKER

Lysozyme is a low-molecular-weight cationic protein which has been detected in high levels in cartilage from various sites in many vertebrate species (Canfield, 1974, Kuettner et al., 1975). Review of the literature and pilot immunoperoxidase studies has shown that most lysozyme localizes in the region of the chondrocyte. Although so far production of more than trace amounts of lysozyme by cultured chondrocytes has not been demonstrable, we hypothesized that substantial amounts of lysozyme are produced by chondrocytes.

Fifteen-day-old chick embryos were killed and cartilage from the distal femora and proximal tibias removed and snap frozen in liquid nitrogen. The cartilage was stored at $-70°C$ for 6 h or less. All glassware and solutions to come in contact with the tissue were treated to eliminate or minimize RNAase contamination. The glassware was baked at $250°C$ for 6 h and all the aqueous solutions were made with diethyl pyrocarbonate (DEPC) treated water ($1\,ml\,l^{-1}$). The tissue was cut at 8 μm on a cryostat at $-15°C$. Sections were collected on poly-D-lysine coated slides and kept frozen for less than 3 h before being fixed. During fixation, the sections were immersed in 4% p-formaldehyde for 4 min. Those sections to be used for in situ hybridization were acetylated with acetic anhydride in fresh 100 mM triethanolamine (pH 7.5). All the slides were then rinsed in 3× phosphate buffered saline (PBS) for 5 min and twice in 1× PBS for 3 min. The slides were then dehydrated in graded alcohols and air dried. They were stored dessicated at $-30°C$.

Sections were incubated with a polyclonal rabbit antichick lysozyme (provided by Dr Eugene Thonar (Thonar et al., 1988)) (1 : 400) and a goat antirabbit IgG using the indirect immunoperoxidase technique of Sternberger.

A small amount of chick lysozyme cDNA in the plasmid pBR322 was kindly provided by Dr Gunther Schutz and coworkers (Institute of Cell and Tumour Biology, German Cancer Research Center, Heidelberg). The DNA was propagated by standard techniques, linearized and transcribed into RNA in the presence of ^{35}S-labeled uridine triphosphate (UTP) (410 Ci $mmol^{-1}$). The transcription mixture included 1× buffer, 10 M DTT, 20 U RNase inhibitor, cold adenosine triphosphate (ATP), cytidine triphosphate (CTP) and guanosine triphosphate (GTP), 100 μCi [^{35}S]-UTP, 1 μg linearized template and 10 U SP6 RNA polymerase. The mixture was incubated at $40°C$ for 45 min, ten more units of SP6 polymerase were added and the incubation was continued for another 45 min.

Pretreatment of the slides to allow access of the probe to mRNA was performed using proteinase

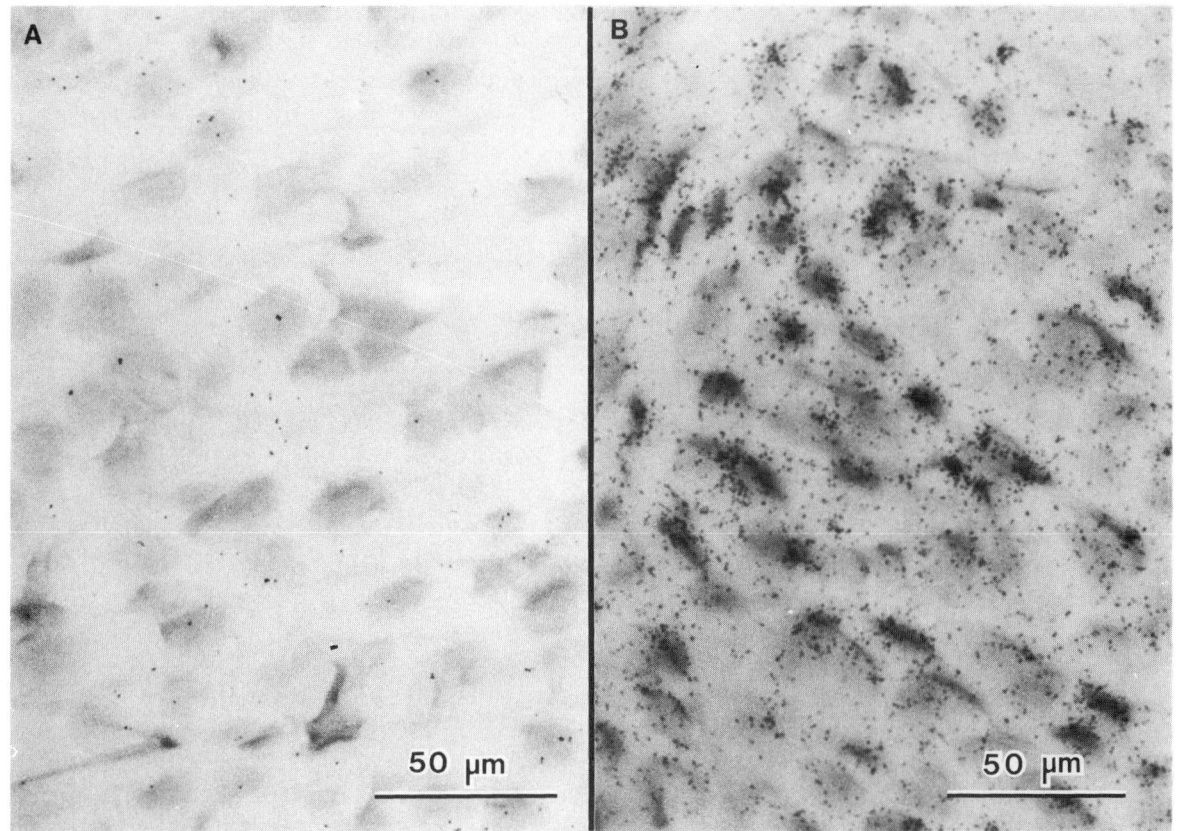

Figure 49.1 *In situ* hybridization with an ^{35}S-labeled antisense riboprobe complementary to lysozyme mRNA (B). There is staining which distinctly localized to the cytoplasm of chondrocytes. (A) Hybridization with the sense RNA probe in which the RNA sequence is identical to the mRNA rather than complementary. Only background levels of staining are observed.

K. The hybridization mixture was as follows: 50% formamide, 0.3 M NaCl, 10 mM (Tris)HCl (pH 7.5), 1 mM EDTA, 1× Denhardt's solution, 250 μg ml^{-1} transfer RNA (tRNA), 250 μg ml^{-1} sheared heterologous DNA, 10% dextran sulfate, 100 mM dithiothreitol (DTT) and 0.2 μg/ml/kilobase of complexity ^{35}S-labeled probe. Probe mixture (20 μl) was put on each section, then the sections were covered with a coverslip and put in a moist hybridization chamber at 55°C for 18 h.

The slides were washed in 2× SSC with 1 μg ml^{-1} RNAase A at 20°C for 10 min, washed twice for 25 min each in 2× SSC at 65°C and wahsed three times for 25 min each in 0.1× SSC at 65°C. The sections were dehydrated with ethanol/0.3 M ammonium acetate and air dried. The slides were dipped into prewarmed Kodak NTB-2 emulsion diluted 1 : 1 with 0.6 M ammonium acetate at 45°C, left to dry for a few hours, placed in slide boxes with dessicant and exposed at −70°C for 2 to 3 weeks. The slides were developed, fixed and stained with hematoxylin and eosin.

The *in situ* hybridization revealed weak but detectable labeling of some chondrocytes (Fig. 49.1). The more centrally located hyperplastic chondrocytes demonstrated a greater density of staining for lysozyme RNA than the smaller chondrocytes found on the articular surface. Our observations demonstrate that at least some of the lysozyme present in chick embryo cartilage is produced endogenously by chondrocytes.

ACKNOWLEDGMENT

The authors would like to thank Dr Janet Rossant and her staff for their advice and assistance.

50

Approaches to studying the regulation of chondrocyte gene expression

W. E. HORTON, JR and S. CHANDRASEKHAR

INTRODUCTION

The expression of gene coding for various cartilage matrix proteins varies dramatically during certain stages of cartilage disease and as a consequence of development. For example, during early osteoarthritis (OA), some authors report an increase in cartilage matrix synthesis and cell proliferation as an apparent attempt to repair the cartilage lesions (Mankin et al., 1971; Thompson and Oegema, 1979). In addition, there is a well-documented activation of expression of the gene coding for cartilage matrix proteins as mesenchymal stem cells undergo chondrogenesis (Kosher et al., 1986a,b). These types of changes suggest that the control of chondrocyte protein expression is regulated very tightly.

The steady-state level of expression of a specific protein by the chondrocyte can be controlled at many levels and studied using several standard techniques (Table 50.1). One level of control involves an interaction between *trans* acting

Table 50.1 Control of protein expression and methods of analysis

Endpoint	Control points	Analysis
Steady-state protein level	Balance between synthesis and degradation	Long-term labeling with radiolabeled amino acids
Newly-synthesized protein	Rate of translation of mRNA	Pulse label with radio-labeled amino acids
Steady-state mRNA level	Balance between mRNA synthesis and turnover	RNA isolation/northern transfer/react with nucleotide probes
Newly-synthesized mRNA	Rate of transcription	Nuclear run-off assay
Activity of regulatory sequences	Balance between + and − *trans* acting proteins	Transfection of regulatory sequences coupled to marker genes

proteins and *cis* acting DNA sequences that up-regulates or down-regulates the rate of transcription. In this chapter approaches to studying regulatory mechanisms are emphasized.

IDENTIFYING REGULATORY DNA SEQUENCES

Figure 50.1 shows the overall concept for identifying regulatory sequences using the type II collagen gene as an example. The gene coding for type II collagen is very large with multiple exons and introns, as well as regions that flank the structural portion of the gene, such as the promoter. In order to simplify the identification of regulatory sequences and regulation of their expression, a marker gene such as chloramphenicol acetyl transferase (CAT) is used. This gene is coupled to the putative regulatory sequences from the gene of interest and this construct is then transfered into cells (see below). In order for the CAT gene to be expressed, the regulatory sequences must interact with general transcription factors (such as RNA polymerase II),

as well as proteins that may be more specific for the gene and the cell type being studied. The level of CAT expression can be monitored either at the RNA level or by determining the ability of cell lysates to acetylate [^{14}C]chloramphenicol which is visualized by thin-layer chromatography. Using this approach, we have previously determined that a sequence in the first intron of the rat type II collagen gene acts as a tissue-specific enhancer for the expression of this gene (Horton *et al.*, 1987).

The two major methods for introducing DNA into cells are electroporation (Toneguzzo *et al.*, 1986) and calcium phosphate precipitation (Graham and Van Der Eb, 1973). Electroporation requires sophisticated equipment and, in our experience, is not necessary for the efficient transfection of chondrocytes. Using the calcium phosphate technique, we have routinely introduced DNA into chondrocytes from different sources (articular, sternal, and costal), species (rabbits, rats and chick) and age (embryonic vs. adult). There are a few modifications to the standard protocols which are worth noting. First, Ham's F-12 is not a suitable medium for forming good precipitates. This may be due to the fact that

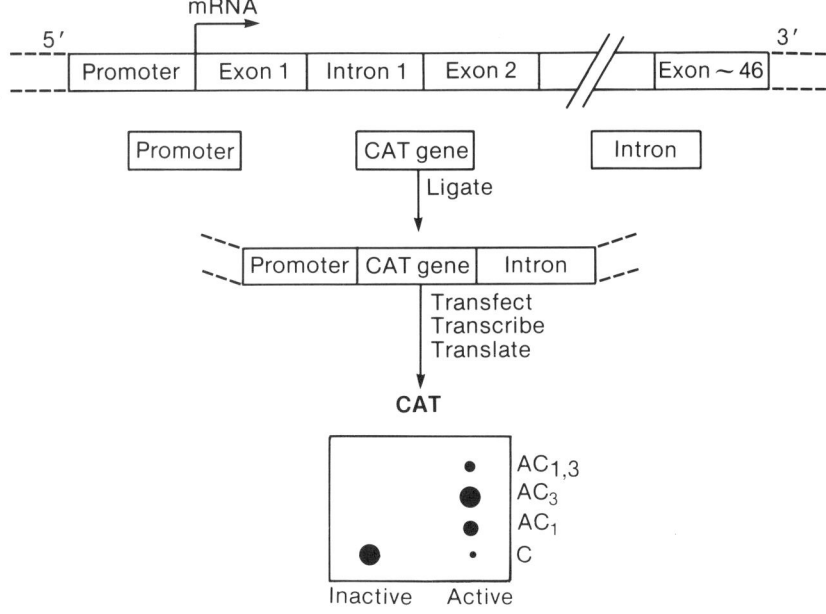

Figure 50.1 Coupling the collagen II promoter to the CAT gene.

the calcium concentration is relatively low (approximately 40 mg ml^{-1}). DMEM medium with a calcium concentration of 200 mg ml^{-1}, is excellent for forming good calcium phosphate precipitates. Second, it is important to incubate the cells with the DNA–calcium phosphate precipitate for only a short time: we have found that 3 h is usually sufficient. Longer incubation times (for example, overnight) results in a change in the chondrocyte phenotype with diminished type II collagen expression. For the same reason, glycerol or dimethyl sulfoxide (DMSO) treatments should be avoided (Horton et al., 1989). An exception to this that we have observed so far is for chondrocytes prepared from the Swarm rat chondrosarcoma. Figure 50.2 shows that, even after an overnight incubation with calcium phosphate precipitate plus the plasmid RSV-CAT (the rous sarcoma viral LRT coupled to CAT), there is negligible CAT activity in lysates of chondrosarcoma chondrocytes. If, however, the overnight incubation with the precipitate is followed by a 2 min glycerol or DMSO treatment, substantial CAT activity is observed. Therefore, it appears that for the transfection of chondrosarcoma cells with foreign DNA, membrane permeabilization may be a prerequisite. With the use of strong, ubiquitous promoters (SV40 promoter/enhancer, RSV promoter, β-actin promoter, etc.) it is possible to determine how well DNA is being taken up for a given cell type or following some type of treatment.

BIOLOGICAL QUESTIONS

With these types of approach it is possible to examine a number of biological questions related to the regulation of chondrocyte gene expression (Table 50.2). When the promoter sequences are identified and coupled to a marker gene, transfection studies can be used to determine the relative strength of the promoter. For example, the collagen II gene has a relatively weak promoter (Horton et al., 1987) and requires an enhancer sequence for high-level expression. Once a high level of expression is obtained in the cell type which expresses the endogenous gene, it is then possible to determine if these sequences are cell-type specific. This is accomplished by transfecting the active constructs into a variety of cell types and determining activity. The chondrocyte responds to a variety of signals by up-regulating or down-regulating the expression of genes coding for matrix proteins. For example, we have shown that a combination of TGF-β and FGF completely

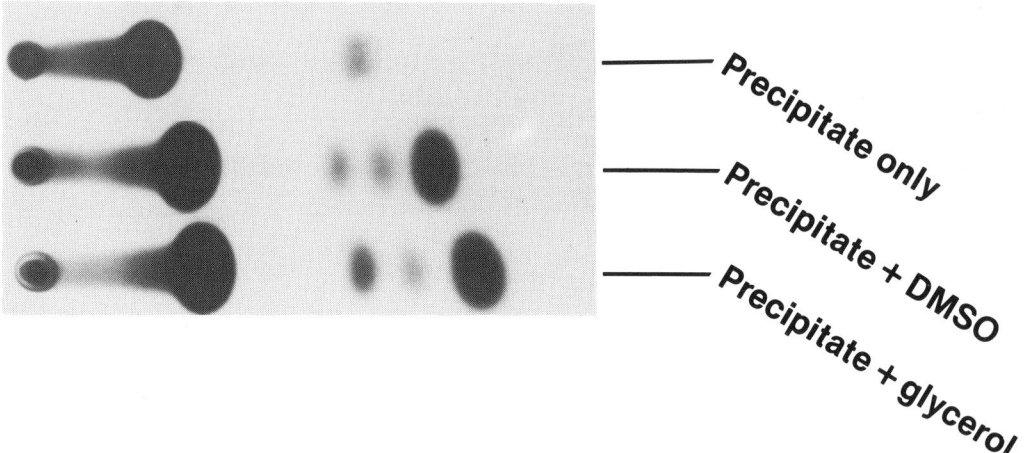

Figure 50.2 Effect of glycerol or DMSO on chondrosarcoma cell transfection.

Table 50.2 Biological questions related to regulation of chondrocyte gene expression

Promoter strength
Enhancer sequences
Cell-type specific activity
Modulation by exogenous signals
   (e.g. growth factors)
Developmental regulation

inhibits the expression of the collagen II gene (Horton *et al.*, 1989). Transfection experiments with different plasmid constructs allow for the determination of which DNA sequences might mediate these types of changes in gene expression. Chondrocytes transfected with plasmid DNA, containing the collagen II promoter/enhancer sequences coupled to CAT, show no CAT activity after treatment with TGF-β and FGF. Thus, treatment with these growth factors probably alters the interaction between DNA-binding proteins and the regulatory sequences that control the expression of the type II collagen gene. Finally, it is possible to examine the molecular basis of differentiation by carrying out transfection studies using mesenchymal cells undergoing chondrogenesis and thus determining at what stage certain DNA sequences are active.

SUMMARY

Identifying important regulatory DNA sequences and determining their activities in transfection experiments is really only the first step toward understanding the molecular mechanism of chondrocyte gene regulation. The next series of studies should focus on the identification and characterization of the proteins that bind to these sequences and result in changes in transcriptional activity. When these proteins are purified and antibodies are made, it is then possible to determine the pattern of expression of these proteins in normal tissues and the way in which these patterns are altered in disease states. It is likely that alterations in the expression of these proteins will correlate with some diseases of cartilage such as OA or chondrodystrophies.

ACKNOWLEDGMENTS

The authors would like to acknowledge the technical assistance of Jill D. Higginbotham and Anita K. Harvey.

51

Detection of type II collagen gene mutations in familial osteoarthritis

SERGIO A. JIMENEZ

INTRODUCTION

It is well established that human osteoarthritis (OA) is a heterogeneous and multifactoral disease, and that multiple pathogenetic mechanisms can be implicated in its development and progression (for reviews see Moskowitz *et al.* (1984), Moskowitz (1985) and Sokoloff and Hough (1987)). Although in most instances OA is an acquired process secondary to various metabolic, mechanical or inflammatory-immunologic events, there is compelling evidence to indicate that several distinct forms of OA are inherited as dominant traits with a Mendelian pattern (Stecher et al., 1953). The most common form of inherited OA is characterized by the frequent development of Heberden's nodes and the premature degeneration of multiple joints, with a concentric or uniform loss of articular cartilage, particularly apparent in the hip and knee joints (Marks et al., 1979). A second type of inherited OA is that associated with familial chondrocalcinosis due to the deposition of calcium pyrophosphate dihydrate (CPPD) crystals in fibrous and hyaline cartilages (Reginato, 1976; Ryan and McCarty, 1987). The observation that the degenerative arthritis occasionally precedes or is not associated with demonstrable deposition of CPPD crystals (Bjelle, 1972) suggests that structural abnormalities in articular cartilage matrix may be a primary common event leading to cartilage degeneration and/or to CPPD crystal deposition. A third familial form of OA is known as Stickler Syndrome (Lieberfarb et al., 1979) or hereditary arthroophthalmopathy (Stickler et al., 1965). This syndrome is characterized by progressive vitreoretinal degeneration, severe myopia and premature degenerative joint disease. Other heritable disorders accompanied by premature OA include hydroxyapatite deposition disease (Marcos et al., 1981) and certain forms of multiple epiphyseal dysplasias (Spranger, 1975).

Analysis of the pattern of inheritance of these diseases suggests the possibility that defects in one or more of the genes encoding for the macromolecular components of articular cartilage may be responsible for the premature and generalized degenerative changes in the tissue. The recent advances in molecular biology make it possible to examine this hypothesis at the molecular level. The abnormal genes could include genes coding for cartilage matrix macromolecules, genes for enzymes involved in the biosynthesis of matrix, genes for chondrocyte hormone and growth factor-receptor proteins, or genes for enzymes involved in the metabolic degradation of the tissue. Identification of mutations in the multiplicity of genes that may be affected would represent a monumental task due to the enormous effort that would be required to determine the sequence of all the possible genes, and to the incomplete knowledge regarding the structure and organization of many of them. Recent evidence, however, suggests that procollagen genes are the most likely candidates. Collagen plays a crucial role in the maintenance of the biomechanical properties of articular cartilage since it is responsible for the remarkable tensile strength and shear stiffness of the tissue. In addition, the normal supramolecular assembly of cartilage collagen serves as a mechanical constraint to prevent the expansion of proteoglycans (PGs) and their tightly-bound water molecules into the large hydrodynamic domains characteristic of PGs in free solution. A failure of this collagenous network would result in swelling of the PGs, increased tissue water, softening of the matrix and eventual cartilage degeneration. The most compelling evidence to suggest that type II procollagen genes may be the genes at fault in heritable OA comes from recent studies on other heritable disorders that cause mechanical failure of the connective tissues such as Osteogenesis Imperfecta and Ehlers-Danlos syndrome. These investigations have established the surprising conclusion that most patients with these diseases have mutations in procollagen genes and not in any of the other genes that encode the large numbers of proteins required for the normal structure and function of the tissues. These studies have also provided a number of strategies that have been successful for the identification of mutations in types I and III procollagen genes. However, as discussed in more detail below, many of these strategies have limitations when applied to the study of mutations in the genes encoding for articular cartilage proteins. Some of these limitations are due to the limited availability of cartilage, the difficulty in expanding chondrocyte populations in vitro, the loss of chondrocyte-specific phenotype during culture, and the difficulty in performing extensive biochemical characterization at the protein level. In the following sections a series of strategies that have been successfully utilized by several groups of investigators to identify type II collagen gene mutations in some of the inherited diseases affecting articular cartilage will be described.

Restriction fragment length polymorphism analysis

The development of recombinant probes that allow the detection of polymorphic sites in human DNA by restriction fragment length polymorphism (RFLP) analysis has made available a vast resource of genetic markers to follow the inheritance of specific DNA sequences in families (Botstein et al., 1980; Willard et al., 1985; Antonarakis, 1989). These polymorphic sequences occur frequently in the flanking regions of most genes as well as in randomly selected genomic DNA. Utilizing cDNAs to detect these polymorphisms, it is now possible to identify abnormal alleles of many genes and to trace their pattern of cosegregation with a given disease phenotype in families. Recently, several polymorphisms in the type II procollagen gene (COL2A1) and surrounding DNA sequences have been identified (Sangiorgi et al., 1984; Väisänen et al., 1988; Weaver and Knowlton, 1989). The identification of these polymorphisms has permitted the application of RFLP analysis to test the possibility that structural mutations in COL2A1 may be responsible for the biomechanical failure of articular cartilage in familial OA.

One of the essential requirements for RFLP analysis is the ability to identify and study families in which the disorder is clearly inherited, and in which blood or tissue samples can be obtained from affected and unaffected members of three or more generations. The premise for RFLP study of such inherited forms of OA is that, despite the heterogeneity and variability of their phenotype, they must have a primary genetic defect that resides at a chromosomal locus. The disease phenotype and the gene responsible must, therefore, map to the same chromosomal location as reflected by their cosegregation in families. Employing appropriate restriction enzymes it becomes feasible to map the inherited trait to a region in the chromosome bracketed by two specific markers.

The potential benefits of utilizing RFLP genetic linkage analysis in heritable forms of human OA is that it will permit the identification of the genes at fault in these disorders. Even the finding of linked genetic markers at some distance from the responsible gene would allow definition of the approximate chromosomal location of the abnormal gene and its cloning and sequencing. In addition, informative RFLPs can be tested in families suffering from diseases with similar phenotypes to determine whether the same genetic defect is present in all cases or whether there is genetic heterogeneity among the various phenotypes. RFLP analysis can also give valuable negative information since the absence of cosegregation (i.e. recombination) with the disease phenotype can exclude the candidate gene as the site of the defect in a given family. The results are analyzed by standard procedures using the probability ratio test or odd ratio with the logarithm of the ratio of probabilities of linkage vs. nonlinkage (LOD score) determined for varying recombination frequencies. Linkage is established when the data yield a LOD score of 3 or greater (odd for linkage of 1000:1).

Several groups of investigators have recently applied RFLP analysis to human OA and related disorders. Francomano et al. (1987) and Knowlton et al. (1989) have recently demonstrated coinheritance of certain polymorphic sites in the type II procollagen gene with the expression of hereditary arthroophthalmopathy or Stickler syndome. Knowlton et al. analyzed three large Stickler syndrome families for clinical manifestations of the disease and for coinheritance of the genetic defect with the Hind III and the variable number tandem repeat (VNTR) polymorphisms in COL2A1. Genetic linkage between the disease phenotype and COL2A1 was demonstrated in the largest family, with a maximum LOD score of 3.52 at a recombination distance of zero. The results from the second family also supported linkage to COL2A1. These observations are consistent with the conclusion that mutations in the COL2A1 gene are responsible for the disease in these two families. In contrast, in the third family, recombination between the clinical expression and COL2A1 was not demonstrated, suggesting, therefore, that the syndrome may be heterogeneous and that in certain families a gene other than COL2A1 may be the defective gene.

In a more recent study, Knowlton et al. (1990) have also demonstrated coinheritance of a phenotype of premature OA and a mild chondrodystrophy in a large family from Cleveland with the Hind III polymorphic site in the type II procollagen gene. The inheritance of the Hind III RFLP in the COL2A1 alleles in a cluster of informative members of this family is illustrated in Fig. 51.1. The autoradiogram shows the Hind III restriction fragments of the COL2A1 genes from each family member. As shown in Fig. 51.1, allelic variants of the COL2A1 gene result from the presence or absence of a Hind III site (H*) halfway between two constant Hind III sites separated by a 14-kb sequence, thus, resulting in two comigrating 7-kb fragments. The mother is homozygous for the 7-kb allele and the father is heterozygous with one 7-kb and one 14-kb allele. The daughter inherited the father's 14-kb allele, and the three sons inherited his 7-kb allele. The three children displaying the clinical phenotype inherited the abnormal 7-kb allele from the father. A high LOD score indicated that a mutation of the COL2A1 gene is responsible for the development of primary OA in this family. A similar study on a large

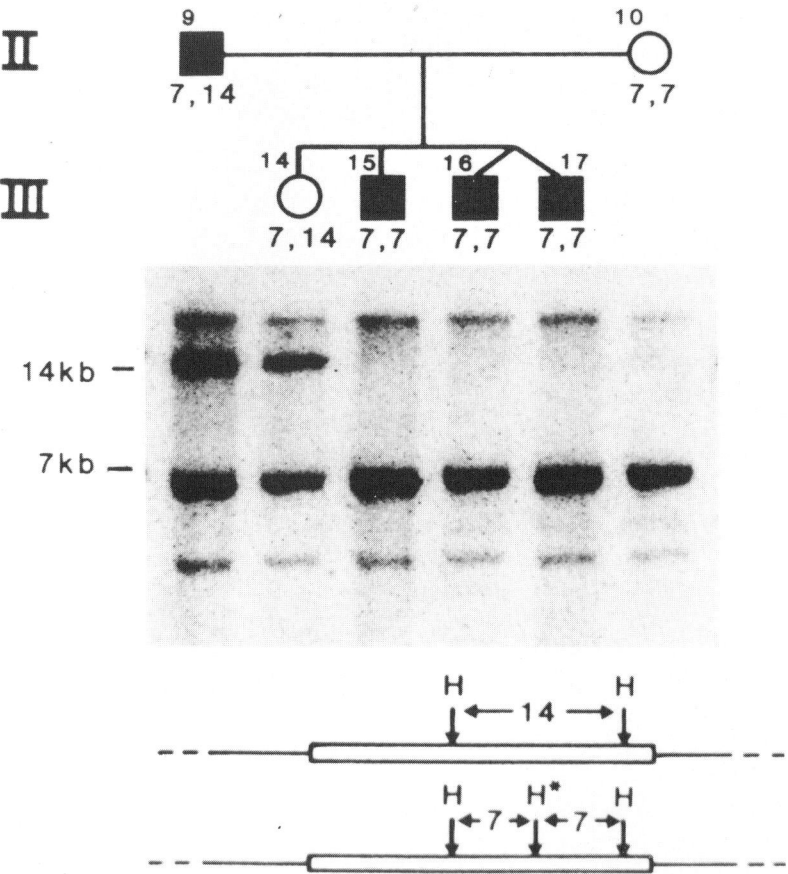

Figure 51.1 Inheritance of COL2A1 RFLP alleles in some members of a large family with premature OA and mild chondrodystrophy.

Finnish family with primary generalized OA also showed coinheritance of the disease with type II procollagen gene polymorphisms (Pelotie et al., 1989).

Identification of type II collagen gene mutations in affected individuals

The recent development of methods for cloning and sequencing cDNAs and genes has already resulted in substantial advances in our understanding of the structure of normal articular cartilage matrix. As the complete nucleotide sequences of the normal genes are determined, it will become possible to identify the mutations in the abnormal genes.

A general approach to identifying these mutations involves the study of those families in which RFLP analysis shows linkage between the phenotype of heritable OA and informative RFLPs. Family members who are heterozygotes for the RFLP should be examined first since the particular RFLP should provide a marker to distinguish the normal from the mutated allele. Once the exact mutation has been defined, other available members of the family can be tested for the presence of the specific mutation.

The identification of mutations in the gene encoding for the structural-connective-tissue components has been accomplished in a large number of families with various forms of osteogenesis imperfecta or the Ehlers–Danlos syndrome and recently in some families with vascular aneurisms. The approach employed in most of these instances has been the determination of the nucleotide sequences of cDNAs prepared by reverse transcription of total cellular RNA from cultured cells from affected individuals. Cultured dermal or amniotic fluid fibroblasts were successfully employed for isolation of RNA which was then submitted to reverse transcription reactions to obtain cDNA libraries. The cDNA libraries were screened with human sequence-specific probes to identify clones containing the inserts of interest. Expansion of these clones followed by their sequencing, usually employing the dideoxy chain termination reaction either manually or with an automatic DNA sequencer, resulted in identification of the mutations. Many of these studies were greatly facilitated by the previous identification and characterization of protein abnormalities which pointed out the likely nature of the mutations and pointed to the approximate regions within the gene containing the mutations. These protein abnormalities included the demonstration of overmodification of posttranslational reactions, 'protein suicide' due to decreased procollagen thermal stability, the finding of disulfide bonded α-chain dimers due to the presence of cysteine residues in the triple-helical domains, or the demonstration of shortened collagen α-chains.

Although this method allowed the identification of a number of mutations affecting types I and III collagen genes, its success depends on the availability of large numbers of cells to obtain sufficient quantitiy of RNA for the abnormal protein, and on the information obtained from structural studies of the mutated protein. This method also requires tedious and time-consuming efforts devoted to cloning the cDNA libraries and sequencing many cDNAs to identify the mutation. This task is made more difficult by the large size of collagen mRNAs and by technical difficulties in obtaining full-length cDNAs from GC-rich nucleotide sequences highly prone to the formation of secondary structures. The availability of cells that express the transcripts from the mutated genes is not a problem for investigations on the mutations affecting genes for types I and III collagens, because cultured dermal fibroblasts can be utilized successfully. In the case of mutations affecting the type II collagen gene, however, it is difficult and often impossible to obtain sufficient amounts of articular cartilage tissue to extract type II collagen mRNA for generation of cDNA libraries. Furthermore, there is an additional complication introduced by the well-known instability of the cartilage-specific phenotype when chondrocytes are isolated and cultured. Under most culture conditions, these cells lose their cartilage-specific phenotype, arresting the synthesis of type II collagen and initiating the synthesis of the soft tissue collagens types I and III. Until these shortcomings are solved, the application of the standard procedure described above to the identification of mutations in the type II collagen gene will have only limited success.

Use of the polymerase chain reaction

The recent discovery of a specific DNA polymerase that is capable of reiterative synthesis of DNA copies from a given template at high temperatures has resulted in the development of one of the most powerful techniques of molecular biology (Saiki et al., 1987). At the present time, most studies of cloning, sequencing, and characterization of normal and altered genes employ the PCR. This procedure involves the use of two oligonucleotide primers that hybridize to specific sequences, one on each strand of the target DNA template. The thermally-stable polymerase from *Thermus aquaticus* is then used to copy the DNA sequences bracketed by the specific nucleotides resulting in the synthesis of a complementary strand of the target DNA. The procedure is automatically repeated by successive cycles of denaturation and annealing at optimal temperatures. After 20–30 cycles, the target DNA sequence is amplified as much as 10^6-fold.

The PCR reaction has been successfully applied to cloning and sequencing cDNAs and genes that were not possible previously either because of the development of secondary structures or because of the lack of available enzyme restriction sites for proper cloning. The possibilities of identifying type II collagen gene mutations employing small amounts of cartilage or chondrocyte cultures have also been improved dramatically by the PCR. The amplification of specific DNA sequences can overcome the limitations introduced by the lack of sufficient amounts of articular cartilage necessary to obtain RNA for generation of cDNA libraries. Using the PCR, minute amounts of RNA can be reverse transcribed to obtain cDNAs. These cDNAs can then be amplified using sequence-specific oligonucleotides based on the known sequence of full-length cDNAs. Since the entire sequence of the type II collagen cDNA has been recently published (Baldwin et al., 1989), it is feasible to amplify the entire coding sequence from the cDNAs.

The PCR products can be sequenced directly or can be cloned into bacterial vectors for standard sequencing procedures. Given the advances in DNA sequencing, as many as 1200 bp can now be read from a single sequencing reaction. Thus, to sequence the entire coding region for the mutant allele is feasible. Single base mutations or small insertions/deletions in coding or regulatory sequences can be identified. Mutations in sequences important for splicing can also be detected utilizing oligonucleotide primers specific for intron sequences at the intron–exon boundaries. Thus, the PCR amplified products will correspond to the coding sequences and to adjacent consensus sequences required for splicing. Despite the extraordinary sensitivity of the PCR, the method requires the availability of at least minute amounts of cartilage or of cultured chondrocytes that maintain their differentiated phenotype. Furthermore, the success of this approach depends on the ability to generate cDNAs that cover the entire coding sequence or of obtaining shorter cDNAs that cover the region where the mutation is located. Since these problems can often be insurmountable, approaches that do not depend on the availability of cartilage will be required in the majority of cases. Two of these approaches are described briefly below.

New approaches to identifying type II collagen gene mutations when articular cartilage tissue is not available

Recent interest has been placed on the possibility of identifying type II collagen gene mutations when cartilage phenotype-expressing cells are not available. These methods have taken advantage of the huge advances made in preparation of cosmid clones. Genomic libraries containing large sections of DNA can be successfully established in cosmid vectors. A recent method developed by Ala-Kokko and Prockop (1990) utilized cosmid clones established from size-fractionated DNA that had been previously digested with specific restriction endonucleases. The cosmid clones were screened to identify those containing type II collagen gene inserts. Clones containing DNA regions displaying the same polymorphism identified by RFLPs were then selected for sequencing.

Large-scale production of cartilage matrix macromolecules in noncartilaginous cells

The ultimate confirmation that a mutation identified at the DNA level is responsible for a given disease phenotype is the finding of the respective mutated protein product and the demonstration that it displays an abnormal function or has an altered structure. The demonstration of abnormalities in the function of the macromolecular components of articular cartilage in OA has been severely hampered by the difficulty in obtaining sufficient amounts of intact molecules in a native state from the tissues. Extraction of collagens and PGs from cartilage usually involves the use of denaturing agents such as guanidinium hydrochloride, lithium salts, etc., and/or limited proteolysis with pepsin or chymotrypsin. Furthermore, purification of these components is difficult and time consuming. Identification of structural defects at the mRNA level has also been limited by the availability of sufficient amounts of type II procollagen mRNA from tissues of chondrocyte cultures from affected individuals. To overcome these difficulties, Ala-Kokko et al. (1989) examined the possibility of obtaining expression of human type II procollagen genes in cultured mouse fibroblasts starting with genomic DNA obtained from either peripheral blood mononuclear cells or cultured fibroblasts. In these studies, a chimeric gene containing a small fragment from the 5'-end of the human proα1(I) gene fused to the entire human proα1(II) gene except for the corresponding 5'-end was constructed. The proα1(I) fragment contained the 5'-promoter region, the first exon and the enhancer in the first intervening sequence. The proα1(II) fragment contained part of the first intervening sequence and the rest of the gene together with 0.5 kb of the 3' flanking region. The construct was transfected into NIH 3T3 mouse fibroblasts using calcium phosphate coprecipitated with a neomycin gene. Several stable clones expressing high levels of type II collagen mRNA as assayed by slot–blot and Northern blot hybridization with a human sequence-specific cDNA were obtained. The system, therefore, makes it possible to obtain mRNA for human type II procollagen in mouse fibroblasts from cosmid clones prepared with genomic DNA from normal individuals and from patients. The expression of human type II procollagen mRNA should, under optimal conditions, result in production of the human protein by the mouse fibroblasts. Large-scale production of the recombinant macromolecule in native and pure form therefore appears feasible. The availability of quantitative amounts of the protein will permit, for the first time, the performance of extensive structural and functional studies. For example, it will be possible to determine the thermal stability of the intact procollagen, the kinetics of procollagen cleavage and collagen fibril formation, the assembly of supramolecular aggregates with PGs, the role of the minor collagens (types IX and XI collagens) in type II collagen fibril size and structure, etc.

CONCLUSION

The approaches described above are directed toward testing the hypothesis that certain inherited forms of OA are caused by mutations in genes expressed in cartilage and specifically in the genes for cartilage procollagens. The hypothesis can now be tested with a number of innovative techniques of molecular biology that will define the exact molecular causes of these diseases. The methods will also permit us to establish whether or not these diseases are single entities at the molecular level and, eventually, will provide simple DNA tests for definitive diagnosis of the molecular defects in individual patients. Extension of the same studies can establish whether or not more common forms of OA are caused by the same mutations.

ACKNOWLEDGMENTS

Supported by Program Project Grant AR 39740-01 from the NIH. The expert assistance of Meredith Billman in the preparation of this manuscript is thankfully acknowledged.

References

Ala-Kokko, L. and Prockop, D.J. (1990). Efficient procedures for isolating and sequencing the gene for type II procollagen from patients with osteoarthritis and related disorders. *Trans. Orthop. Res. Soc.* in press

Ala-Kokko, L., Kontusaari, S., Olsen, A., Hyland, J., Jimenez, S.A. and Prockop, D.J. (1989). Expression of human type II procollagen gene in mouse fibroblasts transfected with a dimeric gene construct containing the promoter of the type I procollagen gene. *Arthr. Rheum.* **32**, 584

Antonarakis, S. (1989). Diagnosis of genetic disorders at the DNA level. *New Engl. J. Med.* **320**, 153

Ausubel, F.M., Brent, R., Kingston, R.E., Moore, D.D., Seidman, J.G., Smith, J.A. and Struhl, K. (1988). *Current Protocols in Molecular Biology*. Wiley-Interscience, New York

Baldwin, C.T., Reginato, A.M., Smith, C., Jimenez, S.A. and Prockop, D.J. (1989). Structure of a cDNA clone coding for human type II procollagen. The $\alpha1(II)$ chain is more similar to the $\alpha1(I)$ chain than two other α chains of fibrillar collagens. *Biochem. J.* **162**, 521

Berger, S.L. and Kimmel, A.R. (1987). *Guide to Molecular Cloning Techniques*. Academic Press, New York

Bjelle, A. (1972). Morphological study of articular cartilage in pyrophosphate arthropathy. *Ann. Rheum. Dis.* **31**, 449

Botstein, D., White, R., Skolnick, M. and Davis, R.W. (1980). Construction of a genetic linkage map in man using restriction fragment length polymorphisms. *Am. J. Human Genet.* **32**, 314

Bourdon, M.A., Krusius, T., Campbell, S., Schwartz, N.B. and Ruoslahti, E. (1987). Identification and synthesis of a recognition signal for the attachment of glycosaminoglycans to proteins. *Proc. Natl. Acad. Sci. USA* **84**, 3194–3198

Canfield, R.E. (1974). In *Introduction, Structure of Lysozymes* (E.F. Osserman, R.E. Canfield and S. Beychok, eds), pp. 3–8. Academic Press, New York

Davies, K.E. (1988). *Genome Analysis: A Practical Approach*. IRL Press, Oxford

Deak, F., Kiss, I., Sparks, K.J., Argraves, W.S., Hampikian, G. and Goetinck, P.F. (1986). Complete amino acid sequence of chicken cartilage link protein deduced from cDNA clones. *Proc. Natl. Acad. Sci. USA* **83**, 3766–3770

Doege, K., Hassell, J.R., Caterson, B. and Yamada, Y. (1986). Link protein cDNA sequence reveals a tandemly repeated protein structure. *Proc. Natl. Acad. Sci. USA* **83**, 3761–3765

Doege, K., Sasaki, M., Horigan, E., Hassell, J.R. and Yamada, Y. (1987). Complete primary structure of the rat cartilage proteoglycan core protein deduced from cDNA clones. *J. Biol. Chem.* **262**, 17 757–17 767

Dublet, B. and van der Rest, M. (1987). Type XII collagen is expressed in embryonic chick tendons. Isolation of pepsin-derived fragments. *J. Biol. Chem.* **262**, 17 724–17 727

Dublet, B., Oh, S., Sugrue, S.P., Gordon, M.K., Gerecke, D.R., Olsen, B.R. and van der Rest, M. (1989). The structure of avian type XII collagen: $\alpha1(XII)$ chains contain 190 kDa non triple-helical amino-terminal domains and form homotrimeric molecules. *J. Biol. Chem.* **264**, 13 150–13 156

Dudhia, J. and Hardingham, T.E. (1989). cDNA sequences to human and porcine cartilage proteoglycan and link protein. *Trans. Orthop. Res. Soc. 35th Meeting*, p. 8. The Orthopaedic Research Society, Park Ridge, Il.

Evered, D. and Whelan, J. (1989). *The Biology of Hyaluronan, Ciba Foundation Symposium 143*, p. 228. Wiley, Chichester

Fosang, A.J. and Hardingham, T.E. (1989). Isolation of the N-terminal globular protein domains from cartilage proteoglycans: Identification of G2 domain and its lack of interaction with hyaluronate and link protein. *Biochem. J.* **261**, 801–809

Francomano, C.A., Liberfarb, R.M., Hirose, T., Maumenee, I.H., Streeten, E.A., Myers, D.A. and Pyeritz, P.E. (1987). The Stickler syndrome: evidence for close linkage to the structural gene for type II collagen. *Genomics* **1**, 293

Glover, D.M. (1985–1987). In *DNA Cloning: A Practical Approach*, Vols I–III. IRL Press, Oxford

Goldstein, L.A., Zhou, D.F.H., Picker, J.L., Minty, C.N., Bargatze, R.F., Ding, J.F. and Butcher, E.C. (1989). A human lymphocyte homing receptor, the hermes antigen is released to cartilage proteoglycan core and link proteins. *Cell* **56**, 1063–1072

Gordon, M.K., Gerecke, D.R. and Olsen, B.R. (1987). Type XII collagen: distinct extracellular matrix component discovered by cDNA cloning. *Proc. Natl. Acad. Sci. USA* **84**, 6040–6044

Gordon, M.K., Gerecke, D.R., Dublet, B., van der Rest, M. and Olsen, B.R. (1989). Type XII collagen: a large multidomain molecule with partial homology with type IX collagen. *J. Biol. Chem.* **264**, 19 772–19 778

Graham, F.L. and Van Der Eb, A.J. (1973). A new technique for the assay of infectivity of human adenovirus 5 DNA. *Virology* **52**, 456–467

Hardingham, T.E. (1981). The role of link protein in the structure of cartilage proteoglycan aggregates. *Biochem. Soc. Trans.* **9**, 489–497

Hardingham, T.E., Beardmore-Gray, M., Dunham, D. and Ratcliffe, A. (1986). Cartilage proteoglycans. In *Functions of the Proteoglycans. Ciba Foundation Symposium* **124**, 30–46

Hogan, B. and Lyons, K. (1988). Gene targeting: getting nearer the mark (news and views). *Nature* **336**, 304–305

Horton, W., Miyashita, T., Kohno, K., Hassell, J.R. and Yamada, Y. (1987). Identification of a phenotype specific enhancer in the first intron of the rat collagen II gene. *Proc. Natl. Acad. Sci. USA* **84**, 8864–8868

Horton, W.E. Jr., Higginbotham, J.D. and Chandrasekhar, S. (1989). Transforming growth factor beta and fibroblast growth factor act synergistically to inhibit collagen II synthesis through a mechanism involving regulatory DNA sequences. *J. Cell. Physiol.* **141**, 8–15

Jaenisch, R. (1988). Transgenic animals. *Science* **240**, 1468–1474

Knowlton, R.G., Katzenstein, P.L., Moskowitz, R.W., Weaver, E.J., Malemud, Ch. J., Pathria, M.N., Jimenez, S.A. and Prockop, D.J. (1990). Demonstration of genetic linkage of the type II procollagen gene (COL2A1) to primary osteoarthritis associated with a mild chondrodysplasia. *New Engl. J. Med.* **322**, 526–530

Knowlton, R.G., Weaver, E.J., Struyk, A.F., Knobloch, W.H., King, R.A., Norris, K., Shambam, A., Uitto, J., Jimenez, S.A. and Prockop, D.J. (1989). Genetic linkage analysis of hereditary arthro-opthalmopathy (Stickler syndrome) and the type II procollagen gene. *Am. J. Human Genet.* **45**, 681–688

Kosher, R.A., Gay, S.W., Kamanitz, J.R., Kulyk, W.M., Rodgers, B.J., Sai, S., Tanaka, T. and Tanzer, M.L. (1986a). Cartilage proteoglycan core protein expression during limb cartilage differentiation. *Dev. Biol.* **118**, 112–117

Kosher, R.A., Kulyk, W.M. and Gay, S.W. (1986b). Collagen gene expression during limb cartilage differentiation. *J. Cell Biol.* **102**, 1151–1156

Krusius, T. and Ruoslahti, E. (1986). Primary structure of an extracellular matrix proteoglycan core protein deduced from cloned cDNA. *Proc. Natl. Acad. Sci. USA* **83**, 7683–7687

Kuettner, K.E., Eisenstein, R. and Sorgente, N. (1975). Lysozyme in calcifying tissues. *Clin. Orth. Rel. Res.* **112**, 316–333

Lasky, L.A., Singer, M.S., Yednock, T.A., Dowbenko, D., Fennie, C., Rodriguez, H., Nguyen, T., Stachel, S. and Rosen, S.D. (1989). Cloning of a lymphocyte homing receptor reveals a lectin domain. *Cell* **56**, 1045–1055

Lieberfarb, R.M., Hirose, T. and Holmes, L.B. (1979). The Wagner–Stickler syndrome — a genetic study. *Birth Defects* **15**, 145

Mankin, H.J., Dorfman, H., Lipiello, L. and Zarins, A. (1971). Biochemical and metabolic abnormalities in articular cartilage from osteoarthritic human hips. *J. Bone Joint Surg.* **53**, 523–537

Marcos, J.C., DeBenyacar, M.A., Garcia-Morteo, O., Malconado-Cocco, J.A., Morales, V.H. and Laguena, R.P. (1981). Idiopathic familial chondrocalcinosis due to apatite crystal deposition. *Am. J. Med.* **71**, 557

Marks, J.S., Stewart, I.M. and Hardinge, K. (1979). Primary osteoarthritis of the hip and Heberden's nodes. *Ann. Rheumat. Dis.* **38**, 107

Moskowitz, R.W. (1985). Clinical and laboratory findings in osteoarthritis. In *Arthritis and Allied Conditions* (D.J. McCarty, ed.), 10th edn, p. 1408. Lea and Febiger, Philadelphia

Moskowitz, R.W., Howell, D.S., Goldberg, V.C. and Mankin, H. (1984). *Osteoarthritis: Diagnosis and Management*, p. 585. W.B. Saunders, Philadelphia

Neame, P.J., Christner, J.E. and Baker, J.R. (1987). The link protein and proteoglycan amino-terminal globular domains have similar structures. *J. Biol. Chem.* **262**, 17 768–17 778

Oldberg, A., Antonsson, P. and Heinegard, D. (1987). The partial amino acid sequence of bovine cartilage proteoglycans, deduced from a cDNA clone, contains numerous Ser–Gly sequences arranged in homologous repeats. *Biochem. J.* **243**, 255–259

Paulsson, M., Morgelin, M., Wiedemann, H., Beardmore-Gray, M., Dunham, D., Hardingham, T.E., Heinegard, D., Timpl, R. and Engel, J. (1987). Extended and globular protein domains in cartilage proteoglycans. *Biochem. J.* **245**, 763–772

Pelotie, A., Vaisaneu, P., Ott, J., Ryhanen, L., Elima, K., Vikkula, M., Cheah, K., Vuorio, E. and Peltonen, L. (1989). Predisposition to familial osteoarthritis linked to type II collagen gene. *Lancet*, 924

Perin, J.P., Bonnet, F., Thurieau, D. and Jolles, P. (1987). Link protein interaction with hyaluronate and proteoglycans: characterization of two distinct domains in bovine cartilage link proteins. *J. Biol. Chem.* **262**, 13 269–13 272

Perkins, S.J., Nealis, A.S., Dudhia, J. and Hardingham, T.E. (1989). The immunoglobulin fold and tandem repeat structures in proteoglycan N-terminal domains and link protein. *J. Mol. Biol.* **206**, 737–753

Ratcliffe, A. and Hardingham, T.E. (1983). Cartilage proteoglycan binding and link protein:

radioimmunoassays and the detection of masked determinants in aggregates. *Biochem. J.* **213**, 371–378

Reginato, A.J. (1976). Articular chondrocalcinosis in the Chiloe Islanders. *Arth. Rheum.* **19**, 395

Rhodes, C., Doege, K., Sasaki, M. and Yamada, Y. (1988). Alternative splicing generates two different mRNA species for rat link protein. *J. Biol. Chem.* **263**, 6063–6067

Ryan, L.M. and McCarty, D.J. (1987). Calcium pyrophosphate crystal deposition disease: pseudo-gout; articular chondrocalcinosis. In *Arthritis and Allied Conditions* (D.J. McCarty, ed.), 10th edn, p. 1515. Lea and Febiger, Philadelphia

Sai, S., Tanaka, T., Kosher, R. and Tanzer, M. (1986). Cloning and sequence analysis of a partial cDNA for chicken cartilage proteoglycan core protein. *Proc. Natl. Acad. Sci. USA* **83**, 5081–5085

Saiki, R.K., Bugawau, T.L., Horn, G.T., Mullis, R.B. and Erlich, H.A. (1987). Analysis of enzymatically amplified beta-globulin and HLA-DQ alpha DNA with allele-specific oligonucleotide probes. *Nature* **324**, 163

Sangiorgi, F.O., Benson-Schanda, V., de Wet, W.J., Sobel, M.E., Tsipouras, P. and Ramirez, F. (1984). Isolation and partial characterization of the entire human proα1(II) collagen gene. *Nucleic Acid Res.* **13**, 1025–1038

Sokoloff, L. and Hough, A.J. (1987). Pathology of osteoarthritis. In *Arthritis and Allied Conditions* (D.J. McCarty, ed.), 10th edn, p. 1377. Lea and Febiger, Philadelphia

Spranger, J. (1975). The epiphyseal dysplasias. *Clin. Orthop. Rel. Res.* **114**, 46

Stecher, R.M., Hersh, A.H. and Hauser, H. (1953). The family history and radiographic appearance of large family. *Am. J. Hum. Genet.* **5**, 46

Stamenkovic, I., Amoit, M., Pesando, J.M. and Seed, B. (1989). A lymphocyte molecule implicated in lymph node homing is a member of the cartilage link protein family. *Cell* **56**, 1057–1062

Stickler, G.B., Belau, P.G., Farrell, F.J., Jones, J.D., Pugh, D.G., Steinberg, A.G. and Ward, L.E. (1965). Hereditary progressive arthro-ophthalmopathy. *Mayo Clin. Proc.* **40**, 433

Sugrue, S.P., Gordon, M.K., Seyer, J., Dublet, B., van der Rest, M. and Olsen, B.R. (1989). Immunoidentification of type XII collagen in embryonic tissues. *J. Cell Biol.* **109**, 939–945

Thompson, R.C., Jr. and Oegema, T.R., Jr. (1979). Metabolic activity of articular cartilage in osteoarthritis. *J. Bone Joint Surg.* **61**, 407–416

Thonar, E.J.M.A., Feist, S.B., Fassbender, K., Lenz, M.E., Matijevitch, B.L. and Kuettner, K.E. (1988). Quantification of hen egg white lysozyme in cartilage by an enzyme-linked immunosorbent assay. *Conn. Tissue Res.* **17**, 181–198

Toneguzzo, F., Hayday, A.C. and Keating, A. (1986). Electric field-mediated DNA transfer. Transient and stable gene expression in human and mouse lymphoid cells. *Mol. Cell. Biol.* **6**, 703–706

Väisänen, P., Elima, K., Palotie, A., Peltonen, L. and Vuorio, E. (1988). Polymorphic restriction sites of type II collagen gene: their location and frequencies in the Finnish population. *Human Hered* **38**, 65

van der Rest, M. and Mayne, R. (1988). Type IX collagen-proteoglycan from cartilage is covalently crosslinked to type II collagen. *J. Biol. Chem.* **263**, 1615–1618

Weaver, E.J. and Knowlton, R.G. (1989). A PvuII polymorphism near the 5' end of the type II procollagen gene [COL2A1]. *Nucleic Acid Res.* **17**, 6429

Westphal, H. (1989). Transgenic mammals and biotechnology. *J. FASEB* **3**, 117–120

Willard, H.F., Skolnick, M.H., Pearson, P.L. and Mandel, J.-L. (1985). Report on the Committee on Human Gene Mapping by Recombinant DNA Techniques. *Cytogenet. Cell. Genet.* **40**, 365

Williams, A.F. and Barclay, A.N. (1988). The immunoglobulin superfamily-domains for cells surface recognition. *Ann. Rev. Immunol.* **6**, 381–405

9

TISSUE COMPOSITION AND ORGANIZATION

COLLATED BY A. MAROUDAS

52

Introduction

A. MAROUDAS

It required only a moment to sever that head (Lavoisier's) and perhaps a century will not be sufficient to produce another like it. (J. Lagrange)

I would like to start this chapter by paying homage to Antoine Lavoisier who 'because of his systematic use of the balance must be regarded as the founder of methods of quantitative analysis' (*Encyclopædia Britannica*, 1971). It is no coincidence that Lavoisier, who introduced quantitative techniques into this hitherto mainly qualitative science, is considered by many to be the father of modern chemistry.

The use of more and more sophisticated methods of analysis to characterize a greater and greater variety of materials has been an essential accompaniment to all other developments in science and technology. The determination of chemical composition has now served for many decades to characterize such diverse materials as domestic fuels, pharmaceutical products, metals and their alloys, rocks, etc. It has been used as a tool for many purposes, from the wish to compare naturally occurring substances and predict their properties to the need for quality control of innumerable manufactured products.

The more complex the substance to be characterized, the more aspects must be considered in order to define adequately its composition. Thus, for a uniform, relatively simple product, such as natural gas, all that is required is a percentage composition in terms of the component gases. On the other hand, an alloy may consist of several phases and components and the chemical compounds themselves may exist under several forms and have different concentrations in the different phases. Sometimes, as in the case of semiconductor materials, it is the trace components, their exact proportions and distribution which determine the final properties.

As far as the application of quantitative analytical techniques to living materials is considered and the definition of their composition in quantitative terms, it is a relatively recent development since biology started out as a qualitative science, with the main stress on morphology: the most important tool initially was the microscope rather than the balance.

The problem of expressing in a meaningful manner the composition of a tissue is intimately linked to the knowledge of the tissue's organization and the latter is seldom known in full detail at present. The difficulty does not end there because, apart from topographical variations, both the composition and the organization of a living tissue may change with time and there is no constant basis to which everything could be referred. Moreover, water — a major constituent of all tissues — is not present in a fixed concentration; its quantity is determined by the particular condition of the tissue, which has to be clearly defined.

In the present section (Chapter 53) I discuss the different ways in which the concentrations of the cartilage constituents can be expressed, with special reference to the tissue's organization, functional properties and metabolism. The appropriateness of the methods of expressing concentrations will be examined in relation to the purpose intended.

The other chapters in the present section will describe different methods for studying the organization of tissues and for distinguishing between the roles of the different components.

Mike Bayliss (Chapter 54) discusses what type of analytical information is required in order to derive meaningful data concerning proteoglycan (PG) structure in cartilage and to determine how this structure varies e.g. with species, age, etc. In particular, he stresses the need to take into account the heterogeneity in size of the PG present as well as the possible existence in adult tissue of poorly glycosylated PG fragments. He also shows the importance of examining the stoichiometric relationships between the different constituents of the PG aggregate such as PG monomer, hyaluronan (HA), binding region and link-protein and he illustrates this with an example relating to the variations with age of the ratio of the binding region to link protein in human articular cartilage.

Frank Meyer (Chapter 55) describes various physicochemical methods for assessing the structure of connective tissues, both intact and after extraction of one or several of the tissue components. The methods he discusses are based on the determinations of excluded volumes of solutes of different size, on the assessment of the mobility of the hyaluronan molecules and on swelling pressure measurements. He used all these methods on a loose connective tissue, *viz.* Wharton's jelly, but similar procedures are applicable to cartilage. Frank Meyer compares the composition of Wharton's jelly with that of human articular cartilage and discusses the differences in some of the functional properties of these two tissues, resulting from the differences in composition. Meyer also mentions some differences in the procedures which have to be used for the two tissues connected with the respective differences in composition and organization.

Both Ellen Wachtel (Chapter 56) and Carmen Berthet-Colominas (Chapter 57) describe methods using low angle X-ray scattering for assessing some structural characteristics of articular cartilage.

Ellen Wachtel describes the use of low-angle X-ray scattering for assessing the mean lateral spacing between the collagen molecules in the different zones of articular cartilage—both native and PG-depleted, as a function of externally applied osmotic pressure. She relates the intercollagen distances to the quantity of intrafibrillar water.

Carmen Berthet-Colominas *et al.* make use of the low-angle X-ray scattering in a different way. They measure the overall projected electron densities in the matrix in a plane parallel to the preferred direction of the axis of collagen fibrils. The meridional X-ray pattern obtained is used by the authors to estimate the density of the 'gap' regions, both in native cartilage and disc and in PG-depleted tissues. Using certain assumptions, Carmen Berthet-Colominas *et al.* attempt to derive from their measurements information about the location of the PG in the matrix in relation to the collagen fibrils.

Robin Stockwell (Chapter 58) discusses various techniques for measuring cell density and cellular volumes in cartilage. He quotes useful figures and tells us how both cell density and cell volume vary, depending on the cartilage thickness and, therefore, on the size of the animal.

53

Different ways of expressing concentration of cartilage constituents with special reference to the tissue's organization and functional properties

A. MAROUDAS

CARTILAGE COMPOSITION ON A 'DRY' BASIS

By and large, particularly in the early years of cartilage research, the concentrations of collagen and glycosaminoglycan (GAG) (or, more recently, proteoglycan (PG)) have been expressed in terms of percentage of dry weight. However, since PG and collagen are the two major cartilage components, accounting for 90–95% of the dry weight (e.g. Maroudas et al., 1980), it is not possible to know, from changes in the percentage composition alone, e.g. with age (see Table 53.1) whether there has been an increase in one component or a decrease in the other: supplementary information is needed.

Tables 53.1 and 53.2 illustrate this point with regard to the variations in the composition of human femoral head cartilage with age. It should be noted in particular that, apart from the percentage composition of cartilage as a whole which changes with age, the composition of the PG itself changes; the protein:uronate ratio increasing from 1.53 in the 10- to 20-year-old age group to 4.9 in the 60- to 90-year-old age group (Bayliss and Venn, 1980; Maroudas et al., 1980). However, one notices (Table 53.1) that the ratio of collagen to chondroitin sulfate (CS) remains practically constant from the first age group to the last. If one assumes that the *absolute amounts* of collagen and CS also remain approximately constant from the youngest age groups onwards and if one calculates the composition of the tissue for, e.g. the oldest age group on that assumption (see Table 53.2), taking into account the increases in the keratan sulfate (KS) and noncollagenous protein (mainly that belonging to PG), one obtains a very similar percentage composition to that obtained experimentally (compare last row of Tables 53.1 and 53.2). It thus seems very likely that our assumption that the collagen content remains constant is correct and that the *decrease* in the concentration of collagen is simply due to the *increase* in the *total dry weight* of cartilage with age. The latter increase is primarily due to the rise in the KS and protein and reflects a change in the number and length of the PG subunits, as reported by Bayliss and Ali (1978) (see also Chapter 54).

Moreover, it should be noted that the increase in the absolute weight of dry tissue with age — assuming, as before, that the quantity of CS and collagen remain constant — is accompanied by a decrease in the water to dry weight ratio. The net result is that the total tissue volume remains substantially unchanged. This is entirely consistent with the independent observation, reported by a number of authors, that the thickness of *normal* cartilage does not vary with age (e.g. Venn, 1978; Roberts et al., 1986).

The above example brings out the point that it is not possible to draw conclusions about increases or decreases in the absolute quantities of a given single component (e.g. collagen) purely on the basis of changes in its percentage concentration. It

Table 53.1 Actual composition on a dry weight basis of human femoral head cartilage for different age groups*

Age range (years)	CS (%)	KS (%)	Protein: uronate ratio	PG protein (%)	Collagen (%)	Other proteins	Mineral (%)	H$_2$O: dry weight ratio	V_T/unit wt collagen[†]
10–20	11.40	5.70	1.53	5.5	73.5	1.0	2.0	3.0	5.0
20–40	10.8	6.2	2.38	8.9	68.3	3.9	2.0	2.7	4.95
40–60	10.1	7.6	4.25	14.6	60.0	5.3	2.0	2.47	5.23
60–90	8.7	10.0	4.9	15.0	55.6	8.0	2.5	2.28	5.28

* Calculated from data of Venn (1978), Bayliss and Ali (1978) and Maroudas et al. (1980).
[†] V_T, Total tissue volume, Maroudas et al. (1980).

Table 53.2 Predicted composition for the 60- to 90-year-old age group, on ther basis of changes in the proportions of certain components. Amounts of collagen and CS are assumed constant throughout the ageing process

	CS	KS	Protein: uronate ratio	PG protein	Collagen	Other proteins	Mineral	Total dry weight
Total weight*	11.4	13.1	4.9	19.2	73.5	10.2	3.2	131
% basis	8.7	10	4.9	14.6	56.1	7.7	1.9	100

* These values are calculated from data in Table 53.1.

is necessary to have detailed information about the other constituents and the overall changes in the volume of the tissue.

It should also be noted that, in view of the variability of the water content (see next section), if one wishes to make comparisons between the concentrations of a particular constituent at different ages or under different circumstances, one should refer the data to the total weight of the dry tissue or, better still, to the weight of collagen, which, according to present evidence, remains substantially constant throughout adult life.

CARTILAGE WATER

Variability in the water content

Although water is an essential and major component of cartilage, its quantity is not a constant for a given tissue but a variable depending on a number of conditions. The quantity of water is affected by the osmotic pressure of the PGs, the tension in the collagen network and the external load on the tissue. Water moves in and out of the tissue and between the different compartments within the tissue, depending on the prevailing pressure gradients. In spite of the above reservations, it is possible to refer to a *characteristic* water content of a cartilaginous tissue, provided its meaning is clearly defined.

Human joints, such as the mature hip or knee, are unloaded *in vivo* when the subject is in a position of rest: the water content of cartilage 'as excised' is consequently determined, at a given site and in a given zone, by purely local factors, i.e. the tensile properties of the collagen network and the PG content. In the above cases, moreover, the collagen network is so stiff that the cartilage has little tendency to swell even when it is separated from the underlying bone or when the osmotic pressure gradients between it and the equilibrating solution are significantly increased. Thus, the value of the water content determined after exposure of the tissue to solution is close to the value 'as excised' and close, therefore, to the value *in vivo* when the cartilage is in an unloaded state.

However, young bovine knee cartilage swells considerably as a result of excision and subsequent exposure to solution: thus its collagen architecture must be different from that in the human adult and its tensile stiffness must be more dependent on attachment to bone and to the remainder of the cartilage sheet.

Plugs of osteoarthritic human cartilage also swell upon excision, a phenomenon which has been attributed to damage in the collagen network and a consequent decrease in its inherent stiffness (Maroudas, 1976; Maroudas and Venn, 1977).

In neither of the latter two cases is the hydration of a cartilage plug, as determined after it had been in solution, a characteristic of the tissue as it was *in vivo*. It is therefore important in such cases to state very clearly whether one is referring to the water content of the tissue as excised or after exposure to normal saline, since the differences in value may be considerable.

In the intervertebral disc, particularly in the nucleus, the collagen network is loose and has little effect in controlling tissue swelling in the range of *in vivo* hydrations: in the absence of an external load, the tissue swells and swells. *In vivo*, the water content is determined only by the relative magnitudes of the osmotic pressure of the PG and the externally applied load. If one is referring to an inherent water content (i.e. 'as cut') as a characteristic of the tissue, one is assuming that the latter is always subject to the same load.

Not all human synovial joints appear to be entirely unloaded *in vivo*. Thus, unlike normal human adult hip cartilage, normal facet cartilage, whether on the joint or excised, imbibes fluid when exposed to saline solutions. It has been shown (Tobias *et al.*, 1990) that the only possible explanation for this behavior is that at least part of the facet joint must always exist *in vivo* in a loaded condition and hence be 'underhydrated'. In this case imbibition of fluid merely returns the tissue to an unloaded condition and is not to be equated with real 'swelling', as is the case for young bovine or human osteoarthritic cartilage.

The above examples show how the factors which determine the water content vary from tissue to tissue and how difficult it is to make generalizations.

Since all physiologically meaningful measurements have to be based on some parameter(s) relating to 'wet tissue' — be it whole tissue weight or volume or thickness, extrafibrillar or intrafibrillar water — it is essential to record in all experiments the water content under the given experimental conditions. Since, unfortunately, the latter water content rarely corresponds to that under the conditions *in vivo* in which we are interested, it is necessary to estimate the properties relevant to the *in vivo* situation by using appropriate conversion factors and formulae.

Changes in the water content lead to alterations in the effective concentrations of the various components, be these macromolecules, small solutes or cells. The changes in the concentrations of the various constituents, as well as in the tissue's volume and dimensions in turn bring about changes in a variety of physicochemical and biomechanical properties, such as osmotic pressure, exclusion volume, solute diffusivities, hydraulic permeability, compressive stiffness, etc. Each of these properties is affected in a different way by the changes in hydration and composition and, therefore, if a quantitative assessment is to be made, the hydration and the composition have to be expressed in an appropriate manner (see Table 53.6).

Cartilage volume — function of hydration

Changes in the overall water content obviously result in changes in the volume and dimensions of the tissue. Thus, tissue volume is given by the formula

$$V_T = V_{H_2O} + V_s \qquad (53.1)$$

where V_s is the volume of solids, V_{H_2O} is the volume of water, and V_T is the total tissue volume. Equation (53.1) was used, for instance, in order to calculate the values of total tissue volume per unit weight of collagen for different age groups (Table 53.1).

An example showing a comparison between normal and osteoarthritic cartilage (Table 53.3) illustrates the fact that what appears to be a relatively small change when the water content is expressed on a percentage basis is in fact a very significant change when the ratio of total tissue volume to dry weight is considered. Tissue dimensions are similarly affected. An important physiological consequence of this is that osteoarthritic (OA) cartilage can become considerably thicker, merely bcause of an increased hydration.

Changes in tissue volume directly affect other parameters, e.g. cell density (e.g. Holm *et al.*, 1981) or diffusion coefficients (e.g. Maroudas and Venn, 1977). These effects will be illustrated later in this section (see Table 53.5).

Changes in the total water content also bring about changes in the relative sizes of the different cartilage compartments, a topic which will be discussed in some detail in the sections which follow.

DIFFERENT CARTILAGE COMPARTMENTS

A schematic view of the matrix of a cartilaginous tissue is shown in Fig. 53.1: the PGs cannot penetrate into the collagen fibril because of their size. The matrix thus consists of two compartments: the space within the collagen fibrils, from which the PGs are excluded and the extrafibrillar space the properties of which are determined chiefly by the presence of the PGs. At physiological pH the intrafibrillar (IF) compartment has no effective charge whilst the extrafibrillar (EF) compartment has a high concentration of negatively charged groups.

It is clearly an oversimplification to consider the matrix as consisting of only two compartments. Other heterogeneities exist: thus there may be differences within the EF compartment with regard to the PG concentration, particularly in the neighborhood of the collagen fibrils. There are also likely to be inhomogeneities with regard to charge distribution within the PG domains themselves. In addition, there is a special milieu around the chondrocyte (see Chapter 21). As more details are learnt about the composition on the molecular scale, more microenvironments will have to be considered.

Extrafibrillar compartment

In order to characterize the extrafibrillar compartment, particularly in relation to its polyelectrolyte behavior, the concentration of the PGs and their fixed charge density must be expressed on the basis of the extrafibrillar water alone (this will be referred to as the 'effective

Table 53.3 Typical changes in water content and tissue volume in OA cartilage

Mean hydration measured after equilibration in saline	Cartilage		% change (increase) in OA over normal cartilage
	Normal	Osteoarthritic	
Hydration after saline (% of total weight)	70	79	13
Ratio of water weight: dry weight	2.33	3.76	61
Tissue volume per unit dry weight	3.0	4.4	47
FCD mEQ			
Per gm wet weight	0.16	0.08	
Per gm dry weight	0.53	0.38	

53. WAYS OF EXPRESSING CONCENTRATION OF CARTILAGE CONSTITUENTS

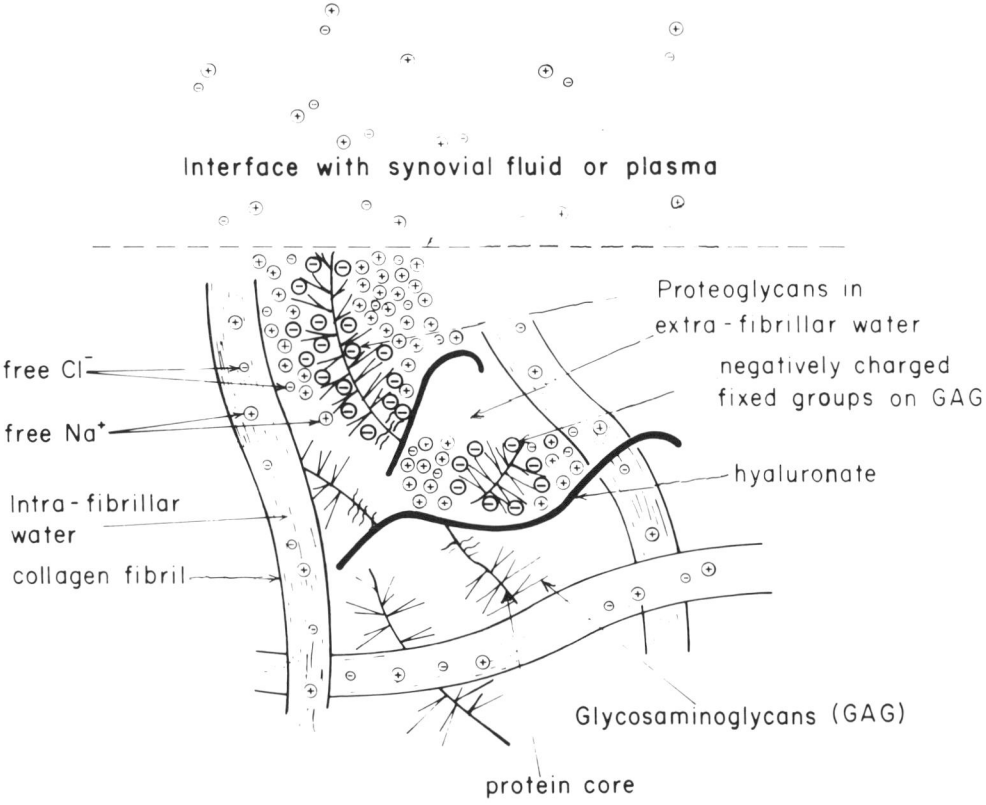

Figure 53.1 Schematic representation of cartilage matrix.

value') rather than on the total tissue water (often referred to as the 'overall value'). It should be noted that, if the concentration of the PG is based on total water in the tissue it will be underestimated, whilst if its effective value is used the properties of the matrix such as osmotic pressure can be deduced directly from the properties of solutions of isolated PG at the same concentration (use of this is illustrated in Chapter 68).

If one wishes to calculate the fraction of EF water corresponding to a given set of conditions, the fraction of IF water must be known. It has been shown recently (Katz et al., 1986; Maroudas et al., 1990) that the latter is not a constant, but itself varies as a function of the osmotic pressure gradient across the surface of the fibrils. The methods of measuring and calculating intrafibrillar water are described in the present volume, (see Chapters 56 and 69).

Table 53.4 shows the differences in the calculated values of a number of parameters when based on total as compared with EF water in uncompressed and compressed femoral head cartilage, respectively. The differences in osmotic pressure and calcium and sulfate partition coefficients are particularly significant. Under pressure, not only is the total hydration reduced, but the proportion of EF to IF water is also reduced, which results in even larger differences in the respective values of the different parameters.

With regard to fluid flow, it is necessary to know not only the relative size of the EF and IF compartments, but also the dimensions of the

Table 53.4 Examples of some calculated parameters: comparison between the values of fixed charge density (FCD), osmotic pressure, ionic partition coefficients and pH as calculated on the basis of total water content and extrafibrillar (EF) water in uncompressed cartilage and in cartilage subjected to a pressure of 7 atm

FCD (meq g^{-1})			H$_2$O per g dry wt		π (atm) based on		Ionic partition coefficient						pH based on	
							Na$^+$		Ca^{2+}		SO$_4^{2-}$		Total H$_2$O	EF H$_2$O
Per total tissue	Per total H$_2$O	Per EF H$_2$O	Total	EF	Total H$_2$O	H$_2$O EF	Per total H$_2$O	Per EF H$_2$O	Per total H$_2$O	Per EF H$_2$O	Per total H$_2$O	Per EF H$_2$O		
Uncompressed cartilage														
0.17	0.23	0.31	2.51	1.84	1.4	2.6	2.1	2.5	4.4	6.25	0.23	0.16	6.68	6.60
0.10	0.14	0.19	2.57	1.86	0.52	0.96	1.6	1.8	2.6	3.3	0.39	0.36	6.80	6.74
Cartilage subjected to a pressure of 7 atm; all values based on measured* H$_2$O														
0.17†	0.37	0.53	1.57	1.11	3.6	7.5	3.17	4.0	10.0	16.0	0.10	0.062	6.50	6.48
0.10†	0.315	0.53	1.11	0.66	2.6	7.5	2.83	4.0	6.7	16.0	0.15	0.062	6.55	6.48

The ionic partition coefficients were calculated from FCD values using the ideal Donnan equations.
* Grushko *et al.* (1989).
† Values in uncompressed state.

component networks. Thus, the extrafibrillar compartment can be pictured as a random assembly of very fine rods (GAG and protein core) — diameter of the order of 5 Å — in which are embedded the very much thicker rods, namely the collagen fibrils (500–1000 Å). Except when the PG concentration is very low, the main resistance to flow is offered by the 'thin' rods, the collagen fibrils acting more or less as a 'dead' volume. The actual flow of fluid and diffusion of solutes takes place through passages between the 'thin' rods. These passages or 'pores' are approximately 2–3 nm in radius (as determined by several methods — see Maroudas (1979) and Byers *et al.* (1983), though some pores are larger than 3 nm, admitting a small fraction of molecules of the size of serum albumin.

It should not be forgotten that fluid exchange does take place between the extrafibrillar and the intrafibrillar compartments and that there is also fluid flow through the intrafibrillar compartment in parallel with that through the extrafibrillar space, though at a very much lower rate (Maroudas *et al.*, 1986; Benaim, 1989; Benaim *et al.*, 1990).

Intrafibrillar compartment

The intrafibrillar compartment contains a small quantity of 'bound' water, the rest consisting of free water the quantity of which is controlled partly by the intermolecular repulsion forces, the precise nature of which is at present not clear, and partly by the osmotic pressure gradients between the outside and the inside of the fibril.

The IF compartment is uncharged at neutral pH. It is possible to investigate the concentrations of various solutes in it by using cartilage from which all PGs have been enzymatically removed (Chun *et al.*, 1986). In such cartilage, the extrafibrillar space is uncharged and can be assumed to have the same properties as the equilibrating solution; thus, any difference between the concentration of a solute in PG-free cartilage as a whole and its concentration in the outside solution is due to the difference existing in the intrafibrillar compartment. It has been found that, whilst the intrafibrillar water is unselective toward monovalent ions such as Na$^+$ and Cl$^-$ (the latter are present in the same concentration as in the solution in which the tissue is equilibrated), Ca^{2+} is present at a much higher concentration in the IF compartment than in the equilibrating solution (partition coefficient approximately 5) (Weinberg and Maroudas, in prep.).

Large solutes such as serum albumin do not penetrate into the intrafibrillar compartment at all and this fact forms the basis of one of the methods for determining the fractional volume of the IF (see Chapter 69; see also Maroudas and Bannon (1981), Weinberg *et al.* (1987) and Maroudas *et al.* (1990)).

Cellular compartment

In adult tissues, particularly in the human, the proportion of the total volume occupied by the cells is very low — around 1% (see Chapter 57). Hence, in the present chapter, which deals chiefly with human cartilage, the error introduced in neglecting cell volume when discussing the composition of the tissue is very small. This may not be so, however, when discussing mouse cartilage which has a cell density of 10–12%.

Cells possess their own mechanisms (ion 'pumps') for maintaining intracellular homeostasis. However, it is obvious that, in the case of the chondrocyte which is surrounded by an environment of high and variable negative fixed charge density, the internal processes and their control mechanisms must be influenced by this very special extracellular environment (see Chapters 30, 31 and 63; see also Schneiderman *et al.* (1986), Gray *et al.* (1988), and Urban and Bayliss (1989)).

The activity of the chondrocytes, e.g. with respect to GAG or protein synthesis, oxygen or glucose consumption or lactic acid production, can be expressed in a number of ways and, again the question arises as to which way is the most appropriate for a particular purpose.

Clearly, one obvious way is to express cellular activity *per cell*, either by determining the amount of DNA or by doing a cell 'count' in the same volume and under the same conditions as those used to estimate the given activity. This will enable one to compare directly the actual activity of the chondrocyte under different circumstances or in different tissues.

In addition to variations in metabolic activities per cell, there are also variations in *cell density*, either intrinsic (e.g. relating to cartilage thickness, see Chapter 16; see also Stockwell (1979)), or accompanying cartilage degeneration. Thus, apart from knowing the activity per chondrocyte, one also needs to find out under a given set of conditions, the number of chondrocytes per unit tissue volume and use both pieces of information to assess the overall cellular activity per unit volume. The knowledge of the latter parameter is necessary for comparative purposes, e.g. with regard to ageing; it is also needed for assessing the balance between cellular requirements and nutrient transport and for computing the concentrations of various metabolites within the tissue matrix. In this connection, one again has to make sure that the volume and thickness of the test specimen is determined under the same conditions as the metabolic rate one is investigating.

Solute concentration profile in the matrix as a function of hydration

One may be interested in assessing both cellular activity and metabolite transport under circumstances *different* from those in the actual experiment. In such a case, calculations based on volume and thickness changes must be carried out.

Let us examine the variation in the concentration profile of a metabolite with the water content of the tissue. As an illustrative example, we shall use a simplified form of the diffusion equation, balancing the rate of diffusion and the rate of consumption of a solute at the plane furthest removed from the source of supply of the solute (i.e. at the midplane in the case of an excised cylindrical plug). The following equation is used (Crank and Park, 1968).

$$\bar{C} = \bar{C}_o - \frac{Ql^2}{8\bar{D}} \qquad (53.2)$$

where l is the cartilage thickness (assumed proportional to volume V), Q is the rate of solute consumption (assumed proportional to cell density), $\bar{D}$ is the diffusion coefficient in the tissue, $\bar{C}_o$ is the solute concentration at the tissue interface with the surrounding medium, and $\bar{C}_o = KC_o$

where K is the solute partition coefficient and C_0 is the solute concentration in solution. $\bar{C}$ is the solute concentration at center of tissue, i.e. $x = l/2$.

If the water content changes, all the parameters in equation (53.2) change in value and the resulting concentration profiles of the metabolites must change accordingly. Table 53.5 lists the formulae used for computing the changes in Q, t and $\bar{D}$ resulting from such changes in water content. An illustrative example is also given in which a decrease in the water content of 50% is assumed.

The actual changes in the concentration profile with hydration will be relatively small, in spite of the relatively large changes in the parameters l, Q and D accompanying loss of water (see Table 53.5) because the decrease in the diffusion coefficient and increase in cell density are compensated for by the decrease in thickness, the latter appearing as a squared term in equation (53.2). The value of K, and hence C_0, depends on the type of solute. For some solutes, e.g. ions (particularly multivalent ions) as well as for larger molecular species, the effect of reduced hydration on K can be dramatic (see Table 53.4 and Chapter 59, see also Schneiderman *et al.* (1986) and Schneiderman (1988).

In the above examples, it was assumed that the intrinsic cellular activity does not alter with hydration and that all effective changes are due to changes in cell density and other tissue parameters as a function of altered composition. However, this is not necessarily so: we know that in many circumstances cellular activity is influenced by the actual changes in the cellular environment; this cannot be predicted at present. However, it can be investigated by creating for the cells *in vitro* the particular environment in the influence of which we are interested (Schneiderman *et al.* (1986); Bayliss *et al.*, 1987; Gray *et al.*, 1988; Urban and Bayliss, 1989).

SUMMARY

Table 53.6 gives a number of examples of how cartilage composition affects the different characteristics of cartilage. It also shows how the concentration should be expressed in different cases under consideration.

In conclusion, as our knowledge advances with regard to both the organization of cartilaginous tissues, as well as to the nature and role of the individual components, it becomes possible to express the concentration of the latter in a more precise and more meaningful manner. In this chapter, we have tried to describe how this can be achieved. In particular, we have shown how the

Table 53.5 Changes in Q, V, l and D as a result of a 50% decrease in cartilage hydration

Ratio of compressed to uncompressed	$\dfrac{V_1}{V_0}$	$\dfrac{l_1}{l_0}$	$\dfrac{Q_1}{Q_0}$	$\dfrac{D_1}{D_0}$
Formula for conversion	$\dfrac{V_1}{V_0} = \dfrac{(V_{H_2O})_1 + V_{s1}}{(V_{H_2O})_0 + V_{s0}}$	$\dfrac{l_1}{l_0} = \dfrac{V_1}{V_0}$	$\dfrac{Q_1}{Q_0} = \dfrac{V_0}{V_1}$	$\dfrac{D_1^*}{D_0} = \left[\dfrac{1 + V_{s0}}{1 + V_{s1}}\right]^2 \left[\dfrac{1 - V_{s0}}{1 - V_{s1}}\right]^{-2}$
Result	0.61	0.61	1.65	0.53

V_s, volume of solids; V_{H_2O}, volume of water; V, total tissue volume. Subscripts 0 and 1 correspond respectively to the initial and altered state ('swollen' or 'compressed').
* Formula due to Mackie and Meares (1955).

variations both in water content and in 'dry' constituents have to be taken into account when one is studying a range of physiological properties and how the manner of expressing composition depends on the purpose for which the information is required.

Table 53.6 Examples of compositional data needed and the manner in which they should be expressed in relation to the calculation of some physiological parameters

Parameters to be calculated and/or compared	Data needed for calculation
Quantity of a given 'dry' constituent; comparison of changes, e.g. with age	Overall composition data based on dry weight
Relative volumes of solids and fluid in cartilage; total tissue volume	Quantities and densities of dry tissue components and quantity of fluid
Cell density (volumetric)	DNA concentration or cell count per unit tissue volume
Metabolic activity per cell	Metabolic activity per amount DNA or per cell number
Metabolic activity per unit volume	Metabolic activity per cell and number of cells per unit volume
Effective GAG concentration and FCD (i.e. in EF compartment)	GAG concentration and FCD based on total tissue water; size of EF compartment relative to total tissue water
Osmotic pressure	Effective FCD and formula for calculating the osmotic pressure of isolated PG solutions*
'Exclusion' volumes† in EF and IF compartments	Experimental measurement of partition coefficients or use of formulae* and data regarding (i) concentration of polymer 'rods' and (ii) their diameters, in both compartments
Overall molal solute concentration in tissue	Concentration in outside solution and partition coefficient based on total tissue water
Solute concentration in EF and IF tissue compartments	(i) Solute-concentration in external medium; (ii) partition coefficient based on total water; (iii) relative volumes of EF and IF water; (iv) partitioning of solute between EF and IF water
pH in EF compartment	External pH and experimental partition coefficient of H^+ (or calculated K_H based on effective FCD)
Solute diffusivity‡	Solute diffusivity in aqueous solution and respective volumes of solids and fluid per unit total tissue volume; in the case of larger solutes, excluded from IF compartment, relative size of latter
Hydraulic permeability§	Relative sizes of EF and IF compartments; concentrations and diameters of polymer rods in both compartments

* See this volume, Chapter 69, contribution by Maroudas and Grushko.
† See this volume, Chapter 64, contribution by Silberberg.
‡ See Table 53.5.
§ See this volume, Chapter 64 and Chapter 68, contribution by Mizrahi et al.

54

Age-related changes in the stoichiometry of human articular cartilage proteoglycan aggregates

M.T. BAYLISS

Of the many factors that influence the composition and extracellular organization of articular cartilage, age is the one that has the most profound effect. Although similar age-related changes have been observed in the articular cartilage of all species that have been studied, the extent to which they occur varies considerably. This is not necessarily a problem when studies are confined to the same animal, but difficulties in interpretation can arise if data from different species are compared.

This dilemma is particularly apparent when considering the complex macromolecular structure formed by aggregating proteoglycans (PGs). The generally accepted model that is used to interpret the aggregation properties and structural heterogeneity of PG monomers has been largely derived from studies of purified, reconstituted PG isolated from immature animal cartilage. Although this relatively simple model is sufficient to explain the changes in composition that occur within the lifespan of most laboratory animals, analysis of ageing in human cartilage illustrates how extreme changes in composition, stoichiometry and stability of PG aggregates can alter our perception of PG organization.

A consistent finding of all studies of ageing, regardless of the source of articular cartilage, is an increase in the content of keratan sulfate (KS); this is usually identified as an increasing molar ratio of GluN : GalN (Fig. 54.1) (Bayliss and Ali, 1978; Roughley and White, 1980). Working on the

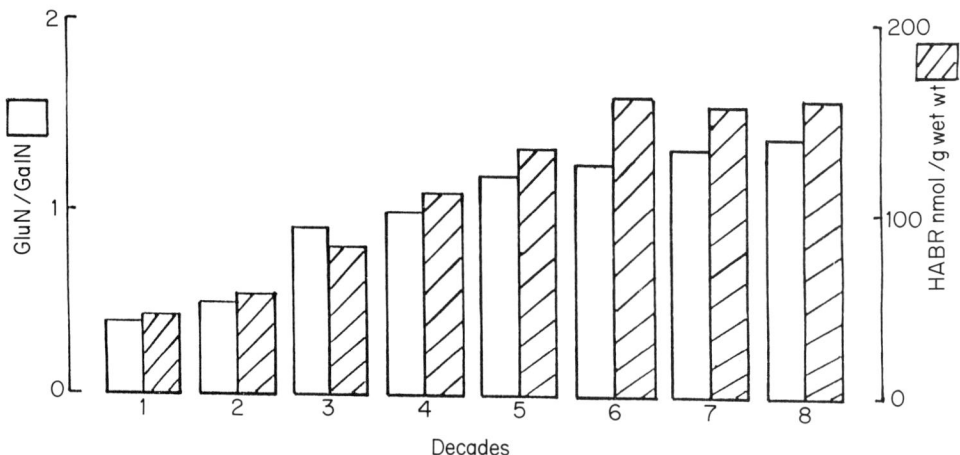

Figure 54.1 Age-related changes in the molar ratio of KS: chondroitin sulfate (GluN/GalN) and the concentration of binding region (HABR) in human articular cartilage.

assumption that all PG monomers have a common region, incorporating the hyaluronan (HA) binding region and the majority of the KS chains, the changes in composition are interpreted as reflecting: (i) an increase in the molar concentration of monomers; and (ii) a decrease in their molecular weight. Indeed, direct analysis of human cartilage extracts for their content of binding region and chromatographic analysis of PG hydrodynamic size, supports both these conclusions (Figs. 54.1 and 54.2) (Bayliss et al., 1984, 1989). However, further consideration of these elution profiles (Fig. 54.2) illustrates how information concerning PG structure, that could potentially be derived from a knowledge of tissue composition, may be severely restricted if traditional methods of analysis are adhered to rigidly. Uronic acid is most often used to monitor column fractions for PG distribution and it can be seen that the age-related decrease in PG molecular weight that was predicted, is observed. Furthermore, an increased polydispersity and heterogeneity in hydrodynamic size is also observed, to the extent that a shoulder appears on the uronic acid profile of adult cartilage extracts. This population of low-molecular-weight PG monomer, has a high KS content (Bayliss et al., 1984) and probably accounts for a large part of the age-related increase in binding region. However, further analysis of the column fractions for binding region content (by radioimmunoassay), shows that the highest concentration does not correspond with either of the uronic acid maxima, but elutes close to the V_t of the column and that adult cartilage is enriched in this component. Consequently, a significant proportion of the binding region in adult human articular cartilage is present in a poorly glycosylated form that probably represents fragments of PG that remain attached to HA after the chondroitin sulfate rich portion of the monomer is released during the process of normal turnover (Roughly et al., 1984; Bayliss and Roughley, 1985). This high concentration of 'free' binding region must influence the packing of PG monomers on the HA chains which may, in turn, modify the local distribution of negatively charged fixed groups and the hydraulic permeability (pore size) of the extracellular matrix.

Aggregation of PGs is an effective way of immobilizing these macromolecules within the extracellular matrix. The PGs are thus able to impart special polyelectrolyte properties on the matrix. For an acellular tissue, such as articular cartilage, this is a fundamental mechanism in the overall process of homeostasis. The stoichiometric relationship of PG monomer, HA and link protein, and the crucial role of the latter in stabilizing the complex that they form, is well known. This interrelationship also means that additional age-related changes in cartilage composition are mandatory if all of the binding region is to be link-stabilized on HA. For example, Holmes et al. (1988) recently confirmed that the

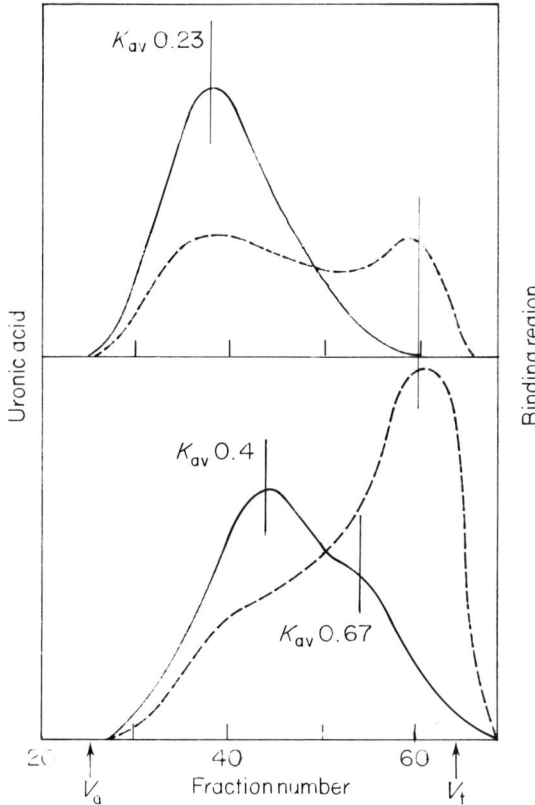

Figure 54.2 Gel chromatography n Sepharose CL-2B of extracts of normal human articular cartilage. The column was eluted under dissociative conditions with 2 M guanidine HCl. (———) Uronic acid; (----) Binding region. (a) 9 years; (b) 76 years.

HA content of human articular cartilage also increases with age and that there is always sufficient to accommodate all of the binding region. However, it is worth stressing that we are probably wrong in assuming that all the binding region, whether monomer or 'free', is bound to HA in articular cartilage. Furthermore, calculations of this kind do not take into account differences in size, and thus steric hindrance, of PG monomers which would undoubtedly influence their assembly on the HA chain. Moreover, our preliminary evidence also suggests that a considerable proportion of the HA is not substituted by PG. Using biotinylated-binding region as a probe, unsubstituted regions of HA were demonstrated in histological sections of cartilage at all ages.

Application of stoichiometric analysis to link protein in extracts of human cartilage has also provided intriguing data. Unlike chondrocyte cultures where newly synthesized components are actively assembled into an extracellular matrix and the binding region and link protein are present in a 1 : 1 molar ratio, in tissue extracts binding region is always in excess of link protein. Even in the youngest specimen investigated (2–5 years) the ratio was 1.5–2.0 to 1 and this increased during maturation to a value of 3.0–4.0 to 1 (Bayliss et al., 1989). These calculations imply that there may be a degree of structural 'instability' in normal human cartilage and that there may be various pools of monomer, binding region, link protein and HA in different stages of extracellular organization. We have recently investigated this hypothesis by sequentially extracting cartilage with buffers of increasing dissociating power. This approach has enabled us to identify age-related changes in the extractability and thus stability of all components of the PG aggregate (Bayliss et al., 1989).

55

The use of enzyme-modified tissues to study selected aspects of tissue structure and function

F.A. MEYER

INTRODUCTION

Enzymatic modification of tissues can be used to assess the contribution of matrix components to selected aspects of a tissue's structure and function (e.g. De Gennes, 1971; Klein and Meyer, 1983; Meyer, 1983; Meyer, 1986). Our particular studies were performed on a relatively simple connective-tissue structure, that of Wharton's jelly of umbilical cord but similar methods are being applied to cartilage (Chun et al., 1986; Maroudas and Bannon, 1981) (see also Chapter 69). Its extracellular matrix, like that of cartilage, is based on a collagen fiber network within which glycosaminoglycans (GAGs) are held (Table 55.1). The relative amounts of the structural macromolecules, however, differ considerably from those in cartilage, and hyaluronan (HA) of high molecular weight rather than sulfated GAGs is the main GAG present. Unlike in cartilage, a minor independent network of glycoprotein

Table 55.1 Compositional data of Wharton's jelly in comparison with femoral head cartilage

Component	% Wet Weight		
	Wharton's jelly	Cartilage	Ref.*
Collagen fibrils	3.6	15–20	1–4
Glycoprotein microfibrils	0.3	—	1, 2
Hyaluronan	0.31	0.03–0.3	1, 2, 9
Sulfated GAGs	0.14	3–6	1–5
Serum proteins	1.2	2×10^{-3}–2×10^{-2}	5, 6
Cellular phase	5†	1†	2, 7
Intrafibrillar water	4.5	20	2, 8
Extrafibrillar water	86.2	55	2, 8
Total water	90.7	65–75	1, 3

* (1) Meyer et al. (1983); (2) Meyer (1983); (3) Bayliss and Venn (1980); (4) Byers et al. (1983); (5) Klein and Meyer (1983); (6) Snowden and Maroudas (1976); (7) Chapter 57; (8) Chapter 53; (9) Holmes et al. (1988).
† % by volume.

microfibrils enmeshed with the collagen fiber network is also present.

ENZYMIC MODIFICATION OF TISSUE

The action of enzymes on tissue slices was monitored by chemical analyses and electron microscopy (Meyer et al., 1983). Treatment with testicular hyaluronidase resulted in the removal of all GAGs while treatment with proteases caused the removal of sulfated GAGs only and the microfibrils. Based on these findings, the following tissue structural variants were produced: (i) intact fibrillar network minus the GAGs (hyaluronidase treatment); (ii) intact collagen fiber network (hyaluronidase followed by protease treatment); and (iii) intact collagen network with hyaluronan (protease treatment).

THE ROLE OF MATRIX COMPONENTS IN DETERMINING TISSUE PORE SIZE AND PENETRABILITY TO GLOBULAR PROTEINS (EXCLUSION BEHAVIOR)

The organization of matrix components in the tissue results in the creation of free spaces of varying sizes which can be occupied by globular proteins depending on their size. As protein size increases, less tissue space is available and there is a progressive exclusion from the tissue with molecular size. Complete exclusion occurs when the molecular size is larger than the limiting pore size of the tissue (Meyer, 1983).

The exclusion behaviors of intact and GAG-free tissues were compared (Fig. 55.1). The solid curves show the exclusion predicted by theory based on the composition of the tissues and the molecular characteristics of the matrix components. The calculation is based on a cylinder/sphere steric exclusion model (Ogston, 1958) which is discussed in detail by Silberberg (Chapter 64). In the case of Wharton's jelly, the above model has been used to describe the interaction between the individual matrix components and globular proteins. It should be noted that we have assumed the GAGs to be confined to the extrafibrillar, extracellular tissue space whose relative size is given in Table 55.1. Good agreement is seen between the experimental data and the predicted curves. Both the GAGs and the fibrillar structures are seen to influence exclusion. The former becomes an increasingly important factor as molecular size increases and is the determining factor as far as the exclusion limit

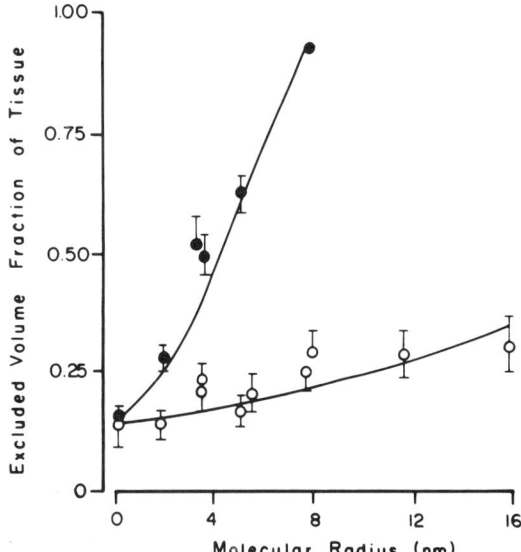

Figure 55.1 Excluded volume fraction for spherical molecules of varying radii in intact tissue (●) and tissue treated with testicular hyaluronidase (○). Equilibration was with sorbitol, myoglobin, albumin, transferrin, catalase and thyroglobulin of hydrodynamic radii (in nm) of 0.36, 1.98, 3.55, 3.82, 5.20 and 8.17, respectively. For hyaluronidase-treated tissue, equilibration was also performed with dextran fractions of radii 5.5, 8.0, 11.7 and 16.0 nm. The solid lines represent the calculated exclusion based on a cylinder/sphere geometric model where the available volume fraction in a network of fibrils, is given by $\exp[-\pi L (r_s + r_f)2]$, where L is the fibril length per unit volume and r_s and r_f are the radii of the sphere and fibril, respectively.

for globular proteins is concerned: this limit is 18 nm diameter. Extrapolation of theoretical curves for enzyme-modified tissue indicates approximate pore sizes of 180 nm and 110 nm for the collagen fibril network and the combined fibrillar network of collagen and glycoprotein microfibrils, respectively.

RELATIONSHIP OF HYALURONAN MOBILITY IN TISSUE TO FIBRILLAR NETWORK PORE SIZE

The role of the collagen fiber network in immobilizing HA was determined by comparing the rate of HA efflux from the collagen network (protease-treated tissue) with that of intact tissue (Klein and Meyer, 1983). Efflux was monitored with time from unswollen thin cylindrical tissue slices held in a stirred buffer solution at 4°C. The rate of efflux obeyed Fickian diffusion kinetics, allowing diffusion coefficients to be calculated (see Chapter 59). The diffusion coefficient for HA translation through the collagen network was 9% of that for unrestricted HA diffusion in free solution, whereas that through intact tissue was lower (1.3%). These results indicate that HA is not completely immobilized in tissue but that its mobility is restricted in part by the collagen network, as well as by other factors.

A theoretical calculation based on the estimated pore size of the collagen network (180 nm) and the molecular weight (15×10^6) and persistence length (5 nm) of the HA molecule is consistent with the translational movement of HA through the collagen network, involving reptational motion, whereby the flexible HA molecular chain threads its way through the pores of the collagen network (De Gennes, 1971; see also Chapter 64).

In the intact tissue, the presence of the glycoprotein microfibril network, in addition to the collagen fibril network, results in a lowering of pore size (110 nm) through which HA diffuses. This would predict a four-fold lowering of the diffusion coefficient relative to that for motion through the collagen network, rather than the seven-fold reduction found experimentally for intact tissue. The latter result would be in better agreement with theory if HA were associated with sulfated GAGs (in proteoglycan (PG) form) as occurs in cartilage. Such PG appendages attached to the HA chain would further impede the reptational movement of HA through the fibrillar networks. The existence of aggregates in Wharton's jelly has not yet been investigated. However, in preliminary experiments with intact tissue, we have found that the rate of PG efflux is compatible with that of HA, suggesting an association between these entities. The above deductions illustrate the way in which one can use transport through tissues in order to study their structure (see Chapters 59 and 64).

MATRIX COMPONENTS AND TISSUE SWELLING PRESSURE

The contribution of GAGs, collagen and microfibrils to tissue swelling pressure was determined using intact and modified tissues (Meyer, 1983). To eliminate any contribution of serum proteins present in tissue, tissue samples were first placed in buffer to allow proteins to diffuse out. Subsequently, tissues were allowed to swell or deswell to equilibrium against an external osmotically active solution. In the case of Wharton's jelly, the tissue-swelling pressure lies in a range which makes it possible to use dilute solutions of HA of high molecular weight as calibrants. Such solutions are convenient to use and their osmotic pressure is known (Silpanta *et al.*, 1968). Although tissue was in direct contact with HA solutions, HA entry from the external solution into tissue did not occur over the time-scale for solvent equilibration. For modified tissues from which GAGs had been removed, some entry of HA was indicated by a superimposed swelling phase. To correct for this the swelling phase was subtracted from the data.

It should be noted that, in contrast to Wharton's jelly, cartilaginous tissues have a much higher osmotic pressure and HA solutions sufficiently dilute to be handled would not be of equivalent osmotic pressure. Therefore, in the case of cartilage, polyethylene glycol (PEG) solutions were employed. However, since PEG is a smaller molecule than HA, its diffusion into the tissue is more rapid and cartilage cannot be placed in direct contact with it (see Chapter 69).

In Fig. 55.2 the swelling pressure of Wharton's jelly as a function of hydration is compared with the osmotic pressure estimated for the GAGs in the extrafibrillar, extracellular tissue space. The osmotic pressure curve was derived using data indicating that the 70% HA/30% sulfated GAG mixture in tissue has osmotic properties similar to those of a solution of pure HA at a concentration 1.26 times higher than that of the total uronic acid present in the extrafibrillar, extracellular space

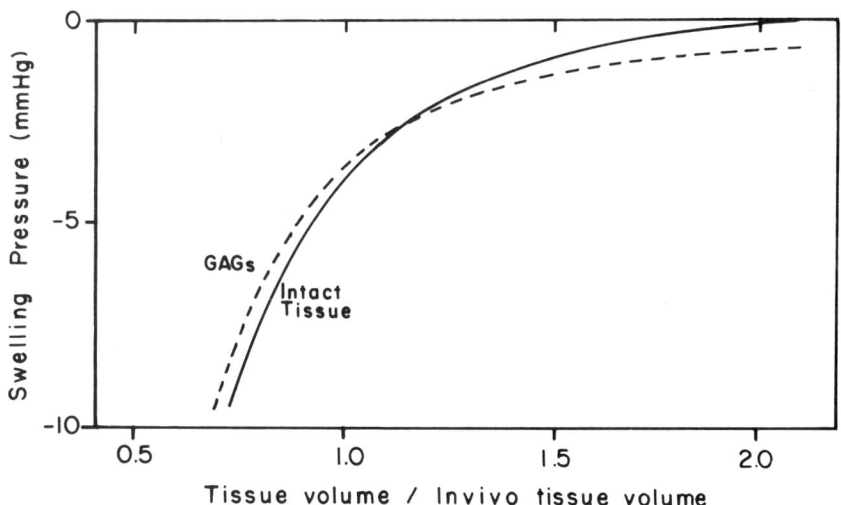

Figure 55.2 Comparison of the swelling pressure of intact tissue with the osmotic pressure calculated for the tissue GAGs, as a function of tissue hydration. The osmotic pressure of the GAGs was determined from their concentration in the extrafibrillar, extracellular tissue space as a function of hydration. Changes in intrafibrillar water content with hydration were not taken into account: in this tissue this effect would not be significant because of the relatively small amount of intrafibrillar water (Table 55.1) and the low osmotic pressure of the tissue GAGs.

(Meyer, 1983). This finding is consistent with there being more charged groups on the sulfated GAGs (per disaccharide) than on HA and made it possible to calculate the osmotic pressure of the GAGs as a function of hydration level using the Silpananta et al. (1968) equation. The results shown in Fig. 55.2 show that the swelling pressure of tissue over much of the hydration range is given mainly by the osmotic pressure of the GAGs. At the point where the curves cross over, which is close to the in vivo tissue volume, the swelling pressure is entirely due to the GAGs. At this tissue volume, therefore, the combined fibrillar network of collagen and glycoprotein microfibrils is in an unstressed configuration (zero net pressure) with no tendency to expand or contract. This observation has been confirmed by swelling measurements on modified tissue (Meyer, 1983). These results suggest a role for the fiber networks in determining tissue shape and volume and for the GAGs in pressurizing this structure to withstand the pressures imposed on it in vivo.

At lower and higher hydration levels the combined fibrillar network contracts and expands, respectively. As a consequence, stresses develop which begin to contribute to tissue-swelling pressure. This leads to a curve for tissue-swelling pressure that deviates from that for the osmotic pressure of the GAGs (Fig. 55.2). The cross-over between the two curves indicates that the stresses developed in the network change direction in going from contraction to expansion and, therefore, always act to return the network to the unstressed configuration close to the in vivo volume of tissue. The stresses developed in the fibrillar networks have been independently determined by swelling-pressure measurements on modified tissues and are found to accord well with the deviations seen between the two curves in Fig. 55.2.

COMPARISON OF THE PROPERTIES OF WHARTON'S JELLY WITH CARTILAGE

Despite marked differences between the tissue properties of Wharton's jelly and cartilage, it is apparent that these differences can be understood in terms of the concentrations and physicochemical properties of their constituent structural macromolecules, especially the GAG components. Relative to cartilage, Wharton's jelly has a lower GAG concentration (and hence fixed charge density) and swelling pressure and a larger pore size, partition coefficient and diffusion rate for globular proteins (Table 55.2). Although the GAG concentration in Wharton's jelly and cartilage differs by approximately one order of magnitude, this leads to much larger differences (two to three orders of magnitude) in swelling pressure and partition coefficients, since square or exponential dependences on GAG concentration are involved. The finding that the fibrillar components may make a contribution in Wharton's jelly (e.g. in protein partitioning) is

Table 55.2 Comparison between Wharton's jelly and cartilage (femoral head) with respect to some structural and transport properties

	Wharton's jelly	Cartilage	Ref.*
Collagen fibril diameter (nm)	3.9	40–100	1, 4
Fixed charge density (M)	0.019	0.2–0.3	1, 2
Swelling pressure	4 mmHg	1–3 atm	1, 2
Pore size (nm)	18	2–6	1, 3
Albumin partition coefficient	0.5	10^{-3}–10^{-2}	1, 4
Albumin diffusion (tissue/free diffusion)	0.7	0.3	5, 6

* (1) Meyer (1983); (2) Grushko et al. (1989); (3) Byers et al. (1983); (4) Snowden and Maroudas (1976); (5) Klein and Meyer (1983); (6) Maroudas (1979).

consistent with the fibers being thinner and present at a higher fiber/GAG ratio as compared with cartilage. Why Wharton's jelly and cartilage are based on different GAG types (mainly HA and PG, respectively) is not apparent from a physicochemical standpoint. It would seem more likely, therefore, that this difference is related to the specific biological properties of HA and PG.

56

Characterization of the packing of collagen in cartilage using X-ray scattering

E. WACHTEL and A. MAROUDAS

INTRODUCTION

Low angle X-ray scattering probes the packing of collagen molecules in cartilage in a nondestructive manner. The method is based on the fact that oriented collagen molecules have characteristic X-ray scattering profiles. During the course of an experiment, the cartilage specimen can be subjected to variations in pH or ionic strength of the surrounding medium, in hydration or in externally applied pressure, and the resulting structural changes determined. Electronic detection techniques permit relatively rapid measurement of the scattering, thereby minimizing problems of specimen lability. The information which may be obtained from such experiments include collagen morphology, degree of packing order and mean intercollagen distances. From the values obtained for the intermolecular distances, the volume of water-filled spaces within the collagen fibril and the spatial dependence of the forces acting between collagen molecules in water may, in principle, be determined. Here we briefly outline the relevant experimental techniques: specimen preparation, scattering measurements and data analysis.

SPECIMEN PREPARATION

Adult human femoral heads, obtained postmortem or at operation for femoral head fracture, are used for X-ray scattering experiments. Bovine specimens consist of patella groove or femoral chondyle cartilage from two- to three-year-old steers. The cartilage should have a completely intact and smooth surface. Tangential slices approximately 400 μm thick are cut parallel to the articular surface. The concentration of negatively charged fixed groups in the extrafibrillar matrix is measured using the radioactive tracer method of Maroudas and Thomas (1970). The osmotic pressure contribution of the proteoglycans (PGs) can be estimated from measurements carried out against a series of polyethylene glycol (PEG) solutions in 0.15 M NaCl of known osmotic pressure (Urban et al., 1979). Osmotic pressure calibration of PEG solutions is also discussed in Le Neveu et al. (1977). To extend the range of PG concentration to very low values, cartilage is treated enzymatically by the method of Chun et al. (1986). This method effectively removes all the negatively charged moieties from the bovine tissue.

The cartilage specimens are kept frozen until use. Upon thawing, care should be taken to ensure that the cartilage is fully rehydrated before preparing specimens for X-ray measurement. As with many biological materials, the dominant constituent elements — carbon, oxygen, nitrogen and hydrogen — determining the X-ray absorption coefficients in an optimum thickness of 1.0–1.5 mm. The slice is easily excised with a scalpel and inserted into a thin-walled X-ray capillary, either lithium glass or quartz (Wolfgang Muller, Berlin), filled with solution. Equilibration time for the specimen in this medium is determined by independent physicochemical experiments or by monitoring the X-ray scattering profile until no further changes are observed. There are some cases in which specimen immersion is not acceptable; for instance, the cartilage from intervertebral disc becomes depleted of PG upon immersion. Also, when the osmotically active polymer PEG is present in the solution, it can penetrate into the extrafibrillar space. There is no evidence, however, that it penetrates into the intrafibrillar space. To try to solve these problems, we have designed and used a dialysis cell which is shown schematically in Fig. 56.1. Because of the cell asymmetry, gradients of hydration (additional to those inherent in tissue composition) may develop across the specimen and in such cases analysis can be difficult. We have checked several specimens after equilibration in two different orientations against a solution containing PEG and have found the same hydration profile in both cases. Furthermore, the hydration was equal to that of an equivalent specimen placed within a dialysis sac totally immersed in the same solution. Nevertheless, caution is advised.

Initial determination of specimen morphology can often be made by examining the cartilage under a polarizing light microscope (Hartshorne and Stuart, 1970; Benninghoff, 1925). The strong birefringence of cartilage observed when the axes of the collagen molecules lie normal to the incident light can assist in estimating the preferred direction of the fibrils. This information will be seen to be important for the scattering experiment.

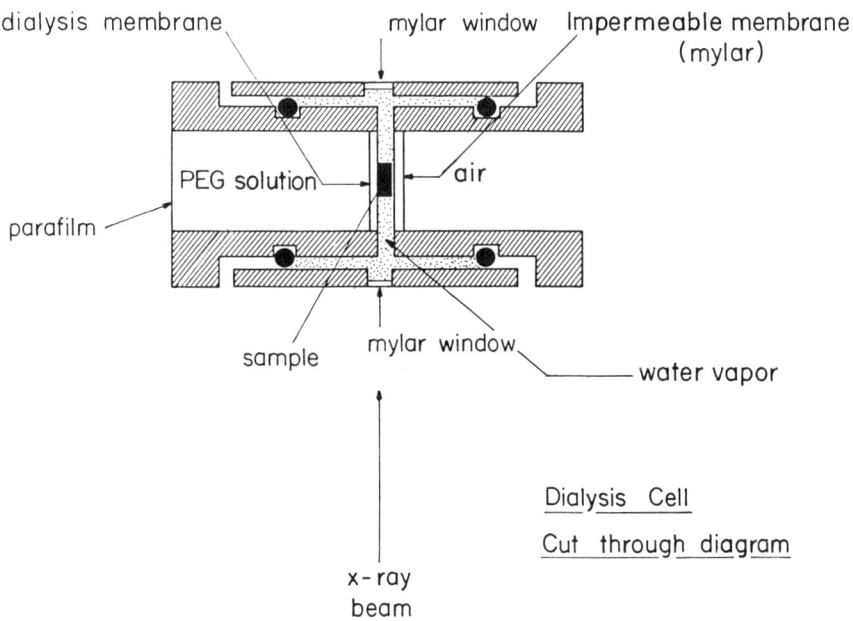

Figure 56.1 Dialysis cell used for X-ray scattering experiments.

SCATTERING MEASUREMENT

In our laboratory, X-ray measurements are made on a low-angle camera (Searle) equipped with Franks' mirror optics (Franks, 1955) and fixed to an Elliot GX6 rotating anode generator operating at 40 kV, 30 mA with a 200-μm focus. A Ni filter and the Franks' mirrors produce nearly monochromatic radiation: the average wavelength (λ) of the Cu K_α doublet is approximately 1.54 Å. Small focal size and high brightness of the X-ray beam are necessary for studying weakly-scattering biological tissues and any generator and optical arrangement which achieves this is satisfactory. A telescope attachment to the Searle camera permits exact positioning and choice of the scattering region. X-ray photographs may be taken using X-ray film of relatively high sensitivity (CEA Reflex 25 or Kodak DEF). A typical photograph is shown in Fig. 56.2. The exposure time for the conditions described above is approximately 16 h. The scattering along the horizontal axis (called the equator) is determined by the side-by-side packing of the collagen molecules. The sharpness of the intensity maxima relates to the degree of packing order—crystalline packing giving sharp reflections and liquid-like packing giving diffuse scattering. The arcing of the maxima off the equator characterizes the disorientation of the axes of the collagen molecules. Calibration of the distances on the film can be made by coating the capillary with a material of known spacing, e.g. cholesterol (34 Å), calcite (3.029 Å), or gypsum (7.56 Å).

We have adopted the Searle camera for use with a single wire position sensitive detector (LPSD) of the delay-line type (Reich et al., 1982). Such a detector is 10–100 times more sensitive to Cu X-rays than is film. In addition, there is no chemical fog. The signal-to-noise ratio is controlled by counting statistics and there is immediate digital (quantitative) output. The detector in use in our laboratory is homemade, but similar systems are also available commercially (Braun, TEC Corp, etc.). Data-collection times with the detector are reduced to about 1–2 h, thereby minimizing specimen deterioration. The principal disadvantage of the detector is that of relatively poor resolution as compared with film. Our experiment cannot resolve scattering features which are more closely spaced than 200 μm in the plane of the detector. A new type of detector has recently become available which acts like supersensitive film with the attendant advantages of homogeneity, linearity and reasonably high resolution. This 'image plate' is coated with a rare-earth emulsion and, after reading with a laser scanner, is reusable (Amemiya et al., 1988).

DATA ANALYSIS

One should photograph a number of specimens in different orientations in order to fix the morphology of the material under investigation. Aspden and Hukins (1979) and Kirby et al. (1988) have developed methods to quantitate the morphological studies of collagen. If a two-dimensional wire detector or an image plate is used, the morphological information and scattering measurements can be obtained at the same time. In our case we use photography as a prelude to systematic series of measurements using the LPSD. The linear detector is aligned parallel to the horizontal axis and consequently samples the equator of the scattering pattern (Fig. 56.3). We vary pH, ionic strength and concentration of

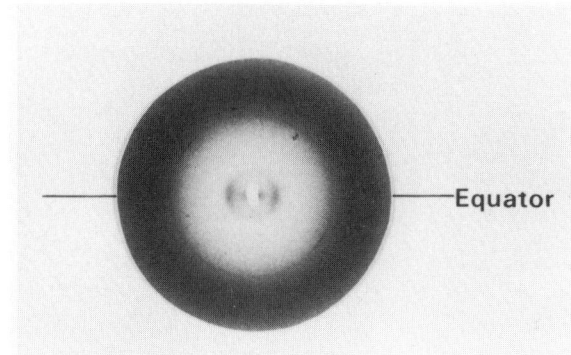

Figure 56.2 X-ray diffraction pattern from the superficial zone of human articular cartilage dialyzed against saline solution containing 30 g PEG per 100 g water. The equatorial plane is noted.

9. TISSUE COMPOSITION AND ORGANIZATION

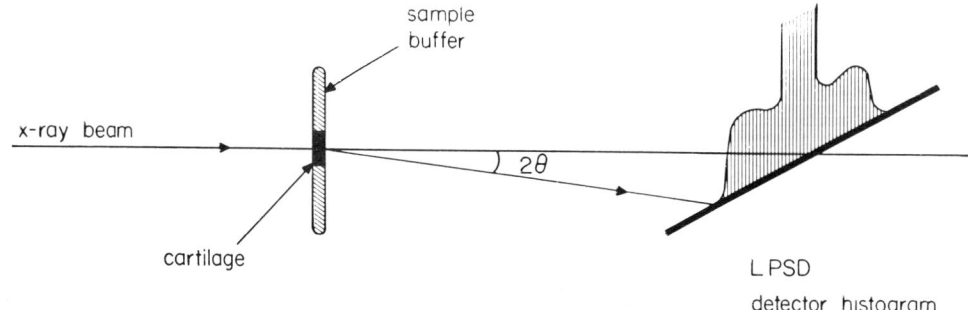

Figure 56.3 Schematic of X-ray scattering experiment. The distance between the sample and detector is approximately 8 cm and the active length of the detector is 5 cm.

osmotically active polymeric molecules. Measurements under conditions of mechanical stress will be made in the future. Data are histogrammed on a Z-80 based microprocessor, and after completion of the experiment, transferred via a hard-wire link to the Weizmann Institute IBM 3090 computer for analysis. Commercial detector systems often include multichannel analyzers for data collection. For time-course experiments, scattering profiles are measured at fixed time intervals and each is stored in predetermined location in the microprocessor memory. At the end of the series all data are transferred for analysis.

As noted above, the collagen molecules in the cartilage specimens are not perfectly aligned. Therefore, the LPSD data must be corrected for disorientation before they may be used for quantitative measurements. Theoretical analysis of disorientation in fibrous specimens (Holmes and Barrington Leigh, 1974; Stubbs, 1974) as well as phenomenological treatment of two-dimensional patterns (Mandelkow, 1973; E. Katz, private communication) indicate that at low angles an appropriate correction consists of multiplication of the intensity at a given point on the pattern by the distance of that point from the origin, after subtraction of the background. We have written a short Fortran program called DISOR to make this correction and typical resulting scattering profiles are shown in Fig. 56.4. The intensity profiles may be compared with the results of theoretical calculations. The real space position (d) of the single intensity maximum is calculated (after calibration as described above) using the relationship $\lambda = 2d\sin\theta$, where 2θ is the relevant scattering angle.

The distance between collagen molecules in fibrils in cartilage may be determined as a function of the environmental parameter to be varied. In those tissues where the collagen molecules exhibit

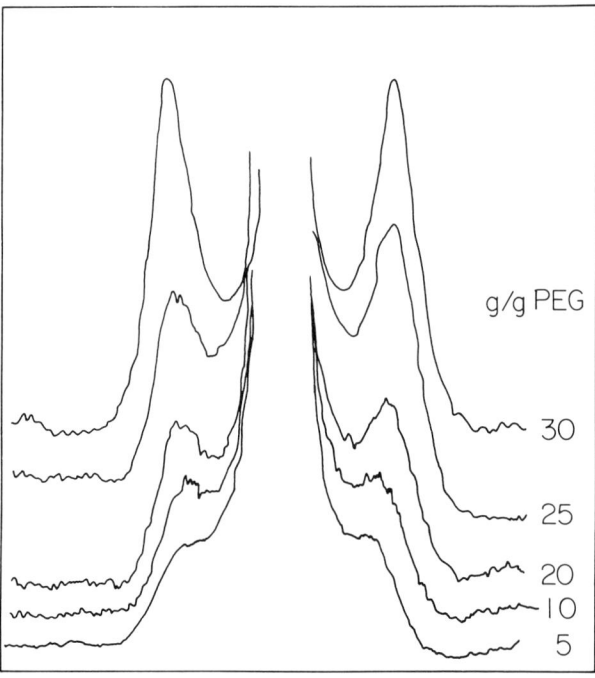

Figure 56.4 Characteristic scattering profiles from bovine articular cartilage, which has been depleted of PGs as a function of PEG content of the dialysis solution.

long-range order, such as in rat-tail tendon, the intermolecular distances are determined directly from the lattice constants. However, in cartilage there is only short-range order. In this case, the low-angle equatorial X-ray scattering is dominated by near-neighbor pair interactions. The measured peak position, d (Å), is related to the intercollagen distance a (Å), by $d c. a/1.11$ (Klug and Alexander, 1974). A plot of distance vs. the pressure difference between the intrafibrillar and extrafibrillar spaces is shown in Fig. 56.5. The main point to note with respect to these results is that, whether the fibrils are surrounded by the PG–water phase as in native cartilage or directly exposed to PEG solutions (as in the case of PG-free specimens), the data all fall on the same curve. This implies that the intercollagen spacing in cartilage is regulated primarily by the magnitude of the pressure gradient (osmotic in this case) existing between the outside and the inside of the fibril.

In addition, the intermolecular space within collagen fibrils in cartilage may be estimated. This parameter is relelvant to a wide range of problems relating to tissue structure, solute and fluid transport. It is the same as the volume of intrafibrillar water. However, because of our incomplete knowledge of cartilage structure some assumptions must be made: (i) the Hodge–Petruska model is valid (Hodge and Petruska, 1963); and (ii) the characteristic coordination number for a two-dimensional array of rods is 6, (Vainshtein, 1966) i.e. pseudohexagonal packing. Then, following Katz and Li (1973), the intermolecular volume per gram of collagen (or, equivalently, grams of water per gram of collagen) is given by

$$V = 5 \cdot D \cdot a^2 \cdot 0.866 \cdot (N_A/M_c) - \varrho_c^{-1}$$

where N_A is Avogadro's number, $D = 670$ Å, $M_c = 283\,000$ Da and $\varrho_c^{-1} = 0.70$ cm^3 g^{-1}. For

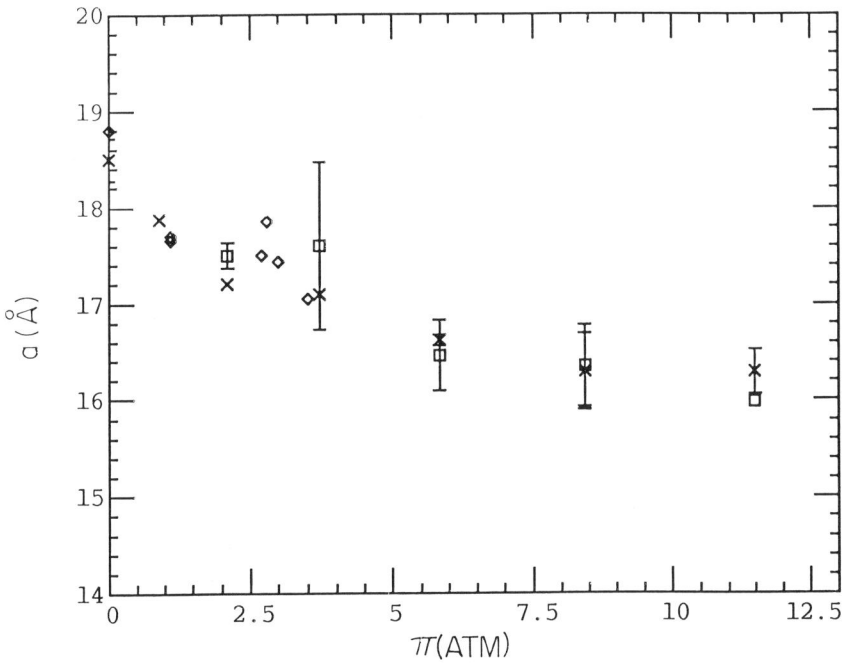

Figure 56.5 Graph of the dependence of the intercollagen distance as a function of pressure. (◇) Native human articular collagen; (X) extracted bovine articular cartilage equilibrated against solutions containing PEG; (□) native human articular cartilage equilibrated against solutions containing PEG. The vertical bars indicate standard deviations when replicate experiments have been performed. In the absence of PEG, equivalent pressures were determined as described by Maroudas *et al.* (1990).

human articular cartilage, the results vary from 1.47 cm³ g⁻¹ for a slice from the superficial zone to 1.09 cm³ g⁻¹ for a slice from the deep zone. At the maximum compression achieved here, the volume is reduced to 0.88 cm³ g⁻¹. The effect of finite fibril size would be to lower the value found for the superficial zone by a few per-cent. Similar measurements can be made as a function of pH, mechanical pressure, etc.

The osmotic-pressure techniques described here have been used in other systems as well: DNA, muscle, TMV, and lipid bilayers (Rand, 1981). There, the work was motivated by an interest in characterizing the intermolecular forces as a function of distance in water. One result is the finding that a so-called 'hydration' force dominates the molecular repulsion at small distances. The force is so named because it is believed to be derived from the work necessary to remove molecules from between the hydrophilic macromolecular surfaces as they approach each other (Le Neveu et al., 1977). Similar measurements could be made on collagen types I and II. The advantages of crystalline packing suggest that lamprey notochord (Eikenberry et al., 1984) would be a better choice for type II collagen than articular cartilage.

ACKNOWLEDGEMENT

This research was supported in part by The Fund for Basic Research Administered by The Israel Academy of Sciences and Humanities.

57

Low-angle X-ray diffraction analysis of cartilaginous tissues

CARMEN BERTHET-COLOMINAS, MARIE-CLAIRE RONZIERE and DANIEL HERBAGE

X-RAY DIFFRACTION AND COLLAGEN STRUCTURE AND ORGANIZATION

X-ray diffraction is the most powerful of the available techniques for studying the structure of large molecules; however, it requires spatial order: the molecules to be studied must be assembled in crystalline form. If the quality of the crystal is good, the X-ray diffraction pattern can reveal the structure and, consequently, interactions at the atomic level.

Natural collagenous molecules have a fibrous form which is not a well-ordered structure. Schematically, high-angle X-ray diffraction provides information on the molecular structure of collagen, and low- and medium-angle X-ray diffraction provides information on the molecular arrangement in collagen fibrils (Fraser et al., 1987). At low resolution, the triple-helix collagen molecule appears as a cylinder of approximately 1.3 nm in diameter and 290 nm in length. Hodge (1967) explained the 67 nm repeat along the fibril axis by using the 'staggered' model: collagen molecules are staggered in parallel to the fibrillar axis at intervals of 67 nm. Consequently, the projected electron density can be studied in one direction, i.e. parallel to the axis of the fibrils. This projected electron density is a step function repeated at a 67 nm periodicity with a well-defined gap/overlap ratio (Table 57.1). Non-collagenous molecules present in a tissue can fill the gap region,

Table 57.1 Interpretation of the meridional low-angle X-ray diffraction pattern from collagenous tissues

Derives from the periodic axial structure of collagen

May be used to produce an axial electron density distribution for the constituent collagen fibrils

The first orders are essentially a function of the step shape derived from the gap-overlap organization

	First- to third-order intensities ratio	Step shape
Annulus fibrosus Tendon	8–10	
Nucleus pulposus Articular cartilage Native	1–2	
+ Hyaluronidase	3	
+ Trypsin	6–7	

Changes in the relative intensities of the reflections (Ex: Cartilage) = regular addition of components along the fibrils at the axial level of the gaps

and interaction with collagen obliges them to have the same periodicity. This phenomenon occurs in calcified collagen, where apatite fills the gap, modifying the electron density of the collagen–mineral complex (Berthet-Colominas et al., 1979). Since the meridional X-ray diffraction pattern is the Fourier transform of the projected electron density, it follows a modification of the relative intensities of the first five orders. Only this region of the pattern is directly related to the step function, the intensities of the higher-order peaks being modulated by the amino acid sequence.

X-RAY DIFFRACTION AND CARTILAGE

In some collagenous tissues, such as rat-tail tendon, all the fibrils are more or less parallel. Therefore, one can obtain a low-angle X-ray pattern from native tendon with enough detail to allow positioning of the amino acids along the fiber (Hulmes et al., 1977). In cartilage, the collagen fibers are disordered in the plane and the information in a diffraction peak is spread over a diffraction circle; the measurement conditions are poor and the statistical errors much higher. Nevertheless, the diffraction pattern from cartilage can give useful information, in particular about possible interactions with noncollagenous material, such as the proteoglycans (PGs) that are present in high concentration in that tissue.

In cartilage, accurate measurement of the intensity of the first-order peak of the meridional pattern is particularly difficult. This peak, which is quite intense in tendon, is weak in cartilage and, therefore, the relative measurement error increases drastically. The reflection is situated very close to the direct beam in a region where the background is higher and varies rapidly.

For this reason, we set up a camera with a long sample–detector distance on account of the background around the direct beam. The apparatus consists of a double-focusing system, with a Frank mirror and a crystal monochromator with a cut angle of 8°. Focus was clearest in the meridional direction, i.e. in the direction parallel to the fibril axis. Four sets of slits — before the mirror, between the mirror and the monochromator, after the monochromator, and the guard slits 40 cm beyond — were used in order to decrease the background as much as possible, the background coming mostly from the crystal. The sample–film distance was about 100 cm. Films were set up at the monochromator focal point, so that the beam was slightly divergent in the direction perpendicular to the fibril axis (Berthet-Colominas et al., 1982).

Low-angle X-ray diffraction studies were carried out on human and bovine intervertebral discs, bovine articular cartilage and reconstituted and native type I and type II collagen fibrils (Berthet-Colominas et al., 1982; Ronziere et al., 1985, 1987). Three regions of bovine lumbar intervertebral discs from two-year-old animals were examined: the external annulus fibrosus, containing type I collagen, the internal nucleus pulposus, containing type II collagen, and a transitional zone, containing both type I and type II collagens in a ratio of 40/60. Articular cartilage from two- to four-year-old steers were obtained from femora. In order to remove non-collagenous components, the samples were treated with trypsin, hyaluronidase or increasing concentrations of $CaCl_2$.

The X-ray diffraction patterns from articular cartilage and the nucleus pulposus were clearly different from those obtained with rat-tail tendon or annulus fibrosus (Berthet-Colominas et al., 1982; Ronziere et al., 1985). The intensities of the first five orders of the meridional X-ray reflections (normalized to the first order), the ratio of the first third order intensities and the PG content of the sample (calculated from the hexosamine level) are compared in Table 57.2 with those obtained with rat-tail tendon. The ratio of the first-order to third-order intensities decreased dramatically in cartilaginous type II collagen-rich tissues: 1.2 for nucleus pulposus and articular cartilage in comparison to 8.5–11.4 for rat rail tendon and annulus. A similar result was obtained by Eikenberry et al. (1984) for type II collagen fibrils in the lamprey notochord sheath. In a model at low resolution constructed to explain the X-ray patterns (Berthet-Colominas et al., 1982) the differences could be interpreted either as a modification of the step function of the collagen itself (not confirmed by electron microscopy of the collagen fibrils) or by the presence of ordered components (PGs or other macromolecules) attached to the collagen specifically at the axial level of the gap region in the collagen fibrils. The latter hypothesis was confirmed by analysis of trypsin-treated articular cartilage and nucleus pulposus. The X-ray diffraction pattern was indeed modified, and the ratio of the first-order to third-order intensities was increased from 1.2 to 6.5. Furthermore, we observed a clear linear relationship between this ratio and the rate of extraction of PGs with increasing concentration of $CaCl_2$ (Ronziere et al., 1985).

These studies provide a direct demonstration of the presence in hydrated nonstained nucleus pulposus and articular cartilage of a component (PG?) that is deposited regularly along the collagen fibrils. This component was extracted by

Table 57.2 Relative intensities of meridional diffraction peaks and percentages of PGs extracted from native and trypsin-treated tissues

Order	Rat-tail tendon	Annulus fibrosus		Nucleus pulposus		Articular cartilage	
	Native	Native	+Trypsin	Native	+Trypsin	Native	+Trypsin
First	1000	1000	1000	1000	1000	1000	1000
Third	118	87	122	846	152	868	154
Fifth	48	40	117	977	112	653	140
First: fifth	8.5	11.4	8.3	1.2	6.5	1.2	6.5
PG extracted (%)	0	0	84	0	91.5	0	90

proteolytic treatment (trypsin) and by $CaCl_2$ extraction (Table 57.1). We confirmed the hypothesis by analysis of the low-angle X-ray diffraction pattern of reconstituted native-like fibrils from purified PG-free type I and type II collagens. Both types of fibril gave similar ratios of first-order to third-order intensities (range 13–22) which where twice and 20 times the values measured for rat-tail tendon and articular cartilage, respectively.

These differences reflect the extent of specific interactions of other components at the gap level along the collagen fibrils in the two tissues. The exact nature of these components remains unclear. Using electron microscopy, Scott (1986) demonstrated a close spatial relationship between type I collagen and PG in skin, tendon and cornea.

Orford and Gardner (1984) observed a similar labeling in articular cartilage. Recently, van der Rest and Mayne (1988) have described the structure of type IX collagen linked to the surface of type II collagen fibrils. In the proposed model, the glycosaminoglycan chain of type IX collagen would be localized at the gap region of the fibril. Direct biochemical determinations and/or electron optical observations are required to interpret the actual biological significance of these findings.

ACKNOWLEDGMENTS

We are indebted to Professor A. Miller for helpful discussion. This work was supported in part by CNAMTS (1984) and INSERM (880.004) grants.

58

Cell compartment in articular cartilage

R.A. STOCKWELL

Cell content can be estimated by either chemical analysis of tissue for DNA or morphometric analysis of histological sections. Both procedures provide an index of cell number (number density) but mean cell size and total cell volume in the cartilage (volume density) are best obtained by morphometry. This also permits analysis of much smaller samples or regions of tissue.

CELL NUMBER

Number density can be estimated using various techiques.

(i) The Abercrombie (1946) method requires all cells or nuclei ($\bar{N}$) to be counted in a quadrant covering the full depth of the cartilage. The section thickness (t) and the nuclear diameter ($\bar{D}$) in a plane at right angles to the plane of section must also be measured. Assuming mononucleate cells, number density $N_V = N_A/(\bar{D} + t)$.

(ii) The disector method (Sterio, 1984) is less biased. In two serial sections a known distance apart (i.e. the section thickness, t), corresponding areas (A) are selected randomly. Those objects (cells) which appear in the first section *only* (and not in both sections) are counted (C). Number density, $N_V = C/(A \times t)$. The disector method does not require measurement of nuclear diameter, but is difficult to use unless the sections are photographed, a disadvantage if the cartilage section is large.

CELL SIZE

Several methods have been tried in the past to measure cell volume.

(i) The oldest method is to cut serial sections of thickness t through the object (the cell) and measure the areas (A) of successive cell profiles. Cell volume = ΣAt. The method is cumbersome but otherwise unbiased.

(ii) Cell-profile diameters ($\bar{d}$) are measured to obtain the true cell diameter ($\bar{D} = 4\bar{d}/\pi$). Strictly speaking, this method applies only to regular spheroids and size/frequency curves should be constructed (Williams, 1977).

(iii) Electron micrographs of randomly selected cell profiles are point counted to give the volume density of nucleus per cell ($V_{v(n)}$). The approximate size of nuclei can be obtained by using method (ii) to calculate the absolute mean nuclear volume. Then, mean cell volume = mean nuclear volume/$V_{v(n)}$.

(iv) A quadrant covering the full depth of the cartilage in a transverse section is point counted to give the volume density of cells ($V_{v(c)}$) per whole tissue. Number density of cells ($N_{v(c)}$) is obtained by either the Abercrombie or disector techniques. Mean cell volume, $V_{n(c)} = V_{v(c)}/N_{v(c)}$ (Paukkonen et al., 1985).

(v) The least biased, truly morphometric method is that of Cruz-Orive and Hunziker (1986); see Chapter 20. In section photographs, cells are point sampled randomly and lengths of intercepts (l_o) through the cells are measured where the random point 'hits' the cell. Mean cell volume, $V_{v(c)} = (\pi/3)\bar{l}_o^3$.

On a single specimen of mouse articular cartilage, the above-described methods gave the following results.

Number density:
Method (i)   578 000 cells mm^{-1};
Method (ii) 578 000 cells mm^{-1}.

Given accurate measurement, it is not surprising that the two methods give the same result, since they are based on similar mathematical principles using different approaches to overcome the problem arising from the chances of profiles of the same transected object appearing in more than one section.

Cell size:
Method (i)   203 μm^3 ($\bar{r} = 3.6\ \mu$m);
Method (ii)   270 μm^3 ($\bar{r} = 4.0\ \mu$m);
Method (iii) 160 μm^3 ($\bar{r} = 3.4\ \mu$m);
Method (iv)   225 μm^3 ($\bar{r} = 3.8\ \mu$m);
Method (v)   186 μm^3 ($\bar{r} = 3.5\ \mu$m).

While these five methods give mean cell volumes that differ enormously, it is noteworthy that the radius (r) of the mean equivalent sphere varies by little more than the extreme limit of optical resolution (0.2 μm, $\lambda = 550$ nm). Apart from purely mathematical considerations of the morphometric methods, it is emphasized that histological requirements, such as absence of shrinkage/swelling during tissue preparation, sharp contrast of the objects measured against the background tissue and high optical resolution to determine object boundaries, are also assumed.

Cell shape, number and size vary within articular cartilage. Cells are discoidal and more numerous near the articular surface with a more spherical profile and a lower number density in the deeper tissue. In the rabbit, the mean cell volume of superficial cells is less than that of deep cells (Paukkonen et al., 1985). Hence, if superficial cells degenerate and atrophy as in early fibrillation, this may have more effect on the number density than on the volume density, expressed per whole tissue.

In the middle zone, cell size appears to increase slightly with increasing cartilage thickness from a radius (mean equivalent sphere) of about 3.65 μm, and mean cell volume 200 μm^3 in thin cartilages, as in the mouse knee, to higher values in larger joints and thicker cartilages. Conversely, number density falls from about 300 000 to 500 000 cells mm^{-3} in mouse cartilage to about 14 000 cells mm^{-3} in the human knee (Stockwell, 1979). Hence the percentage volume of cells in the whole tissue falls from about 10–12% in the mouse, through 7–8% in the rabbit (Paukkonen et al., 1985) to around 1% in the human knee.

References

Abercrombie, M. (1946). Estimation of nuclear population from microtome sections. *Anat. Rec.* **94**, 239–247

Amemiya, Y., Matsushita, T., Nakagawa, A., Satow, Y., Miyahara and Chikawa, J. (1988). Design and performance of imaging plate system for X-ray diffraction study. *Nucl. Instrum. Methods Phys. Res.* **A-266**, 645–653

Aspden, R.M. and Hukins, D.W.L. (1979). Determination of the direction of preferred orientation and the orientation distribution function of collagen fibrils in connective tissues from high angle-X-ray diffraction patterns. *J. Appl. Crystallogr.* **12**, 306–311

Bayliss, M. and Ali, Y. (1978). Age-related changes in the composition and structure of human articular cartilage proteoglycans. *Biochem. J.* **176**, 683–693

Bayliss, M.T. and Roughley, P.J. (1985). The properties of proteoglycan prepared from human articular cartilage by using associative caesium chloride gradients of high and low starting densities. *Biochem. J.* **232**, 111–117

Bayliss, M.T. and Venn, M. (1980). Chemistry of human articular cartilage. In *Studies in Joint Diseases* (A. Maroudas and E.S. Holborow, eds), pp. 2–58. Pitman Medical, London

Bayliss, M.T., Ridgway, G.D. and Ali, S.Y. (1984). Delayed aggregation of proteoglycans in adult human articular cartilage. *Biosci. Rep.* **4**, 827–833

Bayliss, M.T., Urban, J.P.G., Johnstone, B. and Holm, S. (1987). An *in-vitro* method for measuring synthesis rates in the intervertebral disc. *J. Orthop. Res.* **5**, 10–23

Bayliss, M.T., Holmes, M.W.A. and Muir, H. (1989). Age-related changes in the stoichiometry of binding region, link protein and hyaluronic acid in human articular cartilage. *35th Trans. Orthop. Res. Soc., USA* Vol. **14**, p. 32

Benaim, E. (1989). Biomechanical model for cartilage creep in compression. D.Sc. Thesis. Department of Biomedical Engineering, Technion – Israel Institute of Technology, Haifa, Israel

Benaim, E., Mizrahi, J. and Maroudas, A. (1990). Shape and volume changes in cartilage during creep in unconfined compressed. in prep.

Benninghoff, A. (1925). Shape and structure of articular cartilage and its effect on function. II. Effect of structure on function. *Z. Zellforsch. mikr. Anat.* **2**, 783–786

Berthet-Colominas, C., Miller, A. and White, S. (1979). Structural study of the calcified collagen in turkey leg tendon. *J. Mol. Biol.* **134**, 431–445

Berthet-Colominas, C., Miller, A., Herbage, D., Ronziere, M.C. and Tocchetti, D. (1982). Structural studies of collagen fibres from intervertebral disc. *Biochim. Biophys. Acta* **706**, 50–64

Byers, P.D., Bayliss, M.T., Maroudas, A., Urban, J. and Weightman, B. (1983). Hypothesising about joints. In *Studies in Joint Disease* (A. Maroudas and J. Holborow, eds), Vol. 2, pp. 241–276. Pitman Medical, London

Chun, L.E., Koob, T.J. and Eyre, D.R. (1986). Sequential enzymic dissection of the proteoglycan complex from articular cartilage. *Orthop. Res. Soc. Trans. (USA)* **11**, 96

Crank, J. and Park, G.S. (eds.) (1968). *Diffusion in Polymers*. Academic Press, New York

Cruz-Orive, L.-M. and Hunziker, E.B. (1986). Stereology for anisotropic cells: application to growth cartilage. *J. Microsc.* **143**, 47–80

De Gennes, P.G. (1971). Reptation of a polymer chain in the presence of fixed obstacles. *J. Chem. Phys.* **55**, 572–579

Eikenberry, E.F., Childs, B., Sheren, S.B., Parry, D.A.D., Craig, A.S. and Brodsky, B. (1984). Crystalline fibril structure of type II collagen in lamprey notochord sheath. *J. Mol. Biol.* **176**, 261–277

Encyclopaedia Britannica (1971), edition 13, p. 818. Encyclopedia Britannica Inc.

Franks, A. (1955). An optically focussing X-ray diffraction camera. *Proc. Phys. Soc. B* **68**, 1054–1064

Fraser, R.D.B., MacRae, T.P., Chew, M.W.K. and Squire, J.M. (1987). Collagen and elastin. In *Fibrous Protein Structure* (J.M. Squire and P.J. Vibert, eds), pp. 173–191. Academic Press, London

Gray, M.L., Pizzanelli, A.M., Grodzinsky, A.J. and Lee, R.C. (1988). Mechanical and physicochemical determinants of the chondrocyte biosynthetic responses. *J. Orthop. Res.* **6**, 777–792

Grushko, G., Schneiderman, R. and Maroudas, A. (1989). Some biochemical and biophysical parameters for the study of the pathogenesis of osteoarthritis: a comparison between the processes of ageing and degeneration in human hip cartilage. *Conn. Tiss. Res.* **19**, 149–176

Hartshorne, N.H. and Stuart, A. (1970). Crystals and the polarizing microscope. E. Arnold, London

Hodge, A. (1967). Structure at the electron microscopic level. In *Treatise on Collagen* (G.N. Ramachandran, ed.), Vol. 1, pp. 185–205. Academic Press, London

Hodge, A.K. and Petruska, J.A. (1963). Recent studies with the electron microscope on ordered aggregates of the tropocollagen macromolecule. In *Aspects of Protein Structure* (G.N. Ramachandran, ed.), pp. 289–300. Academic Press, London

Holm, S., Maroudas, A., Urban, J., Selstam, G. and Nachemson, A. (1981). Nutrition of the intervertebral disc: solute transport and metabolism. Part 1: Oxygen uptake and lactic acid production in the canine disc. Part 2: Oxygen and lactate concentration profiles. *Conn. Tiss. Res.* **8**, 101–119

Holmes, K.C. and Barrington Leigh, J. (1974). The effect of disorientation on the intensity distribution of non-crystalline fibres. I. Theory. *Acta Crystallogr., Sect.* **30**, 635–638

Holmes, M.W.A., Bayliss, M.T. and Muir, H. (1988). Hyaluronic acid in human articular cartilage: age-related changes in content and size. *Biochem. J.* **250**, 435–441

Hulmes, D.J.S., Miller, A., White, S.W. and Brodsky-Doyle, B. (1977). Interpretation of the meridional X-ray diffraction pattern from collagen fibres in terms of the known aminoacid sequence. *J. Mol. Biol.* **110**, 643–666

Katz, E.P. and Li, S.T. (1973). The intermolecular space of reconstituted collagen fibrils. *J. Mol. Biol.* **73**, 351–369

Katz, E.P., Wachtel, E.J. and Maroudas, A. (1986). Extrafibrillar proteoglycans osmotically regulate the molecular packing of collagen in cartilage. *Biochim. Biophys. Acta* **882**, 136–139

Kirby, M.C., Aspden, R.M. and Hukins, D.W.L. (1988). Determination of the orientation distribution function for collagen fibrils in a connective tissue site from a high angle X-ray diffraction pattern. *J. Appl. Crystallogr.* **21**, 929–934

Klein, J. and Meyer, F.A. (1983). Tissue structure and macromolecular diffusion in umbilical cord. Immobilization of endogenous hyaluronic acid. *Biochim. Biophys. Acta* **755**, 400–411

Le Neveu, D.M., Rand, R.P., Gingell, D., and Parsegian, V.A. (1977). Measurement and modification of forces between lecithin bilayers. *Biophys. J.* **18**, 209–230

Mackie, J.S. and Meares, P. (1955). The diffusion of electrolytes in a cation-exchange resin membrane. *Proc. R. Soc. Ser. A* **232**, 498–509

Mandelkow (1973). Röntgenstrukturuntersuchung am Tabakmosaic Virus. Thesis, University of Heidelberg

Maroudas, A. (1976). Balance between swelling pressure and collagen tension in normal and degenerate cartilage. *Nature* **260**, 808–809

Maroudas, A. (1979). Physico-chemical properties of articular cartilage. In *Adult Articular Cartilage*, (M.A.R. Freeman, ed.), 2nd edn, pp. 215–290. Pitman Medical, London

Maroudas, A. and Bannon, C. (1981). Measurement of swelling pressure in cartilage and comparison with the osmotic pressure of constituent proteoglycans. *Biorheology* **18**, 619–632

Maroudas, A. and Thomas, H.A. (1970). A simple physiochemical micromethod for determining fixed anionic groups in connective tissue. *Biochem. Biophys. Acta* **215**, 214–218

Maroudas, A. and Venn, M. (1977). Swelling of normal and osteoarthritic femoral head cartilage. *Ann. Rheum. Dis.* **36**, 399–406

Maroudas, A., Bayliss, M.T. and Venn, M. (1980). Further studies on the composition of human femoral head cartilage. *Ann. Rheum. Dis.* **39**, 514–534

Maroudas, A., Mizrahi, J., Ben Haim, E. and Ziv, I. (1986). Swelling pressure in cartilage. In *Interstitial Lymphatic Liquid and Solute Movement* (N.C. Staub, J.C. Hogg and A.R. Hargens, eds), *Advances in Microcirculation*, Vol. 13, J. Karger, Basel

Maroudas, M., Wachtel, E., Grushko, G., Weinberg, P.D. and Katz, E. (1990). Osmotic and mechanical pressures alter the spacing of collagen molecules in articular cartilage. *Biochim. Biophys. Acta* in press

Meyer, F.A. (1983). Macromolecular bases of globular protein exclusion and of swelling pressure in loose connective tissue (umbilical cord). *Biochim. Biophys. Acta* **755**, 388–399

Meyer, F.A., Laver-Rudich, Z. and Tanenbaum, R. (1983). Evidence for a mechanical coupling of glycoprotein microfibrils with collagen fibrils in Wharton's jelly. *Biochem. Biophys. Acta* **755**, 376–387

Ogston, A.G. (1958). The spaces in a uniform random suspension of fibers. *Trans. Faraday Soc.* **54**, 1754–1757

Orford, C.R. and Gardner, D. (1984). Proteolgycan association with collagen d band in hyaline articular cartilage. *Conn. Tiss. Res.* **12**, 345–348

Paukkonen, K., Selkainaho, K., Jurvelin, J., Kiviranta, I. and Helminen, H.J. (1985). Cells and nuclei of articular cartilage chondrocytes in young rabbits enlarged after non-strenous physical exercise. *J. Anat.* **142**, 13–20

Rand, R.P. (1981). Interacting phospholipid bilayers: measured forces and induced structural changes. *Ann. Rev. Biophys. Bioeng.* **10**, 277–314

Reich, M.H., Kam, Z. and Eisenberg, H. (1982). Small angle X-ray scattering study of halophilic malate dehydrogenase. *Biochemistry* **21**, 5189–5195

Roberts, S., Weightman, B., Urban, J. and Chappell, O. (1986). Mechanical and biochemical properties of human articular cartilage in osteoarthritic femoral heads and in autopsy specimens. *J. Bone Joint Surg.* **68**, 278–288

Ronziere, M.C., Berthet-Colominas, C. and Herbage,

D. (1985). Low-angle X-ray diffraction analysis of the collagen-proteoglycan interactions in articular cartilage. *Biochem. Biophys. Acta* **842**, 170–175

Ronziere, M.C., Berthet-Colominas, C. and Herbage, D. (1987). Comparative structural studies of reconstituted and native type I and type II collagen fibrils by low-angle X-ray diffraction. *Biochim. Biophys. Acta* **916**, 381–387

Roughley, P.J. and White, R.J. (1980). Age-related changes in the structure of the proteoglycan subunits from human articular cartilage. *J. Biol. Chem.* **255**, 217–244

Roughley, P.J., White, R.J., Poole, A.R. and Mort, J.S. (1984). The inability to prepare high-bouyant density proteoglycan aggregate from extracts of normal HAC. *Biochem. J.* **221**, 637–644

Schneiderman, R. (1988). Regulation of the metabolism of weight bearing tissues. D.Sc. Thesis, Department of Biomedical Engineering, Technion — Israel Institute of Technology, Haifa, Israel

Schneiderman, R., Keret, D. and Maroudas, A. (1986). The effects of mechanical and osmotic pressure on the rate of glycosaminoglycan synthesis in the human adult femoral head. *J. Orthop. Res.* **4**, 393–408

Scott, J.E. (1986). Proteoglycan-collagen interactions. In *Function of the Proteoglycans* (D. Evered and J. Whelan, eds), pp. 104–116. Wiley, Chichester

Silpananta, P., Dunstone, J.R. and Ogston, A.G. (1968). Fractionation of a hyaluronic acid preparation in a density gradient. *Biochem. J.* **109**, 43–50

Snowden, J. McK. and Maroudas, A. (1976). The distribution of serum albumin in human normal and degenerate articular cartilage. *Biochim. Biophys. Acta* **428**, 726–740

Sterio, D.C. (1984). Estimating number, mean sizes and variations in size of particles in 3-D specimens using dissectors. *J. Microsc.* **134**, 127–136

Stockwell, R.A. (1979). *Biology of Cartilage Cells*, pp. 148–163. Cambridge University Press, Cambridge

Stubbs, G.J. (1974). The effect of disorientation on the intensity distribution of non-crystalline fibres. II. Applications. *Acta Crystallogr. Sect. A* **30**, 639–645

Tobias, D., Ziv, I. and Maroudas, A. (1989). Human facet cartilage: swelling and some physical-chemical characteristics as a function of age. Part I. Swelling of human facet joint cartilage. *Spine* in press

Urban, J.P.G. and Bayliss, M.T. (1989). Regulation of proteoglycan synthesis rate in cartilage *in vitro*: influence of extracellular ionic composition. *Biochim. Biophys. Acta* **992**, 59–65

Urban, J.P.G., Maroudas, A., Bayliss, M.T. and Dillon, J. (1979). Swelling pressures of proteoglycans at the concentrations found in cartilaginous tissues. *Biorheology* **16**, 447–464

Vainshtein, B.K. (1966). Diffraction of chain molecules. Elsevier, Amsterdam

Van der Rest, M. and Mayne, R. (1988). Type IX collagen proteoglycan from cartilage is covalently cross-linked to type II collagen. *J. Biol. Chem.* **263**, 1615–1618

Venn, M.F. (1978). Variation of chemical composition with age in human femoral head cartilage. *Ann. Rheum. Dis.* **37**, 168–174

Weinberg, P.D., Maroudas, A., Schneiderman, Katz, E. and Wachtel, E. (1987). Intra-fibrillar water in cartilaginous tissues. In *Current Advances in Skeletogenesis* (S. Hurwitz and J. Sela, eds), Vol. 3, pp. 127–131. Heiliger Publishing Co., Jerusalem

Williams, M.A. (1977). *Quantitative Methods in Biology*. North-Holland, Amsterdam

10

SOLUTE TRANSPORT BETWEEN TISSUE AND ENVIRONMENT

COLLATED BY J.P.G. URBAN

59

Introduction and review of general principles and procedures

J.P.G. URBAN

INTRODUCTION

Knowledge of solute transport in cartilage is important for understanding many of the physiological processes in the tissue since solute transport is involved in the whole process of matrix synthesis and turnover (Fig. 59.1). Nutrients and substrates for synthesis move from the synovial fluid and external blood supply through the matrix to the cells, and then cross the cell membrane by specialized pathways. During intracellular processing, newly synthesized molecules are transported through the compartments of the cell until secreted. The secreted macromolecules then move away from the cell until assembled in the matrix. Finally, metabolic wastes and degraded matrix products are lost from the tissue into the synovial fluid and circulation. In addition, growth factors, cytokines and other substances involved in regulating these processes move through the matrix to their site of action.

Solute transport can also be important in some experimental techniques. For example the rate of extraction of components from cartilage depends partly on their rate of movement through the

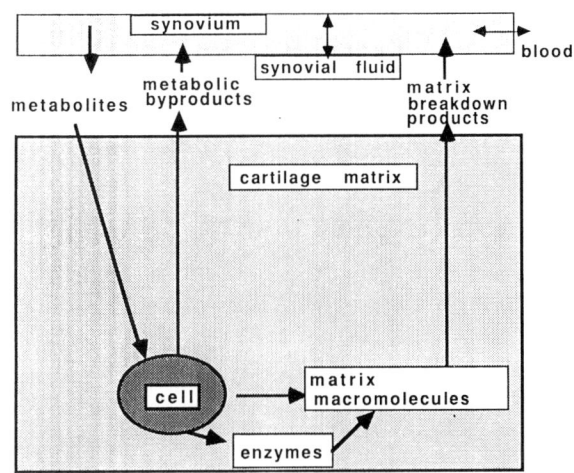

Figure 59.1 A schematic view of the role of solute transport in the processes of matrix synthesis and turnover.

matrix. In labeling studies, movement of radioactive tracers from solutions or from the blood supply through the matrix and into the cells may influence measurements of synthesis. The rate of appearance of degradation products in culture medium depends both on the rate of macromolecule breakdown and on the rate of the loss of breakdown products from the cartilage slice. In studies on the effects of growth factors or drugs on cell behaviour, their degree of penetration into the matrix may affect dose–response behavior. In studies such as these, consideration of factors which govern solute transport may lead to improved experimental design.

The first chapter in this section reviews standard methods of measuring solute transport in cartilage. The following chapters introduce more specialized techniques: A. Silberberg (chapter 64) discusses theoretical methods of estimating transport coefficients, M. Grynpas et al. (chapter 60) show some uses of elemental analysis, B. Preston et al. (chapter 61) and C.P. Winlove and K.H. Parker (chapter 62) describe techniques for obtaining transport coefficients in concentrated proteoglycan (PG) solutions, and A. Hall (chapter 63) reviews methods for measuring membrane transport in isolated cells.

SOLUTE TRANSPORT THROUGH THE MATRIX

Factors influencing transport rate through the matrix

The rate of solute transport through the matrix depends on the properties of both the solute and the matrix. Solute transport is influenced by solute size, by its charge and by its shape (Ogston, 1958; Laurent, 1964; Preston and Snowden, 1973; Maroudas, 1976a; Cumming et al., 1979). It is also affected by the composition of the matrix, particularly by the concentration of PGs, and their charge density (Ogston, 1958; Maroudas, 1970; Ogston et al., 1973; Comper and Laurent, 1978). The properties of the solute and of the matrix determine the maximum concentration of a solute which can exist in the cartilage, i.e. the solute partition coefficient. They also determine how fast the solute is able to move through the matrix, i.e. the solute diffusivity. Since solutes move by diffusion under concentration gradients which are set up by the cells, transport also depends on the rate of utilization or production of metabolites.

Fluid flow, which occurs in response to external loads, may affect movement of larger solutes. In addition to these factors which determine transport within the matrix, external factors such as the size of the cartilage piece, and the concentration of solute in an external solution will determine, for instance, the rate of solute loss from the tissue.

These factors can be related by a transport equation (e.g. Helffrich, 1962; Curry, 1984); a simplified form is shown below. This equation describes transport within the matrix and shows how the concentration of the solute in the matrix, C, and the rate of transport of solute through the matrix, J, depend on the solute diffusion coefficient, D, on the rate of fluid flow, V_s, and on the rate of consumption or production of metabolites, R.

$$J = - D\frac{dC}{dx} + CV_s + R\,dx$$

If values for these constants, and also the solute partition coefficient K, are known, the equation can be solved for any piece of cartilage once the external factors such as the size of the cartilage slice and the concentration of solute in the surrounding fluid are specified. The solutions for most standard cases exist in graphical form (Crank, 1975). A typical solution is shown in Fig. 59.2.

Since the solution to the transport equation depends on both the solute diffusion coefficient and the partition coefficient, most studies of solute transport in cartilage and in other materials have been devoted to determining the relationship between solute size and shape and its diffusion and partition coefficients in the matrix. Thus most of this chapter will be devoted to discussing the methods that are available for determining these coefficients.

The partition coefficient

The measurement of partition coefficients is of interest for several reasons. The first is that knowledge of the partition coefficient is necessary for the solution of the transport equation and thus for determining how solutes move through

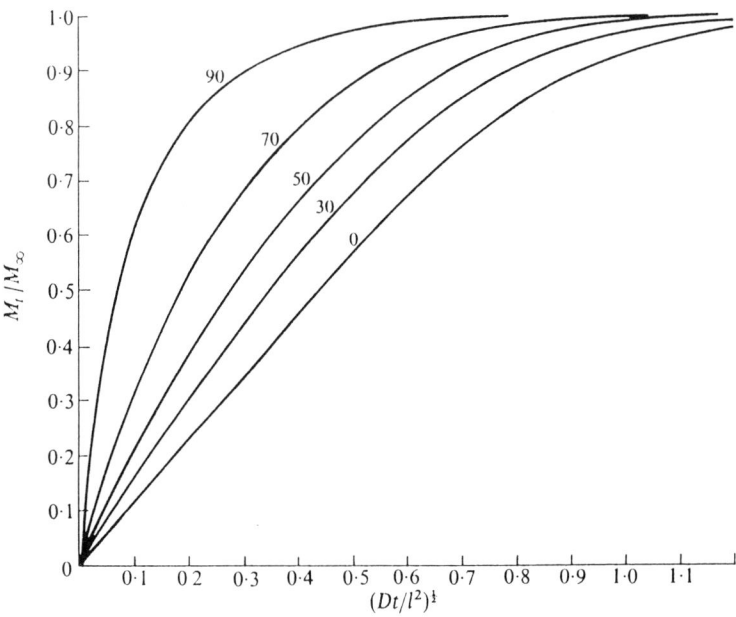

Figure 59.2 Solution to the diffusion equation showing the uptake by a slice of tissue of thickness 2 l from a solution of limited volume in terms of the diffusion coefficient D, and time of exposure to the solution, t. Numbers on the curves show the percentage of the total solute taken up by the sheet relative to the amount at saturation (from Crank (1975), with permission).

cartilage. Secondly, solute partition may affect cartilage behavior; the distribution of ions in cartilage may influence cellular activity (Gray et al., 1988; Urban and Bayliss, 1989) or calcification (Howell et al., 1968), and in load-bearing cartilages the osmotic pressure developed by the distribution of ions influences the mechanical behavior of the tissue (Comper and Preston, 1974; Urban et al., 1979; Grodzinsky et al., 1981).

The partition coefficient of a solute is defined as the concentration of the solute in the matrix relative to its concentration in the external contacting fluid such as synovial fluid or plasma (Maroudas, 1968); it is a measure of the maximum equilibrium concentration of a solute in the matrix. If the molal partition coefficient, K, is 1.00 then the solute distributes equally between cartilage and the external fluid. If K is < 1.00 then the solute is partially excluded from the matrix. The partition coefficient is only unity for small uncharged solutes such as some amino acids or oxygen (Maroudas, 1970). Large solutes are sterically excluded from the matrix (see Chapter 64). Even solutes such as glucose are partially excluded from areas of cartilage where the glycosaminoglycan (GAG) concentration is high, while the partition coefficient of solutes the size of serum albumin ($M_r = 65\,000$) may be as low as 0.01–0.001 (Maroudas, 1976a). If the solute is charged, K depends on the charge density of the matrix; anions are always partially excluded since the GAGs are negatively charged, but cations have a partition coefficient that is greater than unity (Dunstone, 1960; Maroudas and Evans, 1972).

Measurement of partition coefficients

Cartilage. Most information on partition coefficients of solutes in cartilage comes from the use of radioactive tracers. Cartilage (previously frozen to halt cell metabolism) is placed in a solution containing the solute of interest at a known concentration, together with radiolabeled tracer, and is left in the solution until equilibrium.

The cartilage is then removed from the solution and the activity of tracer in the cartilage determined either by digesting the cartilage slice or eluting the tracer from the cartilage. The partition coefficient is calculated from the activity of the tracer in the cartilage and the activity in the solution. For small solutes and for intact articular cartilage (Maroudas and Evans, 1972, 1974) this method presents no problem. However, for disc, or fibrillated cartilage, or any cartilage which swells or loses proteoglycans in solution, the method must be suitably modified (Urban and Maroudas, 1979; Grodzinsky, 1983).

For large solutes there are other problems involved in the measurement of partition coefficients. Firstly, the partition coefficients are very small so the tracer activity in the cartilage tends to be very low. Secondly, if there is some breakdown of radioactive label the results can be misleading. Breakdown is a particular problem if the protein or other solute is labeled with iodine since iodinated compounds break down at a significant rate and it is not possible to remove all traces of free iodine (Snowden and Maroudas, 1976). Free iodine at concentrations as low as 0.5% can cause serious errors in the determination of partition coefficients of solutes such as serum albumin or immunoglobulins where K is 0.01–0.001. Since the partition coefficient for iodide is about 0.5, K for iodide is 50–500 times greater than that of serum albumin. Thus a significant fraction of the tracer in the cartilage will be free iodide, and to measure K very careful separation of the two iodinated species is required (Maroudas, 1976a).

Model systems. As discussed elsewhere, cartilage cannot be considered as a uniform material, but rather as consisting of at least three compartments, *viz.* the intracellular space occupying 1–5% of tissue volume, the space within the collagen fibrils (intrafibrillar space) and the extrafibrillar space containing the PGs (Wells, 1971); solutes do not necessarily distribute evenly between these compartments as discussed by Grynpas *et al.* (Chapter 60) and Maroudas (Chapter 53).

Model systems have been used to clarify the relationship between PG concentration, for instance, and solute partitions. Such model systems have consisted of PGs embedded in gelatine (Meyer *et al.*, 1971); PG solutions encased between membranes (Maroudas *et al.*, 1988; Comper and Preston, 1975); cartilage itself with various components removed enzymatically (Maroudas and Bannon, 1981); and mixtures of dextran and collagen (Bert *et al.*, 1980). The measurement of partition coefficients in such systems can help to relate the dependence of solute partition on concentration of the various cartilage components and, therefore, ultimately enable us to determine the extracellular concentration of solute, i.e. the concentration in the PG space relative to the collagen space. However, in all these systems it is difficult to work at high PG concentrations. Preston *et al.* (Chapter 61) describe a method which they have used to measure the partition coefficients of large solutes at high PG concentrations.

Theoretical models. The equilibrium distribution of a given solute between the cartilage and an external solution depends on the space within the matrix able to accommodate the solute; thus knowledge of the partition coefficient can also give us information on the structure and organization of the tissue. Models have thus been developed which relate the matrix composition to distribution coefficients. The models which are most often used are (i) the Donnan equilibrium condition for relating the composition of small ionic solutes to the cartilage composition (Helfferich, 1962; Maroudas, 1968); and (ii) the models of Curry and Michel (1980) and Ogston (1958) for relating the partition coefficient of large globular solutes to PG concentration. These models are critically reviewed by Silberberg in Chapter 64.

The Donnan equilibrium equations. Since the PGs of cartilage carry fixed negative charges, charged solutes are partitioned between the cartilage and any external solution such that the system is at electrochemical equilibrium. The equilibrium conditions can be described by the Gibbs–Donnan equations (Helfferich, 1962; Maroudas, 1968) which show that the sodium concentration of any ion in cartilage depends both on the molarity of the external solution and on the charge density, i.e. the GAG concentration. While the Gibbs–Donnan equations are only an estimate of the overall distribution of such solutes in cartilage, the results of calculations agree very well with experimental determinations (Maroudas and Evans, 1972). More sophisticated models, which describe the local distribution of ions, such as the Manning condensation model and the Poisson–Boltzman equations (reviewed by Grodzinsky, 1983) have been applied more to model systems than to cartilage (e.g. Wells, 1973; Comper and Preston, 1975; Parker et al., 1988). At the GAG concentration found in cartilages these equations approximate to the Gibbs–Donnan equilibrium conditions.

Large solutes. For large solutes a model developed by Ogston (1958) has been used with reasonable success to calculate partition coefficients in model systems (Ogston et al., 1973; Laurent et al., 1975) as has the partition coefficient of serum albumin in cartilage (Snowden and Maroudas, 1976) and in Wharton's jelly (see Chapter 54). An extension of this theory, the fiber matrix theory developed by Curry and Michel (1980), has been used for some interstitial tissues (Curry, 1984) but has so far not been applied to cartilage.

The diffusion coefficient

Solutes move through the matrix mainly by diffusion and their rate of movement is characterized by the matrix diffusion coefficient, $\bar{D}$; the larger the value of D the faster the rate of diffusion. In general, solute diffusion in the matrix is retarded relative to that in solution, because of 'obstacles' provided by the nonaqueous components of the matrix (Helfferich, 1962). For small solutes such as amino acids or glucose, $\bar{D}/D$ is 0.3–0.5 where D is the diffusion coefficient in solution (Maroudas, 1968, 1970; Bernich et al., 1976); because of frictional effects the degree of retardation increases with increase in solute size, so that $\bar{D}/D \simeq 0.04$–0.08 for Dextran 40. However, for asymmetric large molecules such as polyethylene glycol (Preston and Snowden, 1973) or collagen (Cumming et al., 1979), $\bar{D}/D$ appears to increase rather than decrease, possibly because these long thin molecules can only move along their long axis within the matrix, thus increasing their relative kinetic energy in that direction (de Gennes, 1979a,b). Unlike partition coefficients, diffusion coefficients do not appear to be influenced by charge of solute or matrix except at very low, nonphysiological ionic strengths (Maroudas and Evans, 1972; Comper and Preston, 1975; Maroudas et al., 1988; Parker et al., 1988).

Measurement of diffusion coefficients

Cartilage as a membrane. Most information on the diffusion coefficients of solutes in cartilage comes from treating previously frozen cartilage as a membrane and observing the transport of radioactive tracers across this cartilage membrane. The principles of this method are shown in Fig. 59.3. Here the cartilage slice, of uniform, accurately measured thickness, is clamped between two solutions. The first solution contains the solute at concentration C_1 together with a suitable radioactive isotope of the solute. The second

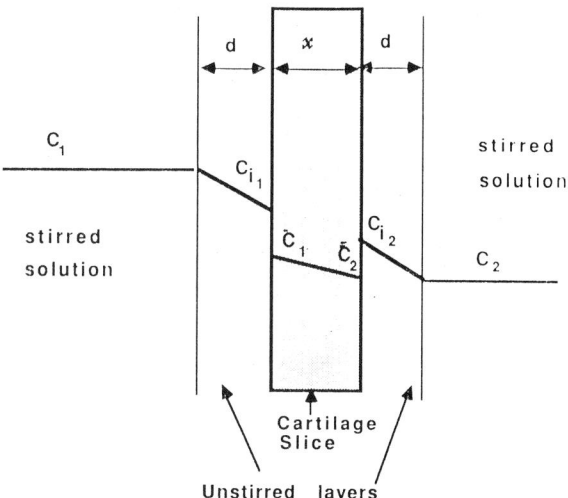

Figure 59.3 A schematic view of the steady-state concentration gradients across a slice of cartilage, showing the effect of the stagnant film.

solution contains no radioactive tracer; but contains solute at concentration C_2. If $C_1 = C_2$, there is only net movement of the radioactive tracer, and the 'self'-diffusion coefficient is obtained. If $C_1 \neq C_2$ then both solute and tracer diffuse and the 'mutual' diffusion coefficient is measured. Crank (1975) discusses the relationship between these diffusion coefficients.

In the situation described in Fig. 59.3, because there is no fluid flow and no reaction, the transport equation reduces to Ficks' first law and the diffusion coefficient can be obtained from measurement of J, the rate of movement of tracer from C_1 into C_2.

The diffusion coefficient can only be measured directly from the concentrations C_1 and C_2, which are not usually known. However, the permeability coefficient, P, can be obtained from the bulk solution concentrations C_1 and C_2, and is related to D by the partition coefficient K.

$$J = -\bar{D}\frac{(C_2 - C_1)}{x} = -P\frac{(C_2 - C_1)}{x}$$

$$P = K\bar{D}$$

In practice, the solution concentration at the interface is usually not the same as that in the bulk even if well stirred, because of the concentration gradient which develops in stagnant fluid film at the interface (Barry and Diamond, 1984). The error introduced by ignoring the stagnant film, depends on the film thickness α relative to cartilage thickness x, on the diffusivity in the liquid relative to that in solution and on the partition coefficient K. Membrane-diffusion controls and film diffusion is negligible when $(D/\bar{D}) \cdot (1/K) \cdot (x/d) \gg 2$ (Helfferich, 1962), i.e. for thick specimens in well-stirred solution and solutes with low values of K and $\bar{D}$. In cartilage, film diffusion is most likely to control for diffusion of divalent cations through thin cartilage slices (Maroudas and Urban, 1983).

If the cartilage 'membrane' strip of thickness l is equilibrated in a radioactive solute, and then placed in a solution containing no tracer, the diffusion coefficient can be obtained from the half-time of tracer desorption, $t_{1/2}$; the solution to the diffusion equation for such a system gives $\bar{D} = 0.49919/(t_{1/2}/l^2)$ (Crank and Park, 1968).

Maroudas and Venn (1977) measured the diffusion coefficient of tritiated water by this method and found the result was the same as that obtained from steady-state fluxes. Maroudas (1976) has also used this technique for measuring diffusion coefficients of large iodinated solutes, and discusses in detail the advantages of this technique over steady-state permeation methods for such solutes.

Concentration distance curves

Diffusion coefficients can also be obtained from concentration vs. distance curves (Crank and Park, 1968; Crank, 1975). In this method a pulse of radioactive tracer is placed at one end of a uniform strip of cartilage cut so that the width : length ratio is 0.1, and allowed to diffuse along the strip for a suitable time. Diffusion is halted by freezing, and the tracer concentration profile obtained by slicing the strip and determining the activity of each slice. Provided that diffusion is halted before the tracer reaches the far end of the strip, the diffusion coefficient can be obtained from the slope of the plot of ln(tracer activity) vs. (distance along the strip)^2, as discussed by Winlove and Parker (Chapter 62). This method has advantages for tissues like intervertebral disc or fibrillated cartilage which would swell if placed in a permeation cell. Diffusion coefficients of small solutes have been obtained in the disc using this technique (Urban and Maroudas, 1981). Concentration vs. distance curves have also been used to obtain diffusion coefficients in the disc nucleus by measuring the change in refractive index as solutes penetrated into the tissue (Paullson et al., 1951): in the latter study, if allowance was made for tissue swelling the results of both methods give values of $\bar{D}$ for the disc which are similar to those found in articular cartilage. These values of $\bar{D}$ give calculated profiles which agree satisfactorily with those measured experimentally (e.g. Urban et al., 1982).

Diffusion coefficients have also been obtained for cartilage plugs from measurements of nonsteady-state concentration profiles (Torzilli et al., 1987). In these studies, tracer diffused from a fluid phase into a cartilage plug. The nonsteady-state profiles were analyzed in terms of time-dependent diffusion and partition coefficients the values of which are difficult to compare with those defined using standard methods of analysis.

Model systems and gels

Solute diffusivities have been measured in PG or hyaluronate acid gels in many studies which are reviewed by Winlove and Parker (Chapter 62). The same authors also describe a capillary technique which is useful for the measurement of diffusion coefficients of large molecules in concentrated gels.

Theoretical models

Various models have been developed to describe the diffusion coefficient in cartilage relative to that in aqueous solution in terms of obstruction effects (Pappenheimer et al., 1951; Mackie and Meares, 1955). An alternative approach views diffusion as a stochastic process with the probability that a diffusional 'jump' will occur being proportional to the probability that a 'pore' of sufficient size lies adjacent to the diffusing solute (Lieb and Stein, 1971; Ogston et al., 1973) (see also Chapter 64).

Preston, Laurent and coworkers (reviewed Preston et al., 1984) in a more exact analysis define the diffusion coefficient in terms of a frictional and a thermodynamic component. The thermodynamic component arises from chemical potential differences, the frictional component can be defined in terms of excluded volume interactions between matrix and diffusing solute. However, none of these models can be used successfully over the whole range of matrix concentrations and sizes. The model of Mackie and Meares (1955) predicts the diffusivity of small solute in cartilage (Maroudas, 1970), while for large solutes the model of Ogston et al. (1973) is more reliable. For asymmetric particles, the possibility of 'end-on' movement or reptation must be considered (de Gennes, 1979a,b; Laurent et al., 1975; see also Chapters 55 and 64).

Effect of fluid flow

Solute transport can also be influenced by fluid flow. Solutes can be carried along with the fluid which flows as the result of the pressure gradients

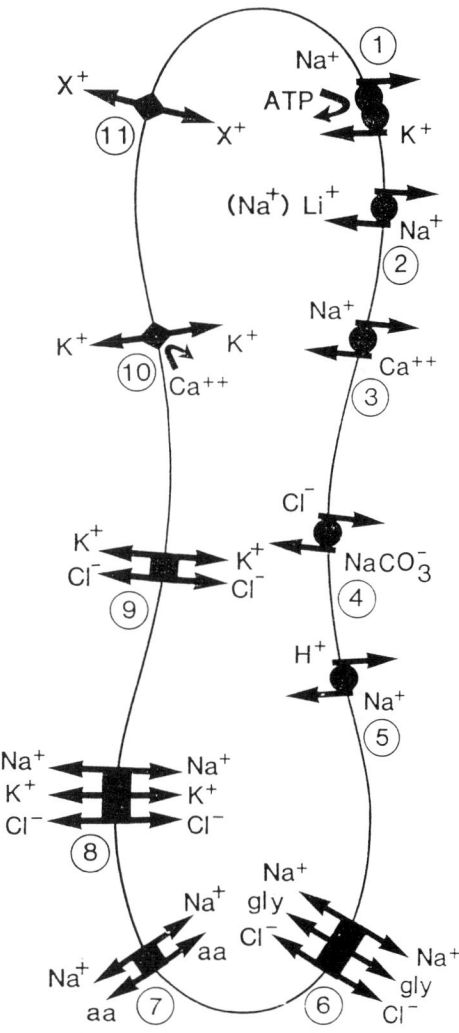

Figure 59.4 The major systems for transport of Na and K across a red cell membrane (stoichiometry not shown) (from Bernhardt et al. (1988) with permission). 1, Na/K pump; 2, Na/Li (Na/Na) exchange; 3, Na/Ca exchange (not present in human red cells); 4, $NaCO_3$/Cl exchange (via band 3); 5, Na/H exchange; 6, Na, Cl dependent glycine transport (gly); 7, Na dependent amino acid transport (ASC) and (N); 8, Na/K/Cl cotransport; 9, K/Cl cotransport; 10, Ca activated K transport; 11, Residual leak.

which arise during loading. Although fluid flow in cartilage has been studied extensively, little work has been done on how fluid-flow velocity influences solute transport. However, calculations show that transport of small solutes is virtually unaffected by fluid flow since their diffusion velocity in cartilage is much greater than the fluid velocity (Maroudas, 1986). However, because of the low diffusivity of macromolecules, the effect of fluid flow may be important in determining their overall rate of transport in cartilage. Although there is some experimental evidence to support these calculations (Urban et al., 1982; Katz et al., 1986; O'Hara et al., 1990), we do not know yet at which molecular weight the effect of fluid flow becomes important.

SOLUTE TRANSPORT ACROSS CELL MEMBRANES

Most of the work on solute transport in cartilage has been directed towards understanding transport of nutrients and other solutes through the matrix. However, nutrients do not only have to reach the cell from an external supply, they also have to penetrate into it. Solutes such as amino acids and glucose can only cross the cell membrane at a significant rate through specialized transport proteins (Yudilevich and Boyd, 1987; Jarvis, 1989). The cell membrane is also virtually impermeable to passive movement of ions, but not to water, and, in order to regulate osmolarity and maintain a constant internal environment, the membrane contains specific proteins which act as pumps, carriers or channels for transport of ions (Thomas, 1988; Glynn, 1989; Jan and Yuh, 1989). Figure 59.4 shows the 11 main transport pathways known to control K and Na transport into a red cell; these pathways have been found in a wide variety of cell types.

Although very little is known about membrane transport in chondrocytes, there is an enormous amount of literature covering the characterization, specificty and modes of actions of these transport proteins (see review by Stein (1986)), several of which have now been sequenced and cloned (e.g. James et al., 1989). In this section Hall (Chapter 63) reviews some of the methods of measuring solute fluxes into cells and shows how these techniques can readily be applied to chondrocytes.

ACKNOWLEDGMENTS

I am grateful to the Arthritis and Rheumatism Council for financial support.

60

Determining the elemental composition of articular cartilage: a comparison between human and non-human primates

M.D. GRYNPAS, J.M.D. CHATEAUVERT and K.P.H. PRITZKER

INTRODUCTION

Knowledge of the concentrations of ions in cartilage, that of calcium (Ca) in particular, may be directly relevant to understanding the pathogenesis of arthritic diseases. The hydrated calcium ion contributes to edema and the physical dissociation of cartilage in vitro (Pritzker et al.,

1981), but the relationship of Ca^{2+} and calcium content to cartilage edema *in vivo* remains to be established. The common forms of degenerative arthritis include osteoarthritis (OA) in which increased hydration of cartilage is a prominent feature (Brocklehurst et al., 1984), and calcium crystal arthropathies such as calcium pyrophosphate dihydrate (CPPD) and calcium apatite deposition diseases (Pritzker, 1980) which may be characterized by relative dehydration; in both cases extracellular ion concentrations will change.

There are very few studies available on the elemental content of articular cartilage. Previous studies on the elemental content of cartilage show a wide range of findings which are due, in part, to the methods by which the samples were obtained and analyzed. Through *in vitro* tracer cation methods, Benderly and Maroudas (1975) predicted that the elemental content of calcium and sodium in cartilage would be greatly increased as compared with synovial fluid or plasma, and that because of the strong interaction between calcium ions and cartilage, this increase in Ca^{2+} concentration can exist without calcium crystal formation. Lin and Sokoloff (1965) studied fluid expressed under controlled pressure from bovine nasal septum and Howell *et al.* (1968) used aspirate of epiphyseal plate cartilage. In both these studies, the contents of calcium and potassium were much lower than those reported by Benderly and Maroudas (1975) and were in the range of the interstitial fluid. Using the technique of neutron activation analysis, Nam and Reddy (1980) found in calf femoral condyle cartilage a Ca content of 2.3% which is several-fold higher than found by others. These differences may be attributed to the difficulty of analysis in the parts-per-million range.

As a first step to understanding the concentrations of elements in cartilage and their variation with disease, we studied the elemental content of articular cartilage from normal and OA human femoral heads and from right knee joints from 41 rhesus monkeys (*Macaca mulatta*) obtained from the Caribbean Primate Research Center (CPRC) in Puerto Rico (Chateauvert et al., 1989) using inductively coupled plasma emission spectroscopy (ICPES), a method capable of assaying simultaneously the content of multiple elements in a single tissue sample (Pritzker et al., 1987). The ICPES method is extremely sensitive, linear over a wide dynamic range, allows the simultaneous determination of many elements with a minimum of matrix interference and has, therefore, become one of the most used analytical techniques for examining the elemental content of biological tissues (Barnes, 1984).

METHODS

The articular cartilage (full depth) was removed by scalpel from the remaining bone. Care was taken to avoid excising the underlying calcified zone of cartilage, subchondral bone, osteophytic cartilage or areas with nonspecific calcifications. The cartilage fragments were immediately weighed, lyophilized overnight and reweighed to obtain wet and dry weights, respectively. The dried cartilage was pulverized into small granules with a mortar and pestle to obtain a homogeneous sample and stored under dessicating conditions at $-20°C$. Approximately 10 mg of dried tissue was wet ashed in 4–6 ml of a 4 : 1 v/v nitric acid : perchloric acid (70%) mixture. A sample-free acid mixture was used as a blank control. External standards included approximately 10 mg of phosphate rock (NBS 120b) and Oyster tissue (NBS 1566). On a low heat setting the mixture was gradually heated to boiling in covered teflon beakers for 1.5 h. The lids were then removed and boiling was allowed to continue until the volume of the digestate was reduced to less than 1 ml (c. 0.5–1 h). The residue was washed with double-distilled water (dH_2O) into accuvettes to a volume of 5 ml; potassium elemental concentrations were determined by using a flame photometer (IL model 943FP). Aspirates of $20 \mu l$ were taken from the 5 ml samples and were autodiluted with 2 ml of $1.5 \, mmol \, l^{-1}$ cesium and read in duplicate. The mean ± standard deviation values (in $mmol \, l^{-1}$) for potassium was obtained. Final concentrations were reported in mmol/kg dry tissue: dry weight values minimized the effects of variability in the initial hydration of the tissues arising from prolonged storage.

Table 60.1 Articular cartilage: elemental composition

Group (N)	[Ca]	[P]	[Mg]	[S]	[K]
Human					
Young normal (9) 29.8 ± 3.1 years*	118.6 ± 20.2†	54.7 ± 11.3	13.2 ± 1.4	407.7 ± 21.3	34.3 ± 3.7
Old normal (13) 75.5 ± 3.2 years	109.5 ± 16.7	46.6 ± 9.9	16.0 ± 1.4	392.2 ± 18.6	21.5 ± 4.2
Osteoarthritic (7) 67.1 ± 1.7 years	271.9 ± 32.7	141.1 ± 17.5	22.8 ± 2.2	335.5 ± 15.0	33.9 ± 7.0
Rhesus macaque					
Young normal (6) 8.0 ± 1.3 years	43.8 ± 8.1	38.1 ± 5.4	12.6 ± 1.9	367.3 ± 19.1	103.9 ± 9.6
Old normal (5) 18.2 ± 1.8 years	66.9 ± 12.7	57.7 ± 9.4	16.2 ± 1.9	439.4 ± 35.3	145.0 ± 18.7
Young OA (9) 12.6 ± 0.5 years	59.8 ± 7.1	42.2 ± 2.8	18.5 ± 1.7	470.7 ± 20.1	154.8 ± 15.6
Old OA (21) 18.7 ± 0.6 years	55.2 ± 5.0	44.1 ± 3.8	14.7 ± 1.2	411.9 ± 20.4	133.1 ± 9.2

* Mean age ± SEM.
† Mean [mmol kg dry weight] ± SEM.

The remainder of the 5 ml volume of sample was further diluted to a final volume of 20 ml with dH_2O and used for ICPES. Analysis by ICPES (Barnes, 1984) was used to determine elemental levels of calcium, phosphorus, magnesium and sulfur (using an ARL 34000 instrument). Aspirates of 6 ml were read in triplicate and a mean ± standard deviation in ppm ($\mu g\ ml^{-1}$) for each element was obtained. Final concentrations were expressed in mmol/kg dry tissue.

RESULTS

Detailed results of these experiments are reported elsewhere (Pritzker et al., 1987; Chateauvert et al., 1989). Of all the elements measured, the calcium and sulfur content can be considered extracellular and potassium as intracellular. The magnesium and phosphorus contents can be considered to be partitioned between cells and extracellular matrix with the intracellular contribution of both elements varying between 10 and 20% of the total (Pritzker et al., 1987).

If we compare the content of the cartilage elements in humans and nonhuman primates using age and OA as group dividers (Table 60.1), we can see that the main differences between humans and rhesus macaques are: (i) calcium concentration is twice as high in humans and (ii) lower cellularity in humans as shown by the lower potassium concentration. In OA the increase in calcium phosphorus and magnesium seen in humans is not reflected in monkeys.

The findings of decreased sulfur content in human OA vs. old normal cartilage holds in the rhesus study, while in the young OA monkeys there is a significant increase in sulfur vs. the young normals (Chateauvert et al., 1989) which confirms the findings of McDevitt and Muir (1976) of an increase in glycosaminoglycan content in early OA of dogs.

Calcium concentrations in monkeys were half those in humans and even lower than in dogs (Eichelberger, 1960), but were still many-fold higher than concentrations of circulating calcium. In contrast to humans, there was no difference between calcium in rhesus OA cartilage and controls. The phosphorus levels were similar in monkeys and humans, but there was no change with OA in the rhesus monkeys. For magnesium there was again a similarity between humans and monkeys; however, the young rhesus monkeys with OA exhibited an increase in Mg, showing the advantage of the monkey model for detecting early chemical changes in a spontaneous model of OA.

In conclusion, the differences in cartilage elemental composition between human and nonhuman primates may reflect the difference in disease progression in the two groups. The population of rhesus monkeys shows various stages of the disease while the human population shows predominantly end-stage disease.

61

Measurement of partition coefficient by gel chromatography

BARRY N. PRESTON, MARIE-PAULE I. VAN DAMME and WILLIAM H. MURPHY

INTRODUCTION

It is reasonable to suggest that many biological reactions take place in concentrated solutions of biopolymers, a situation which readily describes the extracellular environment. A major requirement for an understanding of physiological function of tissues such as cartilage is the quantitative measure of the interactions in such milieu. These interactions arise either from *steric exclusion effects*, due to the expanded domains of macromolecules such as proteoglycans (PGs), or from *electrostatic* interactions which also occur with proteoglycans (PGs). Thus, the composition in a local environment is influenced by the charged nature and concentration of the polymer species. Evaluation of the interactions is thus essential to the understanding of physiological transport processes (Comper and Laurent, 1978; Preston *et al.*, 1984).

A quantitative estimation of the interactions that occur between PGs (or other polymeric species) and other solutes can be made by studying the distribution of the solutes between a PG-rich phase and an adjoining polymer-free phase. The measurement made is the partition coefficient, which is defined as the ratio of the concentration (w/v) of solute in the polymer-rich phase to that in the polymer-free phase.

Until recently, the effects of high concentrations of polymer on the partitioning of a solute between a polymer solution and a polymer-free solution were measured by equilibrium dialysis across a membrane. However, this technique has limitations with regard to the availability of membranes impermeable to the solute under study, e.g. low-molecular-weight solutes ($M_r \leq 10\,000$). This is particularly true when studies are carried out at high polymer concentrations (> 10% w/w). Furthermore, long times are required for attainment of equilibrium (Preston *et al.*, 1972).

In this investigation a frontal gel chromatographic technique (Van Damme *et al.*, 1989), where the gel or other macroporous media replaces the membrane, is described, which provides a faster and more convenient means of obtaining the required partition coefficient. Furthermore, a greater versatility accrues from the fact that the method can be applied to systems in which the larger solute is partially excluded from the gel phase, a situation that is equivalent to a partially permeable membrane.

Application of the gel chromatographic procedure will be illustrated using systems displaying both electrostatic (binding) effects and steric excluded volume effects. The ionic interaction behavior has been measured in systems considered as appropriate models of connective tissues such as dextran sulfate–NaCl and chondroitin sulfate–NaCl. The steric exclusion behavior has been measured in a globular protein–polyethylene glycol (PEG) system. The resultant partition coefficients are compared with those obtained from equilibrium dialysis (Preston et al., 1972) or deduced from phase-separation studies (Atha and Ingham, 1981).

THEORETICAL ASPECTS

In equilibrium dialysis of a mixture of macromolecular solute P and smaller solute S across a membrane impermeable to solute P, the final state may be described in terms of one phase with solute concentrations $\bar{C}_P$ and $\bar{C}_S$ where the bar indicates the phase in presence of polymer and a second phase with concentrations C_S and $C_P = 0$. The partition coefficient of solute S brought about by the presence of the polymer is simply given by

$$\alpha = \bar{C}_S / C_S$$

A similar situation to equilibrium dialysis is observed in frontal gel chromatography if the stationary phase which replaces the dialysis membrane excludes the larger component (polymer) whilst allowing the smaller solute to be distributed between the mobile and stationary phases. The sample containing both polymer and small solute is loaded on the column until the eluate concentration is identical to that of the original sample. Elution is then continued with solvent until both solutes are washed off the column. Various stages of the elution are shown in Fig. 61.1, the profiles being illustrative of systems displaying either steric exclusion properties (Fig. 61.1(A)) or ionic or other associative behavior (Fig. 61.1(B)). The excluded solute is initially

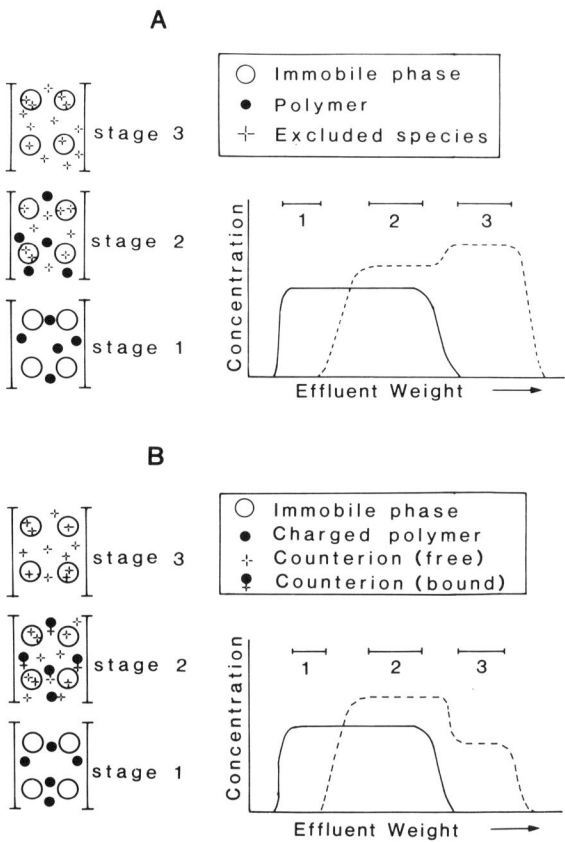

Figure 61.1 Schematic representation showing the stages and the corresponding elution profiles when an interacting mixture containing a macromolecule (○) and small solute (+) is subjected to frontal gel chromatography. (A) Profile of a small solute being excluded by the macromolecule. (B) Associative interaction between a charged polymer and its counterion.

eluted and reaches its original concentration (stage 1). Elution of the small solute follows and also attains its original concentration (stage 2). After changing the eluent to solvent, the polymeric solute is removed from the column. However, the concentration of the small solute in the mobile phase is then changed, being enhanced for steric exclusion effects or reduced for electrostatic, associative effects, thus yielding a new plateau region of higher concentration for steric interactions (stage 3, Fig. 61.1(A)) and a lower concentration for binding (stage 3, Fig. 61.1(B)), which is identified as being the concentration of 'unbound' species. Thus in these studies the partition coefficient of the small solute is simply given by C (stage 2/stage 3); this is equivalent to the term $\bar{C}_S/C_S$ described earlier.

A more detailed theoretical analysis of the techniques has been described recently (Van Damme et al., 1989). In this technique the analysis does allow for quantitative evaluation of the interactions between the two solutes, even if the macromolecular solute is incompletely excluded and/or where the accessibility of the stationary phase to the smaller solute is restricted. Such a situation would correspond to the equilibrium dialysis where the membrane is partially permeable to both solutes.

METHODS AND RESULTS

The columns were packed with either Fractogel TSK or controlled pore glass (CPG 75) as the porous stationary phase. The CPG 75 was coated with PEG ($M_r = 20\,000$) to reduce nonspecific adsorption effects (Hiatt et al., 1971).

The results from three studies, indicative of the diverse uses of the technique, are given here; we report on:

(i) ionic interactions which occur between chondroitin sulfate (CS) and sodium ions;
(ii) similar interactions between dextran sulfate and sodium ions—however, in this case, ionic exclusion is so significant that problems arise in the convective stability of the mobile phase; and
(iii) the steric exclusion of PEG ($M_r = 4000$) by serum albumin—in this case the smaller solute, the PEG, is *partially* excluded from the stationary phase.

The trailing frontal elution profile for both Na$^+$ and CS from a solution of CS (47 mg g^{-1}) in 0.1 M NaCl tagged with radioactive ^{22}Na$^+$ is shown in Fig. 61.2. The Na$^+$ profile displays the two distinct plateau regions as predicted by theory (see Fig. 61.1(A)). The partition coefficient α_{Na^+}, as given

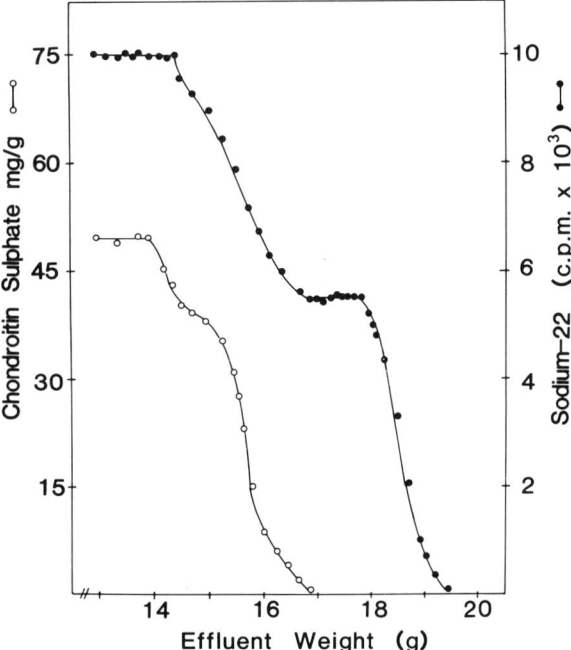

Figure 61.2 The trailing elution profile obtained for ^{22}Na$^+$ (●) and tracheal CS (○) in frontal gel chromatography of CS (50 mg ml^{-1} in 0.1 M NaCl. The column (40 × 0.66 cm) which contained controlled pore glass (CPG-75) pretreated with PEG ($M_r = 20\,000$) was eluted at a flow rate of 0.4 ml h^{-1}. Fractions of 0.32 g were collected until the vicinity of the second plateau for ^{22}Na$^+$ where smaller fractions (0.08 g) were collected in order to obtain a discernible plateau. CS was measured by uronic acid analysis and ^{22}Na$^+$ in a LKB Multigamma counter.

by the ratio of the two plateau regions yields a value of 1.78, which compares favorably with a coefficient of 1.72 as determined by equilibrium dialysis using a benzoylated cellulose membrane (G. Checkley, personal communication). The partition coefficient for Cl$^-$ was 0.67. The charge concentration of CS derived from the electroneutrality condition

$$\bar{C}_{\text{Na}^+} = \bar{C}_{\text{Cl}^-} + C_P$$

(where $\bar{C}_{\text{Na}^+}$ and $\bar{C}_{\text{Cl}^-}$ are calculated from the partition coefficients obtained above) was

0.150 meq ml^{-1} for a 4.7% solution. For a comparable charge concentration Maroudas (1980) obtained partition coefficients for Na$^+$ and Cl$^-$ between cartilage from the femoral head and NaCl solutions of 1.83 and 0.61, respectively, values which are in good agreement with our data.

In a similar experiment on a solution of dextran sulfate (M_r = 45 600) at a concentration of 100 mg ml^{-1} in 0.1 M NaCl tagged with ^{22}Na$^+$, when the elution was carried out with solvent, then no clear plateau region was observed in the trailing elution profile of the Na$^+$; this effect can be seen in Fig. 61.3 (open symbols). It was considered that, under these conditions, the exclusion of the salt by the highly charged dextran sulfate may have reduced the concentration of NaCl in, and hence the density of, the mobile phase. The subsequent addition of 0.1 M NaCl as solvent may have initiated convective flows in the mobile phase due to density inversions (Laurent et al., 1983). This suggestion received support when the eluting solvent was replaced by water and the subsequent trailing profile displayed the two plateaux expected (Fig. 61.3, closed symbols).

The partition coefficient of Na$^+$ (α = 4.6) obtained from these results correlates well with the value obtained using equilibrium dialysis (α = 5.3). Therefore, in all subsequent analyses the solutes were eluted from the column with water, even though the sample was prepared in 0.1 M NaCl and applied on the chromatographic column preequilibrated in this same solvent.

In Fig. 61.4 the corresponding trailing elution profile for the system of bovine serum albumin (30 mg g^{-1}) and PEG 4000 (1.5 mg g^{-1}) is shown. The partition coefficient was calculated as 0.91. The only reported measurement on this system, which may be interpreted in terms of steric exclusion effects, was carried out by phase-separation experiments (Atha and Ingham, 1981). In this case, the measured interaction coefficient is greater than expected from the measurements of Atha and Ingham (1981), but less than that expected on the basis of molecular models (Van Damme et al., 1989).

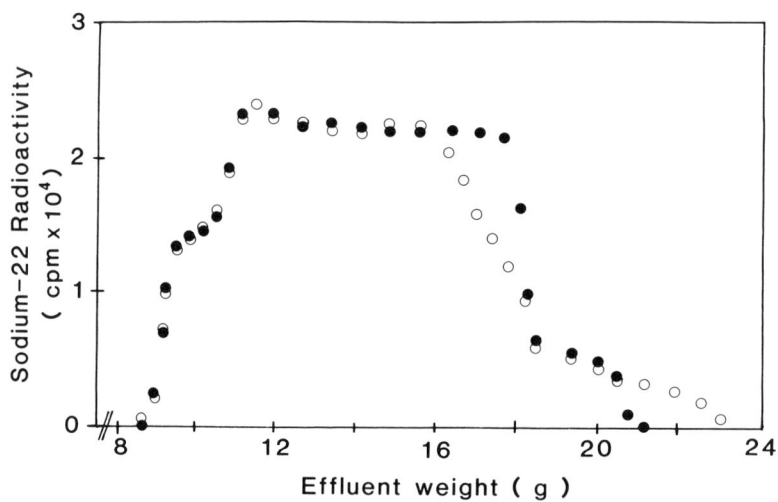

Figure 61.3 The trailing elution profile of ^{22}Na$^+$ in frontal gel chromatography of dextran sulfate (100 mg ml^{-1}) on a column (40 × 0.66 cm) packed with CPG-75. After application of 10 ml of sample in 0.1 M NaCl, the solutes were eluted with either 0.1 M NaCl (○) or water (●) at a flow rate of 0.4 ml hr^{-1}.

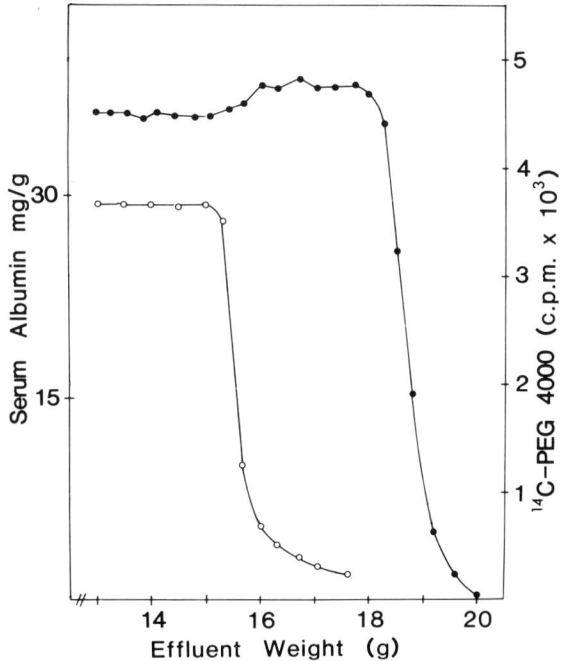

Figure 61.4 Elution profile obtained for frontal gel experiments on mixtures of [^{14}C]PEG-4000 as small solute (●) and the protein (○), bovine serum albumin (10 mg ml^{-1}). The column (48 × 1.2 cm) packed with Fractogel TSK HW40 as the stationary phase was eluted at a flow rate of 18 ml h^{-1}. The fraction size was 0.35 ml. Protein was monitored by absorbance at 280 nm, and [^{14}C]PEG by liquid scintillation spectrometry.

Further examples of the use of frontal gel chromatography in estimating molecular interactions are given in the paper by Van Damme et al. (1989).

CONCLUDING REMARKS

The gel chromatographic technique described offers a simple reproducible procedure for measuring partition coefficients from which interactions occurring between two species may be analyzed. This technique has several advantages over equilibrium dialysis, the method used previously to study molecular interactions. Firstly, the experiments can be performed and analyzed within 2 days, and secondly, the availability of gel chromatographic media with markedly different porosities provide a wide range in the experimental choice of a solute as being 'small'.

The present method is thus not confined to studies where the designated solutes are as small as those considered above. These solutes were chosen only because we were able to compare our findings with previously reported data in order to validate the technique.

62

Measurement of diffusion coefficients in biopolymer solutions and gels

C.P. WINLOVE and K.H. PARKER

Diffusion is an important mechanism for the transport of solutes through the extracellular matrix of connective tissues (Comper and Laurent, 1978; Maroudas, 1980; Preston et al., 1984).

Disturbances in transport are often cited as a factor in connective-tissue pathology and hypotheses have been advanced implicating a whole range of solutes from small nutrients and metabolites to the matrix macromolecules themselves. As our understanding of the structure and biochemical composition of connective tissue develops, it becomes increasingly important to relate these properties to the mass-transport characteristics of the tissue. Only a limited range of measurements are possible in intact tissue and so studies in simple model systems can provide essential information. As we will demonstrate later, a measurement of the diffusion coefficient of a particular solute in a particular matrix can also provide information about interactions between solute and matrix and, conversely, the diffusion properties of well-characterized probe molecules in a particular matrix can provide information about the pore structure of that matrix (Ogston *et al.*, 1973; Meyer *et al.*, 1977; Phillips and Jansons, 1990).

Many methods of measuring diffusion coefficients are available and both they and the rigorous theory of diffusion processes are discussed extensively in the physical-chemistry literature (Vrentas and Duda, 1979; Spragg, 1980; Muhr and Blanshard, 1982; Harding, 1986) and it is not our intention to summarize this material here. We will very briefly note some of the problems which may be encountered in the study of biological molecules and then suggest a very simple, inexpensive technique which seems suitable for use with biopolymers.

One of the classical ways of measuring diffusion coefficients is by means of a diffusion cell (Gosting, 1956). This cell consists of two chambers separated by a membrane containing pores which are sufficiently small to eliminate convective motion between the chambers but large enough not to hinder the passage of solute molecules. The solute is added to one chamber and its diffusivity is determined from its rate of appearance in the second chamber. The method has been applied to a wide range of solutes and is capable of considerable accuracy. However, central to the interpretation of the experimental data is the assumption that the chambers are well mixed and concentration gradients occur only across the membrane. These conditions are extremely difficult to establish for viscous polymer solutions, particularly those which may be broken down by large shear forces. In our experience, they limit the method to solutions no more viscous than, for example, 0.5% (w/v) articular cartilage proteoglycans (PGs) monomer. The choice of membrane is also important and we have experienced difficulty with biopolymers which adsorb either reversibly or irreversibly to the surface and pores of the membrane, thereby altering its permeability characteristics. The volume of solution required to fill the chambers may be a disadvantage in the study of well-characterized biopolymers and the long experimental times needed for large solutes are inconvenient and may pose problems of degradation. Notwithstanding these objections, we have had some success in the study of dilute PGs with very small cells (about 5 ml chamber volume) using Nucleopore membranes, but great care was necessary in calibrating and setting up the cells.

Ultracentrifuge and light-scattering techniques are now widely used in the measurement of diffusion coefficients (Spragg, 1980; Harding, 1986). Without going into detail about the many different methods, we may observe that in some cases the derivation of diffusion coefficients from the experimental data is indirect and depends upon many assumptions concerning, for example, the 'shape' of the diffusing molecule and the homogeneity of the sample. The interpretation of data from heterogeneous mixtures of complex molecules is being actively considered by a number of groups, but the magnitude of the problem has been strikingly demonstrated in recent studies on PGs which found up to an order of magnitude difference between diffusivities measured by light scattering and by ultracentrifugation (Harper *et al.*, 1985). A further problem which has been noted in studies on PGs is that at the high pressures prevailing in the ultracentrifuge the thermodynamic properties of macromolecules and macromolecular assemblies may be different from those under normal conditions (Reihanian *et al.*, 1979). It also seems that at present these methods are best applied to dilute solutions and to single-component systems where matrix and diffusant are identical.

A major constraint in biological investigations is that often only a small amount of the substrate in

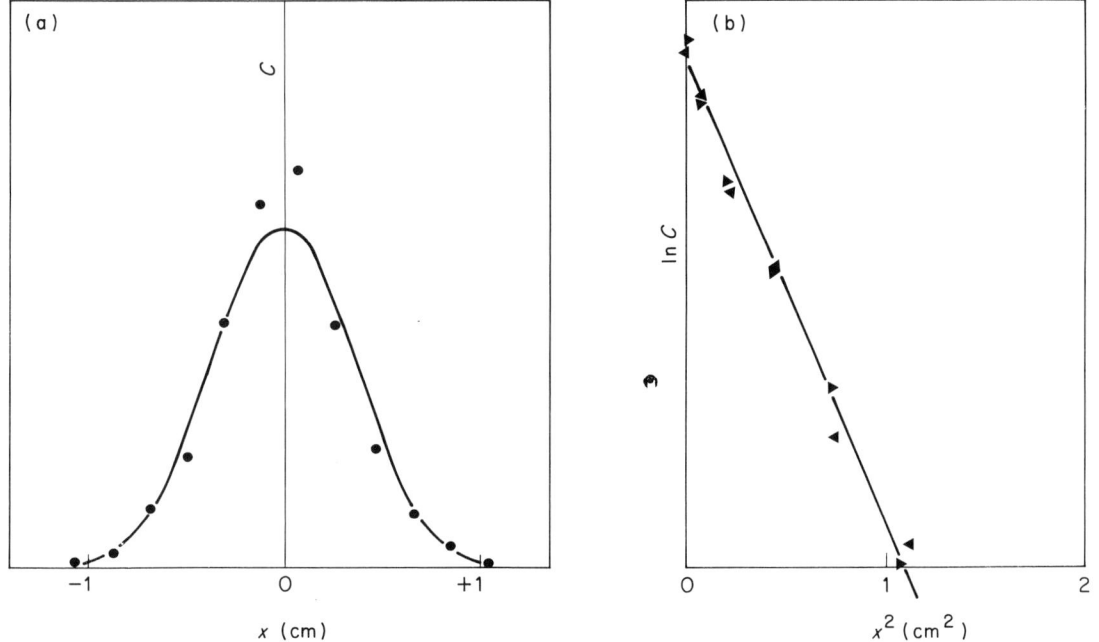

Figure 62.1 The analysis of the diffusion of [^{125}I]albumin in a capillary tube containing 0.5% occipital PG. (a) Tracer radioactivity, C, vs. distance, x, from the injection site determined from the 'centre of mass' of the measured activity. x is calculated for the midpoint of each section. The line is the line of best fit calculated from plot (b). (b) The data of (a) plotted as $\ln C$ vs. x^2. (▶) right-hand-side, (◀) left-hand-side of the curve. Experiments not showing symmetry are rejected. The line was obtained by linear regression and the slope ($= -1/4DT$) corresponds to $D = 3.59 \times 10^{-7}\,\text{cm}^2\,\text{s}^{-1}$. (Incubation time $T = 48\,\text{h}$).

which diffusivity is to be measured is available. This has led a number of workers to study diffusion into or out of open-ended capillary tubes packed with the substrate (e.g. Magdalenat et al., 1974). The major uncertainties in this technique concern the boundary conditions prevailing at the end of the tube. These errors are largest in studies on slowly-diffusing solutes, but even for rapidly-diffusing solutes they have been of sufficient magnitude to lead to errors in interpretation (Hadler, 1980; Norton et al., 1982). Some investigators have immersed the capillaries in solutions during the experiments, but unless the composition of the solution is carefully considered this procedure can lead to large gradients of chemical potential across the boundary and introduces the partition coefficient of the solute between substrate and solution into the calculation of diffusivity.

Realization of these difficulties led us to develop a variant of the capillary-tube technique in which the tube is sealed at both ends and a microinjection of radiolabeled tracer is made through the wall of the plastic capillary. Full details of the technique and method of data analysis have been reported previously (Winlove and Parker, 1984; Maroudas et al., 1988). Briefly, diffusion is allowed to proceed until the tracer has spread a centimeter or two along the tube. The distribution of tracer is then determined by sectioning the tube longitudinally and assaying the radioactivity in each section. In most of our experiments we first froze the tube and cut sections down to 0.5 mm in length in a special jig mounted in a cryostat, though if the matrix is sufficiently viscous, the freezing step may be omitted. For simple Fickian diffusion the distribution of radioactivity should be Gaussian and a plot a ln(concentration) vs.

(distance from injection site)^2 should be linear and of slope $-1/4DT$ where T is the duration of the experiment (see Fig. 62.1). The position of the injection site is determined from the requirement of symmetry of the left- and right-hand branches of the measured curve. This position and the diffusivity are computed from a linear-regression analysis and the improvement in precession which is gained has been found to be very significant. A further advantage of the method is that departures from simple Fickian diffusion are readily detected. These can arise, for example, from heterogeneity of the injected sample or interaction between the injectate and the matrix. In certain favorable cases, the data analysis can provide diffusion coefficients for several components simultaneously or, in other cases, quantitative information about the binding constants (Winlove and Parker, 1984).

In developing this technique we expected that nonuniform packing across the diameter of the capillary or in freezing would give rise to artefacts. However, in a range of investigations covering polymer (principally PGs) concentrations from 0.01% to 10% (w/v) and solutes from small ions to PG aggregates, we have found no evidence for these effects. Nor have we found that injection of the sample leads to the convective instabilities which have been observed in polymer mixtures (Harper et al., 1985) (possibly because of the very small volume injected). Care is required, however, when working with low-viscosity solutions so that convection is not produced either by handling or temperature variations. These effects are readily detected from the asymmetry of the tracer distribution.

We are at present working on a variant of the capillary-tube technique using fluorescent rather than radiolabeled tracers. The distribution of tracer is determined by quantitative fluorescence microscopy with the advantages of higher spatial resolution and the ability to observe the temporal evolution of the tracer distribution.

ACKNOWLEDGMENTS

It is a pleasure to thank Mrs A.R. Ewins and Mr N.E. Birchler who have shared with us many of the trials and frustrations of diffusivity measurements. This work was supported by the BP Venture Research Unit, the SERC, the Wellcome Trust and the Clothworkers Foundation to whom we are grateful.

63

Techniques for studying membrane transport

ANDREW C. HALL

INTRODUCTION

Membrane transport processes play key roles in a number of basic areas of cell physiology and Table 63.1 shows some examples of transport pathways which have been studied. This list is by no means complete since there has been an enormous amount of work in this field and for those interested in more detail there are many comprehensive reviews available (e.g. Hille, 1984; Stein, 1986). In addition, although the movement of ions across the membranes of both excitable and

Table 63.1 Some properties of selected membrane transport pathways in mammalian cells

Pathway	Examples of physiological function	Inhibitor*	Comments	Reference
Active transport				
Na/K pump	Cell volume regulation	Ouabain	Found in almost all animal cells	Glynn and Karlish (1975), Glynn (1988)
	Maintenance of internal environment		Transports 2 K ions into the cell in exchange for 3 Na ions, with the hydrolysis of ATP	
	Generation of Na gradient into cells			
Ca pump	Maintains a very low ($<10^{-7}$ M) intracellular Ca concentration	Vanadate	Found in all eukaryotic cell membranes	Schatzmann (1989); Campbell (1983)
			Ca efflux with hydrolysis of ATP	
Secondary active transport				
Amino acids (e.g. system ASC)	Transport of neutral amino acids (e.g. alanine, serine)	NEM	Driven by the inward Na gradient generated by the Na/K pump	Eddy (1987)
NaKCl cotransport	Cell volume regulation	Bumetanide	Found in many cell types	Chipperfield (1986)
Na:H exchange	Cell pH regulation	Amiloride	Found in many cell types. Uses Na gradient to expel H ions	Hoffmann and Simonsen (1989)
Facilitated diffusion				
Amino acids (e.g. system L)	Transport of leucine, valine, etc.	BCH	Wide species and tissue distribution	Ellory (1987)
Anion transport (Cl, HCO$_3$)	Gas transport in blood. Cell pH regulation	DIDS	Capable of very rapid fluxes of a wide variety of anions	Jennings (1985)
Channels				
Stretch-activated	Mechanoreceptors in endothelial cells? Cell volume control	Gadolinium	Activated by membrane deformation. Found in a wide range of bacterial and animal cell membranes	Kullberg (1987)

* NEM, n-ethylmaleimide; BCH, 2-aminonorborane-2-carboxylic acid; DIDS, 4,4'-diisothiocyanato-2-2'-stilbene-disulfonic acid.

inexcitable cells via specific channels (voltage and ligand-gated) is crucial to the functioning of many cell types and has been studied at the single-channel level using patch-clamp techniques, these will not be discussed further here (see Hille, 1984).

In the present chapter I briefly describe the use of separation techniques which, coupled with radioisotopes, are very versatile methods for studying membrane transport. These experiments can be performed essentially on any isolated cell type (erythrocytes, Ascites tumour cells, hepatocytes, chondrocytes, myocytes, etc.) or membrane preparation (e.g. membrane vesicles) allowing a wide range of substrate concentrations and conditions to be tested. Considering the cells and medium as a two-compartment system, it is generally more sensitive to look at the accumulation of tracer in the empty compartment rather than its depletion in the other. Many transport systems are highly specific and so the tracer under study must have very similar transport characteristics to those of the natural substrate. Intracellular (and rarely extracellular) metabolism must be eliminated, particularly in efflux studies, or nonmetabolized analogs can be used when the permeant substrate is subjected to intracellular metabolism (e.g. 3-*O*-methylglucose for glucose).

UPTAKE STUDIES

Washing techniques

The basic methods used for influx (uptake) studies are shown in Fig. 63.1. Techniques for cell isolation are now well established, however it is important to emphasize that transport studies have to be performed on cells free of extracellular matrix because otherwise there will be problems due to diffusion near the membrane (see Barry and Diamond, 1984). The use of a low cytocrit and relatively short incubation time (sufficient to allow about 5% accumulation of extracellular tracer into the cells) avoids a significant decrease in extracellular tracer which can occur during the course of the experiment and also ensures that the movement of the test substance is unidirectional (i.e. into the cell with no backflow). Ideally, cell suspensions (containing the radiotracer of interest) should be prepared in microcentrifuge tubes (1.5-ml capacity), because the subsequent processing of the cells using any of the small centrifuges available (Eppendorf, Beckman, etc.) is then straightforward. The centrifuges can hold 12–18 tubes, have run-up and run-down times of a few seconds and are ideally suited for use in these experiments.

Oil-separation techniques

For rapid fluxes where there is the possibility of a significant loss of accumulated tracer during washing, or when the cells are fragile and may disintegrate during washing, centrifugation through a denser, water-immiscible layer is a useful technique (Fig. 63.1). The cell pellet will,

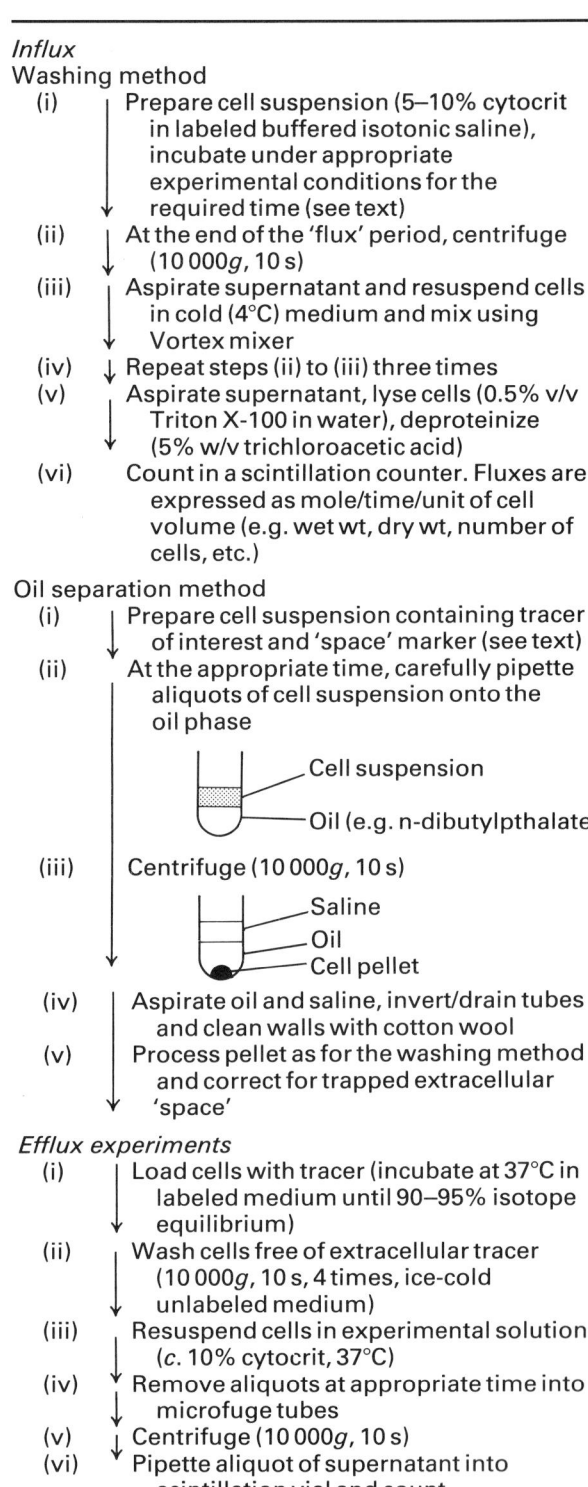

Figure 63.1 Some techniques used for studies on membrane transport.

however, contain some extracellular tracer caused by the passage of the cells through the oil and this is taken into account by the addition of an impermeant radioactive 'space' marker (e.g. [^{14}C]inulin) to the cell suspension. It is important to ensure that the least-dense cells do not remain at the oil–water interface. If the transported substance is subjected to intracellular metabolism, a third (bottom) layer of concentrated formic acid can be included in the centrifuge tube. This allows the cells to be lysed and deproteinized as soon as they pass through the oil. The fastest practicable time for measuring fluxes using this technique is about 5 s, and for fluxes longer than about 1 min there is little to choose between the washing and oil-separation methods. The most suitable method therefore depends to a large extent on the transport rate of the test substance.

FILTRATION TECHNIQUES

Another washing technique which rapidly separates cells from medium, utilizes nitro- or methyl-cellulose filters (pore sizes ranging from 0.2–0.45 µm). Glass-fiber prefilters are used to reduce clogging and lysis. For uptake experiments, cells incubated with the appropriate radioactive medium are rapidly diluted, filtered onto the membrane by suction (e.g. using the Millipore filter system) and washed. The filter is then assayed by dissolving it in scintillation fluid. For efflux experiments, the cell-free filtrates can be collected. Care should be taken with the type of filter used since there can be selective binding of ions or organic molecules. Time courses of about 5 s or more are possible with simple Millipore-Swinnex filters (e.g. Cousin and Motais, 1976); the flow-tube method, which is the ultimate refinement of this technique allows resolution to 5 ms (Brahm, 1976).

EFFLUX EXPERIMENTS

The techniques described above are also used for efflux experiments since in this case it is the appearance of radiotracer in the extracellular space which is determined (see Fig. 63.1). For further details on the methods used for influx and efflux studies see Ellory and Young (1982).

SOME PROBLEMS WITH TRANSPORT EXPERIMENTS

Although isotope flux methods are powerful tools for studying membrane transport processes, they give little information about the *net* movement of the substance of interest. For these experiments, techniques which allow the direct determination of the concentration of the substance (e.g. flame photometry for Na, K, or ion-selective electrodes) can be used in conjunction with the separation techniques outlined above. For some substances there may be intracellular compartmentalization and/or metabolism, surface binding and cell heterogeneity. This can make the interpretation of flux (particularly efflux) data quite complex requiring multicompartmental analysis.

POTASSIUM UPTAKE IN ARTICULAR CHONDROCYTES

The following experiment serves to illustrate the flexibility of membrane transport experiments and the information which can be obtained. For convenience, an experiment is described where radiotracer uptake of K (using ^{86}Rb as a potassium congener) into chondrocytes was studied. It should be noted that, although the concentration gradient for potassium is normally from the cells to medium (because chondrocytes, like most mammalian cells, possess high concentrations of potassium), it is possible to measure the *unidirectional* tracer uptake because for the tracer the concentration gradient is from the extracellular to intracellular compartment.

Bovine articular cartilage from the metacarpophalangeal joint was used and cells isolated using a standard technique (Zanetti et al., 1985). Cell suspensions of $1–2 \times 10^6$ cells ml^{-1} were prepared in saline of the following composition (mM); NaCl 145; KCl 7.5; glucose 5; MOPS (or any good buffer) 15; (300 mOsm, pH 7.4). To assess the contribution of various potassium transport pathways (see Table 63.1) inhibitors of the Na/K pump (ouabain) and (Na + K) cotransporter (bumetanide) were added as required at maximally inhibiting doses (0.1 mM). In addition, the effect of cell shrinkage on potassium transport was studied by measuring fluxes (37°C) in the above medium with 100 mM sucrose added. Control experiments established that potassium uptake was linear over 10 min (i.e. the flux was unidirectional, see above) and, therefore, this was used as the incubation time. Figure 63.2 shows that at 300 mOsm the Na/K pump (i.e. ouabain-sensitive) and (Na + K) co-transport (i.e. bumetanide-sensitive) pathways account for 34% and 12% of the total potassium uptake, respectively. In chondrocytes shrunken by the addition of sucrose to the incubation medium (final osmolality 400 mOsm), the contribution of these transporters to total potassium flux was increased slightly (40% and 17%, respectively), but did not reach the level of significance ($p > 0.05$). The residual flux (i.e. that remaining when ouabain and bumetanide were present) decreased significantly to 43% in the 400 mOsm solution from 55% in the 300 mOsm solution ($p < 0.01$).

These data show that, as with other cell types, potassium transport in chondrocytes is mediated partly by the Na/K pump and (Na + K) cotransport pathways. In addition, there is another pathway (or pathways) which is sensitive to the osmolality of the extracellular medium. The activity of the transporters sensitive to medium osmolality might be particularly relevant in the control of chondrocyte potassium content, since the pericellular environment of the chondrocyte in load-bearing cartilages is constantly changing as fluid is pumped into and out of the tissue (Urban and Bayliss, 1989). Finally, these cells exhibit a relatively large residual potassium flux (i.e. that which remains in the presence of ouabain, bumetanide and hypertonicity) and it would be interesting to determine if, for example, voltage-

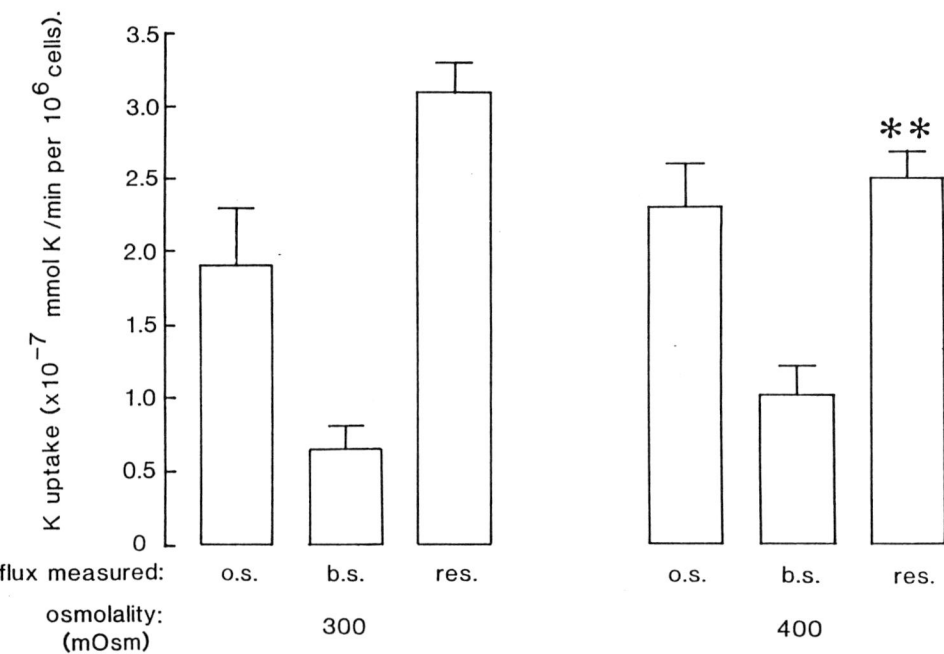

Figure 63.2 Pathways for potassium transport in bovine articular chondrocytes. Fluxes were measured as described in text. o.s., Ouabain-sensitive (i.e. Na/K pump); b.s., bumetanide-sensitive (i.e. NaKCl cotransport); res., residual flux (i.e. that which remains in the presence of ouabain and bumetanide). The results shown are mean ± SEM of at least three independent experiments under the different conditions.

gated potassium channels which might contribute to this flux play a role in the control of cell potassium content and hence chondrocyte biosynthesis.

ACKNOWLEDGMENT

This work was supported in part by the Arthritis and Rheumatism Council.

64

Characterization of networks by the use of molecular probes: static and dynamic methods

A. SILBERBERG

Analysis of the structure and organization of solid, gel-like systems which are heterogeneous on the macromolecular scale is complicated since methods using direct external observation of the intact system are of limited power and resolution. Methods using a more indirect approach, via molecular probes, have thus been extensively used. The methods often involve the determination of the *partition coefficient*, i.e. the determination, in thermodynamic equilibrium, of the effective exclusion of the probe molecule by the structural elements of the system under investigation, or of the *diffusion and/or permeation coefficients* of the tissue, in the hope that measurements of the extent of accessibility as evidenced by a change in diffusion or permeation coefficient can be meaningfully interpreted. In the case of cartilage, as with any other system, molecular probes must obviously be found which are small enough to enter the system, may have to be recognizable when they are inside and must avoid disturbing, or altering, the connections and the structure of the network and its contents. In this chapter I summarize the problems connected with the use of molecular-sized 'investigators' for the purpose of probing connective-tissue structure and the theoretical difficulties associated with a meaningful interpretation of the results.

EQUILIBRIUM DIALYSIS TECHNIQUES

In 1958 Ogston (Ogston, 1958) wrote a very fundamental paper in which he analyzed the distribution of free spaces in a system of infinitely thin rigid rods of length L, n_R rods per unit volume, distributed at random through the system. The probability that a sphere of radius r_S can find a space available to it without any change of the rod system was found to be

$$P(r_S; n_R L) = \exp\{-n_R[\pi L r_S^2 + (4\pi/3)r_S^3]\} \quad (64.1a)$$

which becomes

$$P(r_S; n_R L) \simeq 1 - n_R[\pi L r_S^2 + (4\pi/3)r_S^3]; \quad n_R \to 0 \quad (64.1b)$$

when $n_R L$ is sufficiently small. Ogston also speculated that this formula would still hold if the rods were of finite (but thin) cross-sectional radius $r_R (r_R \ll L)$ and showed that, in that case, formulae equations (64.1a) and (64.1b) would become

$$P(r_S; n_R L, r_R) = \exp\{-n_R[\pi L(r_S + r_R)^2 + (4\pi/3)(r_S + r_R)^3]\} \quad (64.2a)$$

and

$$P(r_S; n_R L, r_R) \simeq 1 - n_R[\pi L(r_S + r_R)^2 + (4\pi/3)(r_S + r_R)^3]; n_R \to 0 \quad (64.2b)$$

respectively. It will be noticed (see Fig. 64.1) that the expression appearing in square brackets in equations (64.2a) and (64.2b) is the volume excluded by infinitely thin rods to spheres of radius $(r_S + r_R)$.

In the case of a network there are no ends, n_R tends to zero, but $n_R L$, the total length of network chains in unit volume of the system remains finite. Equations (64.2a) and (64.2b) then become

$$P(r_S; \phi_R, r_R) = \exp[-\phi_R(1 + (r_S/r_R))^2] \quad (64.3a)$$

and

$$P(r_S; \phi_R, r_R) \simeq 1 - \phi_R(1 + (r_S/r_R))^2; \phi_R \to 0 \quad (64.3b)$$

respectively, where

$$\phi_R = \pi n_R L r_R^2 \quad (64.4)$$

is the volume fraction of the dispersed rods. In a real network the chains are flexible, and not rigid, as assumed by Ogston, but arguments can be presented that this does not matter.

Equation (64.3b) is thus the fraction of space in the network system available to the centers of spheres of radius r_S. Equation (64.3b) is also an expression for the partition coefficient, K, the ratio in equilibrium of the apparent concentration of spheres in the network, calculated on the basis of the total volume of the network phase, to the concentration of spheres in the phase outside.

We can use K to assess the structurally interesting parameter r_R if we can assume, as was done in the above cases, that the spheres and the network substance do not interact energetically and that the fiber, i.e. the rod radius r_R, is the same everywhere. If we measure the distribution of a known amount of spheres inside and out we can then assume that the volume fraction of sphere centers, in the available space inside, equals the volume fraction of the spheres outside. Hence determining the volume of the outside sphere suspension, V_o, and the volume of the network, V_N, and calculating ϕ_S from an analysis of the outside solution we have

$$r_S/r_R = [(1 - K)/\phi_R]^{1/2} - 1 \quad (64.5)$$

where

$$K = 1 - [V_{TOT} \phi_S - V_S]/[V_N \phi_S] \quad (64.6)$$

is the partition coefficient, $V_{TOT} = V_o + V_N$ is the total volume of the system (network plus outside solution) and V_S is the total volume of spheres in the system. All the quantities on the right-hand-side of equation (64.6) and ϕ_R can be evaluated. Hence a plot of the right-hand-side of equation (64.5) vs. r_S should be linear and have the slope $1/r_R$, assuming that a series of nonenergetically interacting spherical probe molecules has been

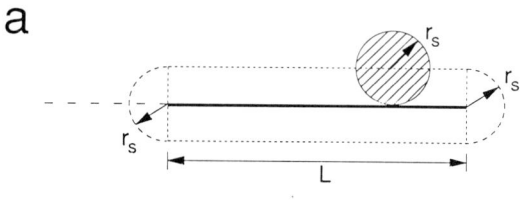

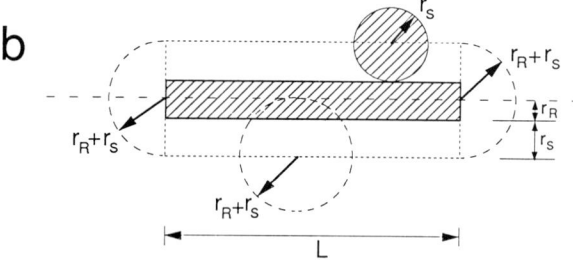

Figure 64.1 Rod/sphere exlusion. L, length of rod; r_R, radius of rod; r_S, radius of sphere. (a) $r_R = 0$; (b) $r_R > 0$.

used. This approach has been applied, for example, with much success by Meyer and Silberberg (1977) in their analysis of the network structure in Wharton's jelly, the structural connective tissue of umbilical cord.

THERMODYNAMIC PROBES

In the Ogston case, a very simple interaction potential was presumed to exist between the network component, the rod, and the probe, the sphere, which assesses the mean thickness of the rod. The potential (Fig. 64.2(a)) has no attractive and no long-range repulsive part. The assumption that the spheres are uniformly distributed at $r > r_R + r_S$ is thus reasonable. Cases where such a potential applies are indeed known. More generally, however, the potential is not flat and most often, in the case of probes which are miscible with the network, it is attractive. The most probable location of the sphere is then close to the minima in the potential curve (Fig. 64.2(b)). There is thus an accumulation of spheres near the rod and the concentration of spheres goes through a minimum half-way between rods. It is the concentration at this minimum which, in general, matches the outside concentration in thermodynamic equilibrium.

It is clear, therefore, that if the uniform distribution model is used to calculate the excluded volume in this case, the radius r_R would be underestimated. A larger available volume, mathematically, is required in order to accommodate the spheres present above the concentration in the region midway between network strands. The radius r_R can even turn out to be negative. It is informative, but structurally meaningless, to use the equilibrium dialysis (Ogston model) approach in these cases unless the potential-energy profile can be calculated in some detail.

In practice, the Ogston approach involves the use of a large number of probes of known radius. The results so obtained are then tested as to whether they conform to a consistent and reasonable value of r_R. Cases that do not agree have to be rejected, although it is useful to study whether the potential that makes them not conform to the general picture can be understood, at least qualitatively (Meyer *et al.*, 1977; Meyer, 1983).

It is not strictly necessary to use compact molecules as 'spheres'. As is well known, linear chain molecules in solution tend to coil into structures that are spherical in the mean and are characterized by root-mean-square-radii of gyration which, though larger than the ideal random-walk prediction in the usual case, can be measured easily. Dilute-solution-viscosity experiments or the angular dependence of light scattering can provide data on the macromolecular coil (Tanford, 1961). Two different species of

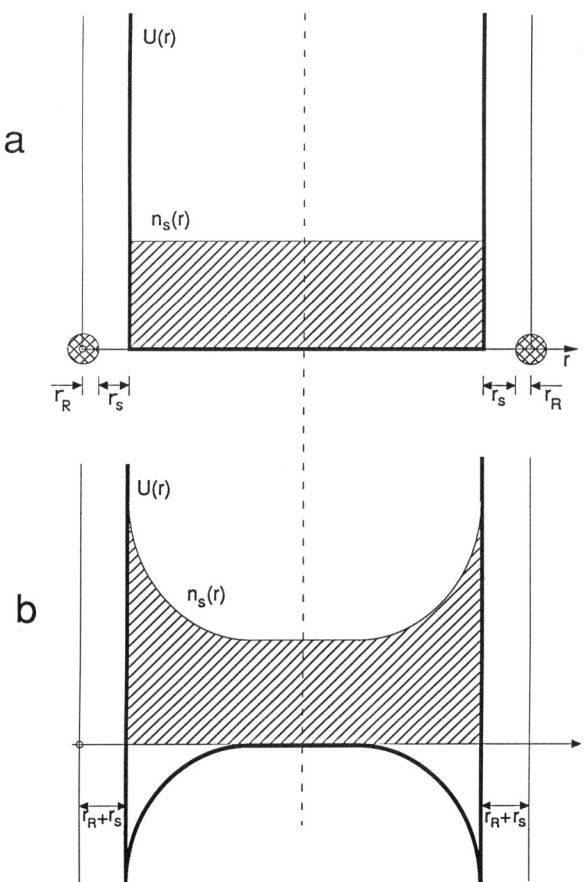

Figure 64.2 Rod/sphere potential $U(r)$. (a) Ideal hard-sphere potential. (b) Ideal hard-sphere potential with rod/sphere attraction. r_R, radius of rod; r_S, radius of sphere; $n_S(r)$, number of sphere centers per unit volume between r and $r + dr$.

moleculary thin, coiling macromolecules, which tend to exclude each other, will, however, not conform to the Ogston model in terms of their coil dimensions. The presence of two different kinds of macromolecules will, in general, induce a phase separation of the system at the point where the coils of the two types of macromolecule begin to overlap, but they will not 'probe' each other sterically in other respects. In the region where they are miscible and mix freely, however, the molecules are represented by two 'rod' systems which interpenetrate each other. An excluded volume can then be measured, but it is the effective excluded volume of the segment composing the chain, i.e. the geometric excluded volume of the segment modified (effectively reduced) by a potential of the type shown in Fig. 64.2(b) (Flory, 1953). The Ogston model does not apply. If, however, much of the exclusion of one of the 'rod' systems is due to the relatively large fibrils of collagen (as in cartilage), the randomly coiled 'rods' of the chain molecule system will act, with respect to these fibers, as spheres in the Ogston sense.

The simplest thermodynamic probe to use and one which is always available is the solvent medium which, in the case of cartilage and other connective-tissue networks, will not be pure water, but a solution of salt and other low-molecular-weight materials. This solution is assumed to distribute uniformly throughout the open network space with exclusion effects which are no more extensive than those of the solvent itself. The presence of the 'solution' of the network substance in the solvent, however, affects (lowers) the solvent chemical potential. Hence, in order for the solvent mixture inside the network to be in equilibrium with that outside, where it is in its 'pure' form, the pressure inside the network phase has to be raised above that outside. (Instead of pressure another system parameter could be altered, e.g. the temperature. There is, however, good thermal contact between the network phase and the surrounding fluid so that a temperature difference could not be maintained. However, the hydrostatic pressure in the network system is easily raised by inducing extra stresses in the network strands.) In order to raise pressure the extra stress must be a tension and the network expands — swells (Silberberg, 1980). The degree of swelling can be measured and the pressure increase can be estimated. Equilibrium swelling is thus an excellent way to characterize the mechanical properties of connective-tissue networks. Further stresses may be applied to the system from outside by mechanical compressive devices and the combination of swelling tendency and mechanical confinement permits the study of the mechanical-response characteristics of the tissue under a variety of conditions (e.g. see Chapters 67 and 68; see also Maroudas (1980)).

Thermodynamic information about the network, i.e. about its interaction with the 'solvent' can also be obtained from swelling equilibrium experiments. In particular, information on the number of charges on the network or on macromolecules not tied to the network but unable to extricate themselves from the network, can be studied by partition, in this case not only of solvent but also of a neutral salt component. The salt (both ions together) is a neutral species whose chemical potential inside and out, must balance in equilibrium much as that of water must be in balance under the same circumstances. Inside the network, and indeed in every volume element of the system, we have to observe electroneutrality. Any local departure from this condition results in enormous fields that would rapidly redistribute the ions until electroneutrality is restored. The fixed charges, however, cannot be displaced. Hence the cation and anion concentration distributions of the added salt inside the network differ from each other and the fixed-charge concentration can be calculated. The equilibrium state which results is the so-called Donnan equilibrium (Tanford (1961); applied to cartilage, Maroudas (1970, 1980); applied to glycosaminoglycan and proteoglycan, Maroudas et al. (1988) and Parker et al. (1988)). Note that, in addition to electroneutrality, two chemical potentials have to match, inside and out, that of 'solvent' and that of the neutral salt. Hence there is both a pressure rise (swelling of the network) and a redistribution of the component ions.

Note that an approach via the Ogston model, even if thermodynamically inactive spherical probes are used, will always occur in swelling equilibrium, when the sample is unconfined. A distorted system is thus analyzed. Only if mechanical restriction of the volume of the tissue sample to its original, i.e. physiological, value is applied will the Ogston approach yield physiological information about the physiologically available space and the physiological network dimensions. Some tissue samples, of course, in cases where the network strands are very stiff springs, need not swell appreciably in order to produce the required pressure increase; this is the case with normal human articular cartilage (see Chapter 53; see also Maroudas (1976b)). In such cases, if only information about r_R is sought, the effect of swelling on the available space can be ignored.

DYNAMIC TECHNIQUES

The partition method and its variants depend upon the system having reached equilibrium with some outside bath. This may be a very slow process. Indeed the time to equilibrium may exceed the survival time of the system or, in the case of *in vivo* experiments, the time for which an animal can be held still for observation. Information about structure and the accessibility of the network interior can, in principle, also be obtained by dynamic, relatively short-time tests using molecular probes. Such tests will generally involve noninteracting molecules whose rate and extent of difficulties or permeation into the network can be studied and assessed.

Diffusion

The distribution of the probe molecule at any instant is usually measured by some optical labeling or radiolabeling technique and the diffusion rates are calculated from the concentration profile as determined by some fast freeze or fixation technique, followed by sectioning and analysis. This is a very painstaking approach and requires good controls before the results can be interpreted with safety (methods along this line, especially applicable to model systems, are discussed in Chapter 62). The probe molecule (e.g. serum albumin) can, however, also be fitted out with a suitable chromophore, preferably a group which fluoresces (e.g. fluorescein isothoicyanate (FITC)), since this very considerably enhances the sensitivity of its detection. It is then possible to analyze samples directly if they are thin enough and light can cross them without serious intensity losses and distortions of the picture. In living systems in particular this is the method of choice, but its use is confined to rather specialized tissues (Fox and Wayland, 1979).

What is usually measured is an apparent diffusion coefficient using the Fick equation. The results are best expressed as the ratio of this diffusion coefficient to the value of the diffusion coefficient in free suspension in the same medium. On the theoretical side in this connection, Ogston *et al.* (1973) expanded the equilibrium distribution model of Ogston (1958) to the case of diffusion of spheres through a fiber system. For the reduced apparent diffusion coefficient they found in analogy to equation (64.3a)

$$D^{APP}/D^{FREE} = \exp[-(1 + (r_S/r_R))\phi_R^{1/2}] \quad (64.7)$$

Agreement with equation (64.7), in the case of model systems, could be established (Preston and Snowden, 1973).

In general, the apparent diffusion coefficient, even of probes whose dimensions are much smaller than the size of the available spaces, is found to be reduced by a large, but constant factor (Maroudas, 1970). When, however, the mean network pore size becomes comparable with the probe dimension, the relative diffusion coefficient drops very rapidly to extremely small values (Fox and Wayland, 1979).

In this connection it should be stressed that diffusion of flexible-chain macromolecules, such as hyaluronan, for example, will not reduce to zero even if the available network spaces have dimensions which are many times smaller than the random coil dimension in free solution. Diffusion occurs in such cases by reptation, i.e. by a snaking through of the chain through the network spaces (de Gennes, 1979a,b; Klein and Meyer, 1983).

In fact, in the absence of external fields and concentration or pressure gradients a large linear macromolecule in a network will gradually adopt a random-walk structure, although each conformation so adopted is prevented from undergoing rapid change except at its ends. These macromolecules can needle in and out of their confinement and thus gradually create a new structure and a new location when it is taken into account that also the entire molecule is moving to and fro along its own contour within the confinement created by the network. The friction association with this movement is proportional to the length l of the linear chain. It is obvious that after a molecule has moved a distance l along its curvilinear path by to-and-fro diffusion the chain has built itself a new environment and a new conformation. Let the time taken for this to occur be τ. In a time τ, therefore, the center of mass of the long chain molecule will have become displaced by the diameter (or radius R_G) of its mean coiled shape. The translational diffusion coefficient will thus be given by (de Gennes, 1979a,b)

$$D \simeq R_G^2/\tau \simeq la/\tau \qquad (64.8)$$

where a is the length of a single step in the random walk. However, we also have the following relationship between the two ways of defining diffusion along the contour length:

$$l^2/\tau \simeq kT/l \qquad (64.9)$$

The left-hand-side of equation (64.9) is the analog of equation (64.8), the right hand side is the Einstein expression for the along-the-contour diffusion coefficient, i.e. kT (k, Boltzmann constant; T, absolute temperature) divided by the frictional resistance encountered by the particle in its random motion. It follows from equation (64.9) that $\tau \simeq l^3$ and that

$$D \simeq l^{-2} \simeq M^{-2} \qquad (64.10)$$

where M is the molecular mass. By comparison, note that in free space

$$D \simeq M^{-1} \qquad (64.11)$$

in a case where the linear chain molecules are freely draining in motion through the solvent and

$$D \simeq M^{-v} \qquad (64.12)$$

if due to strong hydrodynamic interaction between macromolecular segments and solvent the macromolecular coil can be treated as an impermeable (to solvent) 'rigid' sphere of radius R_G, where

$$R_G \simeq M^{-v} \qquad (64.13)$$

Note that in the case of equation (64.8) we assume ideal random-walk statistics and put $v = 0.5$. More generally, in a good solvent environment $v = 0.6$. (de Gennes, 1979a,b). Diffusion rates of long macromolecules are thus enormously reduced once, due to confinement in networks, movement by reptation has become the only possibility.

It is interesting that reptation also occurs in systems of overlapping entangled macromolecular coils, even though no permanent cross-links exist between any of the macromolecules. The reason for this is that the time required for the environment, which traps a particular chain in a particular configuration, to diffuse away and create a new situation is considerably longer than the time of reptational displacement of the macromolecule from out of its 'confinement'. Hence the diffusion coefficient of a long chain macromolecule even in noninterpenetrating chains is determined by reptation and is proportional to M^{-2} (de Gennes, 1979a,b).

Summing up, the interpretation of diffusion experiments is most meaningful in relation to the assessment they provide of the dimensions of transsample passages in cartilage. The friction coefficients involved of course also depend upon 'fiber' dimensions, but the models here, e.g. equation (64.7) are not nearly as good as in the equilibrium case. A better assessment of 'fiber' dimension can, under certain circumstances, be obtained from permeability measurements.

Permeability

The resistance to solvent flux across a network is very sensitively dependent on the organization of the network. If the network and its spaces are homogeneous, then the local distribution of fiber and interfiber spaces will nowhere depart significantly from the average and the overall flow resistance is a good measure of the local structural unit. In such a case the fiber system can with reasonable success be replaced by a system of spheres, one sphere for every four sphere diameters of network strand. Substituting this into the Stokes friction formula, one finds that the overall resistance does not depend upon the sphere diameter, but only upon the length of the fiber system per unit volume (the parameter $n_R L$ in equation (64.4)). Hence if ϕ_R is known, first $n_R L$ and then r_R can be evaluated from the permeability of the network to solvent. Such a model, however, simplifies a number of aspects. It assumes a high degree of homogeneity and ignores higher order (in ϕ_R) hydrodynamic interactions. It will thus tend to overestimate $n_R L$ and underestimate r_R.

If the network is nonuniform in its arrangement, the flow predominantly makes use of any large open spaces and the permeability rate is considerably enhanced. It is indeed immediately possible to detect the presence of highly conducting, essentially open domains since permeability will then be much higher than in a case of a uniform homogeneous distribution of the same amount of network material. The size of the domains and that of the spacings between them can be determined with great sensitivity if other structural information is available, if, for example, their number is independently known (Weiss and Silberberg, 1976; Comper and Zamparo, 1989).

There are a number of problems associated with using a network as a 'membrane', whether it is for the determination of the flux of solvent only, i.e. permeability, or for the flux of dissolved probes, i.e. solute flux. Firstly, the concentration distribution between the outside system and the network has to be known, or must be determined. One can assume that there is equilibrium at the interface itself but the concentration in the outside medium close to the interface is subject to flow-induced concentration-polarization effects which are hard to assess and hard to eliminate. Secondly, the network will swell, i.e. alter structure, unless it is rigidly confined, or composed of very stiff network strands. Thirdly, the network will deform in the flux direction in order to create the required pressure gradient (Silberberg, 1989). Only if these problems have been properly considered will the permeability and the solute transport parameters yield insights into structure. For example, in the case of permeability measurements of unconfined, easily deformable networks only the results obtained by extrapolating the data to zero applied pressure gradient should be used.

In certain cases permeability can be assessed from dynamic mechanical tests, i.e. a determination of the frequency dependence of the complex shear modulus, or the complex compressional modulus, using limitingly small amplitude deformations. Due to the viscoelastic character of the system the real part of the modulus is a measure of the number of deformational mechanisms which respond elastically during the time $1/\omega$, where ω is the circular frequency, and the imaginary part assesses the number of mechanisms which relax during that time and thus respond viscously to the applied stress. The elasticity modulus (whether in shear or compression) gives information about the number of cross-links 'permanently' connected by elastically responding network strands, equivalent often to an assessment of the number of impermeable domains in the system. The viscous-loss modulus, however, is composed of two contributions. One derives from fast stress relaxation, mainly of local deformations of the network strands, and the other from a translative displacement of the network, in shear flow, through the solvent. Hence if the first contribution can be neglected the loss modulus will be a measurement of permeability, i.e. of the frictional interaction between the network and the solvent it contains (e.g. Rosser et al. (1977); see also Chapter 68).

It should be noted that dynamic light-scattering techniques, in principle, also provide this information, but the results are perhaps more difficult to interpret in a highly heterogeneous system such as cartilage (Nossal, 1987).

The interpretation of transmembrane fluxes of probe molecules involves the determination of three transport coefficients. Instead of two components (fiber system and solvent) where there is only one frictional interaction parameter which controls the relative flow, there are at least three components when a probe is used and thus three parameters. A single type of measurement, say of an apparent diffusion constant, will not, except in certain limiting cases, permit a simple interpretation of the data (Zweifach and Silberberg, 1979; Silberberg, 1989).

The use of tracers is particularly open to misinterpretation in this sense. The labeled species has to be seen as an additional component and the number of friction parameters is largely increased. Some of these parameters can of course be equated with each other, but the analysis in the general case is much more complex. Only if conditions are carefully chosen (low tracer concentrations in particular) will the results simplify, but these precautions tend to be ignored. Dynamic measurements, if probes other than the solvent are being used, are thus good mainly in detecting major structural features e.g. the cut-off size.

References

Atha, H. and Ingham, K.C. (1981). Mechanisms of precipitation of proteins by polyethylene glycols. *J. Biol. Chem.* **256**, 12 108–12 117

Barnes, R.M. (1984). Determination of trace elements of biological materials by inductively coupled plasma spectroscopy with novel chelating resins. *Biol. Trace Elements Res.* **6**, 93–103

Barry, P.H. and Diamond, J.M. (1984). Effects of unstirred layers on membrane phenomena. *Physiol. Rev.* **64**, 763–872

Benderly, H. and Maroudas, A. (1975). Equilibria of calcium and phosphate ions in human articular cartilage. *Ann. Rheum. Dis.* **34**, 46–47

Bernhardt, I., Hall, A.C. and Ellory, J.C. (1988). Transport pathways for monovalent cations through erythrocyte membranes. *Studia Biophys.* **126**, 5–21

Bernich, E., Rubenstein, R. and Bellin, J.S. (1976). Membrane transport properties of bovine articular cartilage. *Biochim. Biophys. Acta* **448**, 551–561

Bert, J.L., Pearce, R.H., Mathieson, J.M. and Warner, S.J. (1980). Characterization of collagenous meshworks by volume exclusion of dextrans. *Biochem. J.* **191**, 761–768

Brahm, J. (1976). Temperature-dependent changes of chloride transport kinetics in human red cells. *J. Gen. Physiol.* **70**, 283–307

Brocklehurst, R., Bayliss, M.T., Maroudas, A., Coyte, L. and Freeman, M.A.R. (1984). The composition of normal and osteoarthritic articular cartilage from human knee joints. *J. Bone Joint Surg.* **66A**, 95–106

Campbell, A.K. (1983). *Intracellular Calcium*. Wiley, Norwich, UK

Chateauvert, J.M.D., Pritzker, K.P.H., Kessler, M.J. and Grynpas, M.D. (1989). Spontaneous osteoarthritis in rhesus macaques. I. Chemical and biochemical studies. *J. Rheumatol.* **16**, 1098–1104

Chipperfield, A.R. (1986). The (Na + K) co-transport system. *Clin. Sci.* **71**, 465–476

Comper, W.D. and Preston, B.N. (1974). Model connective tissue systems: a study of polyion-mobile ion and of excluded-volume interactions of proteoglycans. *Biochem. J.* **143**, 1–9

Comper, W.D. and Preston, B.N. (1975). Model connective tissue systems: Measurement of ion flux across gel membranes containing proteoglycan. *J. Colloid Interface Sci.* **53**, 379–390

Comper, W.D. and Laurent, T.C. (1978). Physiological function of connective tissue polysaccharides. *Physiol. Rev.* **58**, 255–315

Comper, W.D. and Zamparo, O. (1989). Hydraulic conductivity of polymers. *Biophys. Chem.* **34**, 127–135

Cousin, J.L. and Motais, R. (1976). The role of carbonic anhydrase inhibitors on anion permeability into ox red blood cells. *J. Physiol.* **256**, 61–80

Crank, J. (1975). *The Mathematics of Diffusion*. Clarendon Press, Oxford

Crank, J. and Park, G.S. (eds) (1968). *Diffusion in Polymers*. Academic Press, New York

Cumming, G.J., Handley, C.J. and Preston, B.N. (1979). Permeability of chondrocyte cultures to solutes of varying size, shape and charge. *Biochem. J.* **181**, 257–266

Curry, F.-R.E. (1984). Mechanisms and thermodynamics of transcapillary exchange. In *Handbook of Physiology, The Cardiovascular System*, Vol. 8, pp. 309–374. American Physiology Society, Baltimore, Md

Curry, F.E. and Michel, C.C. (1980). A fiber matrix model of capillary permeability. *Microvasc. Res.* **20**, 96–99

De Gennes, P.G. (1979a). Diffusion of long chain molecules. *Nature* **282**, 367–370

De Gennes, P.G. (1979b). *Scaling Concepts in Polymer Physics*. Cornell University Press, Ithaca, NY

Dunstone, J.R. (1960). Ion exchange reactions between cartilage and various cations. *Biochem. J.* **77**, 164–170

Eddy, A.A. (1987). The sodium gradient hypothesis of organic solute transport with special reference to amino acids. In *Amino Acid Transport in Animal Cells* (D.L. Yudilevich and C.A.R. Boyd, eds), pp. 47–56. Manchester University Press, Manchester

Eichelberger, L. (1960). Hyaline cartilage: the histochemical characterization of the extracellular and intracellular compartments. *Clin Orthop.* **17**, 77–91

Ellory, J.C. (1987). Amino acid transport systems in mammalian red cells. In *Amino Acid Transport in Animal Cells* (D.L. Yudilevich and C.A.R. Boyd, eds), pp. 106–119. Manchester University Press, Manchester

Ellory, J.C. and Young, J.D. (eds) (1982). *Red Cell Transport — A Methodological Approach.* Academic Press, New York

Flory, P.J. (1953). *Principles of Polymer Chemistry.* Cornell University Press, Ithaca

Fox, J.R. and Wayland, H. (1979). Interstitial diffusion of macromolecules in the rat mesentery. *Microvacu. Res.* **18**, 255–276

Glynn, I.M. (1988). How does the sodium pump work? In *Cell Physiology of Blood* (A. Gunn and D.S. Parker, eds), pp. 2–17. Rockefeller University Press, New York

Glynn, I.M. (1989). The sodium pump. *J. Roy. Coll. Phys. London* **23**, 39–49

Glynn, I.M. and Karlish, S.J.D. (1975). The sodium pump. *Ann. Rev. Physiol.* **37**, 13–55

Gosting, L. (1956). Measurement and interpretation of diffusion coefficients. *Adv. Prot. Chem.* **11**, 429–554

Gray, M.L., Pizzanelli, A.M., Grodzinsky, A.J. and Lee, R.C. (1988). Mechanical and physicochemical determinants of the chondrocyte biosynthetic responses. *J. Orthop. Res.* **6**, 777–792

Grodzinsky, A.J. (1983). Electromechanical and physico-chemical properties of connective tissue. *Crit. Rev. Biomed. Eng.* **9**, 133–199

Grodzinsky, A.J., Roth, V., Myers, E., Grossman, W.D. and Mow, V.C. (1981). The significance of electromechanical and osmotic forces in the non-equilibrium swelling behaviour of articular cartilage in tension. *J. Biomech. Eng.* **103**, 221–231

Hadler, N.M. (1980). Enhanced diffusivity of glucose in a matrix of hyaluronic acid. *J. Biol. Chem.* **255**, 3532–3535

Harding, S. (1986). Applications of light scattering in microbiology. *Biotechnol. Appl. Biochem.* **8**, 489–509

Harper, G.S., Comper, W.D. and Preston, B.N. (1985). Concentration dependence of proteoglycan diffusion. *Biopolymers* **24**, 2165–2173

Helfferich, F. (1962). *Ion Exchange.* McGraw-Hill, New York

Hiatt, C.W., Shelokov, A., Rosenthal, E.J. and Galimore, J.M. (1971). Treatment of controlled-pore glass with poly(ethylene oxide) to prevent adsorption of rabies virus. *J. Chromatogr.* **56**, 362–364

Hille, B. (1984). *Ionic Channels of Excitable Membranes.* Sinauer Associates Inc., Sunderland, MA

Hoffmann, E.K. and Simonsen, L.O. (1989). Membrane mechanisms in volume and pH regulation in vertebrate cells. *Physiol. Rev.* **69**, 315–382

Howell, D.S., Pita, J.C. and Marquez, J.F. (1968). Partition of calcium, phosphate and protein in the fluid phase aspirated at calcifying sites in the epiphyseal cartilage. *J. Clin. Invest.* **47**, 1121–1132

James, D.E., Strube, M. and Mueckler, M. (1989). Molecular cloning and characterization of an insulin-regulatable glucose transporter. *Nature* **338**, 83–87

Jan, L.Y. and Yuh, N.J. (1989). Voltage-sensitive ion channels. *Cell.* **56**, 13–25

Jarvis, S.M. (1989). Uniport carriers for metabolites. *Curr. Opinion Cell Biol.* **1**, 721–728

Jennings, M.L. (1985). Kinetics and mechanisms of anion transport in red blood cells. *Ann. Rev. Physiol.* **47**, 519–534

Katz, M.M., Hargers, A.R. and Garfin, S.R. (1986). Intervertebral disc nutrition: Diffusion versus convection. *Clin. Orthop.* **210**, 243–245

Klein, J. and Meyer, F.A. (1983). Tissue structure and macromolecular diffusion in umbilical cord. Immobilization of endogenous hyaluronic acid. *Biochim. Biophys. Acta* **755**, 400–411

Kullberg, R. (1987). Stretch-activated ion channels in bacteria and animal cell membranes. *TINS* **10**, 387–388

Laurent, T.C. (1964). The interaction between polysaccharides and other macromolecules. 9. The exclusion of molecules from hyaluronic acid gels and solutions. *Biochem. J.* **93**, 106–112

Laurent, T.C., Preston, B.N., Pertoft, H., Gustafsson, B. and McCabe, M. (1975). Diffusion of linear polymers in hyaluronic acid solution. *Eur. J. Biochem.* **53**, 129–136

Laurent, T.C., Preston, B.N., Comper, W.D., Checkley, G.J., Edsman, K. and Sundelof, L.-O. (1983). Kinetics of multicomponent transport by structured flow in polymer solutions. 7. Studies on a poly(vinylpyrrolidone)–dextran system. *J. Phys. Chem.* **87**, 648–654

Lieb, W.R. and Stein, W.D. (1971). Implications of two different types of diffusion for biological membranes. *Nature New Biol.* **234**, 220–222

Linn, F.C. and Sokoloff, L. (1965). Movement and composition of interstitial fluid of cartilage. *Arthr. Rheum.* **8**, 481–494

Mackie, J.S. and Meares, P. (1955). The diffusion of electrolytes in a cation-exchange resin membrane. *Proc. R. Soc. Ser. A.* **232**, 498–509

Magdalenat, H., Turq, P. and Chemla, M. (1974). Study of the self-diffusion coefficients in cations in the presence of an acidic polysaccharide. *Biopolymers* **13**, 1535–1548

Maroudas, A. (1968). Physiocochemical properties of cartilage in the light of ion-exchange theory. *Biophys. J.* **8**, 575–595

Maroudas, A. (1970). Distribution and diffusion of solutes in articular cartilage. *Biophys. J.* **10**, 365–379

Maroudas, A. (1976a). Transport of solutes through cartilage: permeability to large molecules. *J. Anat.* **122**, 335–347

Maroudas, A. (1976b). Balance between swelling pressure and collagen tension in normal and degenerative cartilage. *Nature* **260**, 808–809

Maroudas, A. (1980). Physical chemistry of articular cartilage and the intervertebral disc. In *The Joints and Synovial Fluid* (L. Sokoloff, ed.), Vol. II, pp. 233–291. Academic Press, New York

Maroudas, A. (1986). Mechanism of fluid transport in cartilaginous tissues. In *Tissue nutrition and viability* (A. Hargens, ed.), pp. 47–72. Springer-Verlag, New York

Maroudas, A. and Bannon, C. (1981). Measurement of swelling pressure in cartilage. *Biorheology* **18**, 619–632

Maroudas, A. and Evans, H. (1972). A study of ionic equilibria in cartilage. *Conn. Tiss. Res.* **1**, 69

Maroudas, A. and Evans, H. (1974). In vitro study of sulphate incorporation by adult human articular cartilage. *Biochim. Biophys. Acta* **338**, 265–271

Maroudas, A. and Urban, J.P.G. (1983). *In vitro* methods for studying articular cartilage and intervertebral disc. In *Skeletal Research* A.S. Kunin and D.J. Simmons, eds), 2nd edn. Academic Press, New York

Maroudas, A. and Venn, M.F. (1977). Chemical composition and swelling of normal and osteoarthritic tissues II; Swelling. *Ann. Rheum. Dis.* **36**, 399–406

Maroudas, A., Weinberg, P.D., Parker, K.H. and Winlove, C.P. (1988). The distributions and diffusivities of small ions in chondroitin sulphate, hyaluronate and some proteoglycan solutions. *Biophys. Chem.* **32**, 257–270

Meyer, F.A. (1983). Macromolecular basis of globular protein exclusion and of swelling pressure in loose connective tissue (umbilical cord). *Biochim. Biophys. Acta* **755**, 388–399

Meyer, F.A. and Silberberg, A. (1977). The extravascular space, function of the main structural elements. *Bibl. Anat.* **15**, 213–219

Meyer, F.A., Comper, W.D. and Preston, B.N. (1971). Model connective tissue systems. A physical study of gelatin gels containing proteoglycan. *Biopolymers* **10**, 1351–1364

Meyer, F.A., Koblentz, M. and Silberberg, A. (1977). Structural investigation of loose connective tissue using a series of Dextran fractions as non-interacting macromolecular probes. *Biochem. J.* **161**, 285–291

McDevitt, C.A. and Muir, H. (1976). Biochemical changes in the cartilage of the knee in experimental and natural osteoarthritis in the dog. *J. Bone Joint Surg.* **58B**, 94–101

Muhr, A.H. and Blanshard, J.M.V. (1982). Diffusion in gels. *Polymer* **23**, 1012–1026

Nam, T.L. and Reddy, R.J. (1980). Determination of trace element concentrations in articular cartilage by instrumental neutron activation analysis. In *Trace Element Analytical Chemistry in Medicine and Biology* (P. Bratter, ed.), pp. 351–364. W. de Gruyler, Berlin

Norton, J., Urban, J., Maroudas, A., Parker, K.H. and Winlove, C.P. (1982). A failure to observe enhanced diffusion of glucose in hyaluronate gels. *J. Biol. Chem.* **257**, 14134–14137

Nossal, R. (1987). Dynamic light scattering methods for biorheology. *Biorheology* **24**, 577–584

Ogston, A.G. (1958). The spaces in a uniform random suspension of fibers. *Trans. Faraday Soc.* **54**, 1754–1757

Ogston, A.G., Preston, B.N. and Wells, J.D. (1973). On the transport of compact particles through solutions of chain polymers. *Proc. R. Soc. London A.* **333**, 297–316

O'Hara, B.P., Urban, J.P.G. and Maroudas, A. (1990). Influence of cyclic loading on the nutrition of articular cartilage. *Ann. Rheum. Dis.* in press

Pappenheimer, J.R., Renkin, E.M. and Bossero, L.M. (1951). Filtration, diffusion and molecular sieving through peripheral capillary membranes. A contribution to the pore theory of capillary permeability. *Am. J. Physiol.* **167**, 13–46

Parker, K.H., Winlove, C.P. and Maroudas, A. (1988). The theoretical distributions and diffusivities of small ions in chondroitin sulphate and hyaluronate. *Biophys. Chem.* **32**, 271–282

Paullson, S., Sylven, B., Hirsch, C. and Shellman, O. (1951). Biophysical and physiological investigations on cartilage and other mesenchymal tissues. III. The diffusion rate of various substances in normal bovine nucleus pulposus. *Biochim. Biophys. Acta* **7**, 207–213

Phillips, C.G. and Jansons, K.M. (1990). Flow and diffusion through random rods and applications to proteoglycan solution. *Macromolecules* **23**, 1717–1724

Preston, B.N. and Snowden, J. McK. (1973). Diffusion properties of model extracellular systems. In *Biology of the Fibroblast* (E. Kulonen and J. Pikharainen, eds), pp. 215–230. Academic Press, New York

Preston, B.N., Snowden, J.M. and Houghton, K.Y. (1972). Model connective tissue systems: the effect of proteoglycans on the distribution of small non-electrolytes and micro-ions. *Biopolymers* **11**, 1645–1659

Preston, B.N., Laurent, T.C. and Comper, W.D. (1984). Transport of molecules in connective tissue polysaccharide solutions. In *Molecular Biophysics of the Extracellular Matrix* (S. Arnott, D.A. Rees and E.R. Morris, eds), pp. 115–162. Humana Press, Clifton, NJ

Pritzker, K.P.H. (1980). Crystalline arthropathies. *J. Am. Geriatr. Soc.* **28**, 439–445

Pritzker, K.P.H., Cheng, P.-T. and Omar, S.A. (1981). Calcium pyrophosphate crystal formation in model hydrogel. II. Hyaline cartilage as a gel. *J. Rheumatol.* **8**, 451–455

Pritzker, K.P.H., Chateauvert, J.M.D. and Grynpas, M.D. (1987). Osteoarthritic cartilage contains increased calcium, magnesium and phosphorus. *J. Rheumatol.* **14**, 806–810

Reihanian, H., Jamieson, A.M., Tang, L.H. and Rosenberg, L. (1979). Hydrodynamic properties of proteoglycan subunit from bovine nasal cartilage. Self-association behavior and interaction with hyaluronate studied by laser light scattering. *Biopolymers* **18**, 1727–1747

Rosser, R.W., Roberts, W.W. and Ferry, J.D. (1977). Rheology of fibrin clots. IV. Darcy constant and fiber thickness. *Biophys. Chem.* **7**, 153–157

Schatzmann, H.J. (1989). The calcium pump of the surface membrane and of the sarcoplasmic reticulum. *Ann. Rev. Physiol.* **69**, 315–382

Silberberg, A. (1980). The role of matrix mechanical stress in swelling equilibrium and transport through networks. *Macromolecules* **13**, 742–748

Silberberg, A. (1989). Transport through deformable matrices. *Biorheology* **26**, 291–313

Snowden, J. McK. and Maroudas, A. (1976). The distribution of serum albumin in human normal and degenerative cartilage. *Biochim. Biophys. Acta* **428**, 726–733

Spragg, S.P. (1980). *The Physical Behaviour of Macromolecules with Biological Functions* Wiley, Chichester

Stein, W.D. (1986). *Transport and Diffusion across Cell Membranes* Academic Press, London

Tanford, C. (1961). *Physical Chemistry of Macromolecules* Wiley, New York

Thomas, R.C. (ed.) (1988). Proton passage across cell membranes. *Ciba Foundation Symposium 139* John Wiley, Chichester

Torzilli, P.A., Adams, T.C. and Mis, K.J. (1987). Transient solute diffusion in articular cartilage. *J. Biomech.* **20**, 203–213

Urban, J.P.G. and Bayliss, M.T. (1989). Regulation of proteoglycan synthesis rate in cartilage *in vitro*: influence of extracellular ionic composition. *Biochim. Biophys. Acta* **992**, 59–65

Urban, J.P.G. and Maroudas, A. (1979). Measurement of fixed charge density and partition coefficients in the intervertebral disc. *Biochim. Biophys. Acta* **586**, 166–178

Urban, J.P.G. and Maroudas, A. (1981). Diffusion coefficients of small solutes in the intervertebral disc. *Trans. ORS* **27**, 125

Urban, J.P.G., Maroudas, A., Bayliss, M.T. and Dillon, J. (1979). Swelling pressures of proteoglycans at the concentrations found in cartilagenous tissues. *Biorheology* **16**, 447–464

Urban, J.P.G., Holm, S., Maroudas, A. and Nachemson, A. (1982). Nutrition of the intervertebral disc: effect of fluid flow on solute transport. *Clin. Orthop.* **170**, 296–306

Van Damme, M-P.I., Murphy, W.H., Comper, W.D., Preston, B.N. and Winzor, D.J. (1989). Evaluation of nonideality from gel chromatographic partition coefficients. A technique with greater versatility than equilibrium dialysis. *Biophys. Chem.* **33**, 115–125

Vrentas, J.S. and Duda, J.L. (1979). Molecular diffusion in polymer solutions. *AIChE J.* **25**, 1–24

Wells, J.D. (1971). PhD thesis, Australian National University, Canberra

Wells, J.D. (1973). An empirical extension of the Manning theory to finite salt concentrations. *Biopolymers* **12**, 223–228

Weiss, N. and Silberberg, A. (1976). Permeability as a means to study the structure of gels. In *Hydrogels for Medical and Related Applications* (J.D. Anrade, ed.), pp. 69–79. *ACS Symposium Series*, Vol. 31. American Chemical Society, Washington

Winlove, C.P. and Parker, K.H. (1984). Diffusion of macromolecules in hyaluronate gels. *Biorheology* **21**, 347–362

Yudilevich, D.L. and Boyd, C.A.R. (eds) (1987). *Amino Acid Transport in Animal Cells*. Manchester University Press, Manchester

Zaenetti, J., Ratcliffe, A. and Watt, F.M. (1985). Two subpopulations of differentiated chondrocytes identified with a monoclonal antibody to keratan sulphate. *J. Cell Biol.* **101**, 53–59

Zweifach, B.W. and Silberberg, A. (1979). The interstitial lymphatic flow system. In *International Review of Physiology, Cardiovascular Physiology III*, Vol. 18 (A.C. Guyton and D.B. Young, eds), Vol. 18, pp. 215–260. University Park Press, Baltimore

11

MECHANICAL AND ELECTRICAL PROPERTIES AND THEIR RELEVANCE TO PHYSIOLOGICAL PROCESSES

COLLATED BY A.J. GRODZINSKY

65

Overview

ALAN J. GRODZINSKY

INTRODUCTION

Human articular cartilage functions as a weight bearing, low friction, wear-resistant tissue in synovial joints. Cartilage is subjected to a wide range of mechanical loading forces *in vivo*, which produce time varying and spatially nonuniform compressive, tensile, and shear deformations within the tissue. The ability of cartilage to withstand such deformations and to perform its physiological function depends critically on the structure, composition, and integrity of its extracellular matrix. Methods have therefore been developed to quantify the fundamental mechanical, physicochemical and electromechanical properties of cartilage and to relate these properties to matrix structure and composition.

The objectives of this chapter are to highlight some recent advances concerning measurement of certain *intrinsic material properties* of cartilage. Research in this area has focused on two global issues: (i) the distribution of mechanical stresses at the *surface* of cartilage in *intact* joints during loading, and (ii) the distribution of hydrostatic and osmotic pressure, tissue deformation, fluid flow, and electrical current and potential *within* the tissue during loading. In principle, knowledge of the imposed stress in the intact joint along with the appropriate material properties should enable the prediction of deformations and flows within the tissue. These intratissue fields and flows are also of great interest in recent studies of biophysical mediators of cartilage metabolism.

MEASUREMENT OF MECHANICAL PROPERTIES

Contact pressure and deformation in intact joints

Armstrong *et al.* (1980) measured the deformation of human femoral head cartilage by radiographic means after application of a load equal to five times body weight. Deformation approximately 35 s after loading was found to increase significantly with age. Contact pressures in prepared hip joints have also been measured nondestructively using pressure-sensitive film (see Chapter 66). Hodge *et al.* (1986) used an instrumented femoral head prosthesis for *in vivo* measurements of contact pressures, which revealed local transient pressures as high as 18 MPa during sitting-to-standing transitions. Pressure maps of the acetabulum described in previous *in vitro* studies using such a prosthesis (Rushfeld *et al.* 1979) were interpreted further with the aid of an nondestructive, ultrasonic-based measurement of the cartilage thickness (Rushfeld *et al.*, 1979; Modest *et al.*, 1989).

Intrinsic mechanical properties

The equilibrium stress–strain behavior of cartilage can be conveniently represented for sufficiently small strains by the *equilibrium modulus*, the ratio of the change in stress to the change in strain (see Chapter 67). Figure 65.1 shows schematic configurations that have been used to measure the various equilibrium moduli in confined (Mow *et al.*, 1980) and unconfined (Brown and Singerman, 1986) compression, tension (Simon *et al.*, 1984), and shear (Hayes and Bodine, 1978), respectively. The theory of elasticity for linear, isotropic media requires that a minimum of two independent measurements be made (i.e. two moduli) in order to characterize the material completely. For certain experiments, however, and depending on the questions being addressed, the nonuniform (Maroudas, 1979), anisotropic (Mow *et al.*, 1984), high-strain (Holmes, 1986) behavior of cartilage may also need to be considered.

The nonequilibrium mechanical behavior of cartilage in compression and tension is also significantly affected by the tissue's *hydraulic permeability*. Figure 65.2 shows a schematic of an apparatus for measuring the fluid flux across a cartilage plug in response to an applied pressure drop, from which the permeability can be computed. (As described below, certain electrical properties can also be measured in the same configuration.) Pressure-drop experiments have been used previously to characterize the strain and

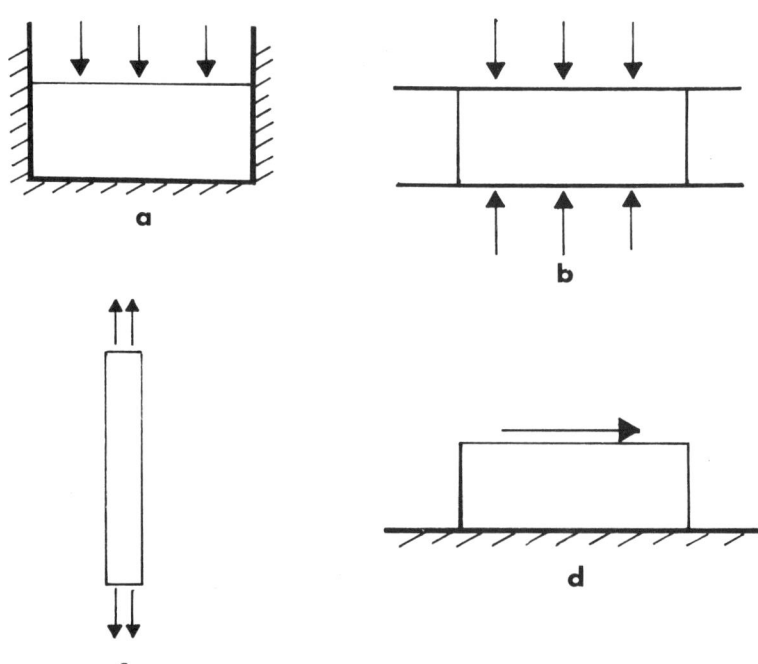

Figure 65.1 Schematic configuration for measurement of equilibrium modulus in (a) uniaxial confined compression, (b) unconfined compression, (c) tension, and (d) shear.

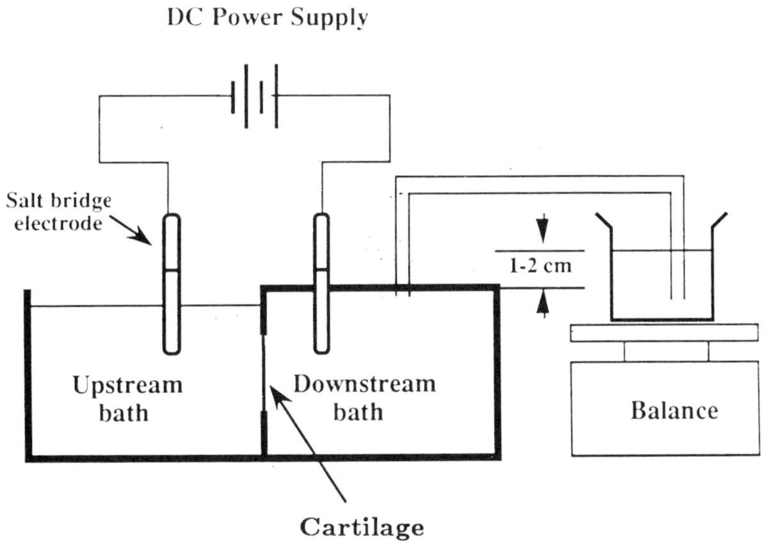

Figure 65.2 Schematic of a system for measurement of cartilage electrokinetic coupling coefficients, k_{12} and k_{21}, as well as tissue hydraulic permeability, k_{11}, and electrical conductance, k_{22}. Electrodes can be used to measure or apply voltage or current; a pressure drop across the tissue can be imposed, and fluid flow across the tissue can be measured continuously by means of a balance.

pressure dependence of the hydraulic permeability (Mow et al., 1984). However, the presence of blood vessels or other large, macroscopic pores in certain cartilages can produce significant errors when using this technique. It is then preferable to infer the permeability from measurements of transient (Mow et al., 1984) creep, stress relaxation or sinusoidal (Frank and Grodzinsky, 1987a,b) compression response of excised specimens, combined with an appropriate model (Mow et al., 1984; Frank and Grodzinsky, 1987a,b) (see Eisenberg and Mizrahi, this chapter).

ELECTRICAL AND ELECTRO-MECHANICAL PROPERTIES

In the one-dimensional (uniaxial) geometry of Fig. 65.2, the fluid velocity relative to the cartilage matrix, $U(z)$, and the current density $J(z)$ at each position z within the tissue are linearly proportional to the gradients in fluid pressure $P(z)$ and electrical potential $V(z)$ (for sufficiently small pressure and potential gradients),

$$U(z) = -k_{11}\frac{\partial P(z)}{\partial z} + k_{12}\frac{\partial V(z)}{\partial z} \quad (65.1)$$

$$J(z) = k_{21}\frac{\partial P(z)}{\partial z} - k_{22}\frac{\partial V(z)}{\partial z} \quad (65.2)$$

where k_{11} is the 'short circuit' hydraulic permeability (i.e. pressure-driven fluid flow with zero potential drop in Fig. 65.2), k_{12} and k_{21} are the electrokinetic coupling coefficients, and k_{22} is the electrical conductivity of the tissue (i.e. voltage-driven current flow with zero pressure drop). The coupling coefficients represent the fundamental electromechanical coupling that is inherent to cartilaginous tissues (Grodzinsky, 1983); these coefficients are equal ($k_{12} = k_{21}$) by Onsager reciprocity. For a tissue with negative fixed charge density, these coefficients are defined as negative.

Figure 65.2 suggests one approach to measuring the intrinsic electrical and electromechanical material properties (k_{ij}): application of a mechanical or electrical stimulus and measurement of the appropriate electrical or mechanical response. For example, the 'streaming potential' produced by a steady applied pressure drop across a disk of tissue is equal to $-(k_{21}/k_{22})$ when the current is constrained to be zero (open circuit). Conversely, the 'electroosmotic' fluid flow produced by an applied current density equals $-(k_{12}/k_{22})$ when the pressure drop is constrained to be zero. An example of the latter measurement (Grimshaw et al., 1989) can be seen in the data of Fig. 65.3 which shows the steady electroosmotic fluid velocity across five disks of adult bovine femoropatellar groove cartilage arranged in parallel and immersed in phosphate buffered saline. In addition, the hydraulic permeability k_{11} can also be calculated from the same measurement, using the ion exchange membrane model that relates electroosmotic flow to permeability (Helfferich, 1962; Frank et al., 1987), $k_{11} = (k_{12}/(\text{fixed charge density}))$. Advantages of this approach are (i) an applied current density of $10\,\text{mA cm}^{-2}$ produces a fluid velocity through cartilage equivalent to that induced by a pressure drop of several atmospheres, and (ii) electro-osmotic fluid flow in the configuration of Fig. 65.2 does not deform or consolidate the matrix (Frank and Grodzinsky, 1987a,b), unlike an applied pressure drop; therefore, the intrinsic permeability in the limit of zero applied strain or pressure (Mow et al., 1984) can be measured.

When cartilage is compressed, deformation of the hydrated matrix causes a flow of interstitial fluid and entrained counterions relative to the fixed charge groups of the matrix. The resulting fluid flow tends to separate counterions from fixed charge groups, producing a local streaming potential proportional to the local fluid velocity (Fig. 65.4(a)). Thus, k_{21} can also be computed from streaming potentials measured in transient or oscillatory uniaxial confined compression (Frank and Grodzinsky, 1987a,b) (see Chapter 67).

Conversely, it was recently discovered that application of a current density across a cartilage disk in uniaxial confinement produces a current-generated stress (proportional to k_{12}) when the tissue is held at fixed thickness (Frank and Grodzinsky, 1987a,b). This phenomenon results from the combination of two electrokinetic effects: (i) an electrophoretic force on the proteoglycan (PG) network in the direction of the positive electrode; and (ii) electroosmotic flow of positively charged interstitial fluid towards the negative electrode (Fig. 65.4(b)). The resulting deformation of the matrix gives rise to the measured stress.

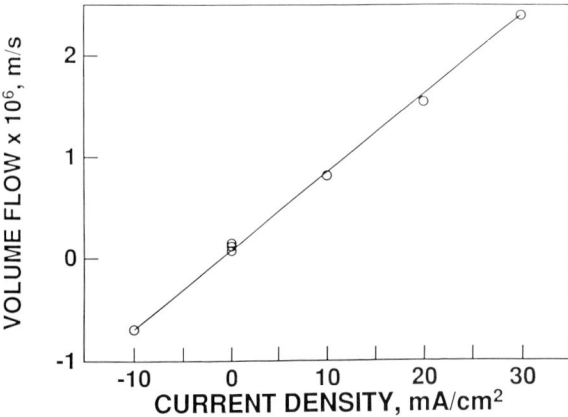

Figure 65.3 Electroosmotic fluid velocity across discs of adult bovine femoropatellar groove cartilage in phosphate buffered saline, versus applied dc current density. The slope of the best-fit line gives $(k_{12}/k_{22}) = 7.5 \times 10^{-9}\,(\text{m}^3\,\text{A}^{-1}\,\text{s}^{-1})$.

SURFACE DETECTION OF BULK MATERIAL PROPERTIES

The electrokinetic measurements described above provide a means for the measurement of bulk mechanical and electromechanical (k_{ij}) properties using a surface electrode configuration (Fig. 65.5). A three-dimensional linearized theory that gives the basis for such measurements has been developed recently (Sachs and Grodzinsky, 1989). When surface electrodes are used to inject a low amplitude, sinusoidal current density into the tissue as depicted in Fig. 65.5, the current will generate a spatially periodic mechanical stress the amplitude of which can be measured at the surface (Salant, 1990). The stress amplitude will depend

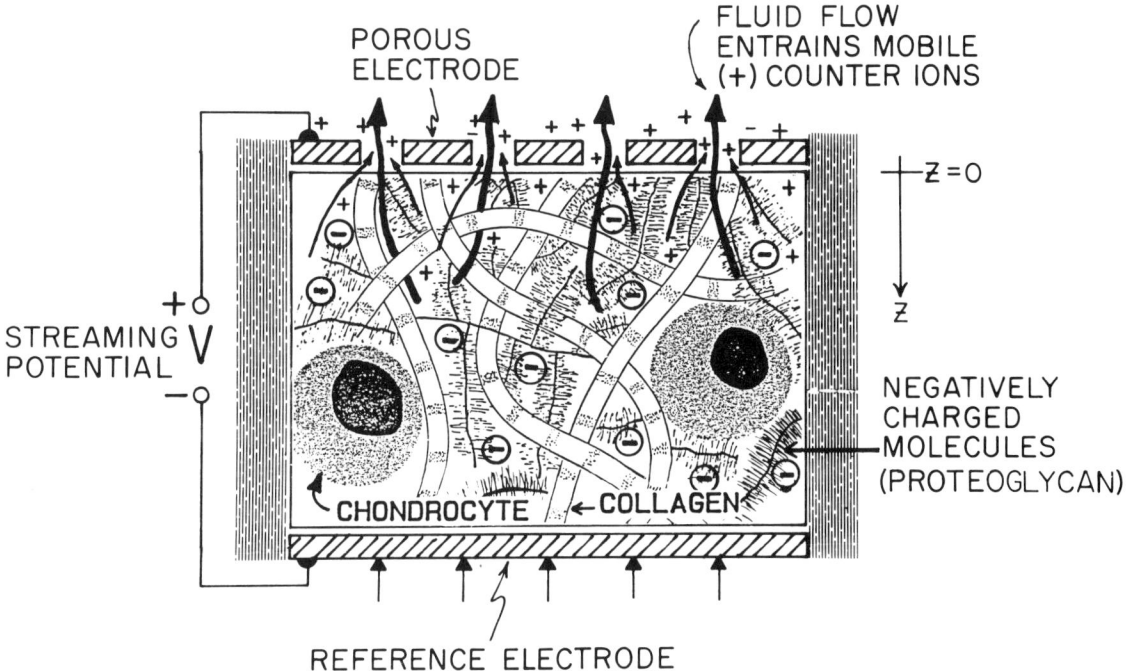

Figure 65.4 Schematic depicting compression-induced streaming potential in cartilage (from Frank and Grodzinsky (1987b), with permission).

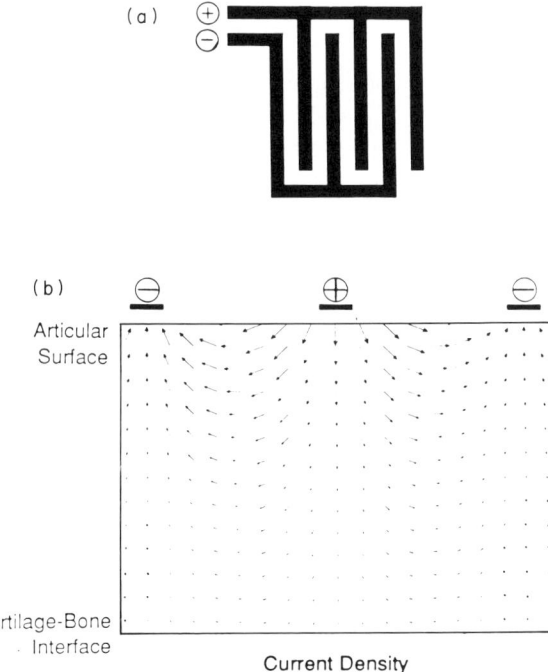

on the tissue's intrinsic material properties which, in turn, can reflect the state of tissue degradation. Thus, such a technique may enable nondestructive probing of cartilage degeneration in intact joints.

For the case of an isotropic, homogeneous tissue layer, Fig. 65.6 shows an example of the predicted matrix displacement in the vertical direction, induced by an applied current (Sachs and Grodzinsky, 1989). The depth of penetration of the tissue displacement decreases with increasing frequency of the current. By appropriate combinations of imposed frequency and wavelength of the applied current, it may be

Figure 65.5 (a) Interdigitated Ag/AgCl electrode structure for use in surface probe measurement of bulk electrokinetic properties of cartilage. (b) Cross-sectional view of current density profile produced in a section of tissue by alternating positive and negative surface electrodes (adapted from Sachs and Grodzinsky (1989) with permission).

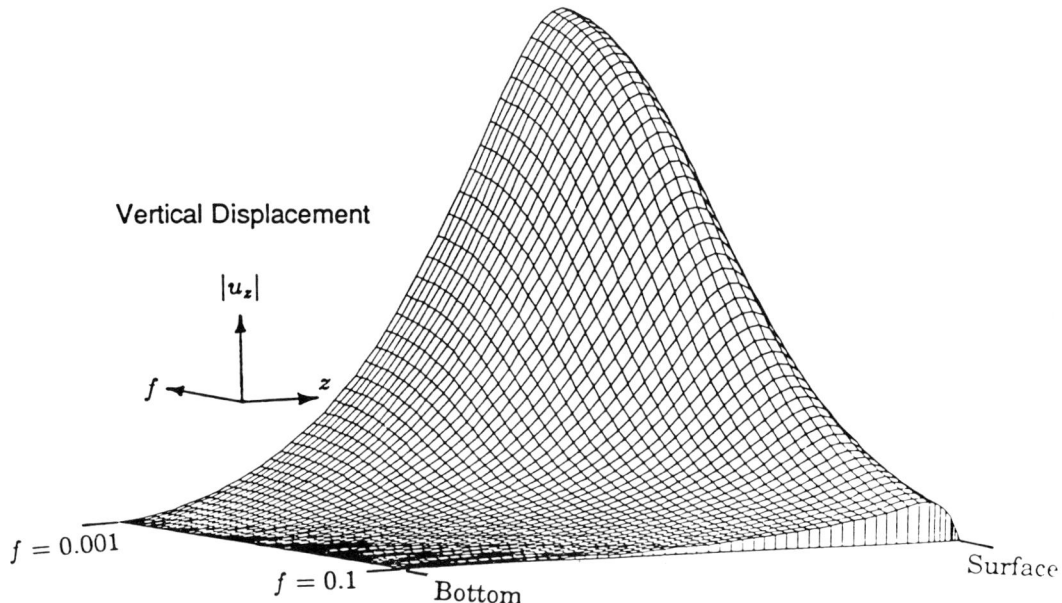

Figure 65.6 Amplitude of the relative vertical displacement as a function of depth within a finite thickness slab of cartilage, plotted for frequencies ranging from 0.001 to 0.1 Hz. Electrode spacing (0.5 mm) corresponds to a spatial wavelength of 1 mm for the imposed current density at the top surface. The electrode structure constrains the tissue displacement to be zero at the articular surface. The electrophoretic force on the matrix, combined with electroosmotic flow of interstitial fluid, produces matrix displacement pattern shown; an imposed current density amplitude of 1 mA cm^{-2} is calculated to produce a maximum displacement amplitude of 0.15 μm, shown as the peak in the curve (from Sachs and Grodzinsky (1989), with permission).

possible to probe the tissue state at various depths and locations. To interpret such measurements, extensions of the model incorporating spatially nonuniform tissue properties (Grodzinsky and Frank, 1990) would need to be included.

PHYSICOCHEMICAL PROPERTIES

Methodologies for characterizing cartilage fixed charge density (Maroudas, 1979; Urban and Maroudas, 1979) hydration, tissue swelling pressure (Staub et al., 1987) (see Chapters 69 and 70) and osmotic pressure of intact cartilage and PG solutions (see Chapter 69) have been studied extensively. The significance of the distribution of water between different tissue compartments has also been investigated recently (see Section 9). It is important to recognize that matrix fixed charge groups provide the basis for many of the tissue's physicochemical, mechanical and electromechanical properties, and the relation between these physical properties and tissue composition and structure.

BRIEF OVERVIEW OF THE CHAPTER

In order to give perspective to the global issue of mechanical stress distribution in intact joints, Afoke et al. (Chapter 66) first describe contact pressures measured using pressure-sensitive film. The advantages and constraints associated with this technique are described. Eisenberg (Chapter 67) and Mizrahi et al. (Chapter 68) then describe the measurement of mechanical and electromechanical properties of excised tissue specimens using, the confined and unconfined compression techniques, respectively. In confined compression, simultaneous measurements of mechanical and electrical properties have been made and interpreted in the context of theoretical models. The effect of the constituents of the bathing medium on these properties is also described.

The unconfined configuration is used to explore important anisotropic and nonhomogeneous behavior of cartilage. These properties are elucidated visually and in terms of creep deformation, and related to physicochemical properties of the matrix such as osmotic pressure of the PG in the extrafibrillar compartment and the hydraulic permeability in both the extra- and intra-fibrillar spaces.

It should be noted that in his approach, Eisenberg associates the tissue's resistance to compressive deformation with microscopic electrical repulsive forces between the double layers surrounding the individual negatively charged glycosaminoglycan (GAG) chains; the resulting macroscopic stress that opposes an applied compressive stress is expressed in terms of two ion-concentration-dependent material properties that can be measured in stress–strain experiments. Mizrahi *et al.* (Chapter 68), on the other hand, consider the negative fixed charge groups as contributing to the tissue's resistance to compression by causing an osmotic pressure gradient due to there being more ions inside the matrix than in synovial fluid, in accordance with the Gibbs-Donnan equilibrium. When normalized appropriately, the electrical repulsion and osmotic pressure approaches can equivalently represent that part of the equilibrium compressive stiffness contributed by fixed-charge groups.

Maroudas and Grushko (Chapter 69) then describe two methods for measuring the osmotic pressure of cartilage by means of equilibration of specimens in poly(ethylene) glycol solutions and by calculation of pressure from independent measurements on PG solutions. Calculations account for the division of water between intra- and extra-fibrillar space. Hargens (Chapter 70) then describes a new osmometer for the measurement of swelling pressure of the nucleus pulposus of the intervertebral disc. Finally, Torzilli (Chapter 71) describes a method for characterizing the compressive properties of thin cartilage slices. He also discusses the use of this method in relation to the variation in cartilage characteristics with distance from the articular surface.

ACKNOWLEDGMENTS

This work was supported by NIH grant AR33236 and NSF grant BCS-8811371.

66

Pressure measurement in the human hip joint using Fujifilm

A. AFOKE, W.C. HUTTON and P.D. BYERS

INTRODUCTION

Difficulties with instrumentation have limited attempts to determine pressure values and their distribution over contact surfaces in synovial joints (Adams and Swanson, 1985). However, the availability of pressure-sensitive film (Fujifilm Prescale) bypasses these difficulties. Fujifilm has been used to obtain contact pressures in apophyseal, patellofemoral and hip joints (Dunlop *et al.*, 1984; Huberti and Hayes, 1984, 1988; Afoke *et al.*, 1987). The following technique has proved successful in the hip joint.

THE PRESSURE-SENSITIVE FILM

The pressure-sensitive film comes in four pressure ranges when used with the standard colour samples provided by the manufacturer for visual comparison: 0.5–2, 2–7, 7–25 and 25–70 MPa. However, with a microdensitometer the working range of the 2–7 MPa pressure film can be extended to 1–10 MPa. The film is 0.2 mm thick and consists of two sheets of polyester film; one coated with a layer of microencapsulated, color-forming material (A sheet) and the other with a color-developing material (C sheet). When the two are pressed together, some of the microcapsules burst and their contents are developed by the material on the C sheet. The density of the red color produced is proportional to the pressure applied, which may be continuous or instantaneous. All our experiments have been studies of instantaneous pressure, meaning that load is applied within 5 s and removed within another 5 s without a dwell.

To convert the pressure imprint to pressure values, the film is first calibrated by applying known pressures, covering the range of the film, to a plane ended cylinder, 12 mm in diameter. The color densities are then read with a double-beam, analog-recording microdensitometer in the reflection mode (Fig. 66.1). The accuracy of pressure measurement using this calibration curve is better than 3.6% for pressures below 7 MPa and ±6% for pressures above 7 MPa.

To compensate for the effects of temperature and humidity, to which the film is sensitive, a calibration curve for the film is obtained for each test.

PREPARATION OF FILM

As the hip joint is a ball and socket, the film must be cut to size to cover the contact area, and to shape so as to invest a sphere without gaps or creases. Lanceolate leaves fill these requirements.

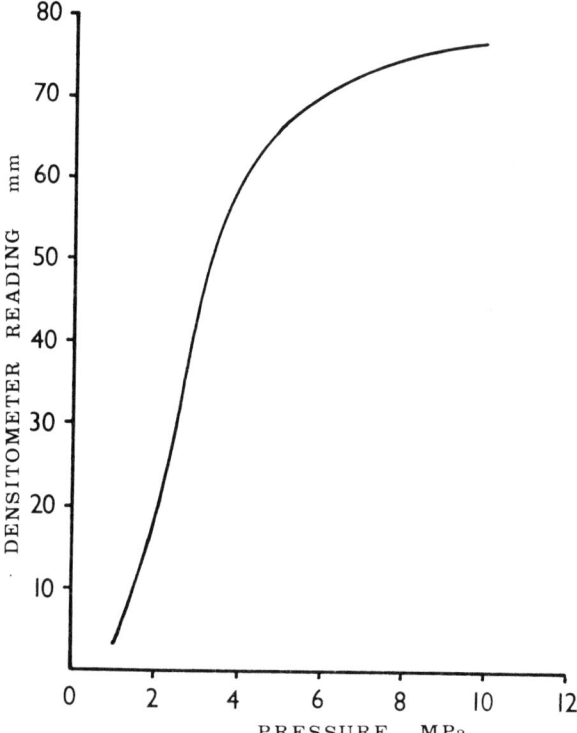

Figure 66.1 A typical calibration curve obtained for the 1–10 MPa film.

Using a punch made for the purpose, the lanceolate shapes are cut into separated strips of the A and C sheets, allowing the leaves to remain attached to the film strip, thereby facilitating handling and storage; when needed, the leaves are detached with scissors.

COVERING THE FEMORAL HEAD

To provide a moisture-free surface and to aid attachment of the film to the head, the latter is covered with cling film. Cling film is ideal for this purpose as it can be stretched tightly over the head and is of negligible thickness. Paired A and C leaves are positioned on the head and held in place by Sellotape at each end. The C sheet (the color-developing sheet) is placed uppermost; this facilitates the extraction of the film after the test is carried out. A second layer of cling film is then

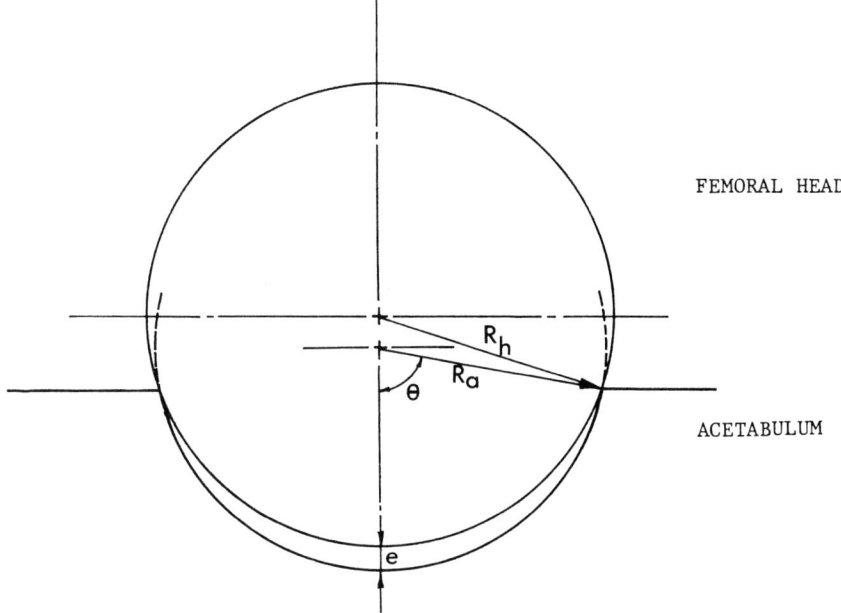

Figure 66.2 Assuming that the radius of the head is the same as that of its acetabulum, covering the head with the film enlarges its radius by 0.2 mm (the film thickness). This creates a gap (e) between the head and the acetabulum and its magnitude will depend upon the angle θ sustained by the acetabular rim in relation to its center. The value of e can be calculated from Walker's (1969) formula: $R_h - R_a = e[(1 - e/2R_a)(1 - \cos\theta - e/R_a)^{-1} - 1]$. If $R_a = 25$ mm, $\theta = 60°$, $R_h - R_a = 0.2$ mm, then $e = 175$ μm. (Reproduced from Afoke *et al.* (1987), with permission).

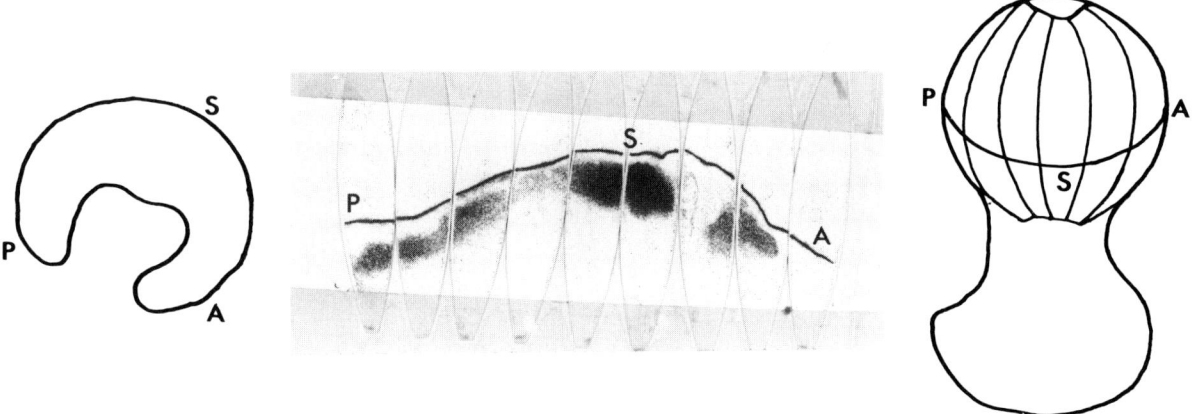

Figure 66.3 (Left) The outline of an acetabulum; (Right) the femoral head covered with the pressure-sensitive film viewed from above. (Middle) The C sheet of the film containing the imprint has been extracted from the head and mounted on paper. A, Anterior; S, superior; P, posterior.

284 11. MECHANICAL AND ELECTRICAL PROPERTIES

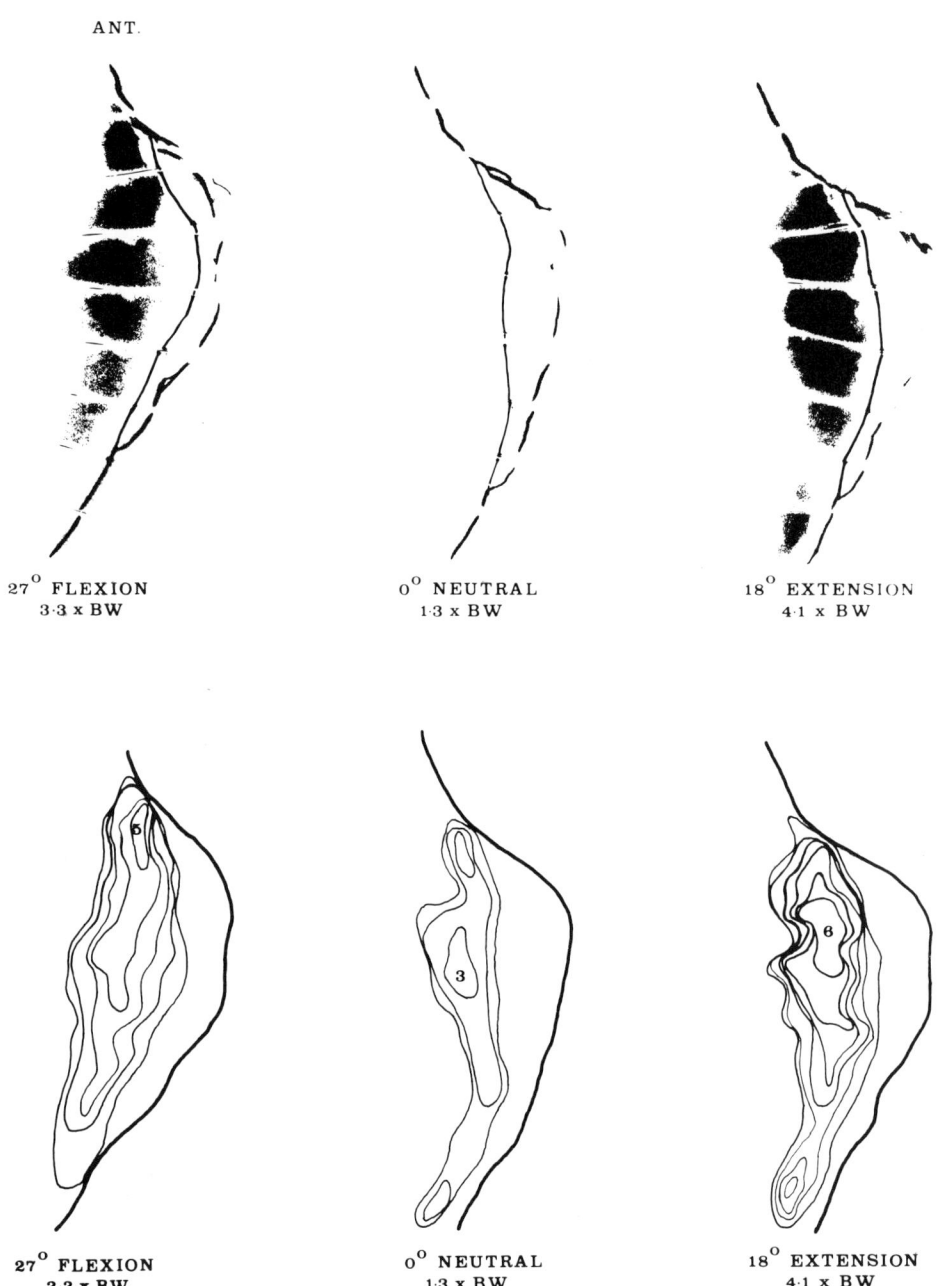

Figure 66.4 Pressure imprint (above) and contour map from a 76-year-old woman for the three positions tested. The contour lines are drawn at 1 MPa intervals. BW, Body weight. (Reproduced from Afoke et al. (1987), with permission).

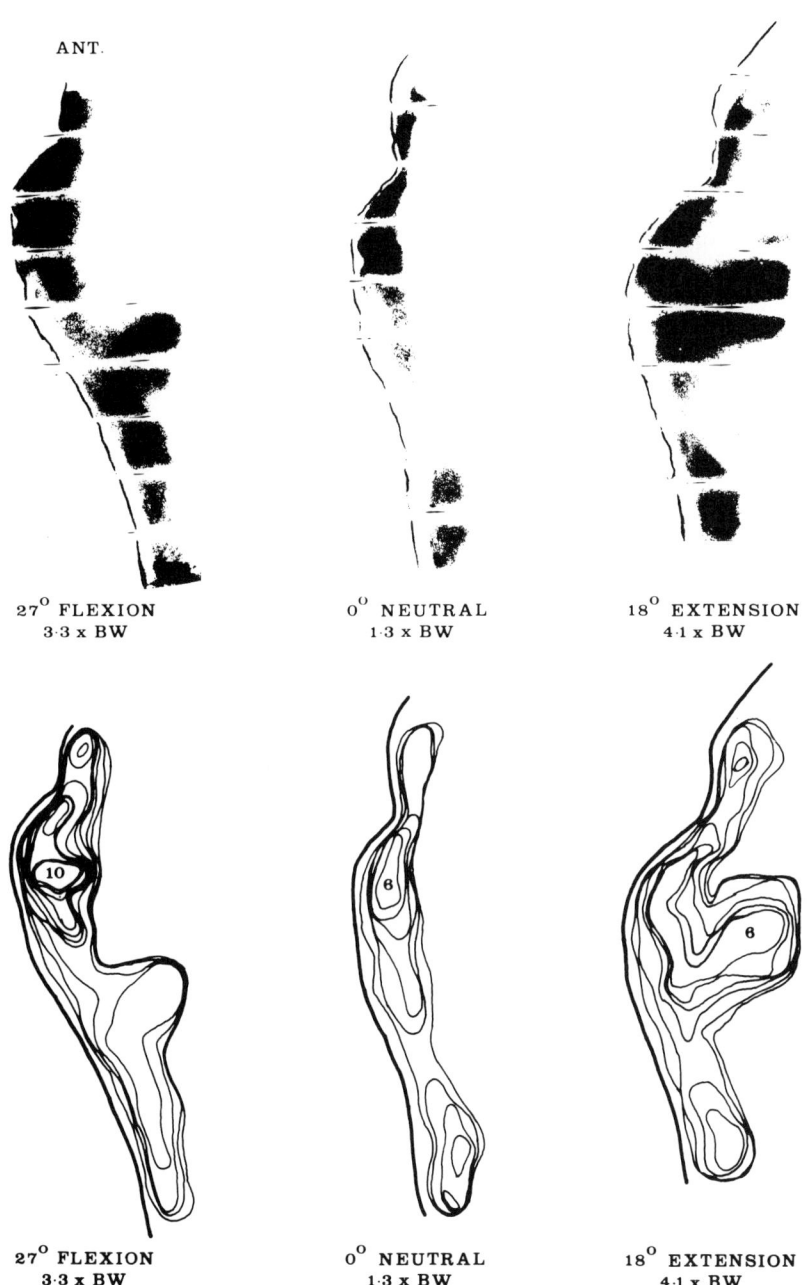

Figure 66.5 Pressure imprint (above) and contour map from a 78-year-old man for the three positions tested. The contour lines are drawn at 1 MPa intervals. BW, Body weight. (Reproduced from Afoke *et al.* (1987), with permission).

applied to complete the protection against moisture.

EFFECT OF THE FILM THICKNESS ON JOINT GEOMETRY

Assuming that the hip joint is congruent, the application of the film to the femoral head produces a gap of 175 μm at the apex between the head and the acetabulum (Fig. 66.2). Preliminary studies have shown that this gap disappears under a small load of about 50 N and that it does not affect the pressure recorded as this load is negligible compared with the test loads.

TEST PROCEDURE

A variable rig was designed for a servo-controlled hydraulic testing machine to set the specimen in any required position and direction of load application (Afoke et al., 1980, 1987). Prepared hip joints are tested in three positions and with loads simulating phases of the walking cycle. These are: heel strike (27° flexion) at 3.3 BW, flat foot (0°) at 1.3 BW, and just before toe off (18° extension) at 4 BW (Paul, 1967).

To obtain a pressure imprint, the specimen is mounted in the rig on the testing machine and set to the required position. The specimen is disarticulated, and the femoral head, after removal from the rig, is then covered with the film and the specimen rearticulated. The load is applied and removed within the specified time and the edge of the acetabulum is inscribed onto the film to provide a reference line. The specimen is disarticulated and the C sheet is extracted and mounted on a sheet of paper. Figure 66.3 shows a typical pressure imprint in relation to the acetabulum and its femoral head.

Table 66.1 Range of contact pressures in normal and pathological joints

Joints	Maximum pressure (MPa)	References
Normal joints		
Apophyseal (Fujifilm)	5.7 at 4° flexion 6.4 at 0° neutral 7.3 at 4° extension	Dunlop et al. (1984)
Patellofemoral (Fujifilm)	2.0 at 20° flexion 4.4 at 90° flexion	Huberti and Hayes (1984)
Hip (Fujifilm)	4.9–10.2 at 27° flexion 2.9–8.6 at 0° neutral 6.0–10.4 at 18° extension	Afoke et al. (1987)
Hip: with acetabulum instrumented with pressure transducers	5.26–8.57	Adams and Swanson (1985)
Hip: using an instrumented endoprosthesis	9.3–11.1	Rushfeld et al. (1981)
Pathological joints		
Patellofemoral (Chondromalacia) (Fujifilm)	1.6 on lesions	Huberti and Hayes (1988)
Hip (Preclinical OA) (Fujifilm)	10.6–13.9 at 27° flexion 4.9–8 at 0° neutral 9–9.8 at 18° extension	Afoke et al. (unpublished)

In between tests the cartilage is allowed to recover in Ringer's solution for 30 mins.

CONVERTING THE PRESSURE PRINTS TO CONTOUR MAPS

The pressure print is scanned by the microdensitometer, with a measuring area of about $1\,mm^2$, which records the whole of each traverse at 2 mm intervals. For each traverse the densitometer output at 2 mm intervals is then reduced to pressure values using the calibration curve. Thus a $2 \times 2\,mm$ grid of pressure values is established, and from this the contour map is drawn, using the acetabular rim as a reference (Figs 66.4 and 66.5).

This nondestructive method provides an assessment of contact pressures in both normal and pathological specimens. Table 66.1 shows the range of contact pressures in different joints recorded by the film and by instrumented specimens.

ACKNOWLEDGMENT

A.A. wishes to acknowledge with thanks the financial contributions from the Institution of Mechanical Engineering, the Fellowship of Engineering and the Bat Sheva Committee.

67

Physical properties of articular cartilage from uniaxial confined compression

SOLOMON R. EISENBERG

INTRODUCTION

Uniaxial confined compression is a simple and effective method for measuring many of the intrinsic mechanical and electromechanical properties of charged poroelastic materials like articular cartilage. The method has been a valuable tool for elucidating and quantitatively assessing the role of the electromechanical interactions between charged matrix constituents determining these intrinsic material properties.

In uniaxial confined compression, a carefully prepared plane parallel disk of cartilage is inserted into a rigid, impermeable confining chamber of the same diameter, as shown schematically in Fig. 67.1. The tissue sample is then compressed in the confining chamber by a freely draining, rigid porous platen. Such an experimental configuration results in tissue deformation and fluid flow only in the axial (z) direction. The one-dimensional nature of the problem allows for a straightforward analysis and interpretation of experimental results.

ELECTROMECHANICAL INTERACTIONS

Electromechanical transduction mechanisms affect the rheological properties of articular

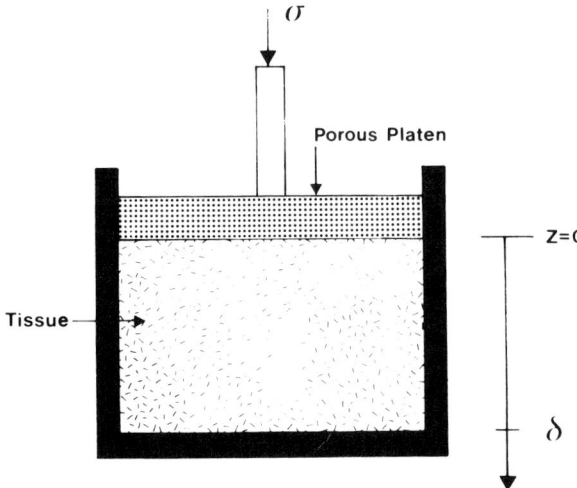

Figure 67.1 Schematic representation of a tissue sample in uniaxial confined compression. Sides and bottom of confining chamber are impermeable. Tissue surface is constrained by rigid, freely draining porous platen. (From Eisenberg and Grodzinsky (1985), with permission.)

cartilage in two distinct ways. The *equilibrium* behavior of the tissue is influenced significantly by interactions between the fixed negative charge groups on the proteoglycan (PG) aggregates and the accompanying mobile counterions that form a diffuse double layer. Neighboring double layers exert repulsive forces against each other over distances of 1–3 nm in physiological saline. These repulsive interactions are manifest macroscopically in the tissue's resistance to compressive deformation. Increasing the salt concentration of the equilibrating bath reduces these electrical repulsive forces by reducing the interaction distance (Debye length) within the tissue and shielding the charged molecules from each other. The reduced electrical interaction results in less tissue resistance to compressive deformation.

The *dynamic* behavior of the tissue is further influenced by electrokinetic coupling when the interstitial fluid flows relative to the charged solid matrix. The convection of the positive mobile counterions in the fluid leaves behind a small fraction of unneutralized negative molecular charge groups in the solid matrix. This charge separation creates an electric field antiparallel to the direction of fluid flow. The microscopic balance between electrical and viscous shear stresses in the double-layer region surrounding the fixed charge groups is the origin of the macroscopically measurable streaming potential, and tends to increase the tissue's resistance to fluid flow.

EQUILIBRIUM MECHANICAL PROPERTIES

In general, the total stress T_{ij} for a homogeneous, isotropic linear poroelastic material can be expressed by a modified form of Hooke's law in terms of the strain ε_{ij}, the chemical stress β, the Lamé constants G and λ, and the fluid pressure $(P - \Delta\pi)$ as

$$T_{ij} = 2G(c)\varepsilon_{ij} + [\lambda(c)\varepsilon_{kk} - \beta(c) - (P - \Delta\pi)]\delta_{ij} \quad (67.1)$$

where P and $\Delta\pi$ are the hydrostatic and osmotic pressures, and the material constants depend on the salt concentration of the equilibrating solution (Eisenberg and Grodzinsky, 1987). In uniaxial confined compression, only ε_{zz} is nonzero, allowing equation (67.1) to be written as

$$\sigma \equiv -T_{zz} = H_A(c)\varepsilon + \beta(c) + (P - \Delta\pi) \quad (67.2)$$

where $H_A \equiv 2G + \lambda$ is the aggregate modulus of the matrix (Mow et al., 1984), and σ and $\varepsilon \equiv -\varepsilon_{zz}$ are positive in compression.

Simple experiments in uniaxial confined compression can be used to examine the role of electrostatic interactions in determining the material properties of articular cartilage in equilibrium when the fluid pressure $(P - \Delta\pi) \equiv 0$ (no fluid flow). As depicted in Fig. 67.2, when a change in uniaxial stress is imposed, a change in the equilibrium deformation results. The ratio of the change in stress $\Delta\sigma$ and the fractional change in thickness $\Delta\varepsilon$ defines the aggregate modulus,

$$H_A = \Delta\sigma/\Delta\varepsilon \quad (67.3)$$

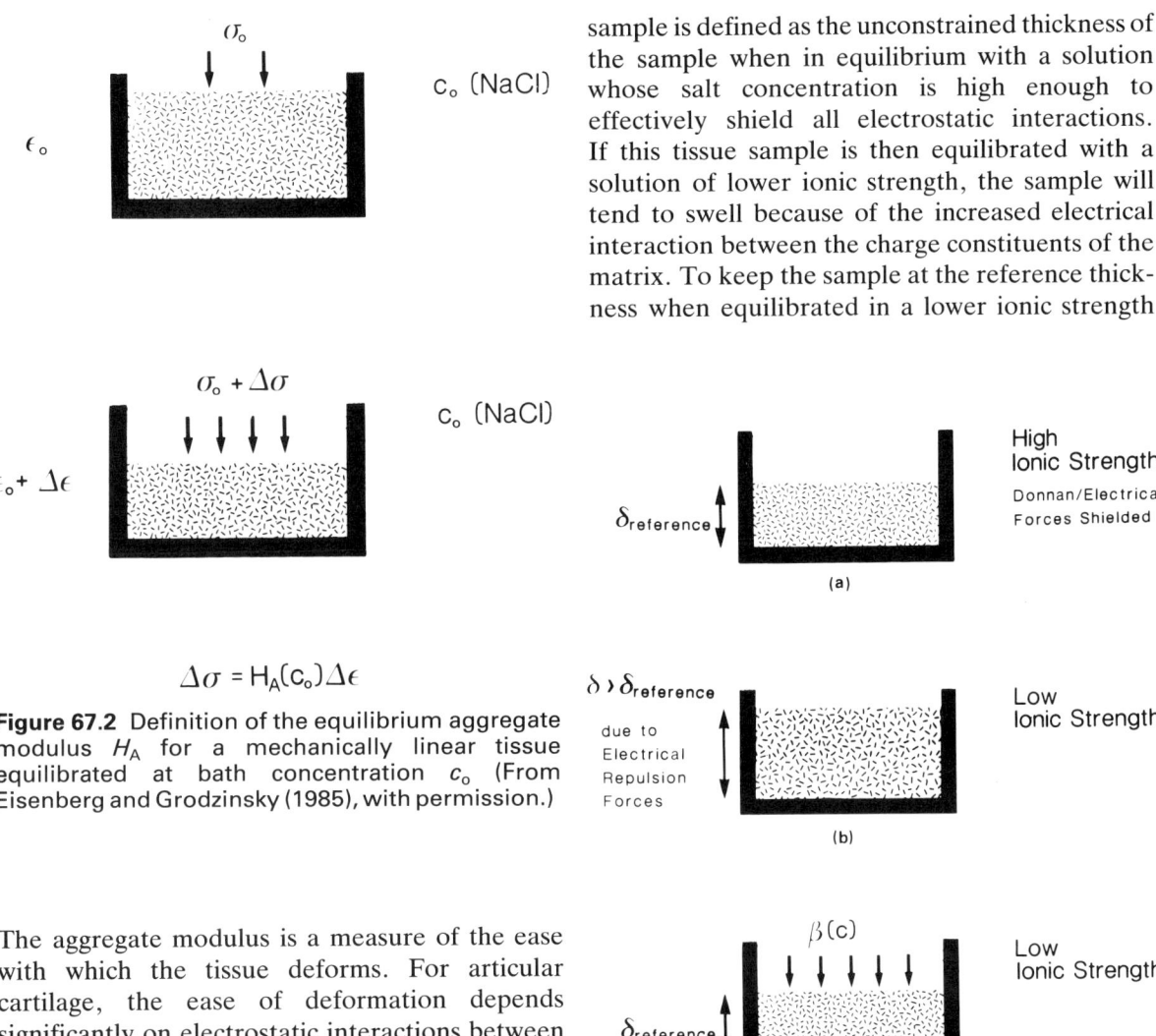

Figure 67.2 Definition of the equilibrium aggregate modulus H_A for a mechanically linear tissue equilibrated at bath concentration c_o (From Eisenberg and Grodzinsky (1985), with permission.)

sample is defined as the unconstrained thickness of the sample when in equilibrium with a solution whose salt concentration is high enough to effectively shield all electrostatic interactions. If this tissue sample is then equilibrated with a solution of lower ionic strength, the sample will tend to swell because of the increased electrical interaction between the charge constituents of the matrix. To keep the sample at the reference thickness when equilibrated in a lower ionic strength

The aggregate modulus is a measure of the ease with which the tissue deforms. For articular cartilage, the ease of deformation depends significantly on electrostatic interactions between matrix constituents. These interactions can be modulated in several distinct ways. Changing the salt concentration of the tissue bathing solution alters the interaction distance (Debye length) between charge groups. For example, increasing the salt concentration in the bath shields the matrix charges from one an other, making the tissue easier to deform (Elmore et al., 1963; Maroudas, 1975). Similar changes can be seen by altering solution pH, thereby titrating matrix charge groups, or by directly altering tissue glycosaminoglycan (GAG) content.

An additional experiment that demonstrates charge–charge interactions is illustrated in Fig. 67.3. The reference thickness of a given tissue

Figure 67.3 Definition of the chemical stress $\beta(c)$ in terms of the stress required to keep a tissue sample at its reference thickness as the concentration of the bath is varied. (a) The reference thickness δ_{ref} is defined as the unconstrained thickness when bath concentration is high enough to shield electrostatic interactions. (b) When allowed to swell in a lower ionic strength solution, the thickness of the sample increases. (c) The stress required to compress the sample back to its undeformed reference thickness ($\varepsilon = 0$) defines the chemical stress. (From Eisenberg and Grodzinsky (1985), with permission.)

solution, a mechanical stress is required. This stress is defined as the concentration-dependent chemical stress $\beta(c)$, which is a second tissue parameter. The total tissue swelling stress $p(c)$ is then

$$p(c, \varepsilon) = H_A(c)\varepsilon + \beta(c) \qquad (67.4)$$

Hence, in equilibrium, a mechanical stress $\sigma = p(c,\varepsilon)$ is required to keep the tissue at a given thickness in the configuration of Fig. 67.1.

By performing a series of stress–strain experiments at different solution ionic strengths, the concentration dependence of the aggregate modulus and chemical stress can be determined (Eisenberg and Grodzinsky, 1985). Figure 67.4 shows the experimentally determined H_A and β of adult bovine articular cartilage over the concentration range 0.005–1.0 M NaCl. The relative insensitivity of H_A to changes in concentration at the highest concentrations tested suggests that in the case of the specific tissue specimens* used in our experiments electrostatic interactions between matrix charge groups are essentially shielded in 1.0 M NaCl. At physiological ionic strength, the aggregate modulus is approximately twice its value at 1.0 M NaCl, suggesting that electrical interactions account for roughly half of this particular tissue's* resistance to deformation at physiological ionic strength.

The role of electrostatic interactions is demonstrated here by varying the salt concentration. However, more generally, the concentration axis can be thought of as the axis along which charge–charge interactions decrease, as physiologically

* *Editors's note*: the dependence of the aggregate modulus on the ionic strength of the external solution is a function of the ratio of the latter to the concentration of the negative charged fixed groups within the tissue and the intercharge distance. It is therefore a function of GAG concentration and chondroitin sulfate: keratan sulfate (CS : KS) ratio and will vary according to species, site depth, etc., from which the cartilage in question originates (see Section 1).

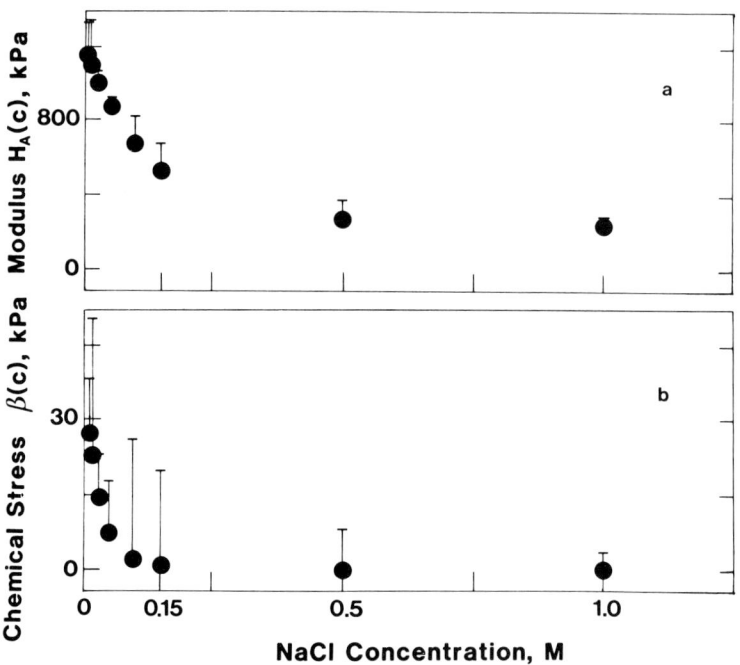

Figure 67.4 (a) Equilibrium aggregate modulus $H_A(c)$ and (b) chemical stress $\beta(c)$ as a function of bath NaCl concentration for adult bovine articular cartilage. (From Eisenberg and Grodzinsky (1987), with permission.)

might occur because of changes in the GAG content of the matrix. The effect of such a reduction in tissue GAG content on the material properties of the matrix would be qualitatively similar (Harris et al., 1972; Kempson et al., 1976; Grimshaw et al., 1983; Li et al., 1984; Frank et al., 1987b).

ELECTROKINETIC TRANSDUCTION IN OSCILLATORY CONFINED COMPRESSION

Oscillatory confined compression has also been used to assess the dynamic mechanical and electrokinetic properties of plane parallel disks of articular cartilage (Lee et al., 1981; Frank and Grodzinsky, 1987a,b; Frank et al., 1987b). Tissue samples were placed in an electrically insulating confining chamber (Fig. 67.5), and compressed to a static offset strain of 10–20% between the lower Ag/AgCl electrode and a porous polyethylene platen that separated the cartilage surface from

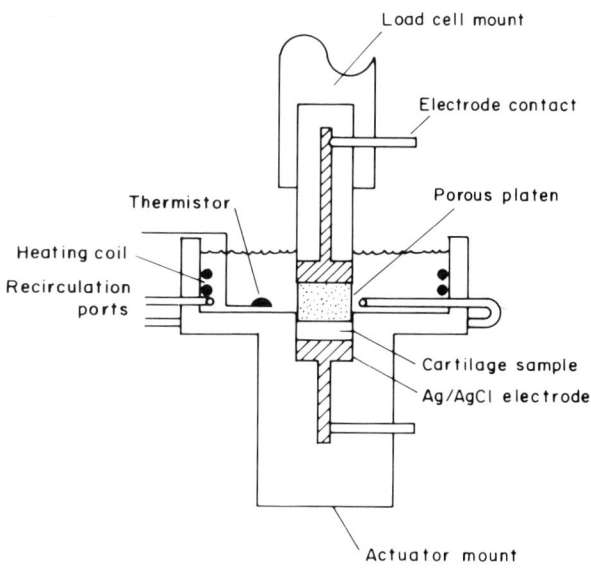

Figure 67.5 Schematic of test chamber for streaming potential and stiffness measurements on adult bovine articular cartilage specimens. (From Frank and Grodzinsky (1987a), with permission).

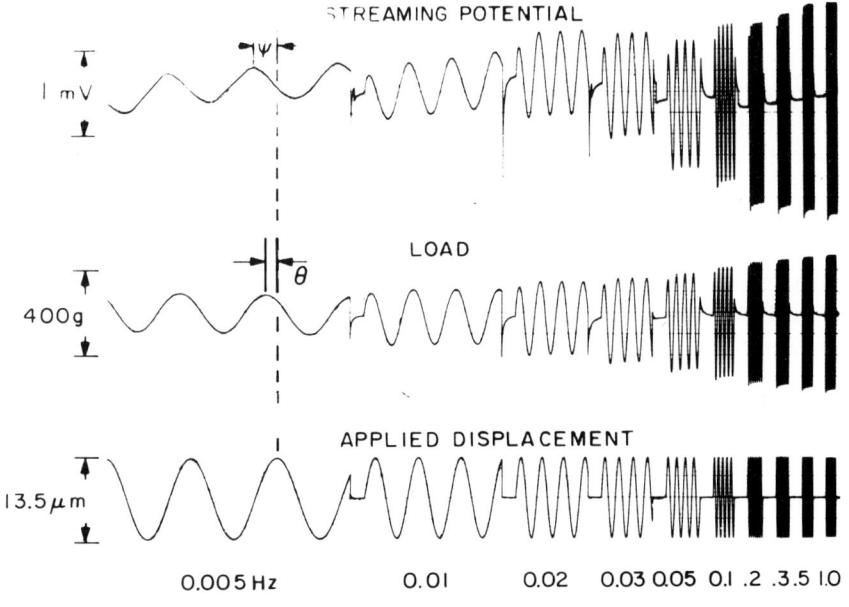

Figure 67.6 Dynamic load and streaming potential response for a specimen equilibrated in 0.05 M NaCl at neutral pH with a static offset strain of 15% and a dynamic strain amplitude of 1%. Stress and streaming potential lead the applied displacement by the phase angles θ and ψ, respectively. (From Frank and Grodzinsky (1987a), with permission).

a similar upper Ag/AgCl electrode. A small-amplitude sinusoidal displacement was superimposed on the static offset strain and the resulting sinusoidal load and streaming potential were measured simultaneously. Figure 67.6 shows the applied displacement and the measured load and streaming potential response for a sample equilibrated in saline and tested over the frequency range 0.005–1 Hz with a dynamic compression amplitude of 1% (Frank and Grodzinsky, 1987a). The stress and streaming potential lead the applied displacement by the phase angles θ and ψ, respectively. In a companion experiment, an applied sinusoidal current has been shown to generate a mechanical stress and strain within the cartilage matrix (Frank and Grodzinsky, 1987a), which is another manifestation of the same electrokinetic coupling mechanism.

Physically based models of the dynamic mechanical and electromechanical behavior have been formulated that combine the KLM biphasic model describing fluid flow in cartilage (Mow et al., 1980) with classical phenomenological models of electrokinetics (Lee et al., 1981; Frank and Grodzinsky, 1987b). These models have been shown to predict mechanical and electromechanical tissue behavior that compares well with experimental observations.

The electromechanical interactions manifest in the streaming potential response can also be altered by changing the tissue's fixed charge density. Figure 67.7 shows the amplitude of the streaming potential and the amplitude of the dynamic tissue stiffness as a function of bath pH (tissue charge) in oscillatory confined compression at 0.5 Hz (Frank et al., 1987b). As solution pH was lowered, the amplitude of the streaming potential decreased until pH $\simeq 2.75$. Further lowering of the pH caused the amplitude of the streaming potential to increase. A distinct minimum in the

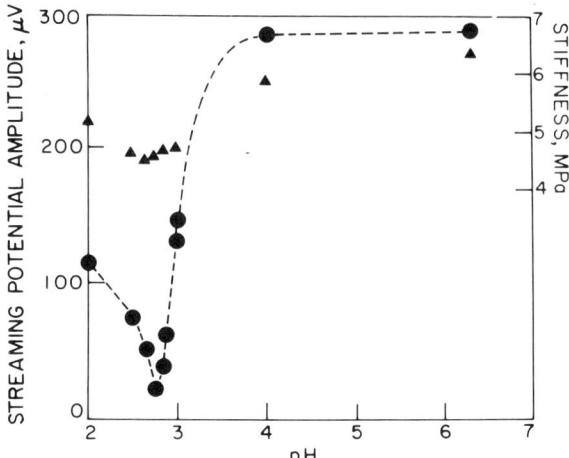

Figure 67.7 Streaming potential amplitude (●) and dynamic stiffness amplitude (▲) as function of equilibrium bath pH for a specimen of adult bovine articular cartilage at 0.05 Hz in 0.05 M NaCl. (From Frank et al. (1987b), with permission.)

amplitude of the streaming potential was observed at pH $\simeq 2.75$, which was accompanied by a reversal in the sign of the measured potential. These observations suggest an isoelectric point at pH $\simeq 2.75$ for the adult bovine femorapatellar groove specimens tested.* The dynamic tissue stiffness behaved similarly, also reaching a minimum at pH $\simeq 2.75$. However, the relative change in the amplitude of the dynamic stiffness was much smaller than the relative change in amplitude of the streaming potential, indicating that changes in tissue charge have a proportionally larger effect on the streaming potential than on the dynamic stiffness.

Editor's note: the isoelectric point is a function of the concentration of *fixed charged groups* in the tissue and will, therefore, depend on the composition of the cartilage sample being tested.

68

Unconfined compression for studying cartilage creep

J. MIZRAHI, A. MAROUDAS and E. BENAIM

INTRODUCTION

Mechanical testing of articular cartilage in compression can be carried out by one of the following methods: indentation, confined compression or unconfined compression. Each of these methods has its own advantages and drawbacks. Testing the cartilage on the joint surface by indentation may be the closest to the physiological loading conditions. However, the results obtained are difficult to analyze and interpret. On the other hand, experiments involving compression of excised plugs of cartilage, whilst further removed from the physiological situation, can yield unambiguous data on the material properties of cartilage.

We have chosen to investigate cartilage plugs in unconfined compression as this method of testing can yield information on both volume change due to fluid loss and lateral shape change due to matrix deformation. As opposed to confined compression, the response is at least two-dimensional, involving a minimum of two independent deformation parameters: one for the thickness and one for the radius (the latter is in itself direction-dependent, due to anisotropy of cartilage (Mizrahi et al., 1986)). These two parameters can be combined to describe volume loss and change in shape. It should be emphasized that in order to obtain the maximum amount of information from unconfined compression tests it is essential to measure not only the changes in thickness—as has been done in the past—but also the changes in surface area and shape. The novelty of the present method lies in introducing the latter measurements.

Thus, we have developed an apparatus and a procedure to determine directly the changes in the lateral dimensions, as well as in the thickness of the cartilage specimen during creep. On the basis of such measurements it is possible to analyze the deformation process and to attempt to clarify the respective roles of the collagen network and the proteoglycan–water solution in resisting the compressive stresses to which cartilage is subjected.

APPARATUS

The experimental system consists of the following components:

(i) loading apparatus, for applying a step-loading compression to the specimen by means of a four-bar mechanism;
(ii) specimen cell and temperature control—during the experiment, the specimen is immersed in saline at 4°C in a transparent glass cell. The top surface of the specimen is compressed against a transparent rigid plunger so that it can be observed throughout the creep phase;
(iii) an optical system which consists of a microscope used to view the deforming top surface and to which a photo camera and a video camera are attached. A second video camera viewing the side of the specimen is used to monitor the changes in the shape and dimensions of the specimen's profile;
(iv) a linear displacement transducer (LVDT) for measuring the thickness of the specimen; and

(v) a computer, used to control the sequence of on-line data collection, to sample and to process the data obtained.

A schematic description of the apparatus is given in Fig. 68.1.

PROCEDURE

Cylindrical cartilage specimens (c. 5 mm diameter) are cut, in our case from human hip and knee joints obtained at postmortem and from operations. Before testing, the initial dimensions are taken. Physicochemical parameters, including effective fixed charge density (FCD), osmotic pressure and permeability are calculated at all stages of creep as well as at final equilibrium by methods described in Chapter 69 and by Benaim (1989) and Benaim *et al.* (1990). The above calculations are based on the volume changes that occur during creep, as well as on supplementary data determined from measurements made before and after the creep tests. These measurements include wet weight, dry weight, and overall FCD, as well as the collagen content.

Creep test

Each specimen is loaded for 24 h, during which period its dimensions are measured continuously. The dimensions measured include the diameters in directions parallel and perpendicular to the prick-line pattern of both the top surface and the 'bulge' contour, the specimen thickness and the specimen profile. Variations in the experimental conditions include: testing with and without the underlying bone as well as with and without the superficial layer of the cartilage; altering the concentration of NaCl in the solution; partial removal of the proteoglycan (PG), etc.

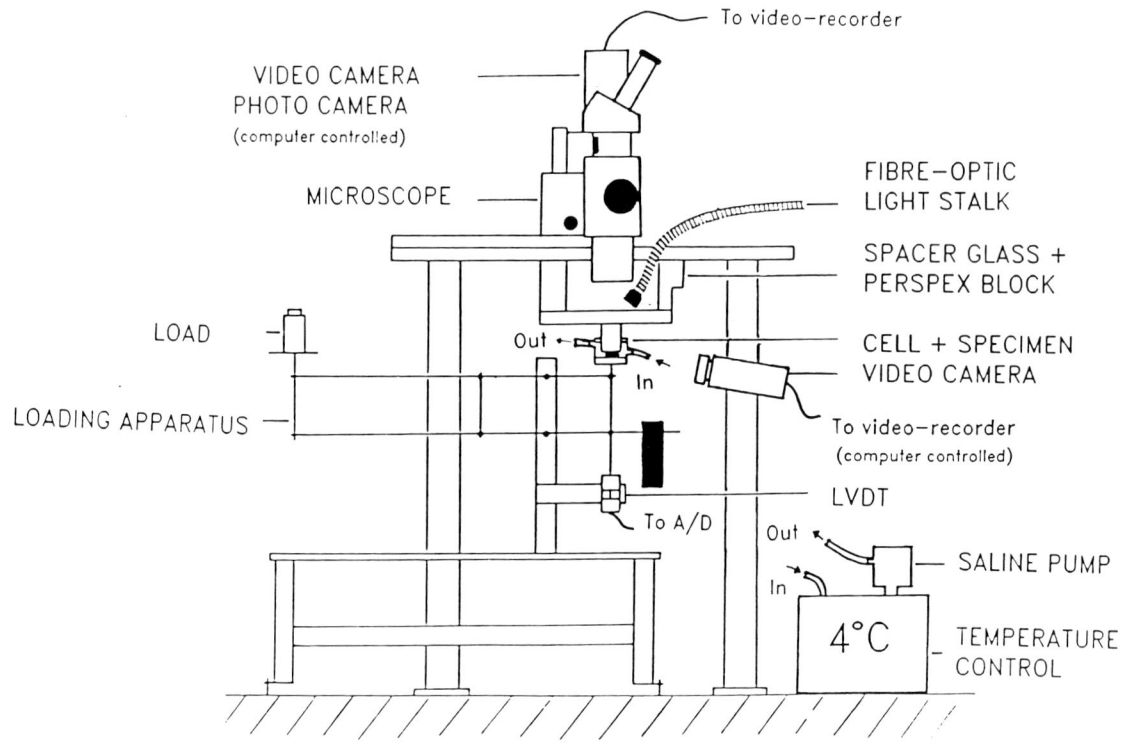

Figure 68.1 A schematic description of the testing apparatus.

'Equivalent' specimen

Due to the anisotropic and nonhomogeneous behavior of cartilage, it was found convenient to analyze the deformation by means of an 'equivalent' specimen, which was defined in such a way as to represent the actual deforming specimen, whilst being of a simpler geometry. Thus, sections parallel to the top surface were first converted into equivalent circles, having the same area as those of the actual specimen, and the resulting solid of revolution was thereafter converted into a cylinder having the same volume and surface area as those of the actual specimen.

ILLUSTRATIVE RESULTS

Diameter deformations and 'bulging'

Two distinct phases characterize the deformation obtained: (i) the instantaneous phase, in which there is a marked change in shape, with no change in volume; and (ii) the creep phase, in which fluid is squeezed out of the specimen. In this phase, the volume decrease is characterized by a significant decrease in thickness, with a minor increase in the surface area of the specimen. The diameter deformation of the specimen is always bigger in a direction perpendicular to the prick-lines as compared with the diameter deformation in a direction parallel to the prick-lines. Diameter deformations of the top surface and of the 'bulge' contour are shown for a typical specimen in Fig. 68.2. The calculated deformation of the radius of the 'equivalent' specimen is also shown in the figure.

We think that, in most cases, the 'bulge' is not due to 'stiction' of the surface to the glass, as might be suspected, but to the presence in the specimen of different zones, with different material properties. Thus, the presence of both the constraining, underlying bone and the superficial

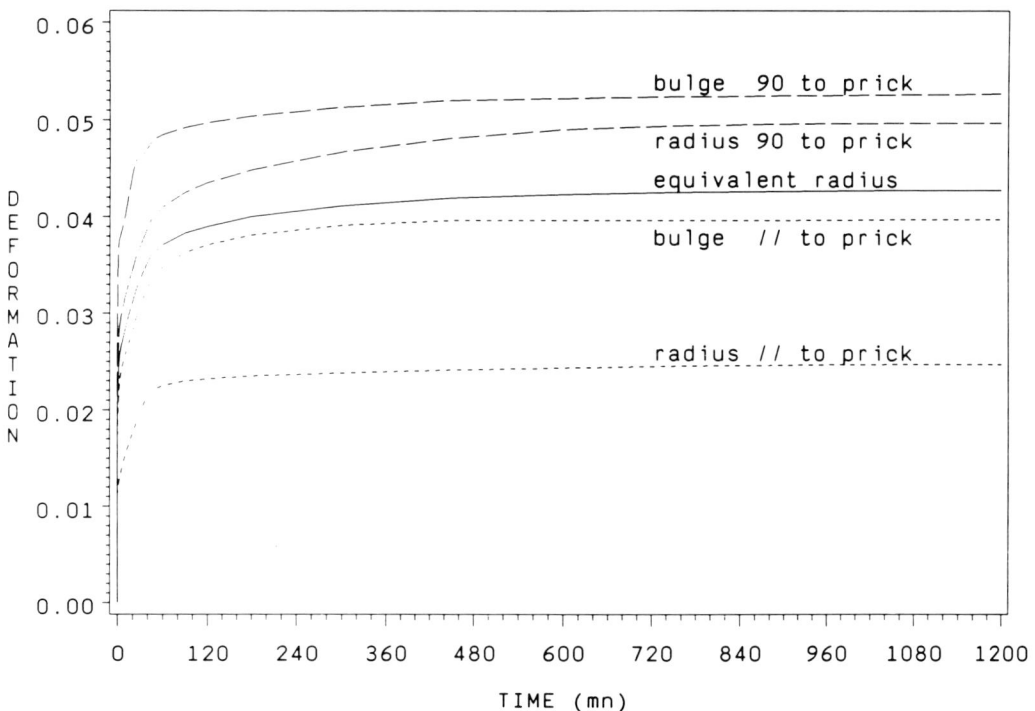

Figure 68.2 Radius deformation of the top surface and of the bulge contour.

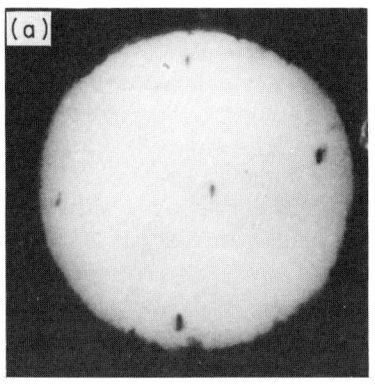 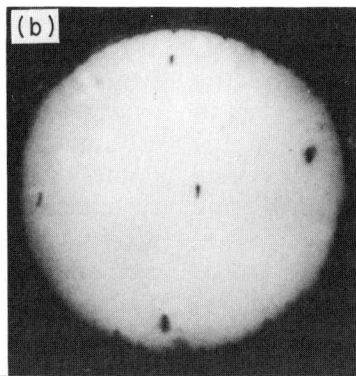 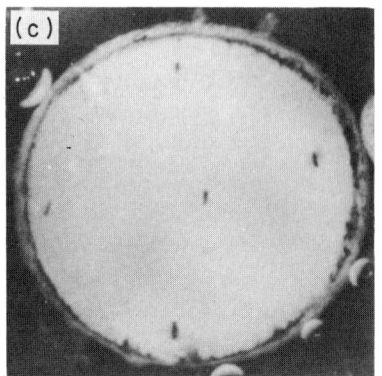

Figure 68.3 Top-view photograph of cartilage sample with its underlying bone and articular surface: (a) before loading; (b) after the instantaneous deformation; (c) at the end of creep.

layer results in bulging of the specimen, i.e. in a barrel-shaped profile. An unconstrained expansion of the specimen with a trapezoidal profile was observed whenever either of these constraints was removed. If *both* constraints were removed, i.e. only the middle zone was present, a practically homogeneous deformation was obtained, *without* bulge.

Figure 68.3 shows a top-view photograph of a cartilage sample with its underlying bone and articular surface in three different stages: (a) before loading; (b) immediately after step-loading, i.e. after the instantaneous deformation; and (c) at the end of the creep phase. The contour of the top surface was initially marked to allow a clear distinction between this surface and bulge formation (see Fig. 68.3(c)).

ANALYSIS OF RESULTS: EXAMPLES OF MODELS WHICH CAN BE USED

Comparison between applied pressure and osmotic pressure of proteoglycan at final equilibrium; physiological implications

In all experiments in which the mechanical loading pressure was higher than the initial osmotic pressure the final values of the osmotic pressure, π, tended to coincide with the applied pressure as shown in Fig. 68.4. This indicates that in the final equilibrium state the applied pressure is resisted only by the osmotic pressure of the PG and that the collagen fibrils do not therefore take part in bearing the compressive load. The fibrils can, however, transmit stress in a direction perpendicular to that of the compressive load.

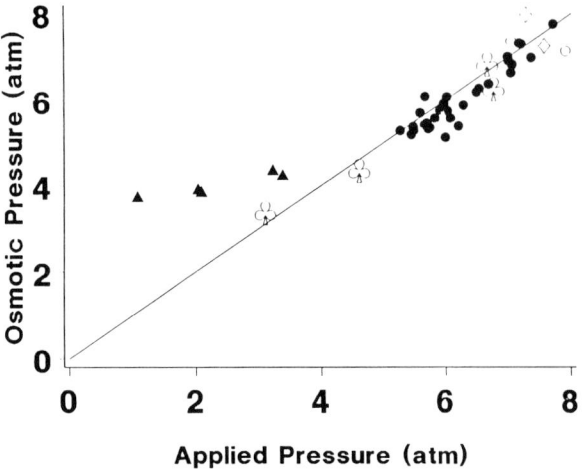

Figure 68.4 Comparison between applied pressure and PG osmotic pressure at final equilibrium. (●) $P_{applied} > P_{osm}$; (◇) hypotonic (0.015 M NaCl); (○) hypertonic (4 M NaCl); (△) partially depleted. (▲) $P_{applied} < P_{osm}$, normal saline (0.15 M NaCl).

Knowing that in the final equilibrium state the compressive stress in the direction of load application is resisted only by the osmotic pressure in the extrafibrillar compartment, we can calculate the amount of water which will remain in the latter compartment for any given applied stress. We also know how the hydration of the intrafibrillar compartment varies with compression and we can, therefore, predict its water content for a given pressure. Hence we can predict the *total* amount of water at final equilibrium for a given applied stress. For instance, at body temperature, for a pressure of 50 atm (5 MPa), corresponding to the physiological pressure range as estimated by modern measurements (see Chapter 66), we estimate that at equilibrium the amount of water retained within human femoral head cartilage will be approximately 90% of its dry weight and the total volume of the tissue will be reduced by some 50% of its initial value.

It should be borne in mind, however, that *in vivo*, except if a person is standing still for a long time, equilibrium is never achieved. Hence, it is essential to be able to provide a description of what happens during the nonsteady-state processes such as the creep phase of the deformation.

Such a description must rely on the knowledge of pressure gradients and hydraulic permeability. Our attempts in this direction are described in the next section.

Derivation of hydraulic permeability from creep measurements

Using Darcy's law, we can derive the hydraulic permeability during the course of creep from fluid flux, and the static *and* the osmotic pressure gradients. Whilst fluid flux is obtainable from volume measurements, determination of the pressure gradients requires additional information, relating to the mechanical properties of the collagen network. A structural model of the collagen network, relating its geometry to the stiffness of the matrix was therefore developed and incorporated into a creep model (Benaim *et al.*, 1990).

Based on the creep results obtained, the hydraulic permeability was derived using two methods: (i) using the solution of the above model (we refer to it as 'our model') for the static pressure gradient; and (ii) using McCutchen's (1962) prediction of a parabolic pressure gradient. The values of permeability thus obtained could be compared with those predicted, for different water contents, by a purely geometrical model based on flow through meshworks of rods (Jackson and James, 1982; Maroudas *et al.*, 1987; also see Chapter 64).

It should be noted that, in the case of cartilage, the latter model has to be based on a two-compartment (extra- and intra-fibrillar) matrix:

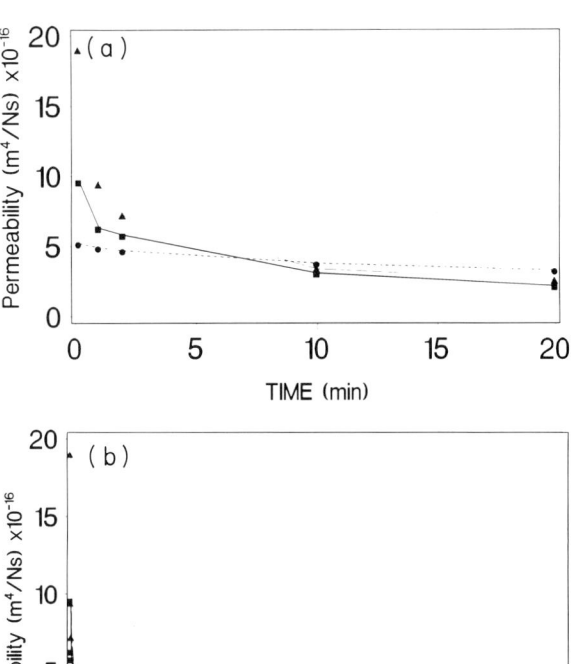

Figure 68.5 Curves of hydraulic permeability versus time (first 20 min of creep) calculated using three different models: (a) first 20 min of creep; (b) total creep period until equilibrium. (●) Geometrical model (Maroudas *et al.*, 1987); (▲) from Darcys law, using 'modified McCutchen' model; (■) from Darcy's law, using present model (Benaim, 1989; Benaim *et al.*, 1990).

flow is assumed to take place in parallel through these compartments, each consisting of rod-like molecules (GAG and collagen, respectively) and each presenting its own resistance to flow, depending on rod diameter and fractional volume of solids (Maroudas et al., 1987).

The curves of permeability calculated from our creep results and those estimated from the geometrical model are shown, as a function of time after load application, in Fig. 68.5. Initially, the values determined from creep lie above the calculated values. The values obtained using the McCutchen model based on a parabolic pressure profile are clearly unrealistically high. The values using our model approach closely those calculated from the geometrical model, especially after the first 30 seconds creep and up to 1 hour. At longer times the permeability results calculated from creep, using either the McCutchen or our model, yield unreliable results because both calculations involve using the difference between the applied and the osmotic pressure, which, at this stage, tends to zero. Thus, any small error in the estimation of the osmotic pressure within the matrix leads to large errors in the calculation of the driving force. Moreover, the very low rate of deformation of the tissue during these late stages means that the responses of the LVDT to dimensional changes in some parts of the apparatus, e.g. due to slight ambient temperature changes, are no longer negligible compared with the tissue response and large errors arise.

CONCLUSION

We have developed an experimental setup for measuring the deformation of cartilage in unconfined compression and have shown that the course of creep can be analysed using independently determined physicochemical parameters and constitutive equations based on a model for the mechanical response of the collagen network.

69

Measurement of swelling pressure of cartilage

ALICE MAROUDAS and GALINA GRUSHKO

INTRODUCTION

It has been found in a number of recent studies that when specimens of cartilage are subjected to a compressive mechanical stress, the decrease in volume at final equilibrium is equal to the decrease in hydration observed during equilibrium dialysis of the same specimen against polyethylene glycol (PEG) solutions, exerting an osmotic pressure equal to the value of the mechanical loading pressure used. Furthermore, it has been shown that the main factor responsible for resisting external compression, be it mechanical or osmotic, is the osmotic pressure of the PG within the cartilage itself (see Chapter 68; Grushko et al., 1989; Benaim, 1989; Benaim et al., 1990). Thus, provided the variation of the osmotic pressure (π) of a given specimen of cartilage with hydration is known, it is possible to predict the decrease in volume of such a specimen under any given external loading pressure.

It should be noted that when cartilage is not

subjected to an externally applied pressure, the swelling tendency of the PG is exactly balanced by the elastic tension in the collagen network. The latter decreases very rapidly as soon as the tissue begins to shrink in volume. When the decrease in volume is equal to or more than approximately 5%, the collagen tension becomes negligible in relation to the osmotic pressure of the PG. Under such conditions, the swelling pressure of cartilage is equal to the osmotic pressure, π, of the constituent PG (Maroudas and Bannon, 1981; Maroudas et al., 1987).

We have employed two methods for determining the swelling pressure of the cartilage matrix at different degrees of hydration: (i) equilibration of cartilage or disc specimens in solutions of PEG of known osmotic pressure (this method can only be used when the initial osmotic pressure of cartilage is inferior to the osmotic pressure of the given PEG solution); and (ii) calculation of the osmotic pressure of cartilage from that of the constituent proteoglycans (PGs).

DETERMINATION OF OSMOTIC PRESSURE BY EQUILIBRIUM DIALYSIS AGAINST POLYETHYLENE GLYCOL SOLUTIONS (METHOD A)

Cartilage (or disc) samples are subjected to different osmotic pressures by immersing them in calibrated solutions of PEG. The procedure is similar to that described by Maroudas and Urban (1983). The solutions are prepared from dialyzed PEG. In order to prevent penetration of PEG into the cartilage specimens, the solutions, after being initially weighed, are placed in fine-pore dialysis tubing (2000). The solutions are allowed to equilibrate in a PEG solution of desired concentration for a period of 24–48 h, depending on specimen thickness. The concentrations of PEG solutions used by us were 15–30 g PEG per 100 g solvent, corresponding to applied pressures of 3–10 atm.

Once equilibrium has been reached, the sacs are lifted out of the PEG solutions, blotted well to remove any adherent moisture and the cartilage samples weighed. From the final and initial weight, it is possible to calculate for each slice the amount of water lost at equilibrium, corresponding to a given applied pressure. The dry-tissue weight is obtained by freeze drying the cartilage to constant weight. The final hydration corresponds to the osmotic pressure of the given equilibrating PEG solution.

One of the difficulties inherent in the method is that, in spite of the very low pore size of the dialysis tubing used, PEG still tends to penetrate into the tissue over long periods of exposure. It is thus necessary to balance carefully the latter risk against the time actually needed to reach osmotic equilibrium. It is recommended to check experimentally whether or not PEG has penetrated by comparing the dry weight of the tissue specimen obtained immediately after incubation in PEG with that obtained, for the second time, after the specimen has been washed for a few hours in a 0.15 M NaCl solution.

Calibration of polyethylene glycol solutions

Urban et al. (1979) calculated the osmotic pressures of PEG solutions using the virial coefficients reported by Edmond and Ogston (1968), at 25°C. These coefficients were used by Urban et al. (1979) for calculations at different temperatures by assuming that the virial coefficient remained constant over a range of 4–37°C. It was mentioned at the time that this assumption may not be exactly correct.

Empirical relations for 7°C and 30°C were recently published by Parsegian et al. (1986), who measured the osmotic pressure of PEG by direct membrane osmometry.

Comparison of the two sets of data (Fig. 69.1) shows considerable differences, especially at low temperatures, and leads to the conclusion that virial coefficients vary with temperature and extrapolation of results obtained at 25°C to other temperatures is not correct.

We ourselves repeated the calibration at 4°C, using a Diaflow cell and air pressure, and obtained the points also shown in Fig. 69.1 (unpublished data). It can be seen that our points fall very close to the curve obtained from Parsegian's data.

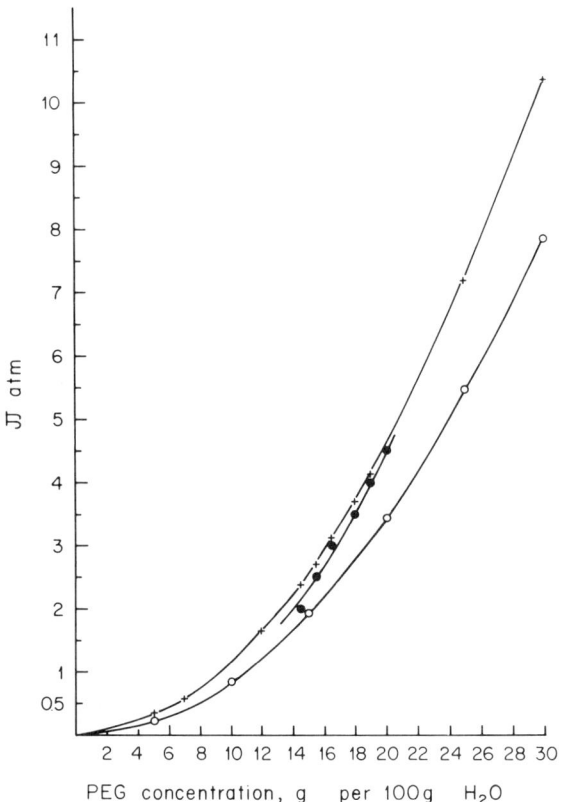

Figure 69.1 Calibration of PEG solutions at 4°C. (+) 4°C data of Urban *et al.* (1979), based on virial coefficients of Edmond and Ogston (1968); (○) 7°C data of Parsegian *et al.* (1986); (●) 4°C unpublished data (Ramon and Maroudas).

CALCULATION OF OSMOTIC PRESSURE OF CARTILAGE BASED ON KNOWLEDGE OF OSMOTIC PRESSURE OF PROTEOGLYCAN AND VOLUME OF EXTRA-FIBRILLAR COMPARTMENT (METHOD B)

The cartilage matrix consists of two compartments: the space within the collagen fibrils, from which the PGs are excluded because of their size, and the extrafibrillar space the properties of which are chiefly determined by the presence of the PGs. Provided the concentration of the PG is expressed on the basis of the extrafibrillar water, within which the PGs are confined, the osmotic pressure of the cartilage matrix can be deduced directly from the osmotic pressure of the PG solution at the same effective concentration, i.e. at the same effective FCD.

In order to calculate the fraction of extrafibrillar water corresponding to a given set of conditions, the intrafibrillar fraction must be known. Recently, it has been shown that the latter fraction is not a constant, but itself varies as a function of the osmotic pressure in the PG compartment (Katz *et al.*, 1986; Maroudas *et al.*, 1990).

The calculations require the knowledge of three parameters: the collagen content, the total water content and the overall FCD. Once the fraction of intrafibrillar water is known, it is possible to calculate the extrafibrillar fraction and, hence, the effective FCD.

Method of calculating effective fixed charge density

In order to calculate the effective FCD of any given specimen we need to know the fraction of extrafibrillar (EF) water. In order to calculate the EF water content, the intrafibrillar (IF) water per gram of collagen has to be determined. The following relations hold:

$$\text{FCD}_{\text{eff}} = \text{FCD}_{\text{overall}} \frac{W_0}{W_{\text{H}_2\text{O}}} \quad (69.1)$$

$$\text{FCD}_{\text{eff}} = \text{FCD}_{\text{overall}} \frac{W_0}{W_{\text{H}_2\text{O}} - W_0 \times C_{\text{coll}} \times W_{\text{IF}}} \quad (69.2)$$

where W_0 is the total initial wet weight of the specimen, $W_{\text{H}_2\text{O}}$ is the weight of total water in the specimen either initially or under pressure, W_{EF} is the weight of EF water, C_{coll} is the weight of collagen per gram of initial specimen weight, $\text{FCD}_{\text{overall}}$ is the fixed charge density based on initial total weight of specimen, and W_{IF} is the weight of IF water per gram of dry collagen.

Furthermore, the relation between the osmotic pressure, π, and PG concentration as expressed by fixed charge density is given by (Urban *et al.*, 1979):

$$\pi = B\,(\text{FCD}_{\text{effective}})^2 \quad (69.3)$$

Table 69.1 Mean osmotic pressure of hip cartilage in different age groups: comparison between measured and calculated values

Age (years)	Region	25% PEG ($P = 7.1$ atm)			30% PEG ($P = 10.3$ atm)		
		n	FCD$_{eff}$	P*	n	FCD$_{eff}$	P*
17–20	Superior	7	0.530	7.50	6	0.668	11.90
	Inferior	4	0.522	7.26	6	0.659	11.58
20–30	Superior	11	0.518	7.15	10	0.603	9.71
	Inferior	5	0.521	7.25	5	0.654	11.4
30–45	Superior	10	0.506	6.84	16	0.616	10.1
	Inferior	4	0.478	6.09	5	0.611	9.97
50–65	Superior	—	—	—	11	0.588	9.22
	Inferior	—	—	—	3	0.618	10.2
70–81	Superior	12	0.513	7.03	11	0.611	9.95
	Inferior	5	0.502	6.72	7	0.618	10.2

* Calculated (method B).

According to recent data on the osmotic pressures of PEG solutions (Fig. 69.1) and the data of Urban et al. (1979) for PG solutions, the value of the coefficient B at 4° is 26.6.

It should be noted that the above empirical equation was determined for solutions of PGs. Therefore, our first assumption is that PG within the tissue behaves in the same way as isolated PG in solution at the same concentration or FCD.

Our second assumption is that the fraction of IF water in PG-free cartilage is affected by an externally applied pressure in the same way as in native cartilage it is affected by the osmotic pressure of the PG present in the EF space (see Chapter 56). Thus, we make use of an empirical equation found as a best fit to the experimental data for PG-free cartilage (Maroudas et al., 1990)

$$W_{IF} = 0.76 + 0.85 \exp(-0.38 \times P) \quad (69.4)$$

where P is the applied pressure (and is equivalent to π in its effect on IF space).

Substituting equation (69.3) into equation (69.4) we obtain:

$$W_{IF} = 0.76 + 0.85 \exp[-0.38 \times (FCD_{eff})^2] \quad (69.5)$$

It can be seen that equations (69.2) and (69.5) contain the same two unknowns, viz, the IF water content and effective FCD, and can be solved for any water content, provided the initial tissue composition and the overall initial FCD are known. For human femoral head cartilage the composition is as follows (e.g. see Chapter 53; Maroudas et al., 1980): collagen 15–20%, water content 70–75%; FCD 0.1–0.2 meq g^{-1}.

EXAMPLE OF COMPARISON BETWEEN OSMOTIC PRESSURE OBTAINED BY METHODS A AND B

A comparison between the measured and the calculated values of osmotic pressure for cartilage of different age groups is given in Table 69.1. It should be noted that the original measurements of osmotic pressure of extracted PGs on which our calculations are based were obtained from a mean curve, not taking into account the systematic changes in the chondroitin sulfate: keratan sulfate: hyaluronan (CS : KS : HA) ratios which occur with age (see Chapters 53 and 54) and which affect the mean interchange distances and hence π. Clearly, it would be desirable to obtain separate curves of osmotic pressure for PG extracted from cartilage obtained from different age ranges. However, considering this shortcoming, the agreement between the two sets of values (usually within 10%) bears out the validity of the assumptions underlying the procedure described for the second method.

70

Osmometer for rapid measurement of swelling pressure of nucleus pulposus from the intervertebral disc

ALAN R. HARGENS

INTRODUCTION

The disc serves an important weightbearing function and its cross-sectional area (Wilder et al., 1988) and internal swelling pressure (Hargens, 1989) increase directly with body mass. Classic studies of lumbar nucleus pulposus in humans document changes in pressure with posture (Nachemson and Elfström, 1970).

Increased loading of the spine during spinal muscle contraction or weightbearing drives fluid from the disc, whereas decreased loading (e.g. sleep or microgravity) pulls fluid into the disc (Urban and Maroudas, 1980, 1981; Urban and McMullin, 1985; Urban, 1987; Hargens and Mahmood, 1989). Thus, compressive stresses are counteracted by the internal swelling pressure of the disc. Swelling pressure is a function of fixed charge density of the proteoglycans (PGs), with a small contribution from excluded-volume effects (Urban et al., 1979); Urban and Maroudas, 1981; Maroudas, 1979).

Disc swelling pressures have been measured by Urban and Maroudas (1981) using equilibrium dialysis against calibrated polyethylene glycol (PEG) solutions (see Chapter 69). This procedure, unfortunately, is rather lengthy and requires relatively large tissue specimens. Standard osmometers, however, are not suitable as they do not cover the required pressure range; moreover, air bubbles tend to form on the side of the membrane opposite the sample of the nucleus pulposus.

We have developed a modified osmometer whose chief advantages are speed of operation and the fact that only very small quantities of disc material are needed for measurement.

DESCRIPTION OF NEW OSMOMETER AND METHOD USED

New osmometer

The new osmometer (Fig. 70.1) (Glover et al., 1988; Hargens and Mahmood, 1989) consists of a screw-down plexiglass top that compresses a 0.45 μm Millipore filter membrane (M) over a circular crimp ring (CR). The filter membrane (M) separates the tissue specimen placed in the sample well (SW) from the saline column that is in contact with the sensing diaphragm of a low-volume displacement arterial pressure transducer (PT). It is important that no leakage occurs across M or across the sealing O-ring (OR). If leakage occurs, the nucleus pulposus sample will not produce a large negative pressure, but the PT can still be calibrated with a water column. The osmometer works on the principle by which the swelling pressure of the nucleus pulposus sample is counterbalanced by compression of the sample by using nitrogen gas (Fig. 70.2).

Sample

In order to minimize drying artifacts, the samples of fresh or recently-frozen nucleus pulposus are removed from the disc by a curet in a humidified chamber just prior to measurement. A sample as

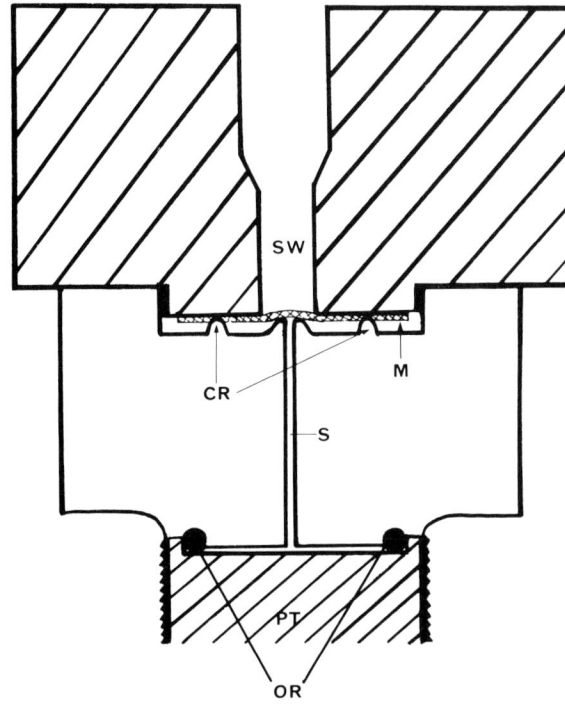

Figure 70.1 Cross-section of new osmometer. See text for description.

(vi) After matrix relaxes and adjusts to compression, negative pressure is again obtained and overrides the nitrogen compression.
(vii) Steps (v) and (vi) are repeated until equilibrium is approached.
(viii) Equilibrium is defined as zero PT recording for at least 1 min.

It should be noted that the higher the swelling pressure of the sample, the longer it takes to reach equilibrium. Our experience indicates that most samples can be measured within 15–20 min. An important precaution is that one should not pressurize the sample too rapidly because nitrogen gas may transfer across the membrane and produce a bubble beneath the membrane so that the swelling pressure is lost.

DISCUSSION

This new technique for measuring swelling pressure has several potential advantages and

small as 3–5 mg can be used to make measurements in the osmometer. This sample size corresponds to the amount obtained from one lumbar disc of a medium-sized rat.

Procedure

The procedure consists of the following steps—the numbers quoted corresponding to the phases on the osmometer recording (Fig. 70.3).

(i) Calibration of PT to +100, 0 and −100 mmHg.
(ii) Recheck zero by applying a few mg of saline to SW.
(iii) Remove all saline and dry membrane to about −10 to −20 mmHg.
(iv) Add 3–5 mg nucleus pulposus sample.
(v) After negative pressure goes off scale, apply nitrogen compression causing zero overshoot and compressing matrix and fluid components of nucleus pulposus.

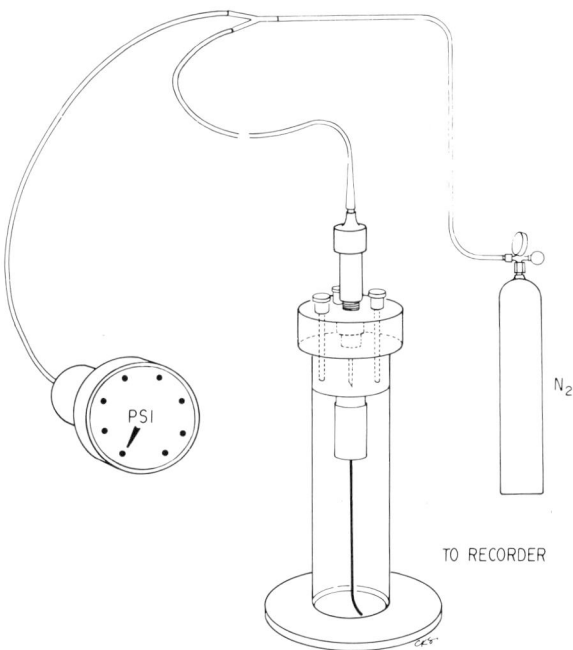

Figure 70.2 Overall set-up of apparatus with osmometer cap, nitrogen gas, precision pressure gauge (0–50 psi or 0–100 psi) and PT connection to recorder.

304   11. MECHANICAL AND ELECTRICAL PROPERTIES

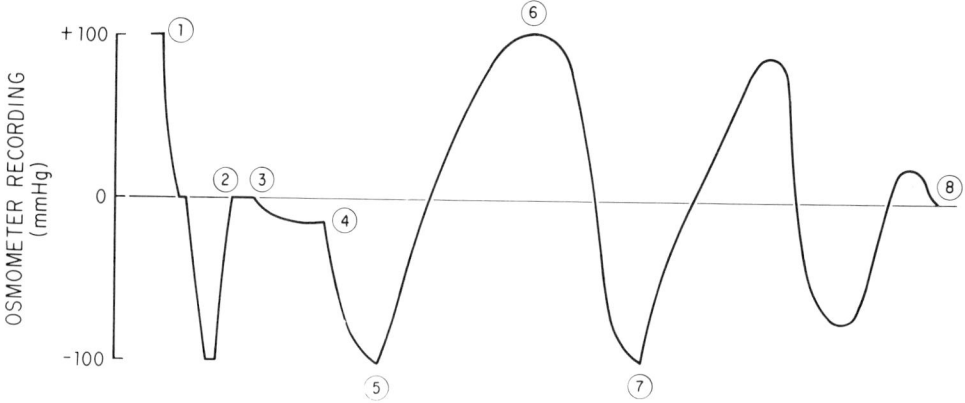

Figure 70.3 Typical osmometer recording. See text for description.

disadvantages. First, an advantage is that equilibrium is rapidly approached using direct compression of relatively small samples. Second, results from this technique agree fairly well with the equilibrum dialysis technique (Glover *et al.*, 1988). Third, it is a nondestructive measurement and samples can be analyzed biochemically, for example. Some of the potential disadvantages or uncertainties are: (i) the filter membrane and PT are not perfectly rigid and small volumes of saline may move in and out of the sample; (ii) the membrane may not completely retain the PGs — the component responsible for the swelling pressure; and (iii) the exact point of fluid equilibrium may not be reached by the whole sample. These uncertainties must be further investigated.

ACKNOWLEDGMENTS

Support from NASA is acknowledged.

71

Measurement of the compressive properties of thin cartilage slices: evaluating tissue inhomogeneity

PETER A. TORZILLI

INTRODUCTION

We are well aware today that articular cartilage is a highly inhomogeneous tissue having a unique spatial morphology (see Sections 1, 3 and 9). It is this unique spatial distribution of tissue constituents that influences mechanical and biological response during normal physiological function.

It is well documented that in cartilage there is a continuous change in constituent morphology and content from the articular surface to the subchondral bone (e.g. Stockwell and Scott, 1967; Maroudas, 1968; Maroudas *et al.*, 1969; Kempson *et al.*, 1970, 1971; Mow *et al.*, 1974, 1980). In the superficial tangential zone collagen fibers are arranged tangential to the articular surface, in the middle zone they are more randomly oriented, while the deep zone contains radially oriented fibers. Collagen content is highest at the articular surface, decreases in the middle zone, and then increases as it becomes embedded into the subchondral bone. On the other hand, proteoglycan (PG) content is lowest at the articular surface and increases with depth. Water content is also higher at the articular surface and decreases with depth, (e.g. Maroudas *et al.*, 1969; Torzilli, 1985).

SPATIAL MECHANICAL PROPERTIES

The spatial variation in both the structural conformation and constituent composition greatly influences the mechanical deformation of articular cartilage (e.g. Kempson *et al.*, 1970; Mizrahi *et al.*, 1986). When articular cartilage is loaded in compression the local tissue deformation (strain) will vary nonlinearly throughout its thickness (e.g. Mow *et al.*, 1980). The nonlinear spatial strain distribution is a result of fluid permeation and the inhomogeneous, anisotropic nature of the tissue. This can be demonstrated using an experimental test to measure the compressive properties of thin

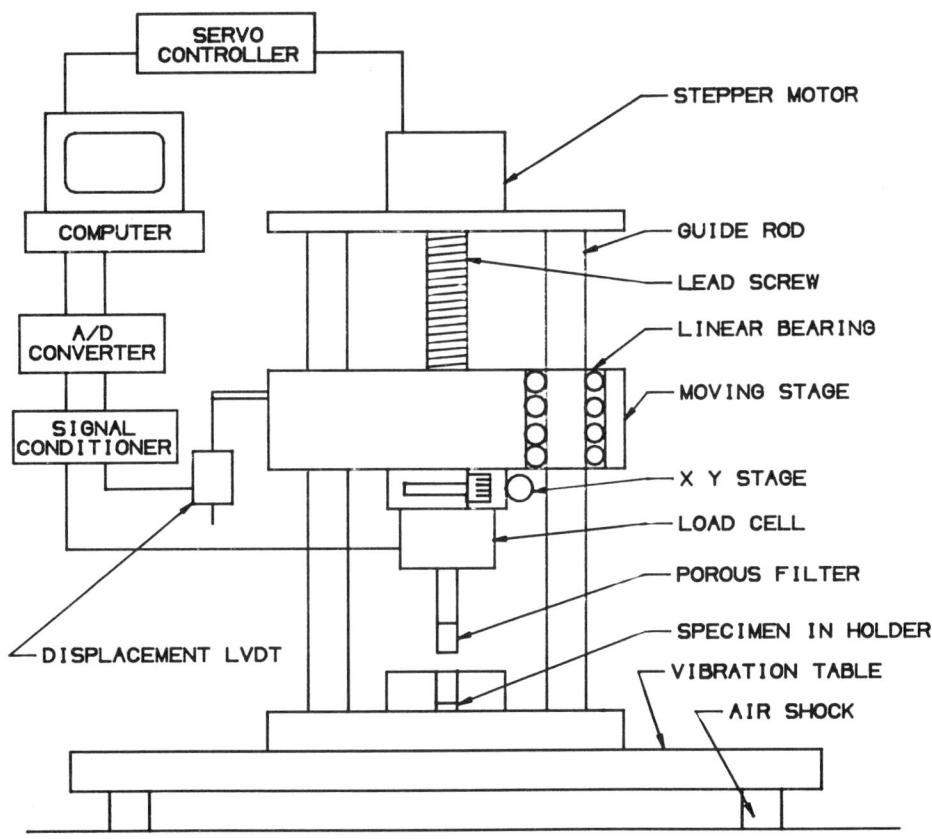

Figure 71.1 The computer-aided slice tester (CAST).

11. MECHANICAL AND ELECTRICAL PROPERTIES

Table 71.1 Capabilities of the computer automated slice tester

	Sensitivity	Resolution	Repeatability	None
Load	0.15 g mV^{-1}	0.18 g bit^{-1}	1 bit	2 bits
Displacement	0.02 μm step^{-1}	0.02 μm	0.02 μm	None
Position (LVDT)	0.15 μm mV^{-1}	0.18 μm bit^{-1}	1 bit	2 bits

slices of cartilage removed from the full layer thickness, which is described below.

A specially designed ultrasensitive servo-controlled test apparatus was developed to compress thin soft tissue specimens (Torzilli et al., 1988). The computer-automated slice tester (CAST) consisted of a 25 000 step per revolution stepper motor coupled to a 50 thread per inch linear screw (Fig. 71.1). Attached to the rotating screw is an XY stage, a 5 lb. load cell and a plane ended porous platen. Displacement and load resolution are 0.02 μm and 0.18 g, respectively. The stepper motor and load cell are coupled to a computer to provide both displacement and load servofeedback control. Linear velocity can be controlled from 0.03 μm s^{-1} to 10.2 mm s^{-1}. The CAST is capable of performing a variety of tests depending on the computer-control program (e.g. creep and relaxation) and specimen fixture (e.g. unconfined and confined compression).

Unconfined compression stiffness tests were performed on thin slices (100 μm) of articular cartilage. Full-thickness plugs of articular cartilage were removed from mature bovine knees, frozen and microtomed frozen parallel to the articular surface. The specimens were immediately transferred to the polished flat base of the CAST (unconfined) and loaded with the porous filter at a strain rate of 20% s^{-1} (Fig. 71.2). All specimens showed a biphasic stiffness with an initial region

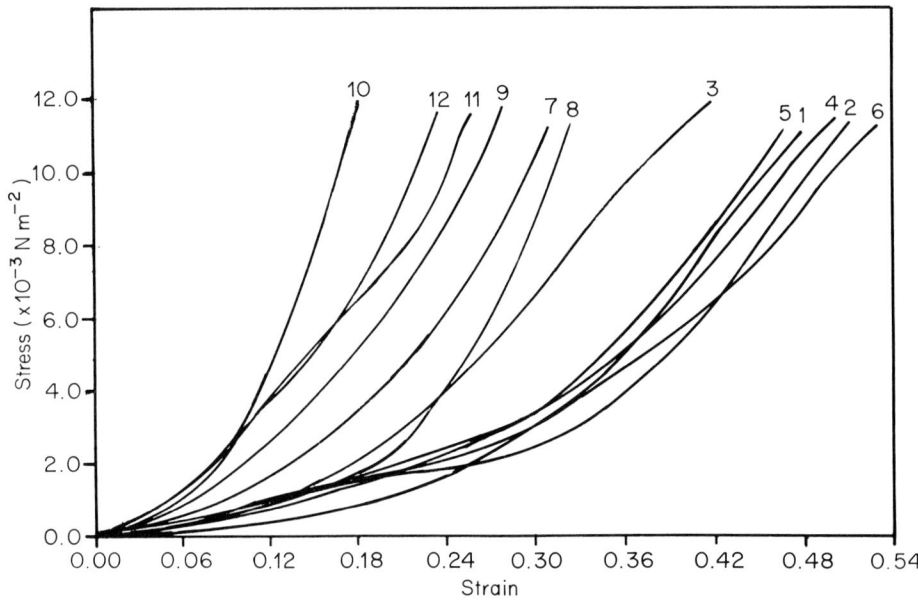

Figure 71.2 Stress–strain curves for slices. $H = 100 \pm 8\,\mu$m; strain rate = 20% per slice. Slices numbered from surface.

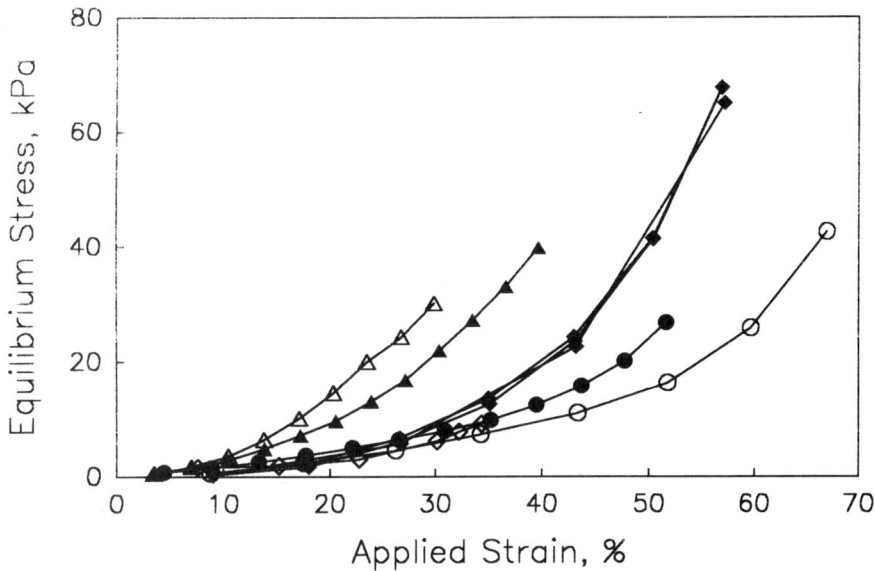

Figure 71.3 Equilibrium stress vs. applied strain: (○) 22-5 slice 1; (△) 22-5 slice 2; (◇) 22-5 slice 3; (●) 23-3 slice 1; (▲) 23-3 slice 2; (◆) 23-3 slice 3.

of low stiffness followed by increasing stiffness as the specimen continued to deform. The most superficial slices (1–6) demonstrated the lowest stiffness or least resistance to deformation, especially in the toe or initial slope region of the stress–strain response.

The unconfined compression tests, performed over 1 to 2 s, represent a transient characteristic of both fluid transport and solid-matrix morphology. To investigate the equilibrium characteristics of the solid matrix, that is, independent of fluid flow, equilibrium compression tests were performed. Step relaxation tests were performed on 200–250 μm thick slices of bovine articular cartilage in confined compression (Fig. 71.3). Small strains (displacements) were applied to each slice and the resulting stress (force) measured until stress equilibrium was achieved (approximately 15–30 min). This procedure was repeated with increasing strains in a step-wise sequence. The resulting equilibrium stress versus applied strain response was nonlinear over the entire strain range. With increasing depth the cartilage matrix became stiffer, as evidenced by a higher tangent modulus. At the end of each loading test the displacements were reversed and the equilibrium stress again determined. The equilibrium response was identical during the unloading phase as compared with the loading phase. This reversibility of tissue deformation was found for each slice and when tests were repeated for more than one cycle.

CONCLUSIONS

The CAST provides a new capability for measuring the spatial variation in mechanical properties of articular cartilage. Tests can be easily performed on very thin slices of tissue under a variety of test configurations. The submicron and subgram measurement capabilities provide the resolution and sensitivity necessary to apply very small loads and displacements, in a stepwise, sequential and reversible mode. This results in better resolution of stress–strain characteristics and allows for measurement of mechanical properties in both a loading and unloading mode. In addition, the computer-controlled feedback allows for the application of complex test conditions which can be monitored on a continuous basis. For instance, real-time correction of system stiffness errors (e.g. load cell deflection) can be made during relaxation tests to maintain constant tissue deformation. To date few difficulties have been encountered. Most notable have been in handling thin tissue specimens and possible artifacts introduced in the tissue structural integrity due to cutting. However, handling problems were overcome by keeping the specimens frozen until positioned within the test device, and preparation artifacts do not appear significant as evidenced by testing variable specimen thicknesses.

The results from these preliminary studies clearly demonstrate yet again the inhomogeneous morphology of the tissue with respect to mechanical properties (e.g. Kempson et al., 1970, 1971). The most superficial slices had the lowest resistance to deformation. This is probably a result of the lower content of the PG compression-resisting component. However, the deeper layers were found to be stiffer and better able to resist compression, again probably a result of the higher PG content.

One consequence of this spatial variability will be in overall tissue mechanical response. The decreased compressive resistance of the surface layer probably influences the overall mechanical deformation of the tissue by controlling fluid transport. When loaded, the surface layer will collapse due to its decreased stiffness, and effectively decrease its porosity resulting in restricted fluid exudation. This phenomenon has been demonstrated using full-thickness cartilage specimens (Torzilli, 1984; Torzilli et al., 1989). It is also interesting to note that in the regions of increased compressibility the chondrocytes are flattened; on the other hand, in areas of high compressive resistance the cells are spheroidal (see Section 3). This may be related to the spatial inhomogeneity in the mechanical properties. The local strain around the chondrocyte is dependent on its spatial position within the tissue and, therefore, local tissue mechanical properties may cause grossly different chondrocyte deformations and different cellular activity (see Chapters 31 and 63).

ACKNOWLEDGMENTS

Supported by National Institutes of Health Grants AR28151 and AR38520.

References

Adams, D. and Swanson, S.A.V. (1985). Direct measurement of local pressures in the cadaveric human hip joint during simulated level walking. *Ann. Rheum. Dis.* **44**, 658–666

Afoke, N.Y.P., Byers, P.D. and Hutton, W.C. (1980). The incongruous hip joint: a casting study. *J. Bone Joint Surg.* **62B**, 55

Afoke, N.Y.P., Byers, P.D. and Hutton, W.C. (1987). Contact pressures in the human hip joint. *J. Bone Joint Surg.* **69B**, 536

Armstrong, C.G., Bahrani, A.S., Gardner, D.L. (1980). Changes in the deformational behavior of human hip cartilage with age. *Trans. ASME* **102**, 214–220

Benaim, E. (1989). Biomechanical model for cartilage creep in compression. D.Sc. Thesis, Department of Biomedical Engineering, Technion–Israel Institute of Technology, Haifa, Israel

Benaim, E., Mizrahi, J. and Maroudas, A. (1990). Shape and volume changes in cartilage during creep in unconfined compression. *Biorheology* in press

Brown, T.D. and Singerman, R.J. (1986). Experimental determination of the linear biphasic constitutive coefficients of human fetal proximal femoral chondroepiphysis. *J. Biomech.* **19**, 597–605

Dunlop, R.B., Adams, M.A. and Hutton, W.C. (1984). Disc space narrowing and the lumbar facet joints. *J. Bone Joint Surg.* **66**, 706–710

Edmond, E. and Ogston, A.G. (1968). An approach to the study of phase separation in ternary aqueous systems. *Biochem. J.* **109**, 569–576

Eisenberg, S.R. and Grodzinsky, A.J. (1985). Swelling of articular cartilage and other connective tissues: Electromechanochemical forces. *J. Orthop. Res.* **3**, 148–159

Eisenberg, S.R. and Grodzinsky, A.J. (1987). The kinetics of chemically induced non-equilibrium swelling of articular cartilage and corneal stroma. *J. Biomech. Eng.* **109**, 79–89

Elmore, S.M., Sokoloff, L., Norris, G. and Carmeci (1963). Nature of imperfect elasticity of articular cartilage. *J. Appl. Physiol.* **18**, 393–397

Frank, E.H. and Grodzinsky, A.J. (1987a). Cartilage electromechanics. I. Electrokinetic transduction and the effects of electrolyte pH and ionic strength. *J. Biomech.* **20**, 615–627

Frank, E.H. and Grodzinsky, A.J. (1987b). Cartilage electromechanics-II. A continuum model of cartilage electrokinetics and correlation with experiments. *J. Biomech.* **20**, 629–639

Frank, E.H., Eisenberg, S.R. and Grodzinsky, A.J. (1987a). Microcontinuum and macrocontinuum models of cartilage electromechanics: theory and experiment. *Proc. 9th IEEE Eng. Mech. Biol. Soc., Boston*, pp. 444–445

Frank, E.H., Grodzinsky, A.J., Koob, T.J. and Eyre, D.R. (1987b). Streaming potentials: a sensitive index of enzymatic degradation in articular cartilage. *J. Orthop. Res.* **5**, 497–508

Glover, J.G., Hargens, A.R., Mahmood, M.M., Gott, S., Brown, M.D. and Garfin, S.R. (1988). A new technique for the *in vitro* measurement of nucleus pulposus swelling pressure. *J. Orthopaed. Res.* submitted.

Grimshaw, P.E., Grodzinsky, A.J., Yarmush, M.L. and Yarmush, D.M. (1989). Dynamic membranes for protein transport: chemical and electrical control. *Chem. Eng. Sci.* **44**, 827–840

Grimshaw, P.E., Eisenberg, S.R., Grodzinsky, A.J., Koob, T.J. and Eyre, D.R. (1983). The kinetics of *in vitro* neutralization and enzymatic extraction of cartilage charge groups: characterization by isometric compressive stress. *Trans. 29th ORS* **8**, 122

Grodzinsky, A.J. (1983). Electromechanical and physicochemical properties of connective tissue. *CRC Crit. Rev. Bioeng.* **9**, 133–199

Grodzinsky, A.J. and Frank, E.H. (1990). Electromechanical and physicochemical regulation of cartilage strength and metabolism. *Connective Tissue Matrix, Vol. II, Topics in Molecular and Structural Biology*, MacMillan, London (in press)

Grushko, G., Schnaiderman, R. and Maroudas, A. (1989). Some biochemical and biophysical parameters for the study of the pathogenesis of osteoarthritis: a comparison between the process of ageing and degeneration in human hip cartilage. *Conn. Tiss. Res.* **19**, 149–176

Hargens, A.R. (1989). Developmental adaptations to gravity. In *Strategies of Physiological Adaptation* (S.C. Wood and C. Lenfant, eds). Marcel Dekker, New York

Hargens, A.R. and Mahmood, M. (1989). Decreased swelling pressure of rat nucleus pulposus associated with simulated weightlessness. *Physiologist* **32**, S23–S24

Harris, E.D., Parker, P.G., Radin, E.L. and Krane, S.M. (1972). Effects of proteolytic enzymes on structural and mechanical properties of cartilage. *Arthrit. Rheum.* **15**, 497–503

Hayes, W.C. and Bodine, A.J. (1978). Flow-independent viscoelastic properties of articular cartilage matrix. *J. Biomech.* **11**, 407–419

Helfferich, F. (1962). *Ion Exchange*, pp. 221–420. McGraw-Hill, New York

Hodge, W.A., Fijan, R.S., Carlson, K.L., Burgess, R.G., Harris, W.H. and Mann, R.W. (1986). Contact pressures in the human hip joint measured in vivo. *Proc. Natl. Acad. Sci., U.S.A. Biophysics* **83**, 2879–2883

Holmes, M.H. (1986). Finite deformation of soft tissue: analysis of a mixture model in uni-axial compression. *J. Biomech. Eng.* **108**, 372–381

Huberti, H. and Hayes, W.C. (1984). Patello femoral contact pressures. *J. Bone Joint Surg.* **66A**, 715–724

Huberti, H. and Hayes, W.C. (1988). Contact pressures in chondromalacia patellae and the effect of capsular reconstructive procedures. *J. Orthop. Res.* **6**, 499–508

Jackson, G.W. and James, D.F. (1982). The hydrodynamic resistance of hyaluronic acid and its contribution of tissue permeability. *Biorheology* **19**, 317–330

Katz, E.P., Wachtel, E.J. and Maroudas, A. (1986). Extrafibrillar proteoglycans osmotically regulate the molecular packing of collagen cartilage. *Biochim. Biphys. Acta* **882**, 136–139

Kempson, G.E., Muir, H., Freeman, M.A.R. and Swanson, S.A.V. (1970). Correlations between the compressive stiffness and chemical constituents of human articular cartilage. *Biochim. Biophys. Acta* **215**, 70–73

Kempson, G.E., Spivey, C.J., Swanson, S.A.V. and Freeman, M.A.R. (1971). Patterns of cartilage stiffness on normal and degenerate human femoral heads. *J. Biomech.* **4**, 597–601

Kempson, G.E., Tuke, M.A., Dingle, J.T., Barrett, A.J. and Horsfield, P.H. (1976). The effects of proteolytic enzymes on the mechanical properties of adult human articular cartilage. *Biochim. Biophys. Acta* **428**, 741

Lee, R.C., Frank, E.H., Grodzinsky, A.J. and Roylance, D.K. (1981). Oscillatory compressional behavior of articular cartilage and its associated electromechanical properties. *J. Biomech. Eng.* **103**, 28–292

Li, J.T., Mow, V.C., Koob, T.J. and Eyre, D.R. (1984). Effect of chondroitinase-ABC treatment on the tensile behavior of bone articular cartilage. *Trans. 30th ORS* **9**, 35

Maroudas, A. (1968). Physicochemical properties of cartilage in light of ion-exchange theory. *Biophys. J.* **44**, 575–595

Maroudas, A. (1975). Fluid transport in cartilage. *Ann. Rheum. Dis.* **34**, 77–82

Maroudas, A. (1979). Physico-chemical properties of articular cartilage. In *Adult Articular Cartilage* (M.A.R. Freeman, ed.), 2nd edn, pp. 214–290. Pitman, Tunbridge Wells

Maroudas, A. and Bannon, C. (1981). Measurement of swelling pressure in cartilage and comparison with the osmotic pressure of constituent proteoglycans. *Biorheology* **18**, 619–632

Maroudas, A. and Urban, J.P.G. (1983). In vitro methods for studying articular cartilage and intervertebral disc. In *Skeletal Research*, (A.S. Kunin and D.J. Simmons, eds), Vol. 2, pp. 135–182. Academic Press, New York

Maroudas, A., Muir, H. and Wingham, J. (1969). The correlation of fixed negative charge with glycosaminoglycan content of human articular cartilage. *Biochim. Biophys. Acta* **177**, 492–500

Maroudas, A., Bayliss, M.T. and Venn, M.F. (1980). Further studies on the composition of human femoral head cartilage. *Ann. Rheum.* **39**, 514–523

Maroudas, A., Mizrahi, J., Ben Haim, E. and Ziv, I. (1987). The role of swelling pressure in fluid transport in cartilage. In *Interstitial Lymphatic Liquid and Solute Movement* (N.C. Staub, J.C. Hog and A.R. Hargens, eds), *Advances in Microcirculation*, Vol. 13, pp. 203–212. J. Karger, Switzerland

Maroudas, A., Wachtel, E., Grushko, G., Weinberg, P.D. and Katz, E. (1990). Osmotic and mechanical pressures alter the spacing of collagen molecules in articular cartilage. *Biochim. Biophys. Crys. Acta.*, (submitted)

McCutchen, C.W. (1962). The frictional properties of minimal joints. *Wear* **5**, 1–17

Mizrahi, J., Maroudas, A., Lanir, Y., Ziv, I. and Webber, T.J. (1986). The instantaneous deformation of cartilage: effects of collagen fiber orientation and osmotic stress. *J. Biorheol.* **23**, 311–330

Modest, V.E., Murphy, M.C. and Mann, R.W. (1989). Optical verification of a technique for in situ ultrasonic measurement of articular cartilage thickness. *J. Biomech.* **22**, 171–176

Mow, V.C., Lai, W.M. and Redler, I. (1974). Some surface characteristics of articular cartilage. I. A scanning electron microscope study and theoretical model for the dynamic interaction of synovial fluid and articular cartilage. *J. Biomech.* **7**, 449–456

Mow, V.C., Kuei, S.C., Lai, W.M. and Armstrong, C.G. (1980). Biphasic creep and stress relaxation of articular cartilage in compression: Theory and experiments. *J. Biomech. Eng.* **102**, 73–84

Mow, V.C., Holmes, M.H. and Lai, W.M. (1984). Fluid transport and mechanical properties of articular cartilage: a review. *J. Biomech.* **17**, 377–394

Nachemson, A. and Elfstrom, G. (1970). In *Intravital dynamic pressure Measurements in Lumbar Discs* (Almquist and Wicksell, eds). Stockholm

Parsegian, V.A., Rand, R.P., Ruller, N.L. and Rau, D.C. (1986). Osmotic stress for the direct measurement of intermolecular forces. In *Methods in Enzymology* (L. Packer, ed.), Vol. 127, pp. 400–416

Paul, J.P. (1967). Forces transmitted by joints in the human body. *Proc. Inst. Mech. Eng.* **181 : 3J**, 8–15

Rushfeld, P.D., Mann, R.W. and Harris, W.H. (1981). Improved techniques for measuring in vitro the geometry and pressure distribution in the acetabulum. II. *J. Biomech.* **14**, 315–323

Rushfeld, P.D., Mann, R.W. and Harris, W.H. (1979). Influence of cartilage geometry on the pressure distribution in the human hip joint. *Science* **204**, 413–415

Sachs, J.R. and Grodzinsky, A.J. (1989). An electromechanically coupled poroelastic medium driven by an applied electric current: surface detection of bulk material properties. *PhysicoChem. Hydrodynam.* **11**, 585–614

Salant, E. (1990). M. Sc. Thesis, M.I.T., Cambridge, MA

Simon, B.R., Coats, R.S. and Woo, S.L.-Y. (1984). Relaxation and creep quasilinear viscoelastic models for normal articular cartilage. *J. Biochem. Eng.* **106**, 159–164

Staub, N.C., Hogg, J.C. and Hargens, A.R., eds. (1987). Interstitial–Lymphatic liquid and solute movement. In *Advances in Microcirculation*, Vol. 13, Karger, Basel

Stockwell, R.A. and Scott, J.E. (1967). Distribution of acid glycosaminoglycans in human articular cartilage. *Nature (London)* **25**, 1376–1377

Torzilli, P.A. (1984). Mechanical response of articular cartilage to an oscillating load. *Mech. Res. Commun.* **11**, 75–82

Torzilli, P.A. (1985). The influence of cartilage conformation on its equilibrium water partition. *J. Orthopaed. Res.* **3**, 473–483

Torzilli, P.A. (1988). Water content and equilibrium water partition immature cartilage. *J. Orthopaed. Res.* **6**, 766–769

Torzilli, P.A., Niver, S.M. and Beaupre, S.R. (1989). Effect of articular cartilage surface compression on cartilage deformation. *Proc. Am. Soc. Mech. Eng.* **BED14**, 29–82

Urban, J.P.G. (1987). Factors influencing the fluid content of intervertebral disc. In *Interstitial–*

Lymphatic Liquid and Solute Movement (N.C. Staub, J.C. Hogg and A.R. Hargens, eds), pp. 160–170. Karger, Basel

Urban, J.P.G. and Maroudas, A. (1979). The measurement of fixed charge density in the intervertebral disc. *Biochim. Biophys. Acta* **586**, 166–178

Urban, J.P.G. and Maroudas, A. (1980). Measurement of swelling pressures and fluid flow in the intervertebral disc with reference to creep. In *Engineering Aspects of the Spine*, pp. 63–69. Institution of Mechanical Engineers, Publications, London

Urban, J.P.G. and Maroudas, A. (1981). Swelling of intervertebral disc *in vitro*. *Conn. Tiss. Res.* **9**, 1–10

Urban, J.P.G. and McMullin, J.F. (1985). Swelling pressure of the intervertebral disc: influence of proteoglycan and collagen contents. *Biorheology* **22**, 145–157

Urban, J.P.G., Maroudas, A., Bayliss, M.T. and Dillon, J. (1979). Swelling pressures of proteoglycans at the concentrations found in cartilaginous tissues. *Biorheology* **16**, 447–464

Walker, P.S. (1969). On the lubrication and wear in human joints. Ph.D. Thesis, University of Leeds, Leeds, UK

Wilder, D.G., Krag, M.H. and Pope, M.H. (1988). *Atlas of Mammalian Lumbar Vertebrae: Pictorial and Dimensional Information*. C.C. Thomas, Springfield, II

12

ARTICULAR CARTILAGE REPAIR AND REMODELING

COLLATED BY B. CATERSON

72

Overview

BRUCE CATERSON and JOSEPH BUCKWALTER

The question as to whether or not cartilage can undergo repair is an open and controversial topic that has been the subject of many clinical and basic research investigations for more than 250 years. In 1743, Hunter (Hunter, 1743) first reported the observation that ulcerated cartilage did not undergo repair processes. A century or so later similar findings were also reported by Paget (Paget, 1853) who described the inability of wounded cartilage to repair itself with new and well-formed tissue. Over the years there have been many published cases reported where cartilage has undergone attempts to repair itself. Detailed descriptions of the current status of research involving studies of articular cartilage injury and repair are provided in three recent review articles (Buckwalter *et al.*, 1989, 1990; Buckwalter and Mow, 1990). These studies have demonstrated that the ability to define cartilage repair is variable and unpredictable for many reasons including our inability to adequately categorize the different types of injury, variations in the age and status of health of the joint of the individual before receiving the injury, and the lack of adequate follow-up studies evaluating the durability of the repair tissue and its overall practicability in the long-term function of the joint. In addition, these studies have indicated that the structure and integrity of the matrix that was being replaced in the joint in response to cartilage injury does not always mimic the macromolecular organization or have the material properties of normal articular cartilage. In this overview we briefly describe what is known about factors that contribute to the acute cartilage injury and we also describe some of the current experimental and clinical approaches being used to initiate and facilitate cartilage repair.

CARTILAGE INJURY

There are several types of insult which result in cartilage injury that in turn initiate a cartilage repair response. Based on experimental work these injuries fall into two general groups (Buckwalter *et al.*, 1989, 1990), one involving situations where there is loss of noncollagenous matrix without mechanical damage to the cartilage fibrillar network or cell death, and the other more severe case where there is mechanical disruption of the matrix as a whole and significant cellular damage. These two situations often overlap with one another since extensive loss of matrix material can compromise the cartilage's ability to resist everyday mechanical stresses which eventually leads to mechanical disruption of the matrix and cell death.

Several events can contribute to the acute and transient loss of noncollagenous macromolecules from cartilage extracellular matrix. These include situations such as infection, joint immobilization, surgical or traumatic disruption of the synovial membrane, acute bouts of inflammatory arthritis, the use of antiinflammatory agents and even joint irrigation and arthroscopy may cause increased proteoglycan (PG) degradation and/or suppression of PG biosynthesis (Curtiss, 1969; Palmoski et al., 1979; Palmoski and Brandt, 1981; Parsons et al., 1982; Reimann et al., 1982; Reagan et al., 1983; Donohue et al., 1983; Hoch et al., 1983; Jurvelin et al., 1986; Kiviranta et al., 1987). It appears that these acute and transient repair situations are capably handled as long as the chondrocytes are viable, the loss of matrix material does not exceed what the cells can rapidly replace, and that the collagen meshwork is still intact. However, if this situation continues and becomes chronic, the articular cartilage damage becomes permanent. It is not known at what point that this irreversibility of repair occurs, but it presumably correlates with situations where there has been considerable cell death and significant mechanical disruption of the matrix.

More severe injuries to cartilage are usually caused by blunt trauma, penetrating injuries and frictional abrasion. These types of mechanical injury to cartilage disrupt the matrix and kill chondrocytes. The response of cartilage to these types of injury is variable and the quality of repair is very much dependent upon factors such as the volume and surface area of the cartilage injury, the depth of the injury and whether or not subchondral bone or other periarticular tissues were involved.

Under normal circumstances, cartilage experiences everyday physiological levels of impact loading that do not appear to produce cartilage injury. However, blunt trauma to cartilage also occurs on a frequent basis and can be classified into two categories: (i) trauma involving greater than 'normal' loading but not sufficient to cause bone or cartilage fracture; and (ii) trauma which causes fracture of bone and/or cartilage (Buckwalter et al., 1989, 1990). In an experimental animal model Donohue et al. (1983) reported that in situations where there was abnormal loading that is insufficient to cause fracture, several changes occur in the cartilage. At the site of injury the cartilage was swollen, there was an increase in the diameter of the collagen fiber meshwork, and histological examination revealed alterations in the extracellular matrix interactions involving PG and collagen. Blunt trauma which results in fracture of bone or cartilage show similar repair responses to penetrating injuries described below.

The response of cartilage to penetrating injuries is also variable and seems to be dependent upon whether or not the defect is restricted to the articular cartilage (i.e. occurs above the zone of calcified cartilage), or whether it extends to the subchondral bone where the involvement of blood vessels and marrow cells can influence the response to injury. Lesions that are restricted to cartilage do not heal; however, they seldom progress to eburnated bone (Meachim, 1963; Mankin and Boyle, 1967; Fuller and Ghadially, 1972; Mankin, 1974a,b, 1982; Ghadially et al., 1977; Mitchell and Shepard, 1987; Buckwalter et al., 1989, 1990). In recent studies, Buckwalter et al. (1989, 1990) examined perpendicular, wedge-shaped injuries to articular cartilage in rabbits that did not involve subchondral bone. Because these lesions do not obtain access to the subchondral vessels, their repair was limited to events involving local chondrocyte proliferation. However, the new matrix they synthesized did not fill the lesion and the state of the injury one year after repair was almost identical to that seen 24 h after the injury.

Repair of 'full-thickness' injuries that involve both cartilage and bone depend on the extent of the injury (volume and surface area) and also the location of the injury in the joint (Convery et al., 1972; Stover et al., 1987; Buckwalter et al., 1989, 1990). Larger injuries are less likely to repair than smaller defects and osteochondral injuries in weight-bearing regions of joints that articulate are less likely to heal than those that do not articulate. The repair response of rabbit cartilage to full-thickness injury has been described recently by Buckwalter et al. (1990). Full-thickness injuries undergo repair processes primarily because they involve bone marrow and vasculature that can participate in inflammation and tissue remodeling. Most full-thickness defects undergo repair through the first few months after injury. However, although histologically the replacement tissue appears normal, the biochemical composition and macromolecular organization of the tissue is not the same as the original normal cartilage. The result of this inconsistency is that the new repair cartilage becomes fissured and fibrillated and extensive degenerative changes occur 6–12 months after the initiation of cartilage repair. These studies also showed that there was a variation in the repair response with the diameter of the injury to the cartilage surface.

Very little is known about the biochemical changes that occur in the matrix macromolecules with full-thickness-penetrating injuries (Cheung et al., 1980; Furukawa, et al., 1980). Furukawa et al. (1980) examined the various collagen types present in rabbit articular cartilage inflicted with 3 mm diameter defects that extended to the subchondral bone. In their follow-up analysis of the repair tissue they observed that type I collagen was the predominant collagen type present in early stages of repair (1 month after injury) and after 2 months it was still 40% of the total collagen in spite of the fact that histological analyses indicated that abundant amounts of PG were present in what appeared to be normal hyaline cartilage. At 6 months after injury, 25–30% of the collagen was still type I and this level persisted even as the defect cartilage became more fibrillated in the later degenerative phase.

These studies demonstrate the inability of cartilage to recover from full-thickness defects. In the initial stages of repair, progenitor cells from the marrow migrate to the site of injury where some of them appear to differentiate into chondrocytes and produce a cartilaginous matrix. The problem that seems to occur is that this 'repair cartilage' does not have the same material properties and composition as the original cartilage or the surrounding tissue (Coletti et al., 1972; Whipple et al., 1985; Nelson et al., 1988; Athanasiou, 1989; Buckwalter and Mow, 1990) and it thus becomes fibrillated and eventually undergoes degeneration (Mitchell and Shepard, 1976; Furukawa et al., 1980; Buckwalter et al., 1989, 1990; Buckwalter and Mow, 1990). This problem may eventually be solved if we learn more about the factors that control the differentiation processes that enable marrow progenitor cells to develop into chondrocytes, and also when we understand better how to fine tune and control how the macromolecular ingredients of cartilage can be deposited to produce functional repair tissue after injury.

ARTICULAR CARTILAGE REPAIR

There are now several well-known limitations to the ability of cartilage to repair itself in terms of restoring a long-term functional diarthrodal joint. In addition, repair of significant defects of articular cartilage is rarely if ever successful (Coletti et al., 1972; Convery et al., 1972; Mitchell and Shepard, 1976; Cheung et al., 1980; Furukawa et al., 1980; Whipple et al., 1985; Stover et al., 1987; Nelson et al., 1988; Athanasiou, 1989; Buckwalter et al., 1989, 1990; Buckwalter and Mow, 1990). For these reasons one questions why investigators still continue to search for methods of inducing the restoration of articular surfaces and why surgeons continue to perform operations intended to stimulate repair of damaged or degenerated joints. One answer to this dilemma comes from the fact that the use of surgical procedures can in some instances stimulate the formation of new joint surfaces that compare favorably with alternative surgical options using artificial joints and arthrodeses (Amadio et al., 1982; Burton, 1983; Sherman et al., 1984; Dell and Muniz, 1987; Richardson, 1987). Another answer is that surgical treatments such as arthrodesis and total joint arthroplasty are frequently not a satisfactory solution for young patients because these procedures have a limited life span (they loosen during skeletal development) and they have a restricted tolerance for heavy loading and vigorous activity. For young patients the option of using a procedure which stimulates cartilage repair, even if it does not restore a normal functional articular surface, is a feasible one. Even if the repair tissue only lasts a few years it can potentially improve their quality of life, allowing them to remain physically active and delaying the option of total joint arthroplasty until they reach skeletal maturity (Buckwalter and Mow, 1990). For these and other reasons, investigators continue to search for a means of stimulating cartilage repair that will create an optimal biological and mechanical environment to produce a functional alternative that will replace the injured cartilage. Some of the current research and clinical methods that are being employed to achieve this goal are described below.

PERFORATION OR ABRASION TO SUBCHONDRAL BONE

Penetration of cartilage to subchondral bone disrupts the intraosseous blood vessels and enables marrow and inflammatory cells access to the cartilage defect which in turn stimulates the synthesis of a repair matrix. Animal and human studies have employed a variety of procedures ranging from the use of multiple 'full thickness' drill holes over the articular surface to complete removal of cartilage from the articular surfaces, and even resection through to the cancellous bone (spongialization) (see Chapter 75; also Buckwalter et al. (1990) and Buckwalter and Mow (1990) for reviews). The results from these procedures have been variable. The use of drill holes promotes healing responses and recovery of an apparently normal articular surface in the initial phase; however, in the long term the holes becomes more collagenous and deteriorate within a year (Coletti et al., 1972). When the total articular surface and subchondral bone was removed and a vitallium cup interspaced between the cancellous bone of the femoral head, a nonuniform articular surface resulted that showed variability between animals: there were differences in the response in different regions of the femoral head and the cartilage of the acetabulum, and in the long term there were abnormal levels of PG and collagen in the repair tissue (Akeson et al., 1969). In spite of these problems, some successes have clearly been achieved in humans using these and other related procedures. Ficat (Chapter 75) describes reasonable success in the use of spongialization to promote cartilage healing. A better understanding of factors that control these processes will diminish the variability observed with this type of methodological approach.

PERIOSTEAL AND PERICHONDRIAL GRAFTS

Periosteal and perichondrial grafts have been used as another method of inducing articular cartilage repair (Cohen and Lacroix, 1955; Skoog et al., 1972; Tonna and Pentel, 1972; Ohlsen, 1978; Engkvist, 1979; Engkvist and Ohlsen, 1979; Engkvist et al., 1979; Rubak, 1982; Rubak et al., 1982; Kulick et al., 1984; O'Driscoll and Salter, 1984, 1986; Amiel et al., 1985; O'Driscoll et al., 1986, 1989a,b; Kleiner et al., 1986; Zarnett et al., 1987; Kwan et al., 1987; Delaney et al., 1989). This method also provides a means of introducing progenitor cell populations to the site of repair, but, unlike drilling and abrasion, this procedure has a potential advantage in that it avoids disruption of the subchondral bone. These grafting procedures are capable of resurfacing relatively large areas of articular surface and provide a surface of hyaline-like cartilage that remains intact for over one year. The influence of passive joint motion upon the success of grafting has also been studied (O'Driscoll and Salter, 1984, 1986; O'Driscoll et al., 1986, 1989a; Zarnett et al., 1987; Delaney et al., 1989) as well as joint immobilization following grafting (Delaney et al., 1989). However, the long-term benefits of these treatments are unclear and review of these studies indicate that there is considerable variability between animals and among regions of the joint. At present the benefits of grafting procedures have not been compared with abrasion treatment of similar defects, but further investigation of these experimental procedures is certainly warranted.

IMPLANTATION OF CHONDROCYTES OR MESENCHYMAL CELLS

Current approaches to the implantation of chondrocytes and mesenchymal cells as a means of inducing cartilage repair are discussed by Robinson et al. (Chapter 76). The isolation of chondrocytes (or undifferentiated mesenchymal cells), their proliferation and maintenance in cell culture, followed by their subsequent implantation into cartilage defects has been studied by several investigators (Moskalewski and Kawiak, 1965; Moskalewski et al., 1966; Moskalewski and Rybicka, 1977; Chesterman and Smith, 1968; Bentley and Greer, 1971; Green, 1977; Bentley et al., 1978; Aston and Bentley, 1986; Grande et al., 1987; Itay et al., 1987, 1988; Wakitani et al., 1988, 1989; Grande and Pitman, 1988; Malejezyk and Moskalewski, 1988; Kawabe et al., 1989; Robinson et al., 1989a,b; and Chapter 76). In addition, some of these preliminary studies have investigated the use of resorbable gels as a means of maintaining the chondrocytes in the cartilage defect (Passl et al., 1976; Widenfalk et al., 1986; Itay et al., 1987; Wakitani et al., 1988, 1989; Robinson et al., 1989a,b). It appears that the cartilaginous matrix produced by these methods more closely resembles normal cartilage than the tissue that forms in defects not treated with chondrocyte or mesenchymal cells. Although this procedure has shown considerable promise, the matrix produced by these implants is still not durable enough to repair large cartilage defects. However, in the future one should expect that there will be significant progress in using this approach as a successful method of inducing cartilage repair.

IMPLANTATION OF NATURAL AND SYNTHETIC MATRICES

One of the limiting factors in the induction of cartilage repair may be the lack of formation of a fibrin clot in the cartilage defect. The formation of the fibrin clot of vascularized tissues promotes healing by stimulating platelets to release growth factors and thereby inducing appropriate cellular migration and proliferation at the site of injury (Nemeth et al., 1988). Fibrin clot implantation has recently been demonstrated as a useful means of facilitating repair in avascular regions of meniscus (Arnoczky et al., 1988). In applications to cartilage healing, studies have suggested that matrix PG might inhibit platelet aggregation and thus suppress the beneficial effects of fibrin clot formation (Mankin, 1982). To overcome this dilemma some investigators have proposed irrigating the defects with saline or enzyme solutions that degrade the PGs and thus facilitate fibrin clot formation (Farkas et al., 1977; Mankin, 1982).

Recent experimentation has also investigated the use of artificial synthetic matrix implantation as an initial repair scaffold that might stimulate mesenchymal cell migration, subsequent cellular proliferation and matrix formation. These studies have used carbon fiber implants, and collagen or fibrin gels to fill cartilage defects and thereby to promote healing (Speer et al., 1979; Hart, 1987; Grande and Pitman, 1988; Wakitani et al., 1988, 1989). In future studies, it may be worthwhile to consider the use of several methodologies based on artificial matrices containing chondrogenic growth factors in combination with undifferentiated mesenchymal cells or chondrocytes.

GROWTH-FACTOR STIMULATION OF CARTILAGE REPAIR

Growth factors directly influence many chondrocyte and mesenchymal cell functions including cellular migration, differentiation, growth and proliferation and extracellular matrix formation (Nemeth et al., 1988). Bone matrix contains many growth factors that are capable of stimulating chondrogenesis and these factors must probably influence both cartilage and bone repair in osteochondral defects (Reddi and Hubbins, 1972; Sampath et al., 1982, 1987; Reddi, 1983, 1985; Sporn et al., 1986; Seyedin et al., 1986; Reddi et al., 1987). At present, discrimination has not been made between combinations of growth factors that promote chondrogenesis as opposed to osteogenesis, but further study in this area has considerable potential as a means of bettering our understanding of factors that control cartilage-repair processes. Further work is needed to identify the most useful factors, to determine their dose–response relationship, and to establish an efficient means of delivering them to the site of cartilage injury.

BIOMECHANICAL AND BIOPHYSICAL APPROACHES TO CARTILAGE REPAIR

The effect of biomechanical influences on cartilage-repair processes is an important component contributing to the apparent success of failure of all the biological approaches to cartilage repair described above. Decreasing or altering the load distribution applied to damaged areas of joints using osteotomy or altering muscle forces to the joint may also allow or stimulate cartilage repair and promote more successful restoration of articular surfaces (Adam and Spence, 1958; Robbins and Piggot, 1960; Harris and Kirwan, 1964; Mensor and Scheck, 1968; Scheck, 1970; Nissen, 1971; Knodt, 1971; Byers, 1974; Radin et al., 1975; Weisl, 1980; Radin and Burr, 1984). In addition, Salter et al. (1980, 1982) have demonstrated that continuous passive motion facilitates healing of osteochondral defects in rabbit articular cartilage, although this approach did not affect repair of injuries when the defect was limited to cartilage alone. Large osteochondral defects treated with periosteal grafts also improve after several weeks of passive motion (Cohen and Lacroix, 1955; Skoog et al., 1972; Tonna and Pentel, 1972; Ohlsen, 1978; Engkvist and Ohlsen, 1979; Rubak, 1982; Rubak et al., 1982; O'Driscoll and Salter, 1984, 1986; O'Driscoll et al., 1986, 1989a,b; Zarnett et al., 1987; Delaney et al., 1989), these studies indicate that controlled early motion may be needed to help restore the function of injured cartilage and joint tissues.

There is also considerable evidence that chondrocytes and other mesenchymal cells respond to electromagnetic field stimulation (Baker et al., 1974a,b; Norton et al., 1977; Brighton et al., 1984; Aaron et al., 1987; Aaron and Plaas, 1987). Studies have indicated that application of electromagnetic fields can stimulate chondrocyte proliferation, PG synthesis and the formation of hyaline-like cartilage in some osteochondral defects. Although electrical stimulation has been successfully applied to bone healing (Brighton, 1984; Brighton et al., 1985; Brighton and Pollack, 1985) its use for repair of articular cartilage injury has not been definitively established. In other studies, application of low dose laser energy to cartilage injury has also been reported as yet another biophysical means of stimulating cartilage repair (Schultz et al., 1985). The underlying mechanism of this effect is at present not known and the long-term follow-up studies using this type of procedure have not been performed.

SUMMARY

In this chapter we have provided an overview of current status of methodological approaches that are being used to better our understanding of cartilage repair in response to injury. For a more comprehensive review of the literature in this field see Buckwalter et al., (1990). The application of these studies to treatment of osteoarthritis has also been reviewed recently (Buckwalter and Mow, 1990).

The contributions following in this section relate to current concepts and methodological approaches to the study of articular cartilage repair and remodeling. Byers and Brown (Chapter 73) discuss factors and criteria that need to be considered when undertaking investigations into the repair of articular cartilage and they put forward their own 'testable' hypothesis about the mechanisms involved. Oegema and Thompson (Chapter 74) describe the methodological approach used in their laboratories to study remodeling mechanisms in the zone of calcified cartilage — a component of articular cartilage that has received very little attention in relation to remodeling and repair. In Chapter 75, Ficat describes results of 90 human cases in which spongialization has been used as a means of promoting articular cartilage repair in humans; this method compares favorably with other methods employing cartilage shaving and abrasion. Robinson et al. (Chapter 76) describe methodology used in their in vivo avian model that uses orthotopic location of chondrocytes to facilitate repair processes in chicken cartilage defects (see also Chapter 4).

Reflections on the repair of articular cartilage

P.D. BYERS and R.A. BROWN

It is generally agreed that damage involving the surface and confined to the cartilage undergoes little restoration; such cartilage has little intrinsic ability to heal itself (Stockwell, 1979; Mankin, 1962b). However, given that there is exposure of underlying bone, fibroblastic tissue will enter the defect and proceed toward reconstituting the lost tissue (Landells, 1957; Calandruccio and Gilmer, 1962; Byers, 1974; Cheung et al., 1978). The reason for this disparity between intrinsic and extrinsic repair is open to speculation.

Seeking a point of entry into the problem has led to the reflection that even though their causal factors and their immediate purposes differ, there are features of each which are common to growth, repair, and remodeling. Most obvious is the formation of new tissue. Since the weakness of intrinsic cartilage repair is the inadequacy of tissue formation there appears to be merit in exploring growth as a first step.

We use the term 'physis' to refer to the growth cartilage lying between metaphysis and epiphysis; the cartilage whereby the epiphysis grows is the inner layer of the articular cartilage. Mankin (1962a), using [^{3}H]thymidine labeling in immature, juvenile and adult rabbits demonstrated two annuli of mitotic activity in growing animals (but none in adults), concluding that during the growth phase there are two anatomically and functionally distinct layers, one for epiphyseal growth and the other for articular growth. We were able to confirm this in a child's metatarsal labeled with [^{3}H]thymidine, through the courtesy of Professor N. Kember. The two layers must grow in tandem; cells of each producing the necessary quantities of matrix. A major difference between the two layers is in the amount of tissue they are required to make. The produce of the epiphyseal layer is consumed in conversion to bone, but the articular layer needs only to add to its substance. In the articular layer the cells have the arrangement usual for articular cartilage. The growth layer has the columnar organization as in the physis. However, instead of mineralization being polarized around the columns, as in the physis, permitting resorption of the nonmineralized septae by perivascular and endothelial cells (Anderson and Parker, 1966; Schenk et al., 1967, 1968), the mineral is distributed as a continuous layer (Byers and Brown, in preparation). This necessitates a prior stage of resorption by 'clastic cells'. This mechanism of articular cartilage ossification persists into adulthood.

The termination of the child's growth is marked by the conversion of all the growth cartilage to bone and the formation of a continuous bone plate beneath the articular cartilage. This leaves in place the articular layer. What of its growth potential? Even though it is held in check, it seems certain that it remains in place. This is evidenced by osteophyte formation; and by the addition of subchondral bone without appreciable loss of articular cartilage substance (Johnson, 1959, 1962; Green et al., 1970; Bullough, 1981; Sokoloff, 1987). Indeed, it must constitute the only practicable addition phase of joint remodeling, a process in which the resorption phase is ossification itself. Given that joint remodeling is a process that is continuous throughout life, albeit ever so slowly, one can postulate that the growth of articular cartilage is never arrested in any final sense (as it is in the physeal growth plate). Since it must by design be extremely slow (i.e. growth is constrained), so the capacity for intrinsic cartilage repair is limited. Although this might seem disadvantageous, it would nevertheless result in the slow renewal of articular cartilage, in effect a form of turnover. This effect must be pertinent to repair of mature cartilage and leads us to consider how growth occurs in cartilage matrix.

The osmotically driven swelling pressure of cartilage is restrained by the organization of a collagen net (Maroudas, 1976; Muir et al. 1970; Clark, 1985; Broom, 1986). Since growth of cartilage is interstitial there must be a mechanism for the controlled expansion of that network. Any hypothesis must meet two conditions:

(i) there must be no loss of structural integrity; and
(ii) the control of expansion, a cellular activity, must extend to all parts of the matrix.

These requirements can be met by postulating a focal, migratory process; the expansion achieved at one focus can only be realized when the neighboring matrix is also expanded. A dynamic image would be of random development of spherical fronts of net expansion, centred on cells, whose coalescence would enlarge the entire net.

A two-stage process is envisaged for net expansion: loosening of existing substance and addition of new. The addition stage must start with collagen synthesis. Fibrils, chiefly of type II collagen with small amounts of IX and XI, are thought to be assembled by a self-regulated process of accretion (Lee and Piez, 1983; Muller-Glauser et al., 1986; van der Rest and Mayne, 1988; Vaughan et al., 1988; Mendler et al., 1989). The weaving of an organized network of collagen fibrils is thought to be an active cellular process, involving, in the tendon, assembly and orientation by the cell membrane (Trelstad and Birk, 1985; Birk and Trelstad, 1986). A similar, through less orderly, process can be envisaged for cartilage, but remains contentious (Trelstad and Birk, 1985). Conventional wisdom, then, explains how new parts for the network could be fabricated by lateral assembly of collagen at the cell surface (Trelstad, 1982), but not how they are inserted, nor how expansion (i.e. the loosening stage) occurs at a distance from the cell. It is difficult to conceive how expansion could be achieved by enzymatic disintegration of part of the net followed by insertion of new collagen:

(i) the necessary precision of proteolytic control is unlikely;
(ii) it would represent an implausibly wasteful mechanism; and
(iii) where they exist, figures for collagen turnover are too low (Fry et al., 1962).

An elegant solution to this problem is supplied by the concept of 'slip' within the network (Fry et al., 1962; Nemetschek et al., 1980; Nimni and Harkness, 1988; Brown and Byers, 1989).

The central point of the slip concept is that the collagen net is built up of 'collagen aggregate units' which are *reversibly* bound together. Harkness and Harkness (1973) have proposed the five molecule 'microfibril' (Miller and Wray, 1971) as a candidate for this unit. Up to the size of a single unit, collagen molecules would be able to form stable intermolecular crosslinks. However, further aggregation of units into the collagen network must be by reversible interactions which do not require that participating collagen molecules are destroyed to achieve slippage. Expansion of the network would involve localized, cell-regulated lysis of the reversible bonds between units. Affected parts of the network would expand by longitudinal slippage of collagen units. The consequential thinning of fibrillar arms of the net would be compensated by addition of new collagen units onto the surface. Finally, cells would reform the reversible bonds between collagen units to leave a functional but expanded network.

Critical to the concept of slippage is the nature of the reversible bonding. Clues to this are available from reports of *in vitro* treatments which expand the collagen network. Three candidates are available to date:

(i) expansion of the network has been reproduced following treatment with water (Veis et al., 1970) or chelation of divalent metal ions, with suspicion falling on Ca^{2+} (Steven, 1967, 1976);
(ii) natural metabolites (notably homocysteine) are said to cleave labile collagen crosslinks (Fry et al., 1962; Harkness and Harkness,

1973; Harkness and Hood, 1984; Nimni and Harkness, 1988); and

(iii) a protease sensitive collagen type (type IX) is incorporated into type II fibrils and could act as a 'disposable' bridge between units (Wu and Eyre, 1984; Eyre et al., 1987).

Swelling (as opposed to solubilization) of polymeric collagen has been achieved by treatment with EDTA (Steven, 1967, 1976) or prolonged soaking in water (Veis et al., 1970). The effect of EDTA suggests that divalent cations are necessary mediators of bonding. Campo (1988) has demonstrated that whole-growth-plate cartilage swells in EDTA and EGTA. Although we have been able to confirm this effect in physeal cartilage, mature articular cartilage, cannot be induced to swell (Brown and Byers, unpublished observations) or to form polymeric collagen (Steven and Thomas, 1973; Steven, 1976), though its tensile properties are modified by the ionic environment (Akizuki et al., 1986).

Harkness and coworkers (Harkness and Harkness, 1973; Harkness and Hood, 1984; Nimni and Harkness, 1988) have drawn attention to the presence of labile crosslinks which 'can be broken by naturally occurring substances'. Such substances include pyridoxal phosphate, cysteamine, homocysteine and glutathione. The underlying nature of the bonds or chemistry of their cleavage has not been detailed.

Type IX collagen is covalently crosslinked into (or onto) type II collagen fibrils, yet it can be degraded by neutral proteases which do not degrade helical collagen. Consequently, Eyre and coworkers (Wu and Eyre, 1984; Eyre et al., 1987) have proposed that type IX collagen acts as an expendable bridge. Chondrocytes would regulate such a mechanism through production, activation and inhibition of suitable neutral protease(s).

Of these three, the cation-dependent model has been chosen for the following working hypothesis since actual swelling of collagen of most tissues can be achieved *in vitro*. Whilst this model can be set out as an example of a plausible mechanism it clearly does not satisfy all aspects of the problem or exclude other additional mechanisms which might coexist.

(i) Chondrocytes perceive the pattern of stimuli which signal expansion of the matrix (for repair or for growth). Synthesis of collagen and PG is increased.
(ii) Simultaneously the cell begins to reduce the matrix Ca^{2+} ion concentration close to its plasma membrane. Potential mechanisms include:
   (a) release of a calcium binding protein (chondrocalcin (Poole and Rosenberg, 1986; Hinek et al., 1987) deserves attention here since it is produced with type II collagen—being the *c*-terminal propeptide);
   (b) initiation of calcific crystal formation; and
   (c) by a membrane-based Ca^{2+} pump. Chondrocytes are particularly adept at manipulating the form and quantity of extracellular calcium.
(iii) Calcium ions would mediate the linkage between collagen molecules, either directly, or through an intermediate molecule: e.g. a specific PG (Scott, 1986) or fibril regulatory protein (Chandrasekhar et al., 1986).
(iv) With the free Ca^{2+} level reduced, charged groups on the collagen would accept alternative counterions such that bonding is progressively lost and slippage occurs, driven by the existing tension within the tissue. After new collagen units are incorporated, the local Ca^{2+} levels are allowed to rise. In this way the enlarged network would regain its functional integrity.
(v) Since adult articular cartilage does not respond to EDTA treatment alone (Steven and Thomas, 1973) we presume that at least one other linkage mechanism exists in the mature tissue, though not in growth-plate cartilage (campo, 1988; Brown and Byers, 1989).

Repair and remodeling are both processes which involve a degree of manipulation of the collagen network by chondrocytes. It seems logical, then, that a mechanism for this form of matrix expansion should be shared by and integral to these processes.

74

Fluorescent-tracer labeling for measuring remodeling in the zone of calcified cartilage

T.R. OEGEMA, JR and R.C. THOMPSON, JR

During the maturation of cartilage a clearly defined zone of calcified cartilage forms and with its formation the nutrients are no longer able to diffuse in from underlying capillaries. Therefore, the mature articular cartilage largely depends on diffusion from the synovial fluid for nutrition and for removal of waste. In addition, the zone of calcified cartilage becomes a key interface as it helps to distribute the force applied during the loading, and it provides the site of attachment of cartilage to bone (Redler et al., 1975).

Duplication of the tidemark is considered to be one of the hallmarks of osteoarthritis (OA), but the zone of calcified cartilage has generally been considered metabolically inert. Recent studies suggest that the zone of calcified cartilage may play a more active role in normal joint remodeling and in the pathogenesis of OA (Johnson, 1959; Green et al., 1970; Lemperg, 1971a,b; Lane and Bullough, 1980; Bullough and Jagannath, 1983). The zone of calcified cartilage makes up a relatively constant proportion (6–8%) of the total cartilage height (Lane and Bullough, 1980; Müller-Gerbl et al., 1987). The thickness of cartilage and the zone of calcified cartilage varies with the force across the joints (Müller-Gerbl et al., 1987). The relative constancy under a wide variety of conditions, of the ratio of the zone of calcified cartilage to cartilage, suggests that the interactions between the remodeling process of subchondral bone and the deposition of mineral in unmineralized cartilage are tightly regulated. As noted by Bullough (Lane and Bullough, 1980; Bullough et al., 1985) and by using a waviness index (defined as length of the tidemark divided by linear length along the joint), the tidemark is relatively smooth. Using the same index, the cartilage–subchondral bone junction is much more irregular. Increased irregularity was seen in the covered or more stressed areas.

Many analogies have been made between the zone of calcified cartilage and that of the growth plate. Originally the cells in the deep layers of the articular surface do have growth-plate characteristics but these are felt to disappear with the formation of the zone of calcified cartilage and the cessation of cell division (Mankin, 1964). However, there may be persistence of the growth-plate characteristics, especially in disease (Johnson, 1959; Lane and Bullough, 1980; Bullough and Jagannath, 1983; Bullough et al., 1985; Einhorn et al., 1985).

On mineralization of the zone of calcified cartilage, each cell retains an unmineralized matrix that can be shown both at the electron-microscopic and at the light level (Schenk et al., 1986). Proteoglycans remain in the mineralized tissue, although at a lower level (50%). In a preliminary report, Lowell and Eyre (1988) found persistence of type X collagen and a unique 45K protein in bovine cartilage. The mineral present in the zone of calcified cartilage appears to be hydroxyapatite with the degree of mineralization approximating that of bone (Lowell and Eyre, 1988). As studied by microradiography, the content of mineralization is unchanged by age but varies by species (Green et al., 1970).

Different aspects of the biology of the zone of calcified cartilage can be studied using the standard methods of bone biology. In order to study the rate of calcification of the zone of calcified cartilage, and to obtain an even labeling of the tidemark, we used an intraarticular injection of either an alizarin red or DCAF, (2,4-bi-N-di[carboxymethyl]aminomethyl)fluorescein, directly into the joint. This method was preferred over the use of intravenous injections of dyes. In our studies the dye was initially dissolved at 30 mg ml^{-1} in 2% sodium bicarbonate diluted to volume in medium and 0.4–1.0 ml of the dye injected intraarticularly at a dose of 9.25 mg kg^{-1}. The rabbits were allowed free access to food, water and cage movement from 2 to 12 weeks after injections and depending on the age of the animal, the cartilage with underlying bone was harvested, fixed in absolute ethanol, defatted with chloroform and embedded in methyl methacrylate. Approximately 100 μm sections were cut on a diamond saw, polished and viewed with a fluorescent microscope (Donohue *et al.*, 1983). The rate of movement between the zone of calcified cartilage–cartilage interface and the center of the fluorescent dye band can be quantitated and measurements can be made using a calibrated ocular (Fig. 74.1).

In mature animals, where the movement precipitously declines the label remains for longer periods of time at the interface, and the dye is slowly lost, especially in the contact region. This is consistent with a process where, when the newly mineralized tidemark area does not become embedded within the zone of calcified cartilage, the crystals of hydroxyapatite can redissolve and reform with a corresponding loss of the fluorescent label. This limits the useful time-frame between label and harvest to about 6 weeks or less. The use of intraarticular injection gave a more uniform staining, especially in the older animals where the

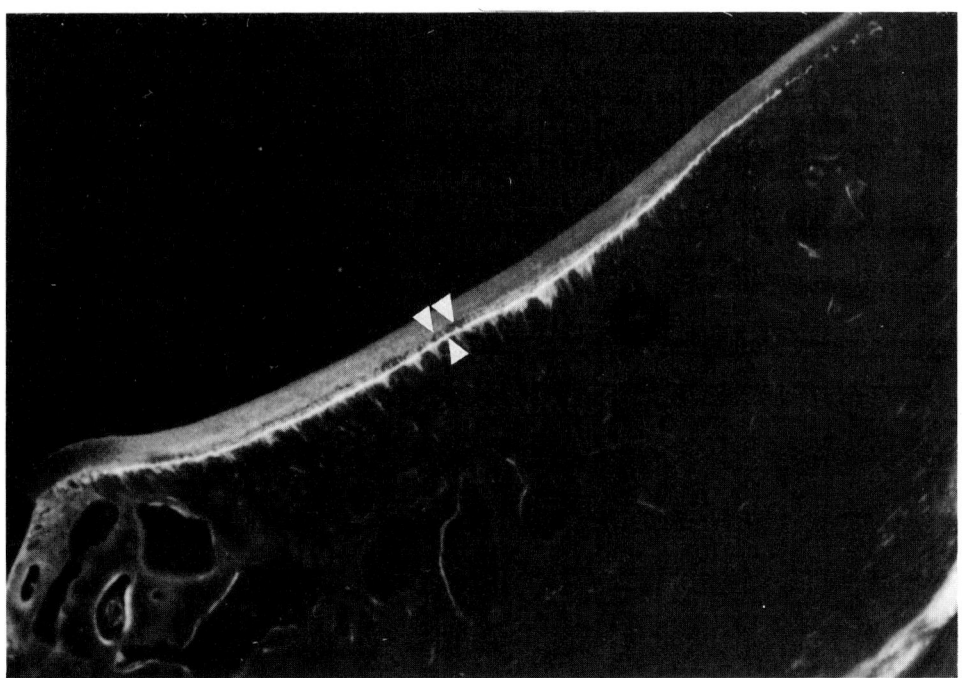

Figure 74.1 Fluorescent photomicrograph of a 100 micron thick section of rabbit patella embedded in methyl methacrylate. The animal had received a single interarticular injection of DCAF at 5 months of age and the tissue was harvested 7 weeks later. The majority of the dye (single arrow) has moved from the tidemark (double arrow) almost to the zone of calcified cartilage-bone interface.

subchondral blood supply is poor and diffusion from the plasma to the synovial fluid into the cartilage did not give adequate labeling. However, there was continued movement even in the adult animals but at a slower rate. This agrees with the observation of Lemperg (1971a,b) who saw some progression of the zone of calcified cartilage in mature rabbits given tetracycline.

The drawbacks of this labeling method include possible poor labeling in some areas of the joint due to too short an exposure to the dye. This can happen when the cartilage surfaces are held in close contact by joint forces or are covered by the meniscus and the limb is not moved while the dye is in the joint. A second problem is a gradual loss of bound dye if the labeled band does not move off the tidemark into the zone of calcified cartilage. Because of the yellow–green autofluorescence of cartilage embedded in methyl methacrylate, faint DCAF staining is difficult to distinguish from background. This problem can be solved by the use of other color dyes such as Alizarin red. The third problem occurs if double labeling is attempted at too close an interval such that the bands overlap and cannot be resolved.

Certain biochemical data (Boskey et al., 1980; Einhorn et al., 1985; Lowell and Eyre, 1988) and many of the morphologic studies (Green et al., 1970; Lemperg, 1971a,b; Bullough et al., 1985) support a strong analogy to the growth plate and similar mechanisms for the regulation of mineralization and resorption, but these are slower processes in the mature tissue (i.e. microns/week or year rather than per hour). The closeness of the analogy is only a matter of speculation. The presence of type X collagen in the zone of calcified cartilage of mature animals certainly adds to the similarity and may provide a means for assaying changes.

Understanding the role of the zone of calcified cartilage in the normal remodeling of the joint and in the progression of osteoarthritis is still in its infancy. While there are tantalizing hints as to possible pathways, very little is known about the biochemistry and biology of this region. With better models and tools such as the type X collagen antibodies and DCAF-tidemark labeling protocols, these questions can now be approached.

ACKNOWLEDGMENT

This work was supported by N.I.H. Grant AR 39255.

75

Spongialization and cartilage healing in the human

CHRISTIAN FICAT

The healing of cartilage lesions when the articular surface is damaged and presents deeply fibrillated areas and ulcerations is difficult to achieve because this tissue is almost incapable of repair by itself. But when the cartilage is completely abraded and the subchondral bone is exposed, buds of fibrocartilage can grow from the medulla of the subchondral bone and, if the mechanical conditions are favorable, they can coalesce and make a new gliding surface.

In some cases the growth of fibrocartilage is dramatic and a complete resurfacing can be

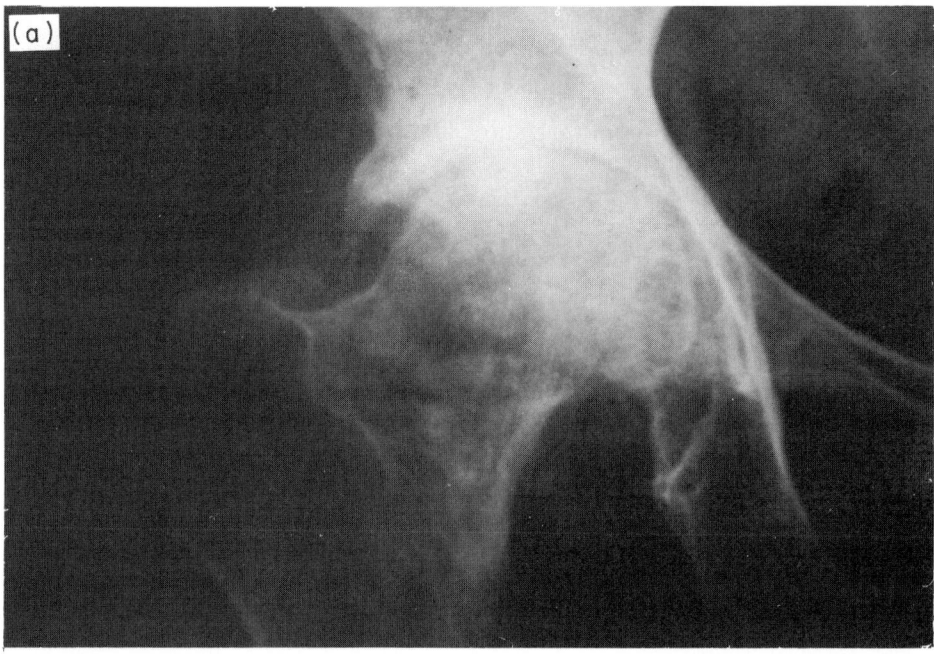

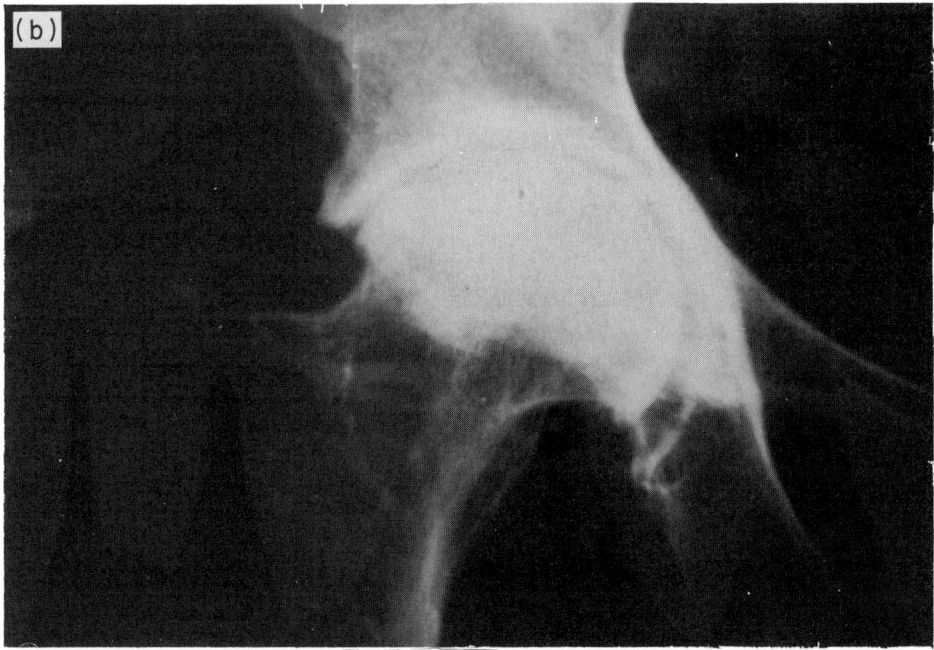

Figure 75.1 (a) X-ray of the hip of a 60 year old woman who had had a one year old Smith-Petersen cup arthroplasty removed. At surgery it was noted that a whitish fibrocartilage surface covered the bony surface of the femoral head which was merely replaced in the acetabulum. (b) X-ray of the same hip 16 years later showing no further progression.

obtained such as in the hip of a 60-year-old woman for whom a Smith–Petersen cup arthroplasty was performed in 1967. One year later the cup had to be removed because of a persistent pain. During the surgical operation it was noticed that the femoral head that was beneath the cup was covered by a whitish tissue looking more or less like fibrocartilage. Nothing more was done at surgery and the femoral head was replaced in the acetabulum (Fig. 75.1(A)). Sixteen years later the hip was examined and was found to be almost clinically normal. X-ray examination of the hip indicated a good joint space and a good congruence with no signs of recurrence of osteoarthritis (Fig. 75.1(B)). The favorable results in this case most probably occurred because the mechanical conditions were good: the head was well covered by the acetabulum, the congruence was good and the anabolic capacities of the medulla of the patient were favorable. This particular case indicates that, in some instances, a biological resurfacing is possible, the preliminary condition being that the joint congruence must be good and that the load is well distributed over a large weight-bearing zone.

In order to stimulate such a resurfacing from the bone marrow Pridie (1959) advocates drilling holes to expose the sclerotic bone. These perforations are convenient to fill a simple cleft or a small defect, but on a large fibrillated area they leave 'in-between' zones of degenerated cartilage and gives an irregular coverage. In the case of bone exposure the perforations also leave dense sclerotic subchondral bone, most of the time necrotic, which is not a good support.

The spongialization procedure (Ficat et al., 1979; Labbé, 1982) consists in excising the deeply fibrillated cartilage which remains on the cartilage surface and to resect the sclerotic subchondral bone plate just under the normal level to promote a better growth of the fibrocartilage. This creates a cavity the bottom of which is the bleeding cancellous bone surrounded by a rim of hard normal (or supposed normal) cartilage which will

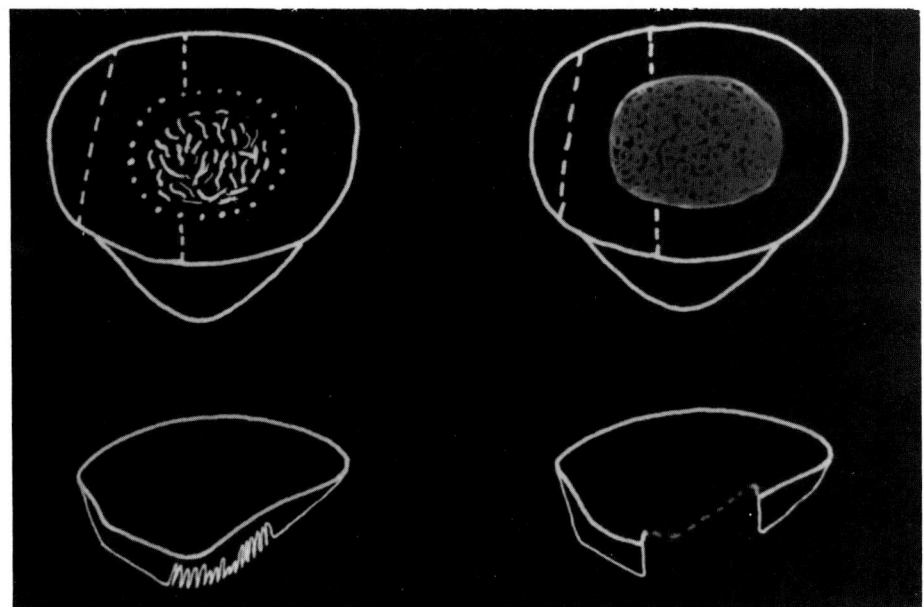

Figure 75.2 Example of the spongialization procedure as applied to a degenerated patella. Spongialization involves excision of the deeply fibrillated cartilage and resection through the subchondral bone to cancellous bone.

protect the growth of the new metaplastic tissue (Fig. 75.2). The removal of the subchondral bone has also an analgesic effect probably by the decompression of the intramedullary spaces and the suppression of nerve endings. If an ulceration is widespread on one facet, the entire facet can be spongialized. Furthermore, all the articular surface of the patella can also be spongialized by a frontal hemipatellectomy which reduces its thickness and thereby has a decompressive effect.

On the rare specimens which have been biopsied during a second operation one can observe a white tissue with an irregular articular surface which is a fibrocartilage with a dense network of collagen fibers that are quite well orientated in the deep zone but disordered and of an irregular diameter and the superficial layer is often fibrillated. In addition, many of the cells look like fibroblasts but some chondrocyte-like cells are seen mainly in the deep zone.

To date, spongializations of the patella on 55 males and 25 females have been performed. The mean age was 40.6 years (range 19–77 years), the mean follow-up was 3 years (range 1–7 years). Trauma was the most common etiology (68.8%), mostly contusions (53.3%). The lesions were situated on the lateral facet in 59.9% of cases, on the medial facet in 17.7% and on the central zone in 22.1%. The results were classified as very good and good in 61.1% (the subjective results were 66.6%) and fair and failures rated in 38.9% of patients. The analysis of the results has shown that the results were better in patients under 35 years old in the degenerative cases (compared with the posttraumatic) and for the medial facet (compared with the lateral facet).

76

Use of cultured chondrocytes as implants for repairing cartilage defects

D. ROBINSON, N. HALPERIN and Z. NEVO

The currently accepted surgical solution to severe joint deterioration is joint replacement by an artificial prosthesis. However, there are several drawbacks to this procedure and this has stimulated researchers to investigate an alternative — a biological resurfacing approach.

Cartilage fragments were the obvious type of biological implant of both autogeneic and allogeneic origin to have been tried experimentally for the repair of articular cartilage. However, fragments of cartilage often deteriorate and lead to the formation of fibrous tissue (Gibson, 1965; Aichroth, 1969; Benum, 1974; Bentley et al., 1978; McKibbin and Ralis, 1978; Aston and Bentley, 1986; Bentley, 1988). The fragments are also difficult to anchor to the implantation site and were frequently dislodged despite the use of various glue-like materials such as fibrin (Passl et al., 1976; Widenfalk et al., 1986; Itay et al., 1987). Osteochondral grafts (a cartilaginous fragment with a sliver of bone) are easier to anchor in place, but tend to invoke a massive immunological rejection reaction, leading to the degeneration of the cartilaginous tissue (Friedlander, 1983; Stover et al., 1989). A newer experimental method involves the use of implants composed of pellets of cultured chondrocytes with or without hormones and/or growth factors (Chesterman and Smith, 1965; Moskalewski and Kawiak, 1965; Moskalewski *et al.*, 1966; Bentley and Greer, 1971; Moskalewski and Rybicka, 1977; Bentley *et al.*, 1978; Helbing, 1981; Yoshihashi, 1983; Grande *et al.*, 1987; Itay *et al.*, 1987; Malejczyk and Moskalewski, 1988; Grande and Pitman, 1988; Brittberg *et al.*, 1989; Kawabe *et al.*, 1989; Osborn *et al.*, 1989; Robinson *et al.*, 1989, 1990; Wakitani *et al.*, 1989). In this article we describe various features (in particular, advantages and disadvantages) characterizing implantation of cultured cells. Our avian model system can serve to measure:

(i) the 'fate' and performance of various chondrocytes cultures used as orthotopic implants *in vivo*;
(ii) the regeneration and repair of injuries in articular cartilage.

It also allows examination of nonimmunological interactions between host and graft, e.g. the effect of the host's age on the implant fate.

THE AVIAN MODEL

Surgery was performed on all chickens under general anesthesia. The area covering the right tibiotarsal joint was plucked, and the skin prepared with Betadine. The tibiotarsal joint was exposed through a lateral longitudinal incision and extended to provide exposure of the condylar articular cartilage. The patella is dislocated. A bone biopsy needle of 1.5 mm diameter was used to create a deep defect, penetrating the subchondral bone, which was then enlarged using a gauge to approximately 3–4 mm in diameter. Four to six such holes were created in the weight-bearing area of each operated joint. In other chickens, large and superficial defects, reaching to, but not penetrating the subchondral bone, were made using a scalpel. The defects could account for up to 40–50% of the total tibial joint surface area.

In the experimental group, the wounds were filled with cultured embryonal chondrocytes embedded in a delivery substance, the initial studies employed fibrin-based adhesive, whereas we now use a hyaluronan based adhesive as described in Chapter 4 and in our recent publications (Robinson *et al.*, 1989, 1990). Animals in the control group were either given the delivery substance alone or received no treatment at all. The contralateral tibiotarsal joint served as a control for histologic comparison with normal chicken cartilage.

This model, utilizing mechanically created lesions, does not imitate any of the common pathological entities of the joints, though it can be closely related to abrasion arthroplasty employed to enhance self-resurfacing in common OA, or in osteochondritis dissicans syndrome. However, certain obvious merits of this model do emerge: it presents an orthotopic natural site of cartilage repair, tissue being bathed by synovial fluid, in contrast to ectopic sites (muscular or peritoneal), with or without an artificial unit (diffusion chamber). At the orthotopic articular site, implants evoke a minimal immunologic response in contrast to the hostile conditions for implanted chondrocytes known to exist in the peritoneal cavity.

The implanted cells are able to proliferate within the lesion, thus filling the whole cavity. Cells in the different zones acquire different characteristics with time. In the surface layers the implanted cells reconstruct the basic histological traits of articular cartilage, including the sphericity of the surface. Between the articular zone and the deeper layers a tide mark is formed, and in the 'reparative' regions underneath the tide mark the process of endochondral ossification takes place and 'Benninghof' arcades are formed.

It should be noted that the rates of these reparative events in the lesions are influenced by the host's age. Three-year-old chickens show an increased rate of cell maturation that is approximately three times that observed in four-month-old chickens (Robinson *et al.*, 1989). Some reparative phenomena are unique to old chickens; these include enhancement of bone density and the formation of hematopoietic centers which surrounded the grafts. The donor's age is also important, as are intrinsic local microenvironmental factors (Nimni *et al.*, 1988b; Robinson *et al.*, 1989). Thus, in order to have standard conditions, we decided to use cells derived from chick embryos in all our experiments. Attempts to utilize older chondrocytes derived from postnatal chicks (even those only three-weeks old) failed to generate cartilaginous tissue, but rather formed a fibrous tissue. This latter observation could be explained by the rapid postnatal decrease in the proliferative ability of the chondrocytes and their increased tendency to dedifferentiate (Stockwell, 1979). An additional cell source, cartilage cells derived from the callus of both normal and vitamin D deficient chick neonates (Lidor *et al.*, 1987a,b), also failed: the cartilage underwent endochondral ossification, even in regions above the tide mark, finally resulting in eburnated bone. In addition to the cell source, the history of cells in culture is of prime importance, as the chondrocyte phenotype is labile and easily lost in monolayer cultures, giving rise to dedifferentiated fibroblast-like cells (Holtzer *et al.*, 1960; Chacko *et al.*, 1969).

In summary, the model we have described presents, we feel, a number of advantages over previous attempts and offers a useful tool for studying the behavior of transplanted chondrocytes in a natural environment.

References

Aaron, R.K. and Plaas, A.A.K. (1987). Stimulation of proteoglycan synthesis in articular chondrocyte cultures by a pulsed electromagnetic field. *Trans. Orthop. Res. Soc.* **12**, 273

Aaron, R.K., Ciomber, D.M. and Jolly, G. (1987). Modulation of chondrogenesis and chondrocyte differentiation by pulsed electro magnetic fields. *Trans. Orthop. Res. Soc.* **12**, 272

Adam, A. and Spence, A.J. (1958). Intertrochanteric osteotomy for osteoarthritis of the hip. *J. Bone Joint Surg.* **40B**, 219–226

Akeson, W.H., Miyashita, C., Taylor, T.K. and LaViolette, D. (1969). Experimental cup arthroplasty of the canine hip. *J. Bone Joint Surg.* **51A**, 149–164

Akizuki, S., Mow, V.C., Muller, F., Pita, J.C., Howell, D.S. and Manicourt, D.H. (1986). Tensile properties of human knee joint cartilage: influence of ionic conditions, weight bearing and fibrillation on the tensile modules. *J. Orthop. Res.* **4**, 385–391

Aichroth, P.M. (1969). Transplantation of joint surfaces by cartilage grafts. *Br. J. Surg.* **56**, 855

Amadio, P.C., Millender, L.H. and Smith, R.J. (1982). Silicone spacer or tendon spacer for trapezium resection arthroplasty. Comparison of results. *J. Hand Surg.* **7A**, 237–244

Amiel, D., Coutts, R.D., Abel, M., Stewart, W., Harwood, F. and Akeson, W.H. (1985). Rib perichondrial grafts for the repair of full thickness articular cartilage defects. *J. Bone Joint Surg.* **67A**, 911–920

Anderson, C.E. and Parker, J. (1966). Invasion and resorption in endochondral ossification. An electron microscopic study. *J. Bone Joint Surg.* **48A**, 899–914

Arnoczky, A., Adams, M., DeHaven, K., Eyre, D., Mow, V. and Meniscus, X.X. (1988). In *Injury and Repair of the Musculoskeletal Soft Tissue* (S.L. Woo and J.A. Buckwalter, eds) Chap. 12, pp. 487–537. American Academy of Orthopeadic Surgeons, Park Ridge, IL

Aston, J.E. and Bentley, G. (1986). Repair of articular surfaces by allografts of articular and growthplate cartilage. *J. Bone Joint Surg.* **68B** 29–35

Athanasiou, K.A. (1989). Biomechanical assessment of articular cartilage healing and interspecies variability. Ph.D. Thesis, Columbia University, OH

Baker, B., Spadaro, J.A. and Becker, R.O. (1974a). Electrical stimulation of articular cartilage. *Ann. NY Acad. Sci.* **238**, 491–499

Baker, B., Becher, R.O. and Spadaro, J. (1974b). A study of electrochemical enhancement of articular cartilage repair. *Clin. Orthop.* **102**, 251–267

Bentley, G. (1988). Transplant potential of the growth plate. In *Behavior of the Growth Plate* (H.K. Uhthoff and J.J. Wiley, eds), pp. 65–71. Raven Press, New York

Bentley, G. and Greer, R.B. (1971). Homotransplantation if isolated epiphyseal and articular cartilage chondrocytes into joint surfaces of rabbits. *Nature* **230**, 385–388

Bentley, G., Smith, A.U. and Mukerjhee, R. (1978). Isolated epiphyseal chondrocyte allografts into joint surfaces. An experimental study in rabbits. *Ann. Rheum. Dis.* **37**, 449–458

Benum, P. (1974). Autogenous transplantation of epiphyseal cartilage to osteochondral defects of joints. *Acta Orthop. Scand.* (Suppl 156)

Birk, C.E. and Trelstad, R.L. (1986). Extracellular compartments in tendon morphogenesis: collagen fibril bundle and microaggregate formation. *J. Cell Biol.* **103**, 231–240

Boskey, A.L., Bullough, P.G. and Droitrovsky, E. (1980). The biochemistry of the mineralization front. *Metab. Bone Dis. Rel. Res.* **25**, 61–67

Brighton, C.T. (1984). The semi-invasive method of treating nonunion with direct current. *Orthop. Clin. North Am.* **15**, 33–45

Brighton, C.T. and Pollack, S.R. (1985). Treatment of recalcitrant non-union with a capacitively coupled electrical field: a preliminary report. *J. Bone Joint Surg.* **67A**, 577–585

Brighton, C.T., Unger, A.S. and Stambough, J.L. (1984). *In vitro* growth of bovine articular cartilage chondrocytes in various capacitively coupled electrical fields. *J. Orthop. Res.* **2**, 15–22

Brighton, C.T., Hozach, W.J., Brager, M.D., Windsor, R.E., Pollack, S.R., Vreslovic, E.J. and Kotwick, J.E. (1985). Fracture healing in the rabbit fibula—when subjected to various capacitively coupled electrical fields. *J. Orthop. Res.* **3**, 331–340

Brittberg, M., Nilsson, A., Peterson, L., Lindahl, A. and Isaksson, O. (1989). Healing of injured rabbit articular cartilage after transplantation of autologous cultivated chondrocytes. *The Bat Sheva Seminar on Methods Used in Research on Cartilaginous Tissues*, Israel

Broom, N.D. (1986). The collagenous architecture of articular cartilage — a synthesis of ultrastructure and mechanical function. *J. Rheumatol.* **13**, 142–152

Brown, R.A. and Byers, P.D. (1989). Swelling of cartilage and expansion of the collagen network. *Calc. Tiss. Int.* **46**, 260–261

Buckwalter, J.A. and Mow, V.C. (1990). Articular cartilage repair in osteoarthritis. In *Osteoarthritis: Diagnosis and Management* (D.S. Howell, H.J. Mankin, R.W. Moskowitz and W.B. Saunders, eds), 2nd edn (in press)

Buckwalter, J.A., Rosenberg, L.C., Coutts, R., Hunziker, E., Reddi, A.H. and Mow, V. (1988). Articular cartilage: injury and repair. In *Injury and Repair of the Musculoskeletal Soft Tissues* (S.L. Woo and J.A. Buckwalter, eds), pp. 465–482. American Academy of Orthopaedic Surgeons, Park Ridge, IL

Buckwalter, J.A., Rosenberg, L.C. and Hunziker, E.B. (1990). Articular cartilage: composition structure, response to injury and methods of facilitating repair. In *Articular Cartilage and Knee Joint Function: Basic Science and Arthroscopy* (J.W. Ewing, ed.), Chap. 2. Raven Press, New York

Bullough, P.G. (1981). The geometry of diarthrodial joints, its physiological maintenance and the possible significance of age related changes in geometry to load distribution and the development of OA. *Clin. Orthop. Rel. Res.* **156**, 61–66

Bullough, P.G. and Jagannath, A. (1983). The morphology of the calcification front in articular cartilage: its significance in joint function. *J. Bone Joint Dis.* **65A**, 72–78

Bullough, P.G., Yawitz, P.S., Tafra, L. and Boskey, A.L. (1985). Topographical variations in the morphology and biochemistry of adult tibial plateau articular cartilage. *J. Orthop. Res.* **3**, 1–16

Burton, R.I. (1983). The arthritic hand. In *Surgery of the Musculoskeletal System* (E.M. Evarts, ed.) pp. 2:621–2:692. Churchill Livingstone, New York

Byers, P.D. (1974). The effect of high femoral osteotomy on osteoarthritis of the hip. *J. Bone Joint Surg.* **56B**, 279–290

Calandruccio, R.A. and Gilmer, W.S. (1962). Proliferation regeneration and repair of articular cartilage of immature animals. *J. Bone Joint Surg.* **44A**, 431–455

Campo, R.D. (1988). Effects of cations on cartilage structure: swelling of growth plate and degradation of proteoglycans induced by chelators of divalent cations. *Calc. Tissue Int.* **43**, 108–121

Chacko, S., Abbott, J., Holtzer, S. and Holtzer, H. (1969). The loss of phenotype traits of differentiated cell. VI. Behaviors of the progeny of a single chondrocyte. *J. Exp. Med.* **130**, 417–442

Chandrasekhar, S., Laurie, G.W., Cannon, F.B., Martin, G.R. and Kleinman, H.K. (1986). *In vitro* regulation of cartilage matrix assembly by a M_r 54,000 collagen-binding protein. *Proc. Natl. Acad. Sci. USA* **83**, 5126–5130

Chesterman, P.J. and Smith, A.U. (1965). Homotransplantation of articular cartilage and isolated chondrocytes. An experimental study in rabbits. *J. Bone Joint Surg.* **50B**, 184–197

Cheung, H.S., Cottrell, W.H., Stephenson, K. and Nimni, M.E. (1978). *In vitro* collagen biosynthesis in healing and normal rabbit articular cartilage. *J. Bone Joint Surg.* **60A**, 1076–1081

Cheung, H.S., Lynch, K.L., Johnson, R.P. and Brewer, B.J. (1980). *In vitro* synthesis of tissue specific type II collagen by healing cartilage. I. Short-term repair of cartilage by mature rabbits. *Arth. Rheum.* **23**, 211–219

Clark, J.M. (1985). The organization of collagen in cryofractured rabbit articular cartilage: a scanning electronmicroscopic study. *J. Orthop. Res.* **3**, 17–29

Cohen, J. and Lacroix, D. (1955). Bone and cartilage formation by periosteum. *J. Bone Joint Surg.* **37A**, 717–730

Coletti, J.M., Akeson, W.H. and Woo, S.L. (1972). A comparison of the physical behavior of normal articular cartilage and arthroplasty surface. *J. Bone Joint Surg.* **54A**, 147–160

Convery, F.R., Akeson, W.H. and Keown, G.H. (1972). The repair of large osteochondral defects: an experimental study in horses. *Clin. Orthop.* **82**, 253–262

Curtiss, P.H. Jr. (1969). Cartilage damage in septic arthritis. *Clin. Orthop.* **64**, 87–90

Delaney, J.P., O'Driscoll, S.W. and Salter, R.B. (1989). Neochondrogenesis in free intra-articular periosteal autografts in an immobilized and paralyzed limb. *Clin. Orthop.* **248**, 278–282

Dell, P.C. and Muniz, R.B. (1987). Interposition arthroplasty of the trapeziometacarpal joint for osteoarthritis. *Clin. Orthop.* **220**, 27–34

Donohue, J.M., Buss, D., Oegema, T.R., Jr and Thompson, R.C., Jr (1983). The effects of indirect blunt trauma on adult canine articular cartilage. *J. Bone Joint Surg.* **65A**, 948–957

Einhorn, T.A., Gordon, S.L., Siegel, S.A., Hummel, G.F., Auitable, M.J. and Carty, R.P. (1985). Matrix vesicle enzymes in human osteoarthritis. *J. Orthop. Res.* **3**, 160–169

Engkvist, O. (1979). Reconstruction of patellar articular cartilage with free autologous perichondrial grafts. *Scand. J. Plast. Reconstr. Surg.* **13**, 361–369

Engkvist, O. and Ohlsen, L. (1979). Reconstruction of articular cartilage with free autologous perichondrial grafts. *Scand. J. Plast. Reconstr. Surg.* **13**, 269–274

Engkvist, O., Skoog, V., Pastacaldi, P., Yormuk, E. and Juhlin, R. (1979). The cartilagenous potential of the perichondrium in rabbit ear and rib. *Scand. J. Plast. Reconstr. Surg.* **13**, 275–280

Eyre, D.R., Apone, S., Wu, J.-J., Ericsson, L.H. and Walsh, K.A. (1987). Collagen type IX: evidence of covalent linkages to type II collagen of cartilage. *FEBS Lett.* **220**, 337–341

Farkas, T., Lippiello, L. and Mitrovic, D. (1977). Papain induced healing of superficial lacerations in articular cartilage of adult rabbits. *Trans. Ortho. Res. Soc.* **2**, 204

Ficat, R.P., Ficat, C., Gedeon, P. and Toussaint, J.B. (1979). Spongialization: a new treatment for diseased patellae. *Clin. Orthop.* **144**, 74–83

Friedlander, G.E. (1983). Immune responses to osteochondral allografts. *Clin. Orthop.* **174**, 58–68

Fry, P., Harkness, M.L.R., Harkness, R.D. and Nightingale, M. (1962). Mechanical properties of tissues of lathyritic animals. *J. Physiol.* **164**, 77–89

Fuller, J.A. and Ghadially, F.N. (1972). Ultrastructural observations on surgically produced partial-thickness defects in articular cartilage. *Clin. Orthop.* **86**, 193–205

Furukawa, T., Eyre, D.R., Koide, S. and Glimcher, M.J. (1980). Biochemical studies on repair cartilage resurfacing experimental defects in the rabbit knee. *J. Bone Joint Surg.* **62A**, 79–89

Ghadially, F.N., Thomas, I., Oryschak, A.F. and LaLonde, J.M. (1977). Long-term results of superficial defects in articular cartilage: a scanning electron-microscope study. *J. Pathol.* **121**, 213–217

Gibson, T. (1965). Cartilage grafts. *Br. Med. Bul.* **21**, 153–156

Grande, D.A. and Pitman, M.I. (1988). The use of adhesives in chondrocyte transplantation surgery preliminary studies. *Bull. Hosp. Joint Dis. Orthop. Inst.* **48**, 140–148

Grande, D.A., Singh, I. and Pugh, J. (1987). Healing of experimentally produced lesions in articular cartilage following chondrocyte transplantation. *Anatom. Record.* **218**, 142–148

Green, W.T. (1977). Articular cartilage repair. Behaviour of rabbit chondrocytes during tissue culture and subsequent allografting. *Clin. Orthop.* **124**, 237–250

Green, W.T., Martin, G.N., Eanes, E.D. and Sokoloff, L. (1970). Microradiographic study of the calcified layer of articular cartilage. *Arch. Pathol.* **90**, 151–158

Harkness, M.L.R. and Harkness, R.D. (1973). Changes with age in some mechanical properties of skin in the rat. In *Connective Tissue and Aging* (H.G. Vogel, ed.), pp. 219–221. Excerpta Medica, Amsterdam

Harkness, R.D. and Hood, J.A.A. (1984). A simple method for testing the effects of reagents on the mechanical properties of sheets of connective tissues. *J. Mat. Sci.* **19**, 339–344

Harris, N.H. and Kirwan, E. (1964). The results of osteotomy for early primary osteoarthritis of the hip. *J. Bone Joint Surg.* **46B**, 477–487

Hart, J.A.L. (1987). The use of carbon fibre implants for articular cartilage defects. Presented at the 47th Annual Meeting of the Australian Orthopaedic Association, Melbourne, 1987

Hinek, A., Reiner, R. and Poole, A.R. (1987). The calcification of cartilage matrix in chondrocyte culture: studies of the C-propeptide of type II collagen (chondrocalcin). *J. Cell Biol.* **104**, 1435–1441

Helbing, G. (1981). Transplantation isolierter chondrozyten in gelenkknorpel defekte. *Med. Habilitat.* 3355–3359

Hoch, D.H., Grodzinsky, A.J., Kobb, T.J., Albert, M.L. and Eyre, D.R. (1983). Early changes in material properties of rabbit articular cartilage after meniscectomy. *J. Orthop. Res.* **1**, 4–12

Holtzer, H., Abbott, J., Lash, J. and Holtzer, S. (1960). The loss of phenotype traits by differentiated cells *in vitro*. I. Dedifferentiation of cartilage cells. *Proc. Nat. Acad. Sci. USA* **49**, 643–647

Hunter, W. (1743). On the structure and diseases of articulating cartilage. *Phil. Trans. R. Soc. (London)* **1743**, 267

Itay, S., Abramovici, A. and Nevo, Z. (1987). Use of cultured embryonal chick epiphyseal chondrocytes as grafts for defects in chick articular cartilage. *Clin. Orthop.* **220**, 284–303

Itay, S., Abramovici, A., Ysipovitch, Z. and Nevo, Z. (1988). Correction of defects in articular cartilage by implants of cultures of embryonic chondrocytes. *Proc. Orthop. Res. Soc.* **13**, 112

Johnson, L.C. (1959). Kinetics of osteoarthritis. *Lab. Invest.* **8**, 1223–1241

Johnson, L.C. (1962). Joint remodeling as the basis for osteoarthritis. *J. Am. Vet. Med. Assoc.* **141**, 1237–1241

Jurvelin, J., Kiviranta, I., Tammi, M. and Helminen, H.J. (1986). Softening of canine articular cartilage after immobilization of the knee joint. *Clin. Orthop.* **207**, 246–252

Kawabe, N., Yoshinao, M. and Hirotani, H. (1989). The repair of full thickness articular cartilage defects. Immune responses to reparative tissue by growth plate chondrocytes implants. *Trans. Orthop. Res. Soc.* **14**, 143

Kiviranta, I., Jurvelin, J., Tammi, M., Saamanen, A.-M. and Helminin, H.J. (1987). Weight-bearing controls glycosaminoglycan concentration and articular cartilage thickness in the knee joints of young beagle dogs. *Arthr. Rheum.* **30**, 801–809

Kleiner, J.B., Coutts, R.D., Woo, S.L.-Y., Amiel, D., Lee, T.Q., Rosenstein, A.D., Harwood, F.L. and Field, F.P. (1986). The short term evaluation of different treatment modalities upon full thickness articular cartilage defects: a study of rib perichondrial chondrogenesis. *Trans. Orthop. Res. Soc.* **11**, 282

Knodt, H. (1971). Pressure reducing effects of hip osteotomies. *Clin. Orthop.* **77**, 105–116

Kulick, M.I., Brent, B. and Ross, J. (1984). Free perichondrial graft from the ear to the knee in rabbits. *J. Hand Surg.* **9A**, 213–215

Kwan, M.K., Woo, S.L.-Y., Amiel, D., Kleiner, J.B., Field, F.P. and Coutts, R.D. (1987). Neocartilage generated from rib perichondrium: a long-term multidisciplinary evaluation. *Trans. 33rd Orthop. Res. Soc. Meeting*, pp. 12–277

Labbé, J.L. (1982). *La Spongialisation de la Rotule*. Thèse, Faculté de Medecine de Toulouse

Lane, L.B. and Bullough, P.G. (1980). Age-related changes in the thickness of the calcified zone and the number of tidemarks in adult human articular cartilage. *J. Bone Joint Surg.* **62B**, 372–375

Landells, J.W. (1957). The reactions of injured human articular cartilage. *J. Bone Joint Surg.* **39B**, 548–562

Lee, S.L. and Piez, K.A. (1983). Type II collagen from lathyritic rat chondrosarcoma: preparation and in vitro fibril formation. *Collagen Relat. Res.* **3**, 89–103

Lemperg, R. (1971a). The subchondral bone plate of the femoral head in adult rabbits. I. Spontaneous remodeling studied by microradiography and tetracycline labeling. *Virch. Arch.* **352**, 1–13

Lemperg, R. (1971b). The subchondral bone plate of the femoral head adult rabbits. II. Changes induced by introcartilagenous defects studied by microradiography and tetracycline labeling. *Virch. Arch. Pathol. Anal.* **352**, 14–25

Lidor, C., Dekel, S., Hallel, T. and Edelstein, S. (1987a). Levels of active metabolites of vitamin D_3 in the callus of fracture repair in chicks. *J. Bone Joint Surg.* **69**, 132–136

Lidor, C., Dekel, S. and Edelstein, S. (1987b). The metabolism of vitamin D_3 during fracture healing in chicks. *Endocrinology* **120**, 389–393

Lowell, T.P. and Eyre, D.R. (1988). Unique biochemical characteristics of the calcified zone of articular cartilage. *Trans. Orthop. Res. Soc.* **13**, 511

Malejczyk, J. and Moskalewski, S. (1988). Effect of immunosuppression on survival and growth of cartilage produced by transplanted allogeneic epiphyseal chondrocytes. *Clin. Orthop.* **232**, 292–303

Mankin, H.J. (1962a). Localization of tritiated thymidine in articular cartilage of rabbits. I. Growth in immature cartilage. *J. Bone Joint Surg.* **44A**, 682–688

Mankin, H.J. (1962b). Localization of tritiated thymidine in articular cartilage of rabbits. II. Repair in immature cartilage. *J. Bone Joint Surg.* **44A**, 688–698

Mankin, H.J. (1964). Mitosis in articular cartilage of immature rabbits. *Clin. Orthop.* **34**, 170–183

Mankin, H.J. (1974a). The reaction of articular cartilage to injury and osteoarthritis: Part I. *N. Engl. J. Med.* **291**, 1285–1292

Mankin, H.J. (1974b). The reaction of articular cartilage to injury and osteoarthritis: Part II. *N. Engl. J. Med.* **291**, 1335–1340

Mankin, H.J. (1982). The response of articular cartilage to mechanical injury. *J. Bone Joint Surg.* **64A**, 460–466

Mankin, H.J. and Boyle, C.H. (1967). The acute effects of lacerative injury on DNA and protein synthesis in articular cartilage. In *Cartilage Degradation and Repair* (A.L. Bassett, ed.), pp. 186–199. National Acad. Sci. National Research Council, Washington DC

Maroudas, A. (1976). Balance between swelling pressure and collagen tension in normal and degenerate cartilage. *Nature* **260**, 808–809

McKibbin, B. and Ralis, Z.A. (1978). The site dependence of the articular cartilage transplant reaction. *J. Bone Joint Surg.* **60B**, 561–566

Meachim, G. (1963). The effect of scarification on articular cartilage in the rabbit. *J. Bone Joint Surg.* **45B**, 150–161

Mendler, M., Eich-Bender, S.G., Vaughan, L.,

Winterhalter, K.H. and Bruchner, P., (1989). Cartilage contains mixed fibrils of collagen types II, IX and XI. *J. Cell Biol.* **108**, 191–197

Mensor, M.C. and Scheck, M. (1968). Review of six years experience with the hanging hip operation. *J. Bone Joint Surg.* **50A**, 1250–1254

Miller, A. and Wray, J.S. (1971). Molecular packing in collagen. *Nature* **230**, 437

Mitchell, N. and Shepard, N. (1976). The resurfacing of adult rabbit articular cartilage by multiple perforations through the subchondral bone. *J. Bone Joint Surg.* **58A**, 230–233

Mitchell, N. and Shepard, N. (1987). Effect of patellar shaving in the rabbit. *J. Orthop. Res.* **5**, 388–392

Moran, M.E., Kreder, H.J., Salter, R.B. and Keeley, F.N. (1989). Biological resurfacing of major full thickness defects in joint surfaces by neochondrogenesis with cryopreserved allogeneic periosteum stimulated by continuous passive motion. *Trans. Orthop. Res. Soc.* **14**, 542

Moskalewski, S. and Kawiak, J. (1965). Cartilage formation after homotransplantation of isolated chondrocytes. *Transplantation* **3**, 737–742

Moskalewski, S. and Rybicka, E. (1977). The influence of the degree of maturation of donor tissue on the reconstruction of elastic cartilage by isolated chondrocytes. *Acta Anat.* **97**, 231–240

Moskalewski, S., Kawiak, J. and Rymaszewska, T. (1966). Local cellular response evoked by cartilage formed after auto- and allogeneic transplantation of isolated chondrocytes. *Transplantation* **4**, 572–581

Muir, H., Bullough, P. and Maroudas, A. (1970). The distribution of collagen in human articular cartilage with some of its physiological implications. *J. Bone Joint Surg.* **52B**, 554–563

Müller-Gerbl, M., Schulte, E. and Putz, R. (1987). The thickness of the calcified layer in different joints of a single individual. *Acta Morphol. Neerl.-Scand.* **25**, 41–49

Muller-Glauser, W., Humbel, B., Glatt, M., Strauli, P., Winterhalter, K.H. and Bruckner, P. (1986). On the role of type IX collagen in the extracellular matrix of cartilage: type IX collagen is localized to intersections of collagen fibrils. *J. Cell Biol.* **102**, 1931–1939

Nelson, B.H., Anderson, D.D., Brand, R.A. and Brown, T.D. (1988). Effect of osteochondral defects on articular cartilage: contact pressure studies in dog knees. *Acta. Orthop. Scand.* **59**, 574–579

Nemeth, G.G., Bolander, M.E. and Martin, G.R. (1988). Growth factors and their role in wound and fracture healing. In *Growth Factors and Other Aspects of Wound Healing: Biological and Clinical Implications* (Barbule, Pines, Caldwell and Hunt, eds), pp. 1–17. Allen R. Liss, New York

Nemetschek, T.H., Riedl, H., Jonak, R., Nemetschek-Gansler, H., Bordas, J., Koch, M.H.J. and Schilling, V. (1980). Functional properties of parallel fibred connective tissue with special regard to viscoelasticity. *Virchows Arch. B Pathol. Histol.* **386**, 125–151

Nimni, M.E. and Harkness, R.D. (1988a). Molecular structure and functions of collagen. In *Collagen* (M.E. Nimni, ed.), Vol. 1, pp. 1–77. CRC Press, Boca Raton, FL

Nimni, M.E., Bernick, S., Ertl, D., Nishimoto, S.K., Paule, W., Strates, B.S. and Villaneuva, J. (1988b). Ectopic bone formation is enhanced in senescent animals implanted with embryonal cells. *Clin. Orthop.* **234**, 255–267

Nissen, K.I. (1971). The rationale of early osteotomy for idiopathic coxarthrosis (epichondro-osteoarthrosis of the hip). *Clin. Orthop.* **77**, 98–104

Norton, L.A., Rodan, G.A. and Bourret, L.A. (1977). Epiphyseal cartilage cAMP change produced by electrical and mechanical perturbations. *Clin. Orthop.* **124**, 59–68

O'Driscoll, S.W. and Salter, R.B. (1984). The induction of neochondrogenesis in free intra-articular periosteal autografts under the influence of continuous passive motion: an experimental study in the rabbit. *J. Bone Joint Surg.* **66A**, 1248–1257

O'Driscoll, S.W. and Salter, R.B. (1986). The repair of major osteochondral defects in joint surfaces by neochondrogenesis with autogenous osteoperiosteal grafts stimulated by continuous passive motion: An experimental investigation in the rabbit. *Clin. Orthop.* **208**, 131

O'Driscoll, S.W., Keeley, F.W. and Salter, R.B. (1986). The chondrogenic potential of free autogenous periosteal grafts for biological resurfacing of major full thickness defects in joint surfaces under the influence of continuous passive motion: an experimental study in the rabbit. *J. Bone Joint Surg.* **68A**, 1017–1035

O'Driscoll, S.W., Kelley, F.W. and Salter, R.B. (1989a). Durability of regenerated articular cartilage produced by free autogenous periosteal grafts in major full thickness defects in joint surfaces under the influence of continous passive motion: a follow-up report at one year. *J. Bone Joint Surg.* **70A**, 595

O'Driscoll, S.W., Delaney, J.P. and Salter, R.B. (1989b). Failure of experimental patellar resurfacing using free periosteal autografts. *Orthop. Trans.* **13**, 294–295

Ohlsen, L. (1978). Cartilage regeneration from perichondrium. *Plastic Reconst. Surg.* **62**, 507–513

Osborn, K.D., Trippel, S.B. and Mankin, H.J. (1989). Growth factor stimulation of adult articular cartilage. *J. Orthop. Res.* **7**, 35–42

Paget, T. (1853). Healing of injuries in various tissues. *Lect. Surg. Pathol.* **T**, 262

Palmoski, M., Perricone, E. and Brandt, K.D. (1979). Development and reversal of a proteoglycan aggregation defect in normal canine knee cartilage after immobilization. *Arthr. Rheum.* **22**, 508–517

Palmoski, M.J. and Brandt, D.K. (1981). Running inhibits the reversal of atrophic changes in canine knee cartilage after removal of a leg cast. *Arthr. Rheum.* **24**, 1329–1337

Parsons, J.R., McManus, E. and Johnson, E. (1982). Time dependent histologic and mechanical alteration of articular cartilage with joint sepsis. *Trans. Orthop. Res. Sco.* **7**, 217

Passl, R., Plenk, H., Radaskiewicz, T., Sauer, G., Holle, J. and Spangler, H.P. (1976). Zum problem der reinen homologen gelenksknorpel transplantation. *Verh. Anat. Ges.* **70S**, 675–678

Poole, A.R. and Rosenberg, L.C. (1986). Chondrocalcin and the calcification of cartilage. *Clin. Orthop. Rel. Res.* **208**, 114–118

Pridie, K.H. (1959). A method of resurfacing osteoarthritic knee joints. *J. Bone Joint Surg.* **41B**, 618

Radin, E.L. and Burr, D.B. (1984). Hypothesis: joints can heal. *Semin. Arthr. Rheum.* **13**, 293–302

Radin, E.L., Maquet, P. and Park, H. (1975). Rationale and indications for the 'hanging hip' procedure. A clinical and experimental study. *Clin. Orthop.* **112**, 221–230

Reagan, B.F., McInerny, V.K., Treadwell, B.V., Zarins, B. and Mankin, H.J. (1983). Irrigating solutions for arthroscopy: a metabolic study. *J. Bone Joint Surg.* **65A**, 629–631

Reddi, A.H. (1983). Extracellular bone matrix dependent local induction of cartilage and bone. *J. Rheumatol.* **10** (Suppl 11), 67–69

Reddi, A.H. (1985). Role of subchondral bone matrix factors in the repair of articular cartilage. In *Degenerative Joints* (G. Verbruggen and E.M. Veys, eds), Vol. 2, pp. 271–274. Excerpta Medica, Amsterdam

Reddi, A.H. and Hubbins, C. (1972). Biochemical sequences in the transformation of normal fibroblasts in adolescent rats. *Proc. Natl. Acad. Sci. USA* **69**, 1601–1605

Reddi, A.H., Wientroub, S. and Muthukumaran, N. (1987). Biologic principles of bone induction. *Orthop. Clin. North Am.* **18**, 207–212

Redler, I., Mow, V.C., Zimny, M.L. and Mansell, J. (1975). The ultrastructure and biomechanical significance of the tidemark of articular cartilage. *Clin. Orthop.* **112**, 357–362

Reimann, I., Christensen, S.B. and Diemer, N.H. (1982). Observations on reversibility of glycosaminoglycan depletion in articular cartilage. *Clin. Orthop.* **168**, 258–264

Richardson, E.G. (1987). The foot in adolescents and adults. In *Campbell's Operative Orthopaedics* (A.H. Crenshaw, ed.), 7th edn, Chap. 35, pp. 829–988. C.V. Mosby, St. Louis

Robbins, R.H. and Piggot, J. (1960). McMurray osteotomy with a note on the 'regeneration' of articular cartilage. *J. Bone Joint Surg.* **42B**, 480–488

Robinson, D., Halperin, N. and Nevo, Z. (1989). The influence of the host's age on the fate of implants of embryonal chondrocytes into articular surfaces. *Mech. Aging Dev.* **51**, 71–80

Robinson, D., Halperin, N. and Nevo, Z. (1990). The repair of mechanically created defects in articular cartilage using embryonal chondrocytes' containing implants. *Calc. Tissue Int.* **46**

Rubak, J.M. (1982). Reconstruction of articular cartilage defects with free periosteal grafts: an experimental study. *Acta Orthop. Scand.* **53**, 175–180

Rubak, J.M., Poussa, M. and Ritsila, V. (1982). Chondrogenesis in repair of articular cartilage defects by free periosteal grafts in rabbits. *Acta Orthop. Scand.* **53**, 181–186

Salter, R.B., Simmonds, D.F., Malcolm, B.W., Rumble, E.J., MacMichael, D. and Clements, N.D. (1980). The biological effect of continous passive motion on healing of full thickness defects in articular cartilage: an experimental study in the rabbit. *J. Bone Joint Surg.* **62A**, 1232–1251

Salter, R.B., Minster, R.R., Bell, R.S., Wong, D.A. and Bogoch, E.R. (1982). Continuous passive motion and the repair of full thickness articular cartilage defects: a one-year follow-up. *Trans. Orthop Res. Soc.* **7**, 167

Sampath, T.K., DeSimone, D.P. and Reddi, A.H. (1982). Extracellular bone matrix-derived growth factor. *Exp. Cell Res.* **142**, 460–464

Sampath, T.K., Muthukumaran, N. and Reddi, A.H. (1987). Isolation of osteogenin, an extracellular matrix-associated, bone-inductive protein, by heparin affinity chromatography. *Proc. Natl. Acad. Sci. USA* **84**, 7109–7113

Scheck, M. (1970). Roentgenographic changes of the hip joint following extra-articular operations for degenerative arthritis. *J. Bone Joint Surg.* **52A**, 99–104

Schenk, R.K., Spiro, D. and Weiner, J. (1967). Cartilage resorption in the tibial epiphyseal plate of growing rats. *J. Cell Biol.* **34**, 275–291

Schenk, R.K., Weiner, J. and Spiro, D. (1968). Fine structural aspects of vascular invasion of the tibial epiphyseal growth plate of growing rats. *Acta Anat.* **69**, 1–17

Schenk, R.K., Eggli, P.S. and Hunziker, E.B. (1986). Articular cartilage morphology. In *Articular Cartilage Biochemistry* (K. Kuettner, R. Schleyerbach and V.C. Hascall, eds), pp. 3–22. Raven Press, New York

Schultz, R.J., Krishnamurthy, S., Thelmo, W., Rodriguez, J.E. and Harvey, G. (1985). Effects of varying intensities of laser energy on articular cartilage: a preliminary study. *Lasers Surg. Med.* **5**, 577–588

Scott, J.E. (1986). Proteoglycan-collagen interactions, in *Functions of the Proteoglycans, Ciba Foundation Symposium No. 124* pp. 104–124. Wiley, Chichester

Seyedin, S.M., Thompson, A.Y., Bentz, H., Rosen, D.M., McPherson, J.M., Conti, A., Siegel, N.R. Gelluppi, G.R. and Piez, K.A. (1986). Cartilage-inducing factor-A: apparent identity to transforming growth factor-B. *J. Biol. Chem.* **261**, 5693–5695

Sherman, K.P., Douglas, D.L. and Benson, D.A. (1984). Keller's arthroplasty: Is distraction useful? *J. Bone Joint Surg.* **66B**, 765–769

Skoog, T., Ohlsen, L. and Sohn, S.A. (1972). Perichondral potential for cartilagenous regeneration. *Scand. J. Plast. Reconstruct. Surg.* **6**, 123–125

Sokoloff, L. (1987). Osteoarthritis as a remodeling process. *J. Rheumatol.* **14** (Suppl. 14), 7–10

Speer, D.P., Chvapil, M., Volz, R.G. and Holmes, M.D. (1979). Enhancement of healing in osteochondral defects by collagen sponge implants. *Clin. Orthop.* **144**, 326–335

Sporn, M.B., Roberts, A., Wakefield, L.M. and Assoian, R.K. (1986). Transforming growth factor-B: biological function and chemical structure. *Science* **233**, 532–534

Steven, F.S. (1967). The effect of chelating agents on collagen interfibrillar matrix interactions in connective tissue. *Biochim. Biophys. Acta* **140**, 522–528

Steven, F.S. (1976). Preparation of macromolecular collagen. In *Methodology of Connective Tissue Research* (D.A. Hall, ed.), pp. 19–27. Joynson-Bruvvers, Oxford

Steven, F.S. and Thomas, H. (1973). Preparation of insoluble collagen from human cartilage. *Biochem. J.* **135**, 245–247

Stockwell, R.A. (1979). *Biology of Cartilage Cells*, pp. 232–240. Cambridge University Press, Cambridge

Stover, S.S., Pool, R.R. and Fischer, A.T. (1987). Healing in osteochondral defects: a comparison of articulating and non-articulating locations. *Trans. Orthop. Res. Soc.* **12**, 275

Stover, S.M., Pool, R.R. and Lloyd, K.C.K. (1989). Repair of surgically created osteochondral defects with autogenous osteochondral grafts. *Trans. Orthop. Res. Soc.* **14**, 543

Tonna, E.A. and Pentel, L. (1972). Chondrogenic cell formation via osteogenic cell progeny transformation. *Lab. Invest.* **27**, 418–426

Trelstad, R.L. (1982). Multistep assembly of type I collagen fibrils. *Cell* **28**, 197–198

Trelstad, R.L. and Birk, D.E. (1985). The fibroblast in morphogenesis and fibrosis: cell topography and surface-related functions. In *Fibrosis. Ciba Foundation Symposium No. 114*, pp. 4–19. Pitman, London

van der Rest, M. and Mayne, R. (1988). Type IX collagen proteoglycan from cartilage is covalently crosslinked to type II collagen. *J. Biol. Chem.* **263**, 1615–1618

Vaughan, L., Mendler, M., Huber, S., Bruckner, P., Winterhalter, K.H., Irwin, M.I. and Mayne, R. (1988). D-periodic distribution of collagen type IX along cartilage fibrils. *J. Cell Biol.* **106**, 991–997

Veis, A., Bhatnagar, R.S., Shuttleworth, C.A. and Mussell, S. (1970). The solubilization of mature, polymeric collagen fibrils by lyotropic relaxation. *Biochim. Biophys. Acta* **200**, 97–112

Wakitani, S., Kimura, T., Hirooka, A., Ochi, T., Yoneda, M., Yasui, N. and Ono, K. (1988). Repair of rabbits' articular surfaces by allograft of chondrocytes embedded in collagen gels. *Proc. Orthop. Res. Soc.* **13**, 440

Wakitani, S., Kimura, T., Hirooka, A., Ochi, T., Yoneda, M., Natsuo, N., Owaki, H. and Ono, K. (1989). Repair of rabbit articular surfaces with allograft chondrocytes embedded in collagen gel. *J. Bone Joint Surg.* **71B**, 74–80

Weisl, H. (1980) Intertrochanteric osteotomy for osteoarthritis. A long-term follow-up. *J. Bone Joint Surg.* **62B**, 37–42

Whipple, R.R., Gibbs, M.C., Lasi, W.M., Mow, V.C., Mak, A.F. and Wirth, C.R. (1985). Biphasic properties of repaired cartilage at the articular surface. *Trans. Orthop. Res. Soc.* **10**, 340

Widenfalk, B., Engkvist, O., Ohlsen, L. and Segerstrom, K. (1986). Perichondrial arthroplasty using fibrin glue and early mobilization. *Scand. J. Plast. Reconstr. Surg.* **20**, 251–258

Wu, J.-J. and Eyre, D.R. (1984). Cartilage type IX collagen is crosslinked by hydroxypyridinium residues. *Biochem. Biophys. Res. Commun.* **123**, 103–109

Yoshihashi, Y. (1983). Tissue reconstitution by isolated articular chondrocytes *in vitro*. *Nippon Seikeigeka Gakkai Zasshi* **57**, 629–641

Zarnett, R., Delaney, J.P., O'Driscoll, S.W. and Salter, R.B. (1987). Cellular origin and evolution of neochondrogenesis in major full thickness defects of a joint surface treated by free autogenous periosteal grafts and subjected to continous passive motion in rabbits. *Clin. Orthop.* **222**, 267–274

13

OSTEOARTHRITIS: MAN, MODELS AND MOLECULAR MARKERS

COLLATED BY L.S. LOHMANDER

77

Introduction

L.S. LOHMANDER

Osteoarthritis (OA) is a slowly progressive condition of heterogeneous presentation and obscure pathogenesis. It is a major cause of disability and early retirement in the industrialized countries and thus of great socioeconomic significance (Kramer et al., 1983). The criteria for diagnosis and classification on the basis of clinical or radiological presentation of even the overt stages of the disease are under dispute (Kellgren and Lawrence, 1957; Ahlbäck, 1968; Altman et al., 1986, 1987; McAlindon and Dieppe, 1989). It is indeed remarkable, as pointed out by McAlindon and Dieppe (1989), that some sets of criteria neglect to mention damage to the joint cartilage itself, a central issue of the disease. This omission is a reflection of the lack of methods available for monitoring the state of the joint cartilage in vivo. There are no routinely available methods for diagnosing the preclinical stages of the condition and there is no way of determining the ongoing disease activity or the prognosis for the individual patient threatened by joint cartilage destruction. Moreover, we are still faced with uncertainty with regard to the effects of either pharmacological or surgical treatment on the long-term outcome of OA; many of the drugs that are used for the treatment of this condition efficiently reduce pain and inflammation but may in fact have no effect on, or may even accelerate, the continuing tissue destruction. Finally, in the absence of universally applicable criteria for the clinical or radiological diagnosis of OA, epidemiological data are difficult to interpret (Mankin et al., 1986; Bergström et al., 1986; Felson, 1988).

One of the reasons for these difficulties is that we currently lack the means to monitor the in vivo metabolism of joint cartilage in the patient or an experimental model animal. We are thus unable to measure with any precision or specificity the effects of pharmacological or surgical intervention, but have to await for months or years to discover the final outcome of the clinical or experimental trial. The development of new molecular markers and imaging techniques for joint disease that could be used together with improved disease models would be a critical step which should aid us in better ways of defining, monitoring and diagnosing OA. The essays contained in this section describe recent advances in research on experimental and human models and molecular markers in OA research.

MODELS

Direct biochemical investigations of joint cartilage in early OA have so far been possible only with the use of animal models. The anterior cruciate ligament lesion of the dog or rabbit knee has been extensively investigated as a model for posttraumatic OA (Hulth et al., 1970; Pond and Nuki, 1973; McDevitt et al., 1977; Muir, 1977; Carney et al., 1984, 1985) and has demonstrated early increases in cartilage hydration and proteoglycan (PG) synthesis and degradation as well as changes in PG structure. Interestingly, recent work has demonstrated the appearance of novel chondroitin sulfate (CS) epitopes in the early OA cartilage of this model (Caterson et al., 1989a,b; Hardingham et al., 1989; see also Chapter 79). Other frequently used animal models are 'blunt trauma' to the knee of the rabbit or dog (Ficat, 1976; Donohue et al., 1983) or lesion of the meniscus of the rabbit knee (Moskowitz et al., 1979; Hoch et al., 1983) which result in the later development of cartilage changes characterized as OA. Prolonged immobilization of the animal knee joint also leads to degenerative cartilage changes (Eronen et al., 1978; Caterson and Lowther, 1978; Palmoski et al., 1979; Palmoski and Brandt, 1981). Finally, the observation of naturally occurring OA in free-living colonies of Rhesus monkeys may provide another useful model for comparison with the human disease (Chateauvert et al., 1989, 1990; see also Chapter 78). Continued experimentation with these models, using improved methods such as those discussed in this volume will continue to yield important information on basic issues of the OA enigma.

However, a major drawback with these large animal models for OA is that, although they are rapidly progressive by human standards, they still require several months or years to develop fully. This makes it difficult and costly to accomplish experiments directed toward prevention of OA development in these models, as well as very difficult to implement *in vivo* examination of metabolic changes by radioactive tracer labeling of cartilage components. These problems can be surmounted by using one of several strains of laboratory mouse which spontaneously develop OA, such as the C57 Black or STR/ORT mouse (Sokoloff, 1956; Walton, 1979). Tracer experiments and intervention trials are more easily done with these models than with larger animals.

It should be noted that one of the animal OA models currently used should be expected to duplicate precisely all the aspects of the human disease. However, the purpose of the model is not to mirror the complete picture but to isolate only one or a few facets of a complex disease, so that these aspects may be manipulated and analyzed more easily. In this context, it may also be fruitful to consider the possibility of using subgroups of the heterogeneous human OA population as models which can be more easily monitored and interpreted than the whole group (Lohmander, 1988). One such human subgroup is the posttraumatic knee OA occurring after lesions of the menisci or cruciate ligaments with ensuing mechanical instability of the joint (McDaniel and Dameron, 1980; Doherty et al., 1983; Funk, 1983; Holden et al., 1988; Graham and Fairclough, 1988; Kannus and Järvinen, 1988; Odenbring et al., 1989; Morrey, 1989). Another interesting model is the knee OA resulting from malaligned fractures of the femur or tibia (Kettelkamp et al., 1988). These human models have the advantage that the time of the initiating trauma is known, the initiating lesion can be precisely mapped by magnetic resonance imaging (MRI), radiography and arthroscopy and, consequently, the patients can be followed from the very earliest stages of the disease. Such groups of patients may be studied both retrospectively and prospectively (Lohmander et al., 1989). Difficulties certainly may arise in obtaining samples of blood, joint fluid or joint cartilage from patients and the prospective studies require a high degree of perseverance. However, human models are greatly needed to compared with and validate the animal data; they should, after all, be the best models for the human OA. It also should be pointed out that investigation of the early stages of the disease, as opposed to advanced stages, will not be confounded by secondary cascade phenomena likely to occur later in the development of OA. Finally, any therapeutic strategy aimed at limiting cartilage damage in OA is most likely to be successful in the early phase of the disease.

MARKERS

As explained, we currently lack routinely applicable methods to monitor the *in vivo* metabolism of normal or diseased joint cartilage in the patient or experimental animal. One possible solution to this difficulty would be to utilize the degradation products of joint cartilage matrix as markers of turnover activity.

A number of cartilage matrix components have been identified and characterized and immunoassays are available for several of them (Heinegård and Oldberg, 1989). However, it should be remembered that probably only about 1/10 of the cartilage mass of the adult is present in the joint, the majority of the remainder in the costal, discs and tracheobronchial tissues. A further complication is presented by the fact that no matrix component specific for the cartilage in joints has been identified with certainty, as differentiated from the extraarticular cartilage.

Any fragment of a joint cartilage matrix component released from the tissue would be expected to appear first in the synovial fluid and be eliminated from this compartment mainly via the lymphatic drainage. Some fragments will be eliminated by the lymph nodes, while the surviving fragments would appear in the blood stream and probably be eliminated largely by the liver (Fig. 77.1). The concentration of fragments in the synovial fluid will therefore depend on both the rate of release from the cartilage and the rate of elimination from the joint space (see Chapter 82). The half-life for elimination of PG fragments from the normal joint has been estimated to be about 8–12 h in the rabbit (Page-Thomas *et al.*, 1987), but may well vary with the disease activity in the joint (Wallis *et al.*, 1987).

Once the molecular fragments are released to the circulation, the remaining half-life is short and will probably vary with the structural characteristics of the fragment. For example, hyaluronan (HA) in joint fluid is eliminated

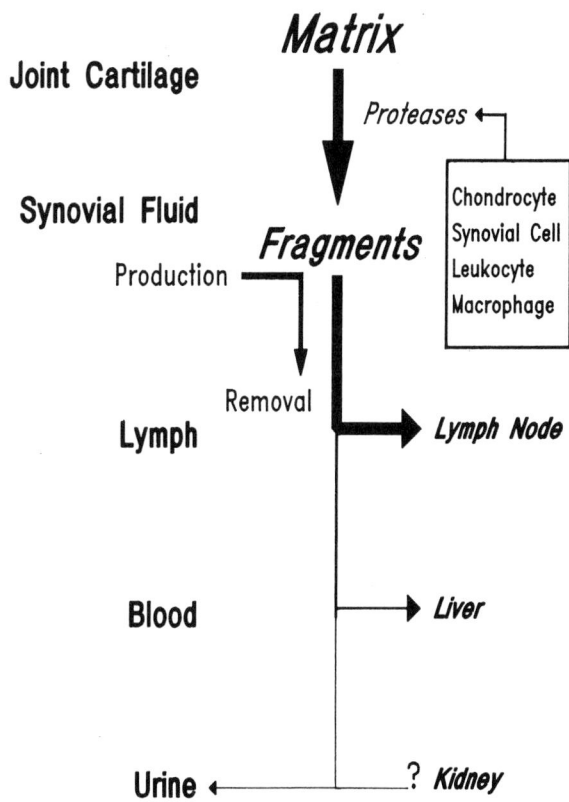

Figure 77.1 Cartilage marker turnover in joint fluid and serum.

efficiently in the nearby lymph nodes and the half-life in the blood circulation for the surviving molecules is a few minutes long (Fraser *et al.*, 1984, 1988). Similarly, the half-life of keratan sulfate (KS) bearing PG fragments in the blood circulation is short and varies from 6 to 50 min and with the structure of the fragment (Maldonado *et al.*, 1989). The influence of liver or kidney disease on the elimination rates for cartilage matrix components is as yet undetermined, but a marked influence on HA levels in the circulation has been observed in patients with, e.g., liver cirrhosis (Engström-Laurent and Laurent, 1989).

Some molecular fragments apparently escape uptake and metabolism and are excreted in the urine, for example, HA, KS and collagen cross-links. Collagen cross-links are resistant to endogeneous metabolic breakdown and are concentrated in the urine, making them attractive candidates as markers of bone, cartilage and connective-tissue turnover (Robins et al., 1986; Eyre et al., 1988; Seibel et al., 1989; Black et al., 1988, 1989; see also Chapter 81). The possibility of developing specific and sensitive immunoassays to cross-links in peptide linkage is intriguing, since this would facilitate the monitoring of turnover of cartilage-specific collagens, including the 'minor' species in joint cartilage, such as type IX collagen.

In general, the concentration of matrix fragments released from the joint cartilage should be expected to be highest in joint fluid and lower in serum and urine, with the exception noted above. Furthermore, some fragments may be eliminated selectively and rapidly by the lymph nodes or liver and, therefore, be very difficult to detect in the blood stream, while other fragments may still be present in serum but may lose their antigenicity by metabolic action. The ratios among different types of markers therefore should not be expected to be the same in joint fluid and serum, but may vary independently at different stages of the disease.

The markers present in joint fluid will be representative of the cartilage-turnover activity within that single joint, while markers present in serum or urine will represent an integrated measure of the turnover activity in all joints and possibly all body cartilage, whether affected by disease or not. The presence of KS epitope in serum is perhaps one example of a cartilage marker which may serve as an indicator of general body cartilage metabolism, which in turn may be correlated to the development of a subgroup of OA (Sweet et al., 1988; see also Chapter 80).

It may be argued that, if at all possible, initial marker studies in joint cartilage diseases should be made at the joint fluid level. When promising disease markers have been identified at this source, serum samples taken at the same time from the same patients should be investigated and compared with synovial-fluid data.

We take it for granted that animals in experimental work are carefully characterized with regard to age, sex, disease, time after surgical or pharmacological intervention, treatment, etc. We should apply no less rigorous standards when investigating patient groups; the criteria for diagnosis should be defined, the stage of the condition should be characterized by clinical and/or radiological parameters, the length of history, the treatment, etc., must be carefully recorded to facilitate meaningful interpretations of marker determinations. A final example will serve to underscore the importance of careful staging of the joint condition in OA studies: the joint fluid concentration of cartilage PG epitope decreases with an increasing degree of joint cartilage destruction as staged by arthroscopy and radiology (Lohmander et al., 1990).

CONCLUSIONS

Future investigations on molecular markers for OA ideally should be interdisciplinary in that laboratory marker data should be correlated carefully with state-of-the-art imaging data, joint biomechanical data and clinical outcome. Marker analysis in each patient series should include markers in joint fluid, serum and urine. Currently, we are able to assay, e.g., different PG epitopes in joint fluid and serum (Carroll, 1987; Witter et al., 1987; Sweet et al., 1988; Ratcliffe et al., 1988; Lohmander et al., 1989) and collagen cross-links in urine (Seibel et al., 1989). With the very rapid current developments in marker assay technology (Caterson et al., 1989b), the establishment of collections of joint fluid, serum and urine samples from carefully characterized series of patients with joint disease at different stages would be of significant value by allowing correlation between present and future markers without the need to procure new series of patients.

ACKNOWLEDGMENTS

This work was supported by the Swedish Medical Research Council, the King Gustaf V 80th Birthday Fund, the Ax:son Johnson Foundation, and the Medical Faculty of Lund University.

78

Studies of naturally occurring degenerative arthritis in rhesus macaques as a model for degenerative arthritis in man

K.P.H. PRITZKER, J. CHATEAUVERT, M.D. GRYNPAS and M.J. KESSLER

Degenerative arthritis, principally osteoarthritis (OA) and the crystal associated arthropathies, particularly calcium pyrophosphate dihydrate (CPPD) crystal deposition disease, are amongst the major sources of pain, reduced joint mobility and general musculoskeletal disability in the ageing human population. Despite the importance of these two diseases, little is known about their pathogenesis and the specific interactions of these diseases with ageing processes in articular cartilage and subjacent bone. Although there are many models to study the reaction of cartilage to injury, some of them, most notably the model of anterior cruciate ligament transection in the dog, have been studied extensively (Pond and Nuki, 1973; Muir, 1986). An understanding of the processes that lead to degenerative arthritis and of the systemic factors that regulate these processes has not yet been developed in part because of the lack of a suitable experimental model for these diseases. Previous spontaneous models, such as the C57 B1 mouse or spontaneous occurrence of degenerative arthritis in large animals, have foundered because of limitations of the amount of tissue available, differences in metabolism from humans or limited availability of the animals (Moskowitz, 1984).

DEVELOPMENT OF THE MODEL

The rhesus macaque colony at the Caribbean Primate Research Center was established on Cayo Santiago in 1938. All animals on the island are descendants of the original 409 monkeys which were released onto Cayo Santiago at that time. Since 1956, the matrilineage of all animals in this population, as well as many other demographic and sociometric factors, have been analyzed. These animals are free ranging, feed on commercial chow of defined composition and are observed daily by primatologists. As the population grew, the animals were culled and a colony composed of social group M was established at a 2 acre hill corral in the Sebana Seca facility of the Primate Center. Further, the bones are conserved post mortem and stored in osteological collections for further studies. Recognition by Dr Matt Kessler that this animal population could be afflicted by CPPD arthropathy similar to that described in the Barbary Ape by Kandel et al. (1983) led to a pilot study of this animal population. Of the first 30 animals examined, calcium pyrophosphate dihydrate arthropathy was found in the articular cartilage of the knee, menisci and intervertebral discs of four animals, three of which were older than 20 years. At the same time, in an additional six animals histological changes of OA characterized by cartilage fibrillation, erosion and osteophyte formation were found (Renlund et al., 1986). Subsequent studies have demonstrated that a degenerative arthritis similar to OA in man is common in these animals, that onset of the disease occurs with maturation and that the histological and biochemical features are similar to those observed in man (Chateauvert et al., 1989, 1990).

ADVANTAGES OF THE RHESUS MACAQUE MODEL

The advantages of this model for the study of degenerative arthritis are:

(i) Common forms of degenerative arthropathies in ageing humans. OA and CPPD crystal arthropathy occur with a high frequency in this population. The population is sufficiently large (*c.* 2000 animals) that population studies can be performed. Of equal importance, there is a subpopulation of animals which is spared this disease so that a control population is available. The animals are free ranging, the environment is well controlled and the animals are observed regularly thereby facilitating accurate observations.
(ii) Matrilineage of these animals is known. It is becoming feasible to determine genetics of these animals, thereby permitting gene-linkage studies.
(iii) The ageing process in rhesus macaques is markedly accelerated (life span 15–25 years) compared with man, thereby facilitating studies on ageing and diseases associated with ageing.
(iv) Preliminary studies have demonstrated that the disease processes appear histologically and biochemically similar to those in man. In particular, the onset of the disease appears at a comparable age to that of man. Similar joints are involved in the case of the OA; this is characterized by fibrillation, erosion, chondrocyte proliferation and osteocyte formation similar to the human disease.
(v) The knee joint of these animals is sufficiently large to permit arthroscopic studies. Therefore, longitudinal studies of cartilage and synovial fluid constituents are feasible.

APPLICATION OF THE MODEL

The model has the following applications:

(i) Identification of the sequence of biochemical and histological changes of arthritis in this animal population.
(ii) Identification of systemic factors which contribute to the pathogenesis of the disease.
(iii) Possible identification of systemic markers for the onset and progression of the disease.
(iv) Identification of clinical subsets of the arthritic disease which may be reflected in different histological and biochemical patterns.
(v) In the future, the model may be useful for studying the effects of therapeutic or chemopreventive drugs on these arthritic-disease processes.

79

Proteoglycan components in synovial fluid as markers of experimental and natural joint disease

TIMOTHY E. HARDINGHAM

The appreciation that degenerative joint diseases such as osteoarthritis (OA) may involve active cellular processes in joint tissues rather than arising merely as the passive consequence of wear and tear has provided the impetus for the search for markers of the processes that are involved, such as those leading to cartilage damage and loss (Hascall and Glant, 1987; Lohmander, 1988).

Articular cartilage is a specialized tissue with an important biomechanical function and it is the proteoglycans (PGs) that are responsible for its ability to withstand compressive loading. PGs are present at high concentration (up to 100 mg g^{-1}; see Chapter 53) in the tissue and are constantly turned over, even in mature cartilage. The chondrocytes continuously synthesize and secrete PGs into the matrix and also control extracellular processes of proteolytic degradation. Normal turnover thus results in the slow release of partially degraded PGs from articular cartilage into synovial fluid (Hardingham, 1988).

When articular cartilage is maintained in explant culture, PG turnover continues and the degraded components are released into the culture medium. The rate of matrix degradation has been reported to be increased greatly by agents such as interleukin-1 (IL-1) which cause a rapid depletion of the cartilage content of PGs (see Chapter 29). The size of PGs released from normal cartilage showed that only limited degradation occurs and, although in the presence of IL-1 the average size of fragments was smaller, the pattern of degradation was similar and far from complete (Ratcliffe *et al.*, 1986). All the glycosaminoglycans (GAGs) released into the culture medium were thus attached to large PG fragments. Link protein was also released and the binding region released was free of PG. The results showed that, although matrix degradation involved proteolytic activity, the extent of PG cleavage was small and many of its protein structural features were retained in the released products. The results from explant cultures thus suggest that *in vivo* articular cartilage will release large PG components into synovial fluid and this has been confirmed by analysis of synovial fluid (Witter *et al.*, 1987; Carroll, 1987). Investigation *in vivo* of a model of inflammatory joint disease, antigen-induced arthritis in the rabbit, showed a good correlation between the depletion of PG content in articular cartilage and its appearance in synovial fluid (Pettipher *et al.*, 1989). Following the intraarticular challenge with the antigen, ovalbumin, there was 50% loss of PG over 2–4 days and a transient rise in PG concentration in synovial fluid, but this had returned to normal by 7–14 days even though the tissue content remained low. An elevated PG level in synovial fluid thus accompanied the acute stage of PG loss but did not remain high, even though the cartilage content of PG continued to be low over several weeks.

Investigation of a model of noninflammatory joint disease showed rather different results. In the canine model of experimental OA in which laxity of the joint is created by section of the anterior cruciate ligament, there are progressive changes in the cartilage over several months that resemble those of early natural OA (McDevitt *et al.*, 1977; Carney *et al.*, 1984, 1985). There is an increase in cartilage water content, a sustained increase in the biosynthesis and turnover of PGs and some induction of chondrocyte cell division. There is not, however, any net loss of cartilage PG and thus no acute stage of cartilage depletion. Analysis of synovial fluid showed the PG components to be at higher concentration in that from the operated joint compared with the contralateral control (Ratcliffe *et al.*, 1989). Link protein, as well as binding region, keratan sulfate (KS) epitope and total GAGs were all constantly raised, although there was considerable variation amongst animals.

Analysis of the synovial fluid from patients with clinically defined joint diseases showed some interesting parallels between the clinical and experimental studies (Ratcliffe *et al.*, 1988). Those patients in which the synovial fluid contained greatly elevated levels of PGs were those with the most acute joint diseases, pseudogout and Reiters syndrome; whereas amongst more chronic joint diseases, rheumatoid arthritis and OA, the levels were lower and did not fall into distinct groups. These results suggest that, without contralateral control synovial fluid for comparison, it is more difficult to detect elevated levels in patients with chronic joint conditions. This may be because the rise in levels is not large compared with the range of variation amongst patients. However, this problem may be minimized by sequential measurements on patients, which may detect periods of greater loss and may be useful in monitoring treatment for its effect on articular cartilage.

The techniques used for the determination of PGs in synovial fluid in these studies have measured total sulfated GAG chains by a dye-binding assay, or KS by radioimmunoassay (Ratcliffe et al., 1988). There was found to be reasonable agreement between the two assays, although it is known that the KS epitope does vary in abundance in KS from different sources (Caterson et al., 1989a). However, both methods are aimed at detecting the increased release of normal PGs as a result of turnover or degradation in cartilage. An alternative approach is now possible as some structural differences in the PGs in experimental OA cartilage have been detected that are recognized by monoclonal antibodies (Caterson et al., 1989b; Hardingham et al., 1989). The use of these antibodies may, therefore, permit more sensitive detection of the processes involved.

The basis of the structural changes detected is in the chondroitin sulfate (CS) chains of the large aggregating PG. Previous work had established that in experimental canine osteoarthritis the PGs were synthesized at an increased rate and their ability to aggregate was undiminished (McDevitt et al., 1977). A slight increase in length of CS chains was noted and a lower KS content (Carney et al., 1984, 1985). However, using monoclonal antibodies, specific structural changes in CS chains have been detected in PGs from all regions of articular cartilage in operated joints. The change in structure has been detected with three different monoclonal antibodies and it is most likely that it reflects a different pattern of sulfation within the chain and at its nonreducing terminal end.

The specificity of one of the monoclonal antibodies used, 3B3, has been reported previously (see Chapter 41; see also Caterson et al., 1989b). It recognizes a terminal chain structure with a glucuronate residue adjacent to a 6-sulfated N-acetyl galactosamine. This appears to be uncommon at the end of native CS chains in mature cartilage, but increases in cartilage from operated joints. It may reflect a change in chain termination that accompanies the high rate of synthesis in the operated tissue. The monoclonal antibodies 7D4 and 6C3 do not appear to recognize terminal chain structures, but their epitopes are variably expressed in CS from different sources and probably consist of chain sequences with particular patterns of sulfation involving 4-, 6- or non-sulfated disaccharides and possibly some more heavily sulfated disaccharide residues. The antigen used for their preparation was the PG from chicken bone marrow, which is highly sulfated and has a high content of 7D4 and 6C3 epitopes. These epitopes are also abundant in shark cartilage CS.

The differences in structure were detected by comparing immunoblots of PGs electrophoretically separated on composite agarose–polyacrylamide gels (Hardingham et al., 1989). The results showed increased expression of epitopes in all regions of joint cartilage and at all depths from the surface and, although the absolute intensity varied, there was a consistent increase in operated compared with contralateral control in all 23 animals tested. With cartilage explants maintained in culture, the epitopes were detected in PGs released into synovial fluid. It thus seems possible that with suitable assays they can be determined in synovial fluid.

Preliminary investigation of PGs from osteoarthritic and normal human articular cartilage showed a general low expression of 3B3 epitope in the older age group as a whole (over 60 years), but the majority of osteoarthritic specimens of similar age contained an increased abundance of the epitope. Detecting changes in these CS structures in PGs released into synovial fluid may, therefore, offer a method for identifying adaptive processes in cartilage that accompany joint disease.

80

Measurement of serum keratan sulfate provides important information about the metabolism of cartilage proteoglycans *in vivo*

EUGENE J.-M.A. THONAR, JAMES WILLIAMS, MARY ELLEN LENZ,
M. BARRY SWEET, LORI OTTEN, GILES CAMPION, THOMAS J. SCHNITZER
and KLAUS E. KUETTNER

The majority of newly-synthesized cartilage proteoglycans (PGs) contain a core protein to which are covalently attached numerous chains of chondroitin sulfate, keratan sulfate (KS) and O-linked as well as N-linked oligosaccharides (Lohmander, 1988). Many PG monomers interact extracellularly with molecules of link protein and a single strand of hyaluronan (HA) to form an aggregate which because of its size becomes firmly entrapped in the insoluble collagenous fiber network (e.g. Fessler, 1960; Lohmander, 1988). When the core protein of a PG molecule is cleaved by a proteolytic enzyme derived from chondrocytes during normal turnover, the PG fragments produced are rapidly lost from the tissue and appear in the body fluids where they may be further degraded before being eliminated from the circulation via the liver and kidneys (Sweet et al., 1988).

Since almost all the KS in the human body is present in the PGs of hyaline, fibrous and elastic cartilages (Thonar et al., 1988), measurement of KS in body fluids provides important information about the catabolism of cartilage PGs. We have developed a sensitive enzyme-linked immunosorbent assay (ELISA) inhibition assay to quantify KS on PG fragments present in small amounts in the circulation (Thonar et al., 1985, 1986; Williams et al., 1988). The assay, which is described in Chapter 43 makes use of a monoclonal antibody (1/20/5-D-4 or ET-4-A-4) specific for a sulfated carbohydrate moiety present only on the longest KS chains (Mehmet et al., 1986; Thonar et al., 1986). It is important to note that because KS in the serum samples and the KS standard may have different ratios of antigenic KS/total mass KS, the concentration of KS in the samples is expressed in terms of equivalents of the KS standard purified from pig costal cartilage. KS-bearing fragments in human blood have relatively long half-lives (50 min) (Maldonado et al., 1989) and are small, consisting of a short peptide to which are attached one or a few KS chains (Thonar et al., 1985).

The concentration of serum KS varies predictably with age (Thonar et al., 1988). In children, levels of KS correlate with rate of growth (Pachman et al., 1987; Thonar et al., 1988). For example, children who are growth-hormone deficient have lower than normal levels of KS in serum, indicating slow cartilage metabolism and impaired growth (Pachman et al., 1987). Recently, we have observed that administration of growth hormone to these children causes a marked rise in levels of serum KS in addition to the expected rise in serum insulin-like growth factor-1 (IGF-1) levels and the concomitant increase in the rate of growth (Pachman et al., 1987). In adults, levels also vary from individual to individual, presumably reflecting differences in rates of cartilage PG metabolism (Thonar et al., 1985; Sweet et al., 1988). However, it is possible that differences in the ratio of antigenic KS/total mass of KS or in the pathway or rate of elimination of KS-bearing fragments also contribute to the exhibited differences in serum levels.

Levels of serum KS do not fluctuate diurnally (Block et al., 1989) and are relatively stable over long periods of time (Campion et al., 1989a). This makes it possible to study the effect of various factors on the rate of catabolism of cartilage PGs. We have shown already that levels in normal adults are not affected by strenuous exercise, i.e. running a marathon (M.B.E. Sweet and E. Thonar, unpublished results). Furthermore, levels in patients with osteoarthritis (OA) do not change significantly following treatment with some nonsteroidal antiinflammatory agents (Campion et al., 1989b). In contrast, levels fall rapidly and remain depressed for several weeks following treatment of asthma patients with oral prednisone for 4 days (Campion et al., 1989b), strongly suggesting that this drug suppresses the rate of catabolism of cartilage PG during normal turnover.

Several other studies have provided support for the contention that levels of serum KS provide a measure of the rate of catabolism of cartilage PGs. For example, the injection of chymopapain in a single joint or intervertebral disc in man (Block et al., 1989), rabbit (Williams et al., 1988) or dog (Oegema et al., 1988) causes a 3–5 fold rise in the level of serum KS. These findings indicate that measurement of the concentration of PG derived fragments in blood can be used to monitor marked acute degradation of cartilage PGs in individual joints. Interestingly, levels return to preinjection values during the successful replenishment of PGs in the cartilage matrix (Williams et al., 1988). This supports the contentions that: (i) changes in levels of serum KS do not always reflect changes in rates of synthesis; and (ii) newly synthesized PGs are effectively incorporated and retained in the matrix until they are degraded by proteolytic enzymes during normal turnover or by pathologic processes which are a feature of diseases such as osteoarthritis and rheumatoid arthritis. Measurements of serum KS can, however, provide indirect but valuable information about the rate of anabolism of cartilage PGs in vivo. For example, the increase in the level of serum KS following transection of the anterior cruciate ligament in the dog is not accompanied by a concomitant loss in PG content of the cartilages in the affected joint, suggesting that the increase in PG catabolism is balanced by an increase in anabolism (Brandt and Thonar, 1989). In this animal model, therefore, this serum marker is a useful indicator not only of changes in the rate of catabolism of cartilage PGs but also of alterations in the rate of synthesis.

The significance of the original observation (Thonar et al., 1985) that patients with OA have elevated levels of serum KS (Table 80.1) was at first unclear. Because OA is heterogeneous in regard to etiology, severity of degenerative changes and number of joints involved, some subsequent studies (Sweet et al., 1988; Campion et al., 1989a) focused on more homogeneous patient subpopulations. In patients with hypertrophic OA, a definite subset of OA characterized by joint narrowing, subchondral sclerosis and marginal osteophyte formation, serum levels were considerably higher in 31 patients with this form of OA than in 41 adults without joint disease (Sweet et al., 1988) (Table 80.1). Of these patients 77% had serum levels which were more than one standard deviation above the mean of the control group, but the corresponding figure for the control group was 12%. Importantly, there was a significant linear relationship between serum levels and joint score ($r = 0.370$, $p = 0.041$), although the relationship was not very strong since only 13.7% of the variations in KS was the result of a variation in joint score. The higher levels did not correlate well with the amount of cartilage destruction in these individuals. This is not surprising since KS-bearing fragments in serum also originate from apparently normal cartilages; OA cartilages probably only represent a small fraction of the total amount of cartilage in the human body.

The findings from our most recent studies are consistent with the contention that individuals with polyarticular OA have elevated rates of cartilage PG metabolism. We have hypothesized that the cartilages of young normal adults with high levels

Table 80.1 Serum levels (mean ± SD) of KS in different groups of patients with osteoarthritis (OA) and controls

	N	Mean age (years)	KS (ng ml^{-1})
Osteoarthritis			
Primary OA (no other selection factor) (Thonar et al., 1985)	24	65	357 ± 73
Primary OA (no other selection factor) (Thonar et al., 1987)	43	66	381 ± 107
Hypertrophic OA of the hip (Sweet et al., 1988)	31	71	475 ± 178
Osteoarthritis of the knee (Campion et al., 1989a)	125	65	393 ± 123
Control groups			
Hospital inpatient population (no evidence of joint disease) (Thonar et al., 1985)	136	60	268 ± 133
Hospital outpatient population (no evidence of joint disease) (Sweet et al., 1988)	42	62	261 ± 51
Normal volunteers (no evidence of joint disease) (Thonar et al., 1985, 1987))	45	30	251 ± 78

of serum KS become more rapidly enriched in nonfunctional GAG-poor PG fragments which have been found to accumulate with age in the articular cartilage matrix (Roughley et al., 1986; Bayliss et al., 1989). These fragments, which have been shown to represent the HA-binding region of the PG molecules (Roughley et al., 1986; Bayliss et al., 1989) may be bound to HA, thereby interfering with aggregate formation and the orderly organization of newly synthesized PG in the cartilage matrix. In patients with high rates of metabolism, this excessive accumulation could cause with time the destabilization and failure of the cartilage matrix in load-bearing regions. Future studies should help address the contention that high rates of cartilage PG turnover in younger adults without any evidence of clinical signs of osteoarthritis predispose to the development of polyarticular degenerative changes.

ACKNOWLEDGMENTS

This work was supported in part by the William Noble Lane Foundation and by grants AG-04736 and 1-P50-AR-39239 from the National Institutes of Health.

81

Collagen markers in urine in human arthritis

SIMON P. ROBINS, MARKUS J. SEIBEL and ALISON M. McLAREN

INTRODUCTION

For many years hydroxyproline measurements have been the most widely used urinary marker of collagen degradation and these methods have been applied to arthritic disease to give an indication primarily of bone involvement (Mbuyi et al., 1982). As approximately 90% of the hydroxyproline released from collagen is metabolized, this marker lacks sensitivity and the presence of hydroxyproline in other proteins, notably the complement component C1q which has a high turnover rate, contributes to the poor selectivity of the method (Robins, 1982b). The use of hydroxylysine glycosides as indices of collagen metabolism has been shown to have some advantages in sensitivity and tissue specificity (Krane et al., 1977) and recent experiments have centered on the use of the monosaccharide galactosylhydroxylysine as a marker for bone resorption (Moro et al., 1988).

As both hydroxylation and glycosylation of collagen are intracellular modifications, the realization that considerable proportions of collagen are degraded intracellularly (Bienkowski et al., 1978) provided additional complications, since both types of marker would reflect degradation at all stages of the extensive processing of newly synthesized collagen. These considerations led to the development of methods based on the cross-linking compounds (Fig. 81.1) pyridinoline (Pyd) and deoxypyridinoline (Dpd), formed during maturation of collagen, as potential markers only of mature, insoluble collagen degradation.

Pyridinoline, initially discovered by Fujimoto et al. (1978), is formed by maturation of the bifunctional cross-link that is the initial product of the lysyl oxidase mediated reaction scheme (Robins, 1988). The component is the predominant cross-link of cartilage but is also present in several other tissues. Deoxypyridinoline, formed by reaction of a lysyl rather than a hydroxy-lysyl residue (Ogawa et al., 1982), appears to be specifically located in bone collagen (Eyre et al., 1984; Robins and Duncan, 1987). Both cross-links are totally absent from normal skin.

Following identification of Pyd and its precursor in urine (Gunja-Smith and Boucek, 1981), an immunoassay for pyridinoline was developed (Robins, 1982b) and its application to arthritic disease showed significantly increased concentrations of the cross-link in urine compared with a control group (Robins et al., 1986).

METHOD DEVELOPMENT

The initial polyclonal antibody preparation against Pyd showed no cross-reactivity with Dpd and, in order to realize the potential tissue specificity of measuring both markers, a high-performance liquid chromatography (HPLC) technique for quantifying both cross-links in urine was developed (Black et al., 1988). These techniques have now been applied to osteoarthritis (OA) and to other arthritis diseases, but evaluation of these methods necessarily involves obtaining extensive background information on normal values and variations. In particular, cross-link concentrations

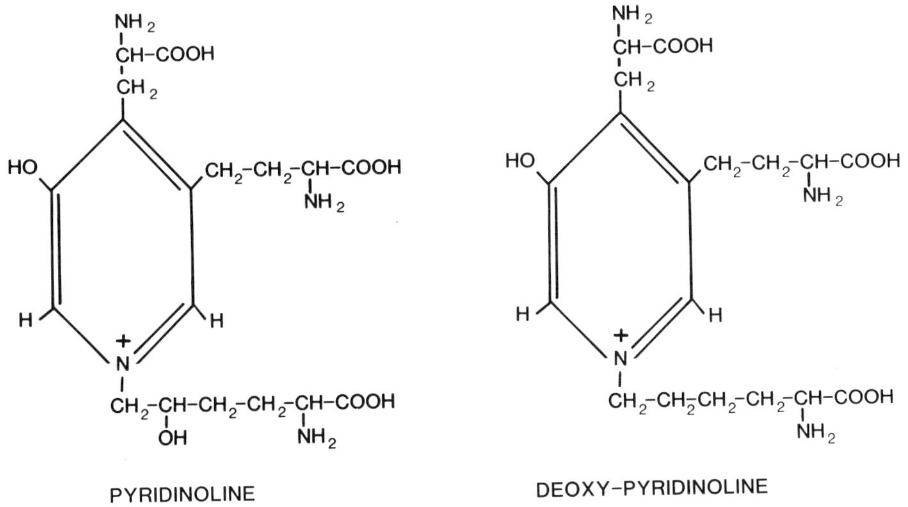

Figure 81.1 Structure of the pyridinium cross-links.

are generally expressed relative to urinary creatinine and may, therefore, be subject to alterations in renal function.

EFFECTS OF PHYSIOLOGICAL VARIABLES ON CROSS-LINK EXCRETION

Age and sex

In a series of 118 healthy individuals aged between 22 and 74 years, values for Pyd and Dpd (nmol/mmol creatinine; mean ± SD) were 25.2 ± 11.9 and 7.2 ± 3.8, respectively. Overall, there were no sex differences and no consistent age-related changes, although recent studies have shown that for more restricted groups of volunteers some statistically significant changes emerge. Thus, there was a 10% increase in the concentrations of both cross-links (relative to creatinine) in male athletes over the age range 25–40 years. A similar increase was noted in males aged 63–87 years, but this trend was not significant for a similarly aged female group. Further studies of control individuals are in progress, particularly for women of perimenopausal age, to assess the contribution of changes in bone metabolism.

Day-to-day and diurnal variations

Cross-link measurements relative to creatinine for urine samples collected daily over a 3-week period in three postmenopausal women showed a variation of about 15% (Fig. 81.2). The total Pyd output level over this period showed a very similar pattern (Fig. 81.2), indicating that changes in creatinine contribute very little to the overall variation.

Diurnal variations in pyridinium cross-link excretion are slight and measurements relative to creatinine in both groups of normal individuals and in OA patients showed less than 10% difference between early-morning and late-afternoon samples. Exercise appears also to have little effect on cross-link excretion: in a group of healthy male volunteers the urinary concentrations of cross-links were unaffected by acute severe strenuous exercise (30 min at 60% of maximal VO_2) and there was no correlation between the level of athletic training and cross-link excretion. In studies of arthritic diseases, cross-link excretion in an age-matched control group was not significantly different from that for a similar group of hospitalized patients without arthritis, although the latter were not completely restricted to bed without exercise (Robins et al., 1986).

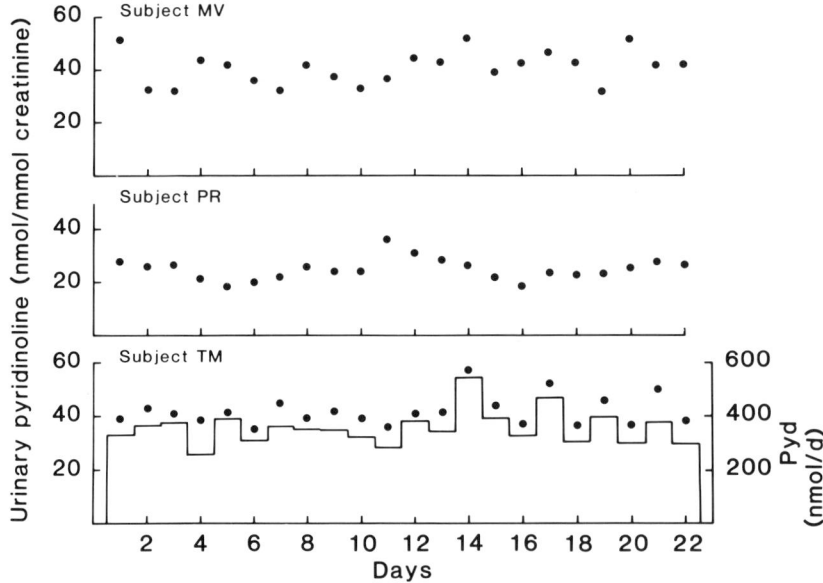

Figure 81.2 Day-to-day variations in pyridinoline excretion. The points show daily Pyd/Cr values for three healthy postmenopausal volunteers over a 3-week period. The lines for subject TM indicate the total daily Pyd output.

Renal function

The effects of renal impairment on cross-link excretion was investigated initially by measuring cross-link excretion in a series of 37 kidney transplant patients having no signs of arthritis but with a wide range of glomerular filtration rates (GFR); there was no correlation between Pyd excretion and GRF. For a group of 88 patients with OA and rheumatoid arthritis (RA), some of whom were receiving drug therapy, there was no correlation between the Pyd : creatinine ratio and creatinine clearance values (Fig. 81.3).

This same group of patients also showed no correlation between the Pyd : creatinine ratio and the marker of renal tubular damage, N-acetylglucosaminidase (Fig. 81.3). These results show, therefore, that renal impairment, either at the glomerular or tubular level, has little effect on pyridinoline excretion.

CROSS-LINK EXCRETION IN OA

Although previous studies showed elevated urinary Pyd concentrations in OA, a more detailed study of both pyridinium cross-links has recently been reported (Seibel et al., 1989). The results for 45 OA patients are shown in Fig. 81.4 in comparison with 41 RA patients, together with values for 118 healthy controls.

The concentrations of both Pyd and Dpd were significantly increased relative to the controls for the groups as a whole: values for Pyd and Dpd exceeded the upper limit of normal (+ 2 SD) in 41% and 50% of cases, respectively. In any study of the efficacy of markers in reflecting the clinical condition, careful description of the patient groups is clearly vital and more extensive details of these patients have been given (Seibel et al., 1989). It was clear, however, that patients presenting with polyarticular and advanced degenerative joint

In comparison with OA patients, those with RA similarly had increased Dpd values, but significantly increased ($p < 0.01$) Pyd excretion (Fig. 81.4).

TISSUE OF ORIGIN OF THE CROSS-LINKS

In interpreting the changes in values for cross-link excretion, elucidating the tissue of origin of the cross-links is clearly an important factor. As Dpd is only present in significant quantities in bone collagen, the increases in this component in urine in OA reflect increases in bone resorption and, since the amounts of this cross-link are correlated with a radiological index of joint destruction, it is likely that a large proportion of the increased Dpd emanates from increased bone turnover associated with the joint lesions. It is noteworthy, however, that urinary Pyd also increases in the same proportion and that the urinary Pyd : Dpd ratio in both the OA group and the healthy control group was within the range of 3–4 found in normal human bone, irrespective of age (Eyre *et al.*, 1988). These facts suggest that in normal individuals and in the OA patients studied the urinary excretion of both Pyd and Dpd cross-links were derived predominantly from bone collagen. This interpretation is strengthened by the dramatic increases in cross-link excretion in a wide range of metabolic bone diseases (Robins *et al.*, 1989).

The origin of the relative increase in Pyd in RA is unclear. This cross-link is present in a higher concentration in cartilage than in any other tissue and cartilage erosion could contribute to the increased amounts appearing in the urine. Another possibility is an increased turnover of synovial tissue, as collagen from this source has recently been shown to contain appreciable amounts of Pyd (S.P. Robins and M.J. Seibel, unpublished results).

In conclusion, measurements of the pyridinium cross-links in urine provide markers primarily of bone degradation. In OA, the concentrations of the cross-links are related to severity of the disease and may provide useful markers for monitoring

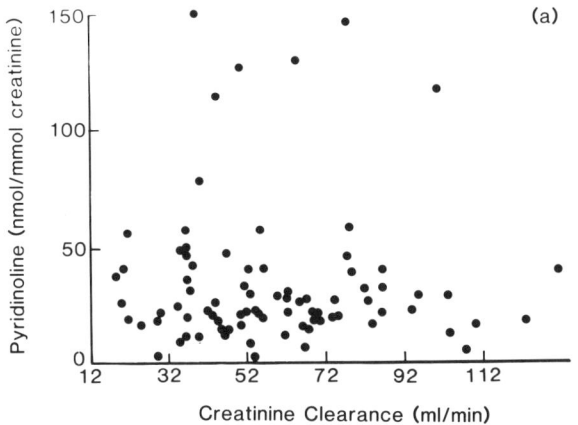

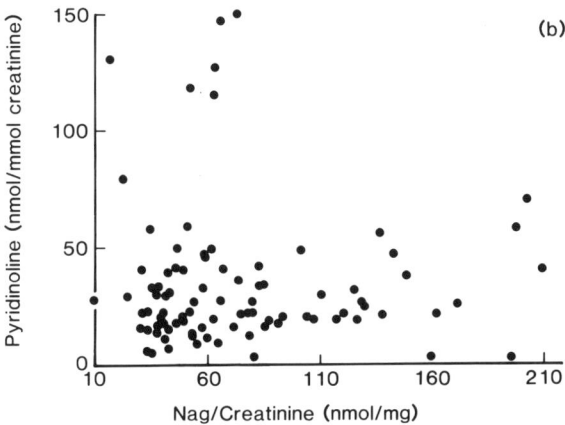

Figure 81.3 Relationships between pyridinoline excretion and renal function. The results for OA and RA patients show a lack of significant correlation between Pyd excretion and either (a) creatinine clearance of (b) N-acetylglucosaminidase.

disease (group OA1, Fig. 81.4) showed significantly higher urinary Pyd concentrations than did patients with pauciarticular and less pronounced evidence of joint damage. Indeed, for the severely affected group (OA1), 78% of Pyd and 89% of Dpd values were above the normal range. Few systematic studies of treatment effects have been carried out, but NSAIDs appear to have little effect on cross-link excretion (Black *et al.*, 1989; Seibel *et al.*, 1989).

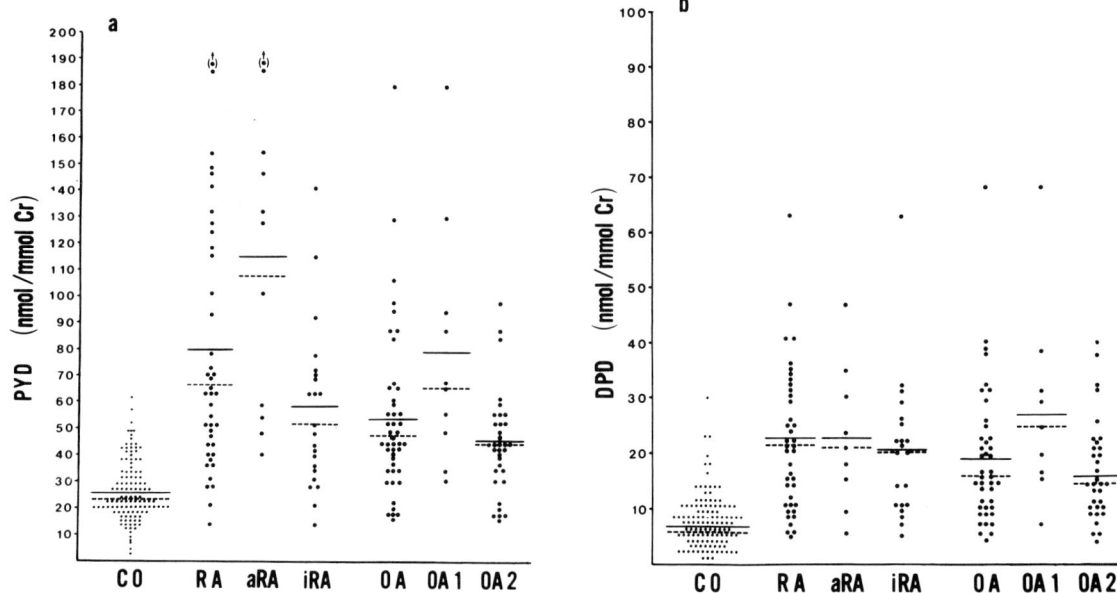

Figure 81.4 Urinary concentrations relative to creatinine of (a) pyridinoline and (b) deoxypyridinoline in patients with OA and RA compared with healthy controls (CO). Individual values are shown for the total OA and RA groups and for subgroups of different severity (OA1 and OA2) or activity (aRa and iRA). Solid bars indicate mean values, broken lines indicate median values. (From Seibel *et al.* (1989), with permission.)

progression of the disease and therapy. Further information on the tissues of origin of the Pyd excretion is necessary to utilize fully the different patterns of excretion in other arthritic conditions.

ACKNOWLEDGMENT

The support of the Arthritis and Rheumatism Council, UK, for part of this work is gratefully acknowledged.

82

The 'clearance' of macromolecular substances such as cartilage markers from synovial fluid and serum

J.R. LEVICK

If we are to use the synovial fluid concentration of a cartilage or synovial marker as an index of disease activity, it is evident that we must understand the kinetics which determine marker concentration. Although we do not have a full understanding at present, some fundamental principles can nevertheless be outlined.

PATHWAYS INVOLVED IN MACROMOLECULAR REMOVAL

Synovial fluid is in contact with two tissues: cartilage and synovium (Fig. 82.1). Synovium, the highly cellular lining of the cavity, possesses a rich superficial capillary bed and, deep to this, a system of lymphatic capillaries (Davies, 1946). In between the lining cells, there are interstitium-filled gaps 1–2 μm wide (Knight and Levick, 1984). The composition of the interstitial matrix is of major importance because it is the main route through which macromolecules leave the joint cavity and reach the lymphatic system and it is composed of a fibrous complex of collagen fibrils, microfibrils and glycosaminoglycans (Levick and McDonald, 1989). The lymphatics are the major pathway for macromolecule removal from normal joints (Bauer et al., 1933) and arthritic joints (Simkin, personal communication). In addition, many synovial lining cells are phagocytic (Henderson

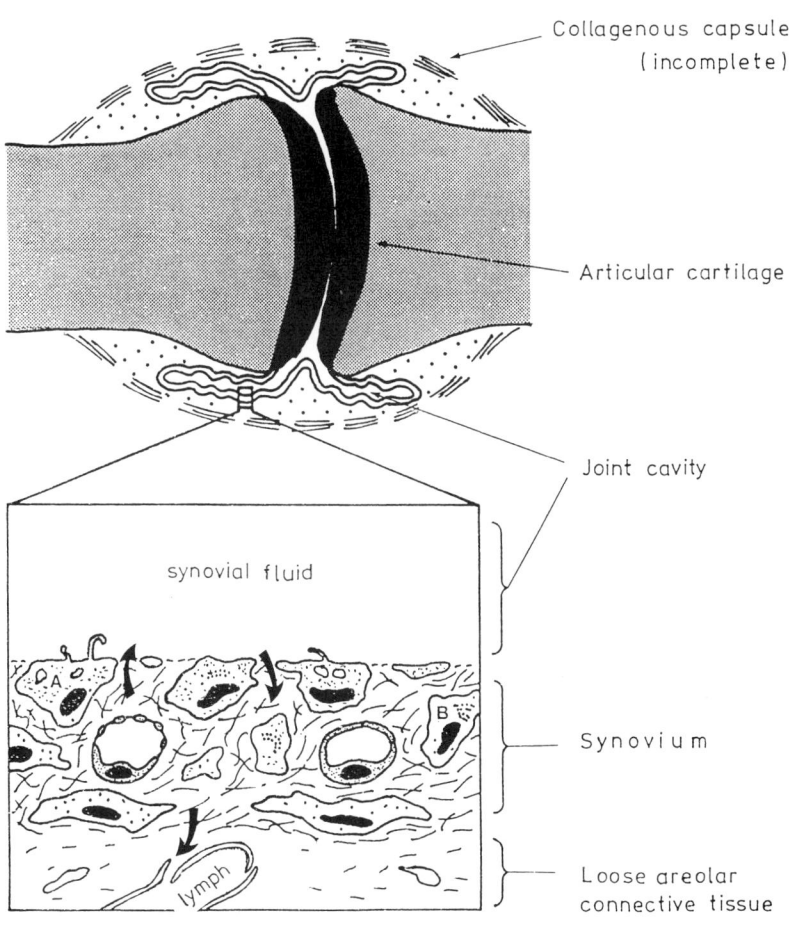

Figure 82.1 Sketch of key features relevant to macromolecule kinetics in a synovial joint cavity. Inset: enlargement of synovial lining based on Knight and Levick (1984) and Levick and McDonald (1989). Arrows indicate filtration of fluid from fenestrated capillaries into the joint cavity and drainage of fluid from the cavity through synovial interstitium into synovial lymph vessels.

and Edwards, 1987) and can degrade macromolecules *in situ* but whether this process occurs at a rate comparable with lymphatic drainage is not known.

'CLEARANCE' AND ITS RELATION TO THE REMOVAL RATE CONSTANT

The modern approach to studying macromolecular kinetics appears, on the surface, to be delightfully simple. A radiolabeled macromolecule, such as a proteoglycan (PG) fragment or protein, is injected into the joint cavity and its disappearance from the knee segment is followed by external γ-counting. A plot of log (counts) vs. time proves linear (Fig. 82.2), indicating that removal is monoexponential (first-order kinetics) and the slope of the line is called the removal rate constant, k. This constant represents the fraction of solute removed per minute and its units are min^{-1}. This is not, however, the same thing as 'clearance' which is defined as the solute removal rate, dm/dt (g min^{-1}), divided by solute concentration, C (g ml^{-1}): clearance = $-(dm\,dt)/C$ (Clark and Smith, 1986). The units of clearance are ml min^{-1}; clearance represents the *virtual volume* of fluid cleared of solute per unit time. To evaluate clearance (ml min^{-1}) from the removal rate constant (k) one must multiply the latter by the volume of fluid in which the solute is distributed, V_d (ml); clearance = $k \cdot V_d$ (Wallis *et al.*, 1985; Levick and Thompson, 1988). V_d is not synonymous with synovial fluid volume because macromolecules are excluded from a fraction of the synovial fluid volume by the molecular web of hyaluronan (HA) chains (see Chapter 64; see also Ogston and Phelps, 1961; Levick, 1981) and because the solute also distributes in the tissues around the joint (synovium, menisci, etc.).

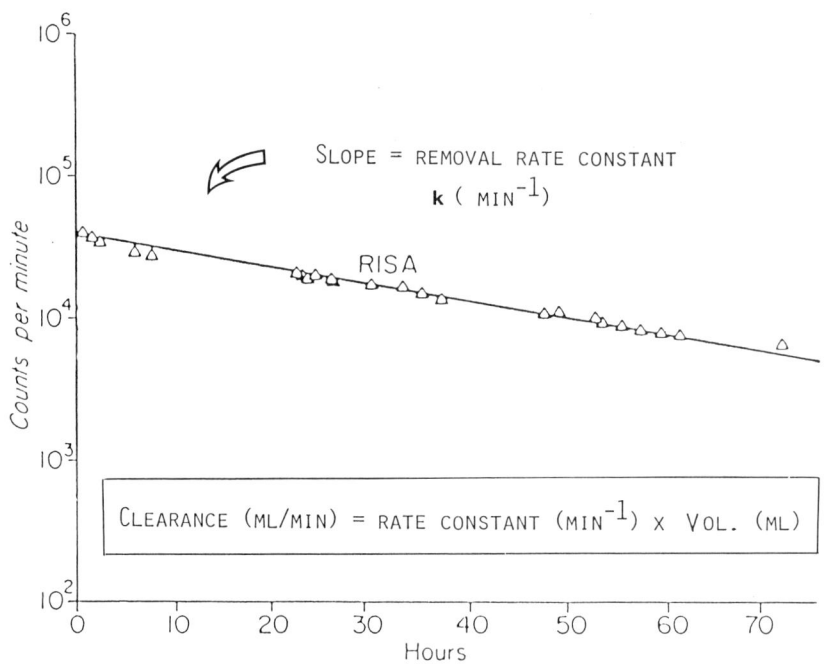

Figure 82.2 Semilogarithmic plot of disappearance of radiolabeled albumin (RISA) from stable knee effusion of an individual with osteoarthritis, monitored exernally and corrected for Compton scatter and isotope decay. In this study the intraarticular volume of distribution of albumin was also measured so that clearance (ml min^{-1}) could be assessed. (Data from Wallis *et al.* (1985).)

IMPORTANCE OF MARKER'S VOLUME OF DISTRIBUTION

The importance of taking volume into consideration is illustrated by the results of a study of PG removal from rabbit knees (Page-Thomas et al., 1987). It was found that the removal rate constant (or its close cousin the half-life) for a radiolabeled PG fragment was not significantly different between normal knees and those with experimental inflammatory arthritis. On the face of it this seems odd, but the anomaly disappears when one recalls that the volume of fluid and synovium in the inflamed joint would be many times greater than in the control joint and that the clearance rate in the diseased joint ($k \times V_d$) would therefore be much higher than in the control joint. Raised clearance in arthritis is due to the increased rate of synovial capillary fluid filtration and concomitant increased lymph flow, as indicated by albumin clearance rates (Wallis et al., 1985). The important point here is that a rate constant can be quite misleading unless intraarticular volume is also measured.

RELATION OF SYNOVIAL FLUID CONCENTRATION TO MARKER RELEASE RATE

It would be very convenient for clinical practice if the concentration of marker in synovial fluid could serve as a quantitative measure of the rate of the marker release and, therefore, of disease activity. The relation between marker release rate (dm/dt) and synovial fluid concentration (C_{sf}) can be assessed with the help of Fig. 82.3, which illustrates the *simplest* possible case — a time-averaged steady state where the removal of the macromolecule occurs exclusively via lymph vessels, the rate of local destruction being negligible. Synovial fluid volume is kept in a steady state by filtration across the capillary wall at a rate equal to lymph flow (Levick, 1987a). The rate is normally 2–4 μl h^{-1}cm^{-2} synovium and this increases in both osteoarthritis (OA) and rheumatoid arthritis, up to four-fold in the latter case (Wallis et al., 1987). In a compartment which is continuously turning over in this fashion, the incoming marker is diluted continuously in a

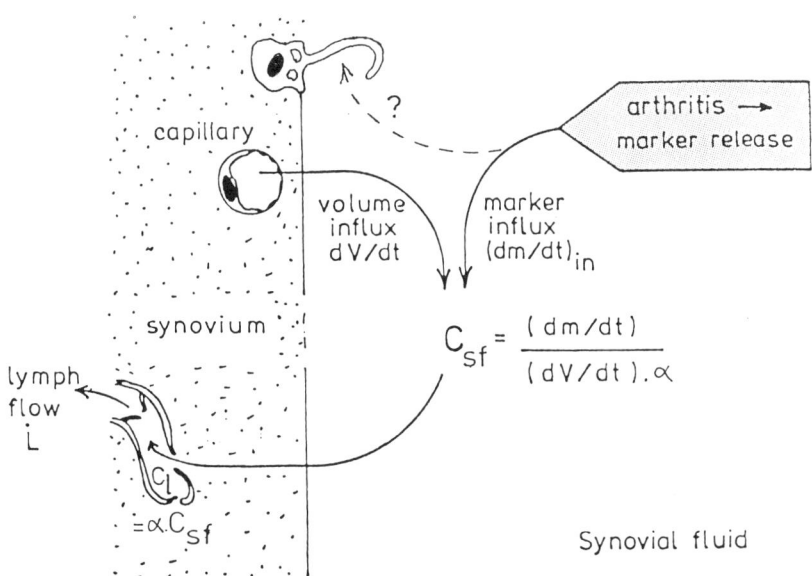

Figure 82.3 The steady-state situation over a period of time in a joint cavity. Concentration of a macromolecular marker depends on the relative rates of marker input into the joint dm/dt (minus any local phagocytic uptake/degradation (----)) and the rate of fluid turnover (capillary input dV/dt, lymph outflow ($\dot{l}$)). The concentration of marker in lymph is not necessarily equal to that in synovial fluid (α).

stream of fluid and the concentration of marker is set primarily by the ratio of marker entry rate (dm/dt) to fluid entry rate (dV/dt). Both fluid and marker are removed together by the synovial interstitial–lymphatic system (lymph flow L).

If the concentration of marker in lymph (C_l) equals that in synovial fluid (C_{sf}), we would simply write

$$C_{sf} = (dm/dt)/(dV/dt) = C_l.$$

However, it is improbable that macromolecular concentration in synovial fluid is identical to that in lymph owing to: (i) the exlusion of marker from part of the synovial fluid water by HA (Ogston and Phelps, 1961); and (ii) the effect of synovial interstitium on macromolecular movement. Indirect evidence based on hydraulic permeability (Levick, 1987b) indicates the synovial interstitial matrix may be quite dense, dense enough to partially reflect and restrict macromolecules without stopping them completely. While the latter effect may be slight for small proteins like albumin, it is probably significant for larger macromolecules. Page-Thomas et al. (1987) found for example that the half-life of PG fragments in a given joint was longer than that of albumin, while Knox et al. (1988) found evidence that hyaluronate turnover in synovial fluid may be substantially slower than protein turnover. We need to know far more about the quantitative composition and permeability of synovial interstitium, but in the meantime, we can take account of the interstitial effect empirically by introducing a correction factor, α, which is the ratio of marker concentration in lymph to that in synovial fluid; $\alpha = C_l/C_{sf}$. The rate of removal of marker by lymph remains $C_l \times L$, but, in terms of synovial fluid concentration, the removal rate becomes $\alpha C_{sf} L$.

Since marker removal rate equals marker input rate in a steady state (dm/dt) and since fluid input rate equals lymph drainage rate, we can write: $dm/dt = C_l L = \alpha C_{sf} \cdot dV/dt$. This rearranges to define the marker concentration in synovial fluid:

$$C_{sf} = \frac{(dm/dt)}{\alpha(dV/dt)} = \frac{\text{marker influx rate}/\alpha}{\text{volume turnover rate}}$$

It is emphasized that α is not a constant; it will vary with marker size, volume flow, interstitial composition and synovial hyaluronate concentration, but the treatment of these aspects is beyond the scope of this article.

IMPORTANCE OF FLUID TURNOVER RATE IN INTERPRETING MARKER CONCENTRATION

One major point is clear from this very simple analysis, i.e. the concentration of a marker in synovial fluid depends not only on its net rate of production by the disease process but also on the rate of turnover of synovial fluid. Phagocytosis and interstitial effects (α) introduce further weaknesses in the link between disease activity and marker concentration, but the fact that disease activity alters fluid turnover (Wallis et al., 1985, 1987) is the single most important confusing fact. Because of this, the synovial fluid concentration of marker cannot be accepted as a direct quantitative measure of marker-release rate.

The need to consider fluid turnover rate is illustrated vividly by the synovial transferrin concentrations given in Table 82.1. Transferrin, of course, enters from inflamed synovial capillaries rather than cartilage, but the same principles govern its synovial fluid concentration. Synovial fluid transferrin concentration was not

Table 82.1 Comparison of concentration and flux of a 'marker' of capillary inflammation in arthritic human knees

	RA	OA	p
Transferrin concentration in synovial fluid (C_{sf}, mg ml^{-1})	1.22	0.96	N.S.
Lymph flow (albumin clearance rate) ($\bar{L}$, ml min^{-1})	0.071	0.039	<0.01
Solute flux ($C_{sf} \times \bar{L}$, mg min^{-1})	0.095	0.033	<0.01

Data from Wallis et al. (1987).

Table 82.2 Comparison of marker concentration in synovial fluid and plasma

	Synovial fluid	Plasma
Detection	Easier	Lower concentration
Access	Specialized	Routine
Type of measure	Single joint	Integrated: all joints
Relation to disease activity	Depends on volume flux through joint, which is changed by the disease	Independent of local joint volume flux
Governing expression	$C_{sf} = \dfrac{(dm/dt)}{\alpha(dV/dt)}$	$C_p = \dfrac{\Sigma(dm/dt)\cdot\tau}{V_p}$

C_{sf}, concentration of marker in synovial fluid; $\Sigma(dm/dt)$, net influx of marker; (dV/dt), net synovial fluid inflow; C_p, concentration of marker in plasma; τ, elimination time constant (plasma); V_p, plasma volume; α, ratio of marker concentration in lymph to synovial fluid.

significantly greater in rheumatoid fluid than in OA fluid, even though the former disease has a greater inflammatory component. The volume turnover, however, is much higher in rheumatoid knees and, by multiplying the volume turnover by the concentration, Simkin found that the marker flux, the true index of disease severity, was in fact three times higher in the rheumatoid knee. Here then is a well-documented example where measurement of synovial fluid concentration alone would have been quite misleading. There is clearly a need for great caution in using synovial fluid concentration as a quantitative guide to disease severity, unless fluid turnover is also measured.

PLASMA CONCENTRATION OF MARKER

Many markers are removed very rapidly from the plasma by the liver (and perhaps lymph nodes too), so their plasma levels are very low (Revell and Muir, 1972; Engström-Laurent and Laurent, 1989). While this presents technical problems for measurement, there are nevertheless real interpretational advantages in looking at plasma rather than synovial fluid. The major advantage is that the plasma marker level is independent of local variations in fluid volume and volume turnover rate within the joint. It can be shown that plasma marker concentration, C_p, is related to the total release of marker into the plasma pool from all joints, $\Sigma(dm/dt)$, thus:

$$C_p = \Sigma(dm/dt)\cdot\tau/V_p$$

where τ is the removal rate constant from plasma (due chiefly to hepatic uptake and degradation) and V_p is plasma volume (Levick, 1988). Thus provided that τ, V_p and any lymph node uptake are not significantly altered by the disease (and it is conceivable that there might be 'upregulation' of τ), then C_p should be a valid measure of overall disease activity. Table 82.2 summarizes the practical merits of plasma and synovial concentrations of marker as a measure of disease activity.

References

Ahlbäck, S. (1968). Osteoarthritis of the knee, a radiographic investigation. *Acta Radiol.* (Suppl) **277**, 7–72

Altman, R., Asch, E., Bloch, D., Bole, G., Borenstein, D., Brandt, K., Christy, W., Cooke, T.D., Greenwald, R., Hochberg, M., Howell, D., Kaplan, D., Koopman, W., Longley, S.I., Mankin, H., McShane, D.J., Medsger, T.J., Meenan, R., Mikkelsen, W., Moskowitz, R. and Murphy, W. (1986). Development of criteria for the classification and reporting of osteoarthritis. *Arthr. Rheum.* **29**, 1039–1049

Altman, R.D., Fries, J.F., Bloch, D.A., Carstens, J., Cooke, T.D., Genant, H., Gofton, P.G.H, McShane, D.J., Murphy, W.A., Sharp, J.T., Spitz, P., Williams, C.A. and Wolfe, F. (1987). Radiographic assessment of progression in osteoarthritis. *Arthr. Rheum.* **30**, 1214–1225

Bauer, W., Short, C.L. and Bennett, G.A. (1933). The manner of removal of proteins from normal joints. *J. Exp. Med.* **57**, 419–433

Bayliss, M.T., Holmes, M.W. and Muir, H. (1989). Age-related changes in the stoichiometry of binding region, link protein and hyaluronic acid in human articular cartilage. *Trans. Orthop Res. Soc.* **14**, 32

Bergström, G., Bjelle, A., Sundh, V. and Svanborg, A. (1986). Joint disorders at ages 70, 75 and 79 years—a cross-sectional comparison. *Br. J. Rheum.* **25**, 333–341

Bienkowski, R.S., Cowan, M.J., McDonald, J.A. and Crystal, R.G. (1978). Degradation of newly synthesized collagen. *J. Biol. Chem.* **253**, 4356–4363

Black, D., Duncan, A. and Robins, S.P. (1988). Quantitative analysis of the pyridinium crosslinks of collagen in urine using ion-paired reversed-phase high-performance liquid chromatography. *Anal. Biochem.* **169**, 197–203

Black, D., Marabani, M., Sturrock, R.D. and Robins, S.P. (1989). Urinary excretion of the hydroxy-pyridinium crosslinks of collagen in patients with rheumatoid arthritis. *Ann. Rheum. Dis.* **48**, 641–644

Block, J.A., Schnitzer, T.J., Andersson, G.B.J., Lenz, M.E., Jeffery, R., McNeill, T.W. and Thonar, E.J.-M.A. (1989). The effect of chemonucleolysis on serum keratan sulfate levels in humans. *Arthr. Rheum.* **32**, 100–104

Brandt, K.D. and Thonar, E.J.-M.A. (1989). Lack of association between serum keratan sulfate concentrations and cartilage changes of osteoarthritis after transection of the anterior cruciate ligament in the dog. *Arthr. Rheum.* **32**, 647–651

Campion, B., McCrae, F., Schnitzer, T., Lenz, M., Dieppe, P. and Thonar, E. (1989a). Serum and synovial fluid keratan sulfate levels in osteoarthritis of the knee. *Arthr. Rheum.* **32** (Suppl. 4), S-105

Campion, G., Schnitzer, T., Zeitz, H. and Thonar, E. (1989b). The effect of oral administration of Prednisolone and of the non-steroidal anti-inflammatory drug NSAID Piroxicam on serum keratan sulfate. *Arthr. Rheum.* **32** (Suppl. 4), S-105

Carney, S.L., Billingham, M.E.J., Muir, H. and Sandy, J.D. (1987). Demonstration of increased proteoglycan turnover in cartilage explants from dogs with experimental osteoarthritis. *J. Orthop. Res.* **2**, 201–206

Carney, S.L., Billingham, M.E.J., Muir, H. and Sandy, J.D. (1985). Structure of newly synthesized [^{35}S]proteoglycans and [^{35}S]proteoglycan turnover products of cartilage explant cultures from dogs with experimental osteoarthritis. *J. Orthop. Res.* **3**, 140–147

Carroll, G.J. (1987). Spectrophotometric measurement of proteoglycans in osteoarthritic synovial fluid. *Ann. Rheum. Dis.* **46**, 375–379

Caterson, B. and Lowther, D.A. (1978). Changes in the metabolism of the proteoglycans from sheep articular cartilage in response to mechanical stress. *Biochim. Biophys. Acta* **540**, 412–422

Caterson, B., Brooks, K., Sattsangi, S., Ratcliffe, A., Hardingham, T. and Muir, H. (1989a). Factors effecting the determination of keratan sulphate using monocolonal antibodies in immunoassay procedures. In *Keratan Sulphate: Chemistry, Biology, Chemical Pathology* (H. Greiling and J.E. Scott, eds). Biochemical Society, London

Caterson, B., Mahmoodian, F., Sorrell, J.M., Bayliss, M.T., Hardingham, T.E. and Muir, H. (1989b). Monoclonal antibodies that recognize novel chondroitin sulfate structures that are specifically expressed during development and in disease. *Trans. Orthop. Res. Soc.* **14**, 12

Chateauvert, J.M.D., Pritzker, K.P.H., Kessler, M.J. and Grynpas, M.D. (1989). Spontaneous osteoarthritis in Rhesus Macaques: I. Chemical and biochemical studies. *J. Rheumatol.* **16**(8), 1098–1104

Chateauvert, J.M.D., Grynpas, M.D., Kessler, M.J. and Pritzker, K.P.J. (1990). Spontaneous osteoarthritis in Rhesus Macaques: II. Characterization of disease and morphometric studies. *J. Rheumatol.* **17**, 73–83

Clark, B. and Smith, D.A.S. (1986). *An Introduction to Pharmacokinetics*, 2nd edn. Blackwell, Oxford

Davies, D.V. (1946). The lymphatics of the synovial membrane. *J. Anat.* **80**, 21–23

Doherty, M., Watt, I. and Dieppe, P. (1983). Influence of primary generalised osteoarthritis on development of secondary osteoarthritis. *Lancet* **8340**, 8–11

Donohue, J.M., Buss, D., Oegema, T.R. and Thompson, R.C. (1983). The effects of indirect blunt trauma on adult canine articular cartilage. *J. Bone Joint Surg.* **65A**, 948–957

Engström-Laurent, A. and Laurent, T.C. (1989). Hyaluronan as a clinical marker. In *Clinical Impact of Bone and Connective Tissue Markers* (E. Lindh and J.I. Thorell, eds), pp. 235–252. Academic Press, London

Eronen, I., Videman, T., Friman, C. and Michelsson, J.E. (1978). Glycosaminoglycan metabolism in experimental osteoarthrosis caused by immobilization. *Acta Orthop. Scand.* **49**, 329–334

Eyre, D.R., Koob, T.J. and Van Ness, K.P. (1984). Quantitation of hydroxypyridinium crosslinks in collagen by high-performance liquid chromatography. *Anal. Biochem.* **137**, 380–388

Eyre, D.R., Dickson, I.R. and Van Ness, K.P. (1988). Collagen cross-linking in human bone and articular cartilage. Age-related changes in the content of mature hydroxypyridinium residues. *Biochem. J.* **252**, 495–500

Felson, D.T. (1988). Epidemiology of hip and knee osteoarthritis. *Epidemiol. Rev.* **10**, 1–28

Fessler, J.H. (1960). A structural function of mucopolysaccharide in connective tissue. *Biochem. J.* **76**, 124–141

Ficat, C. (1976). The reaction of articular cartilage to mechanical trauma: an experimental study. *Rev. Chir. Orthop.* **62**, 493–500

Fraser, J.R.E., Laurent, T.C., Engström-Laurent, U.B.G. (1984). Elimination of hyaluronic acid from the blood stream in the human. *Clin. Exp. Pharm. Physiol.* **11**, 17–25

Fraser, J.R.E., Kimpton, W.G., Laurent, T.C., Cahill, R.N.P. and Vakakis, N. (1988). Uptake and degradation of hyaluronan in lymphatic tissue. *Biochem. J.* **256**, 153–158

Fujimoto, D., Moriguchi, T., Ishida, T. and Hayashi, H. (1978). The structure of pyridinoline, a collagen crosslink. *Biochem. Biophys. Res. Commun.* **84**, 52–57

Funk, F.J. (1983). Osteoarthritis of the knee following ligamentous injury. *Clin. Orthop.* **172**, 154–157

Graham, G.P. and Fairclough, J.A. (1988). Early osteoarthritis in young sportsmen with severe anterolateral instability of the knee. *Injury* **19**, 247–248

Gunja-Smith, Z. and Boucek, R.J. (1981). Collagen cross-linking compounds in human urine. *Biochem. J.* **197**, 759–762

Hardingham, T.E. (1988). Biosynthesis, assembly and turnover in cartilage proteoglycans. In *The Control of Tissue Damage* (A.M. Glauert, ed.), pp. 41–54. Elsevier, Amsterdam

Hardingham, T.E., Caterson, B., Bayliss, M.T., Carney, S.L., Ratcliffe, A. and Muir, H. (1989). Appearance of novel chondroitin sulfate structures in the articular cartilage from experimental canine osteoarthritis joints. *Trans. Orthop. Res. Soc.* **14**, 505

Hascall, V.C. and Glant, T.T. (1987). Proteoglycan epitopes as potential markers of normal and pathologic cartilage metabolism. *Arthr. Rheum.* **30**, 586–588

Heinegård, D. and Oldberg, Å. (1989). Structure and biology of cartilage and bone matrix non-collagenous macromolecules. *FASEB J.* **3**, 2042–2051

Henderson, B. and Edwards, J.C.W.S. (1987). *The Synovial Lining*. Chapman & Hall, London

Hoch, D.H., Grodzinsky, A.J., Koob, T.J., Albert, M.L. and Eyre, D.R. (1983). Early changes in material properties of rabbit articular cartilage after meniscectomy. *J. Orthop. Res.* **1**, 4–12

Holden, D.L., James, S.L., Larson, R.L. and Slocum, D.B. (1988). Proximal tibial osteotomy in patients who are fifty years old or less. *J. Bone Joint Surg.* **70-A**, 977–982

Hulth, A., Lindberg, L. and Telhag, H. (1970). Experimental osteoarthritis in rabbits: preliminary report. *Acta Orthop Scand.* **41**, 522–530

Kandel, R.A., Renlund, R.C., Cheng, P.-T., Rapley, W.A., Mehren, K.G. and Pritzker, K.P.H. (1983). Calcium pyrophosphate dihydrate crystal deposition disease with concurrent vertebral hyperostosis in a Barbary ape. *Arthr. Rheum.* **26**, 682–687

Kannus, P. and Järvinen, M. (1988). Age, overweight, sex and knee instability: their relationship to the posttraumatic osteoarthrosis of the knee joint. *Injury* **19**, 105–108

Kellgren, J.H. and Lawrence, J.S. (1957). Radiological assessment of osteo-arthrosis. *Ann. Rheum. Dis.* **16**, 494–502

Kettelkamp, D.B., Hillberry, B.M. Murrish, D.E. and Heck, D.A. (1988). Degenerative arthritis of the knee secondary to fracture malunion. *Clin. Orthop.* **234**, 159–169

Knight, A.D. and Levick, J.R. (1984). Morphometry of the ultrastructure of the blood–joint barrier in the rabbit knee. *Quart. J. Exp. Physiol.* **69**, 271–288

Knox, R., Levick, J.R. and McDonald, J.N. (1988). Synovial fluid — its mass, macromolecular content and pressure in major limb joints of the rabbit. *Quart. J. Exp. Physiol.* **73**, 33–45

Kramer, J.S., Yelin, E.H. and Epstein, W.V. (1983). Social and economic impacts of four musculoskeletal conditions. *Arthr. Rheum.* **26**, 901–907

Krane, S.M., Kantrowitz, F.G., Byrne, M. Pinnell, S.R., Singer, F.R. (1977). Urinary excretion of hydroxylysine and its glycosides as an index of collagen degradation. *J. Clin. Invest.* **59**, 819–827

Levick, J.R. (1987a). Flow through interstitium and

other fibrous matrices. *Quart. J. Exp. Physiol.* **72**, 409–437

Levick, J.R. (1987b). Synovial fluid and trans-synovial flow in stationary and moving joints. In *Joint Loading* (H.J. Helminen, I. Kiviranta, M. Tammi, A.-M. Säämänen, K. Paukkonen and J. Jurvelin, eds). Wright & Sons, Bristol

Levick, J.R. (1981). Permeability of rheumatoid and normal human synovium to specific plasma proteins. *Arthr. Rheum.* **24**, 1550–1560

Levick, J.R. (1988). Determinants of macromolecular marker concentration in synovial fluid and plasma in the steady state. In *Laboratory Markers of Joint Inflammation and Destruction* (P.W. Thompson, J.R. Kirwan, S.R. Rudge, B.J. Houghton and H.L.F. Currey, eds). Arthritis and Rheumatism Council, London

Levick, J.R. and McDonald, J.N. (1989). The microfibrillar meshwork of the synovial lining and associated broad-banded collagen — a clue to identity. *Ann. Rheum.* **49**, 31–36

Levick, J.R. and Thompson, P.W. (1988). Intra-articular volume as an important factor governing macromolecular half-life in synovial fluid. *Ann. Rheum. Dis.* **47**, 701–702

Lohmander, L.S., Dahlberg, L., Ryd, L. and Heinegård, D. (1989). Increased levels of proteoglycan fragments in joint fluid after knee injury. *Arthr. Rheum.* **32**, 1434–1442

Lohmander, L.S., Dahlberg, L., Ryd, L. and Heinegård, D. (1990). Joint cartilage markers in synovial fluid in human osteoarthritis. *Trans. Orthop. Res. Soc.* **15**, 212

Lohmander, S. (1988). Proteoglycans of joint cartilage: structure, function turnover and role as markers of joint disease. *Baillière's Clin. Rheumatol.* **2**, 37–62

Maldonado, B.A., Williams, J.M., Otten, L.M., Flannery, M., Kuettner, K.E. and Thonar, E.J.-M.A. (1989). Differences in the rate of clearance of different KS-bearing molecules injected intravenously in rabbits. *Trans. Orthop. Res. Soc.* **14**, 161

Mankin, H.J., Brandt, K.D. and Shulman, L.E. (1986). Workshop on etiopathogenesis of osteoarthritis. Proceedings and recommendations. *J. Rheumatol.* **13**, 1127–1160

Mbuyi, J.-M., Dequeker, J., Teblick, M. and Merlevede, M. (1982). Relevance of urinary excretion of alcian blue–glycosaminoglycans complexes and hydroxyproline to disease activity in rheumatoid arthritis. *J. Rheumatol.* **9**, 579–583

McAlindon, T. and Dieppe, P. (1989). Osteoarthritis: definitions and criteria. *Ann. Rheum. Dis.* **48**, 531–532

McDaniel, W.J. and Dameron, T.B. (1980). Untreated ruptures of the anterior cruciate ligament. *J. Bone Joint Surg.* **62A**, 696–705

McDevitt, C.A., Gilbertson, E.M.M. and Muir, H. (1977). An experimental model of osteoarthritis; early morphological and biochemical changes. *J. Bone Joint Surg.* **59B**, 24–35

Mehmet, H., Scudder, P.T.P.W., Hounsell, E.F., Caterson, B and Feizi, T. (1986). The antigenic determinants recognized by three monoclonal antibodies to keratan sulphate involve sulphated hepta- or larger oligosaccharides of the poly(N-acetyllactosamine) series. *Eur. J. Biochem.* **157**, 385–391

Moro, L., Mucelli, R.S.P., Gazarrini, C., Modricky, C., Marotti, F. and de Bernard, B. (1988). Urinary β-1-galactosyl-O-hydroxylysine as a marker of collagen turnover of bone. *Calcif. Tiss. Int.* **42**, 87–90

Morrey, B.F. (1989). Upper tibial osteotomy for secondary osteoarthritis of the knee. *J. Bone Joint Surg.* **71B**, 554–559

Moskowitz, R.W. (1984). Experimental methods of osteoarthritis. In *Osteoarthritis* (R.W. Moskowitz, D.S. Howell, V.M. Goldberg and H.J. Mankin, eds). W.B. Saunders, Philadelphia

Moskowitz, R.W., Howell, D.S., Goldberg, V.M., Muniz, O. and Pita, J.C. (1979). Cartilage proteoglycan alterations in an experimentally induced model of rabbit osteoarthritis. *Arthr. Rheum.* **22**, 155–163

Muir, H. (1977). Heberden oration 1976. Molecular approach to the understanding of osteoarthrosis. *Ann. Rheum. Dis.* **36**, 199–208

Muir, H. (1986). Current and future trends in articular cartilage research and osteoarthritis. In *Articular Cartilage Biochemistry* (K.E. Kuettner, R. Schleyerbach and V.C. Hascall, eds). New York, Raven Press

Odenbring, S., Tjörnstrand, B., Egund, N., Hagstedt, B., Hovelius, L., Lindstrand, A. Luxhöj, T. and Svanström, A. (1989). Function after tibial osteotomy for early medial gonarthrosis in patients below the age of 50. *Acta Orthop. Scand.* **60**, 527–531

Oegema, T.R.J., Swedenburg, S.M., Bradford, D.S. and Thonar, E.J.-M.A. (1988). Levels of keratan sulfate-bearing fragments rise predictably following chemonucleolysis of dog intervertebral discs with chymopapain. *Spine* **13**, 707–711

Ogawa, T., Ono, T., Tsunda, M. and Kawanishi, Y. (1982). A novel fluor in insoluble collagen: a crosslinking moiety in collagen molecule. *Biochem. Biophys. Res. Commun.* **107**, 1252–1257

Ogston, A.G. and Phelps, C.F. (1961). The partition of solutes between buffer solutions and solutions containing hyaluronic acid. *Biochem. J.* **78**, 827–833

Pachman, L.M., Green, O.C., Hayford, J.R., Lenz, M.E., Thonar, E.J.-M.A. (1987). The effect of growth hormone on plasma levels of keratan sulfate, Somatomedin-C and height in children with growth hormone deficiency. *Clin. Res.* **35**, 916A

Page-Thomas, D.P., Bard, D., King, B. and Dingle, J.T. (1987). Clearance of proteoglycan from joint cavities. *Ann. Rheum. Dis.* **46**, 934–937

Palmoski, M.J. and Brandt, K.D. (1981). Running inhibits the reversal of atrophic changes in canine knee cartilage after removal of a let cast. *Arthr. Rheum.* **24**, 1329–1337

Palmoski, M., Perricone, E. and Brandt, K.D. (1979). Development and reversal of a proteoglycan aggregation defect in normal canine knee cartilage after immobilization. *Arthr. Rheum.* **22**, 508–517

Pettipher, E.R., Henderson, B., Hardingham, T.E. and Ratcliffe, A. (1989). Cartilage proteoglycan depletion in acute and chronic antigen-induced arthritis. *Arthr. Rheum.* **32**, 601–607

Pond, M.J. and Nuki, G. (1973). Experimentally-induced osteoarthritis in the dog. *Ann. Rheum. Dis.* **32**, 387–388

Ratcliffe, A., Tyler, J.A. and Hardingham, T.E. (1986). Articular cartilage cultured with interleukin 1: increased release of link protein, hyaluronate-binding region and other proteoglycan fragments. *Biochem. J.* **238**, 571–580

Ratcliffe, A., Doherty, M., Maini, R.N. and Hardingham, T.E. (1988). Increased concentrations of proteoglycan components in the synovial fluids of patients with acute but not chronic joint disease. *Ann. Rheum. Dis.* **47**, 826–832

Ratcliffe, A., Billingham, M.E., Muir, H. and Hardingham, T.E. (1989). Experimental canine osteoarthritis and cartilage explant culture: increased release of specific proteoglycan epitopes. *Trans. Orthop. Res. Soc.* **14**, 507

Renlund, R.C., Pritzker, K.P.H., Cheng, P.-T. and Kessler, M.J. (1986). Rhesus monkeys (*Macaca Mulatta*) as a model for calcium pyrophosphate dihydrate crystal deposition disease. *J. Med. Primatol.* **15**, 11–16

Revell, P.A. and Muir, H. (1972). The excretion and degradation of chondroitin 4-sulphate administered to guinea pigs as free chondroitin sulphate and as proteoglycan. *Biochem. J.* **130**, 597–606

Robins, S.P. (1982a). An enzyme-linked immunoassay for the collagen cross-link pyridinoline. *Biochem. J.* **207**, 617–620

Robins, S.P. (1982b). Turnover and crosslinking of collagen. *Collagen in Health and Disease* (J.B. Weiss and M.I.V. Jayson, eds). Churchill Livingstone, Edinburgh

Robins, S.P. (1988). Functional properties of collagen and elastin. *Baillière's Clin. Rheumatol.* **2**, 1–36

Robins, S.P. and Duncan, A. (1987). Pyridinium crosslinks of bone collagen and their location in peptides isolated from rat femur. *Biochim. Biophys. Acta* **914**, 233–239

Robins, S.P., Stewart, P., Astbury, C. and Bird, H.A. (1986). Measurement of the cross linking compound, pyridinoline, in urine as an index of collagen degradation in joint disease. *Ann. Rheum. Dis.* **45**, 969–973

Robins, S.P., Duncan, A., Reid, D.M., Paterson, C.R. (1989). Urinary hydroxypyridinium crosslinks of collagen as markers of resorption in a range of metabolic bone diseases. *J. Bone Mineral Res.* **4**, S397

Roughley, P.J., Poole, A.R., Campbell, I.K. and Mort, J.S. (1986). The proteolytic generation of hyaluronic acid-binding regions derived from the proteoglycans of human articular cartilage as a consequence of ageing. *Trans. Orthop. Res. Soc.* **11**, 209

Seibel, M.J., Duncan, A. and Robins, S.P. (1989). Urinary hydroxy-pyridinium crosslinks provide indices of cartilage and bone involvement in arthritic diseases. *J. Rheumatol.* **16**, 964–970

Sokoloff, L. (1956). Natural history of degenerative joint disease in small laboratory animals. *AMA Arch. Pathol.* **62**, 118–128

Sweet, M.B., Coelho, A., Schnitzler, C.M., Schnitzer, T.J., Lenz, M.E., Jakim, I., Kuettner, K.E. and Thonar, E.J.-M.A. (1988). Serum keratan sulfate levels in osteoarthritis patients. *Arthr. Rheum.* **31**, 648–652

Thonar, E.J.-M.A., Lenz, M.E., Klintworth, G.K., Caterson, B., Pachman, L.M., Glickman, P., Katz, R., Huff, J. and Kuettner, K.E. (1985). Quantification of keratan sulfate in blood as a marker of cartilage catabolism. *Arthr. Rheum.* **28**, 1367–1376

Thonar, E.J.-M.A., Meyer, R.F., Dennis, R.F., Lenz, M.E., Maldonado, B., Hassell, J.R., Hewitt, A.T., Stark, W.J.J., Stock, E.L., Kuettner, K.E. and Klintworth, G.K. (1986). Absence of normal keratan sulfate in the blood of patients with macular corneal dystrophy. *Am. J. Ophthal.* **102**, 561–569

Thonar, E.J.-M.A., Schnitzer, T.J. and Kuettner, K.E. (1987). Quantification of keratan sulfate in blood as a marker of cartilage metabolism. *J. Rheumatol.* **14** (Suppl.), 23–24

Thonar, E.J.-M.A., Pachman, L.M., Lenz, M.E., Hayford, J., Lynch, P. and Kuettner, K.E. (1986). Age related changes in the concentration of serum keratan sulphate in children. *J. Clin. Chem. Clin. Biochem.* **26**, 57–63

Wallis, W.J., Simkin, P.A., Nelp, W.B. and Foster, D.M. (1985). Intraarticular volume and clearance in human synovial effusions. *Arthr. Rheum.* **28**, 441–449

Wallis, W.J., Simkin, P.A. and Nelp, W.B. (1987). Protein traffic in human synovial effusions. *Arthr. Rheum.* **30**, 57–63

Walton, M. (1979). Patella displacement and osteoarthrosis of the knee joint in mice. *J. Pathol.* **127**, 165–172

Williams, J.M., Downey, C. and Thonar, E.J.-M.A. (1988). Increase in levels of serum keratan sulfate following cartilage proteoglycan degradation in the rabbit knee joint. *Arthr. Rheum.* **31**, 557–560

Witter, J., Roughley, P., Webber, C., Roberts, N., Keystone, E. and Poole, A.R. (1987). The immunologic detection and characterization of cartilage proteoglycan degradation products in synovial fluids of patients with arthritis. *Arthr. Rheum.* **30**, 519–529

Index

Acrylamide *see under* Agarose gel
Affinity, chromatography, of proteoglycans fragments, 174–5
Agarose gel
  agarose–acrylamide electrophoresis, 166–7
    of proteoglycans and large protein complexes, 40–3
  articular chondrocytes cultured in, 90–2
  submerged, electrophoresis of proteoglycan monomers in, 44–6
Age-related changes
  in cartilage cell density, 9–11
  in cartilage composition, 211–2
  in cartilage fixed charge density, 9–11
  in cartilage hydration, 9–11
  in IL1 effect on cartilage degradation, 115
  in proteoglycan composition, 220–2
  in proteoglycan extractability from cartilage, 37–9
  in sulfate incorporation by cartilage, 13–4
Albumin
  diffusion coefficient by capillary technique, 257
  partition coefficient, difficulties in measurement, 244
  partition coefficient, use of for determination of extra-fibrillar space, 218
Analysis of matrix constituents *see* Extraction, separation and analysis
Anatomical aspects, sampling of articular cartilage, 4–5
Anatomical location of articular cartilage samples, 7–8
Antibodies
  monoclonal
    against proteoglycans, characterization of, 164–7
    and immunochemical methods, 156–7

    to carbohydrate epitopes, keratan sulfate, 161–2
    chondroitin sulfate, 161–2
    to native or denatured protein structures, 160–1
  polyclonal
    and immunochemical methods, 156–7
    to collagen, characterization and use of 168–9
  sulfate, anti-keratan, and quantitation of keratan sulfate epitope, 173–7
Antigenic keratan sulfate measured by enzyme-linked immunosorbent assay, 170–2
Antigen-specific T-lymphocyte clone as new tool for proteoglycans research, 177–81
Anti-keratin sulfate antibodies and quantitation of keratan sulfate epitope, 173–7
Arthritis *see* Osteoarthritis
Articular surface
  absence of in degenerate cartilage, 11
  fixed charge density of, 11
  measurement of compressive properties of, 306–7
  measurement of cell size, number and shape in, 236
  morphology of,
    general, 61–2
    study of using low temperature SEM, 64-7
  nature of,
    study of using cationized ferritin, 67–9
  structure of,
    study of using micronotch stressing technique, 72–3
  sulfate incorporation in, 13
    effect of FCS in long-term culture, 15–7
  water content of, 11
Articular chondrocytes, 62–3
  cultured in agarose gel, 90–2

  immortalization of, 96–7
  studies of membrane transport in, 261–2
Associative extraction centrifugal methods, 48
Avian model of implants, 328–9

Baboon tibial condylar cartilage, 66
Biomechanical approaches to cartilage repair, 318
Biomechanics of cartilage, 274–311
Biopolymer solutions and gels, measurement of diffusion coefficients in, 255–8
Biosynthesis *see* Synthesis
Bone, collagen metabolism measured in, 140–2
Boundary sedimentation centrifugal method, 47

Calcified cartilage, fluorescent-tracer labeling for measuring remodeling in, 322–4
Calf serum, fetal, and sulfate incorporation, 14–17
Carbohydrate epitopes, monoclonal antibodies to, 161–2
Cationized ferritin labeling, electron microscopy of articular sufface, 67–9
Cell, *see also* Chondrocyte
  compartment, 215–19, 235–6
  counting using disector method, 76
  granulosa, rat ovarian, 133–6
  measurement of numbers and size, 74–7, 235–6
  membranes, transport across, 248, 258–62
  multiplication, analysis of, 93

364 INDEX

Centrifugal methodologies
  centrifugation density gradient, 39
  for studying proteoglycans, 46–9
Cesium sulfate gradients, 48
Chickens
  embryo cartilage, lysozyme source in, 194–6
  implants in, 328–9
Chondrocytes, 62–3, see also Cell
  articular, studies of membrane transport in, 261–2
  culture, 85–104
    immortalization of, 95–8
    for implantation, 98–100, 317–19
    subpopulations of articular chondrocytes cultured in agarose gel, 90–2
    techniques for, 85–9
    three-dimensional culture model for studying, 93–5
  gene expression, regulation of, 196–9
  growth-plate proliferating, 22
  hypertrophic, electron microscopy of, 21
  implantation, 316–17
Chondroitin sulfate
  concentration in femoral head cartilage, 211
  monoclonal antibodies to, 161–2
Chondrons, extracted from articular cartilage, 78–80
Chromatography
  affinity, of proteoglycan fragments, 174–5
  gel, partition coefficients measured by, 251–5
  of proteoglycan aggregates, sepharose CL-2B chromatography of, 37–8
Classification of tissue, 4–6, 7–9
Clearance of macromolecular substances from synovial fluid and serum, 352–7
Cloning
  cDNA, 191
  T-lymphocyte, as new tool in proteoglycan research, antigen-specific, 177–81
Coefficients
  diffusion,
    in biopolymer solutions and gels, measurement of 255–8
    general methods of measurement, 245–7

partition,
  and characterization of networks, 263–6
  general methods of measurement, 242–5
  measured by gel chromatography, 251–5
Collagen
  cross-linking interactions between type II and type IX, 28–33
  fibril organization, 62
  gene mutations (type II) and familial osteoarthritis, 199–205
  inter-molecular cross-linking in, 29
  mammalian, identification of forms, 33–6
  markers of arthritis in human urine, 348–52
  metabolism, in cartilage and bone, measurement of, 140–2
  packing studied using X-ray scattering, 227–32
  polyclonal antibodies to, characterization and use of, 168–9
  structure and organization and X-ray diffraction, 232–3
  synthesis, 140–2
  types in mammalian cartilage and their identification, 33–6
  type II, radioimmunoassays, 93
  types II and IX, cross-linking and interactions, 28–33
  type XII
    discovered, 190–4
    stoichiometry of, 54–5
  turnover, see Metabolism
Compartment see under Cell; Extra-fibrillar; Intra-fibrillar
Composite agarose–acrylamide electrophoresis of proteoglycans and large protein complexes, 40–3
Composition of tissue see Tissue composition
Compression
  chamber, dynamic, 117
  confined, for studying physical properties of cartilage, 287–92
  and cartilage metabolism, 116–22
  and osmotic, and cartilage metabolism, 119–22
  oscillatory confined, 291–2
  structural response of articular cartilage to, 71–2

unconfined,
  measurement of thin slices in, 305–8
  for studying physical properties of cartilage, 293–8
  see also Osmotic pressure; Pressure
Concentration of cartilage constituents, 211–19
Connective-tissue proteoglycans, monoclonal antibodies against, 164–7
Continuous labeling under steady-state conditions, 149–50
Contour maps of pressure, 284–5, 287
Creep, unconfined compression for studying cartilage, 293–8
Cross-linking
  in collagen, inter-molecular, 29
  excretion, 348–52
  interactions, collagens, cartilage, 28–33
Cultures
  chondrocytes, as implants for cartilage defects, 327–9
  tissue, cartilage explant, 112–13
  see also Chondrocyte culture
Cysteines, analysis of, 51
Cytokine activity, effect on matrix synthesis and degradation, 113–15

Defects, cartilage
  cultured chondrocytes as implants for, 98–100, 327–9
  see also Osteoarthritis
Degenerative arthritis see Osteoarthritis
Degradation
  fragments, characterization of, 115–16
  matrix, 112–116, see also 313–35
Denatured protein structures, antibodies to, 160–1
Density
  fixed charge see Fixed charge density
  gradient centrifugation, 39
Depth
  from articular surface vs. sulfate uptake, 11–12
  variations in fixed charge density and water content with, 10–11

Dialysis
  equilibrium, to determine osmotic pressure, 299
  techniques in molecular probes, 263–5
Diameter deformations, 295–6
Differential interference contrast light microscopy of articular cartilage, 71
Diffraction analysis of tissues, low-angle X-ray, 232–5
Diffusion
  coefficient, general methods of measurement, 245–7
  coefficients in biopolymer solutions and gels, measurement of, 255–8
  of molecular probes and characterization of networks, 267–8
  see also Solute transport
Disc see Intervertebral disc
Disease, joint see Osteoarthritis
Disector method, cell counting using, 76
Dissection of articular cartilage samples, 5
DNA see Recombinant DNA
Domain structure and sequence homologies in proteoglycans, 187–90
Dynamic
  compression chamber, 117
  methods of network characterization, 266–70

Efflux experiments, techniques and membrane transport studies, 261
Electrical properties see Mechanical and electrical properties
Electromechanical interactions, 287–8
  see also Mechanical and electrical properties
Electron microscopy
  of articular surface, 68
    using cationized ferritin labeling, 67–9
  of bovine collagen, 35
  of growth-plate proliferating chondrocyte, 22
  of hypertrophic chondrocyte, 21
  low temperature, 63–7
  molecular imaging by, 162–4

  of terminal determinant, 169
  three-dimensional ultrastructural studies, 73
Electrophoresis of proteoglycan
  agarose–acrylamide, 40–3
  monomers in agarose submerged gels, 44–6
Elution profiles, 253–5
End-plate, intervertebral disc, 17–9
Enzyme
  -linked immunosorbent assay, measurement of antigenic keratan sulfate, 170–2
  -modified tissues used to study structure and function, 222–7
Epitopes
  carbohydrate, monoclonal antibodies to, 161–2
  keratan sulfate, in quantitation of proteoglycans, 173–7
  proteoglycan protein, 155 et seq.
Equilibrium
  centrifugation method, 47
  dialysis techniques in molecular probes, 263–5
  dialysis to determine osmotic pressure, 299
  mechanical properties, 288–91, 296
Ex vivo tissues see Sampling
Exclusion behaviour, 223–4, 243–5, 263 et seq.
Excretion, cross-link, 348–52
Explant culture of cartilage, short- and long-term, 14–7, 105–29
  of intervertebral disc, 123–6
  mechanical compression and cartilage metabolism, 116–19
  mechanical and osmotic pressure and glycosaminoglycan synthesis, 119–22
  model system for analysis of matrix degradation, 112–16
  steady-state metabolism of proteoglycans, 108–12
Extraction, separation and analysis of matrix constituents, 27–60
  associative centrifugal methods, 48
  collagens
    cross-linking interactions, 28–33
    mammalian, identification of forms, 33–6
    composite agarose–acrylamide electrophoresis of proteoglycans and large protein complexes, 40–3

  electrophoresis of proteoglycan monomers in agarose submerged gels, 44–6
  extraction of proteoglycan and hyaluronan, 36–9
  microsequencing of cartilage components, 50–5
Extrafibrillar compartment, 216–17, 244, 297
  osmotic pressure determination, 299–301

Familial osteoarthritis and collagen gene mutations (type II), 199–205
Femoral head cartilage (human)
  composition of, 111 et seq.
  glycosaminoglycan synthesis in, 119–22
  pressure measurement using Fuji film sampling and topographical variations, 9–17
Ferritin labeling, cationized, electron microscopy of articular surface, 67–9
Fetal calf serum, and sulfate incorporation, 14–17
Fibril organization, collagen, 62 et seq., 70–3
Fibrillar
  network pore size and hyaluronan mobility, 224
  see also Extrafibrillar; Intrafibrillar
Filtration techniques and membrane transport studies, 261
Fixed charge density, variations in, 9–11
Fluid flow,
  effects of on solute transport, 247–8
  and cartilage deformation, 287–98
  see also Solute transport; Synovial fluid; Water
Function of tissues studied in enzyme-modified tissues, 222–7
Functional properties of cartilage constituents, 211–19

Gel
  and biopolymer solutions, measurement of diffusion coefficients in, 255–8

Gel (*cont.*)
  chromatography, partition coefficients measured by, 251–5
  filtration of proteoglycan fragments, 174–5
  see also Agarose gel
Genes
  expression, chondrocyte, regulation of, 196–9
  mutations, collagen (type II), and familial osteoarthritis, 199–205
  SV40 early, immortalization by, 96–7
Glycosaminoglycan
  concentration
    in human femoral head cartilage, 119–122
    profile in disc end-plate, 17–9
    in synovial fluid, 343–4
  synthesis rate
    effect of compression, 116–22
    effect of growth factors on zonal variations in, 15–7
    measurement in intervertebral disc, 123–6
    normal vs. osteoarthritic cartilage, 13
    topographical variations, 12
    traced by radioactive sulfate, 143–8
Grafts, periosteal and perichondrial, 316
Granulosa cells, rat ovarian, 133–6
Growth-factor
  effect on proteoglycan synthesis and degradation, 112–16
  effect on sulfate uptake in different cartilage zones, 15–17
  stimulation of cartilage repair, 317–18
Growth-plate cartilage, rat, 20, 75

Head cartilage *see* Femoral head cartilage
Healing and spongialization in human articular cartilage, 324–7
Hips, human
  contour maps of pressure, 284–5, 287
  healing, 325
Human articular cartilage
  compared with non-human primates, 248–51
  extraction of proteoglycan and hyaluronan, 36–9
  proteoglycan aggregates, age-related changes in, 220–2
  repair and remodeling, 324–7
  selection and classification, 7–9
  cartilage proteoglycans, quantitation of keratan sulfate epitope in, 173–7
  chondrocytes, three-dimensional culture model for studying, 93–5
  defects, *see* Defects
  femoral head cartilage
    age-related changes in composition, 211–2
    effect of pressure on glycosaminoglycan synthesis in, 119–22
    topographical variations in properties of, 9–13
  hip *see* Hips
  link proteins, natural proteolysis of, 53–4
  synovial fluid, analysis of, 175
  urine, collagen markers of arthritis in, 348–52
Hyaluronan
  concentration in Wharton's jelly, 233
  extraction from human articular cartilage, 36–9
  metabolism in articular cartilage explants, 136–7
  mobility and fibrillar network pore size, 224
  synthesis, radiolabeled glucosamine used as precursor for measuring, 132–7
Hydration
  of cartilage
    control of, during sample preparation, 5
    factors determining level of, 212–3
    topographical variations in, 10–1
  of disc
    controlled by dialysis against ethylene glycol, 123–126
    topographical variations in, 17–19
  effect of on
    ionic partition coefficients, 213–9
    rate of glycosaminoglycan synthesis in cartilage and disc, 122–6
    solute concentration profiles, 213–9
    solute diffusion coefficients, 213–9
    tissue volume and thickness, 213–9
  see also Water
Hydraulic permeability, 297–8
Hypertrophic chondrocyte, electron microscopy of, 21

Immortalization of chondrocytes in culture, 95–8
Immunoassay procedures in quantitation of keratan sulfate epitope, 173–7
Immunochemical methods in cartilage research, 155–84
  antigen-specific T-lymphocyte clones as new tool in proteoglycan research, 177–81
  cartilage proteoglycans, characterization, 156–64
  characterization and use of polyclonal antibodies to collagen, 168–9
  and discovery of type XII collagen, 191–2
  measurement of antigenic keratan sulfate by enzyme-linked immunosorbent assay, 170–2
  production and characterization of monoclonal antibodies against proteoglycans, 164–7
  quantitation of keratan sulfate epitope in cartilage proteoglycans, 173–7
Immunosorbent assay, enzyme-linked, measurement of antigenic keratan sulfate by, 170–2
Implantation
  chondrocyte cultures for, 98–100, 327–9
  of chondrocytes or mesenchymal cells, 316–17
  of natural and synthetic matrices, 317
In vitro
  cytokine activity, 113
  glycosaminoglycan synthesis compared with *in vivo*, 143–8
  labeling protocols and biosynthesis of proteoglycans, 148–52

In vivo
    glycosaminoglycan synthesis compared with *in vitro*, 143–8
    identification of mammalian cartilage collagens, 33–6
    serum keratan sulfate measurement and proteoglycan metabolism, 345–7
Injection, pulse *see* Radioisotopes
Injury, cartilage, 313–15
Inter-molecular cross-linking in collagen, 29
Intervertebral disc explant culture of cartilage, 123–6
    measurement of pressure of nucleus pulposus of, 302–4
    sampling, 17–19
    variations in composition of, 17–19
Intrafibrillar compartment, 217–18
Isotopes *see* Radioisotopes

Joint disease *see* Osteoarthritis

Keratan sulfate
    antigenic, measured by enzyme-linked immunosorbent assay, 170–2
    epitope in proteoglycans, quantitation of, 173–7
    measurement, and proteoglycan metabolism, 345–7
    monoclonal antibodies to, 161–2

Labeling
    fluorescent-tracer, for measuring remodeling, 322–4
    radioisotope-tracer *see* Radioisotopes
Light microscopy of articular cartilage, 71
Link protein *see* Protein, link
Localization and characterization of cartilage proteoglycans, 162
Long-term culture of cartilage *see* Explant culture
Low temperature scanning electron microscopy, 63–7
Low-angle X-ray diffraction analysis of tissues, 232–5
Lymphocytes *see* T-lymphocyte

Lysozyme source in chick embryo cartilage, 194–6

Macromolecules
    from synovial fluid and serum, clearance of 352–7
    production of, 205
Mammals
    cartilage collagens, identification of forms, 33–6
    see also Human; Primates; Rabbits; Rat
Markers, collagen, in human urine, 348–52
Matrix
    components
        pore size, penetrability and globular proteins, 223–4
        and tissue swelling pressure, 225–6
    constituents *see* Extraction, separation and analysis
    degradation
        in cartilage explant cultures, model system for, 112–16
        enhanced by cytokine activity, 113–15
    macromolecule production, 205
    solute transport through, 241 *et seq.*
    synthesis and turnover, 143–8
    synthetic, implantation of, 317
    see also Recombinant DNA
Membranes, cell, transport across, 248, 258–62
Mesenchymal cells, implantation of, 316–17
Metabolism
    collagen, in cartilage and bone, measurement of, 140–2
    hyaluronan, in articular cartilage explants, 136–7
    and mechanical compression, 116–19
    proteoglycans, and serum keratan sulfate measurement and, 345–7
    steady-state, of proteoglycans in bovine articular cartilage explants, 108–12
    study of *see* Radioisotopes
Micronotch/stressing techniques, 72–3
Micro-rate zonal sedimentation, 48
Microsequencing of cartilage components, 50–5

Model system for analysis of matrix degradation in cartilage explant cultures, 112–16
Molecular imaging by electron microscopy, 162–4
Molecular probes, network characterization by, 263–70
Monoclonal antibodies
    against proteoglycans, characterization of, 164–7
    and immunochemical methods, 156–7
    to carbohydrate epitopes, keratan sulfate and chondroitin sulfate, 161–2
Monolayer culture and chondrocyte culture, 87
Morphology of cartilage, 61–83
    articular cartilage
        chondrons extracted from, 78–80
        structure–function relationships, 70–3
    electron microscopy of articular surface using cationized ferritin labeling, 67–9
    low temperature scanning electron microscopy, 63–7
    morphological studies, preservation of samples for, 19–23
    stereological methods in articular cartilage research, 74–7
Mutations, collagen gene (type II), and familial osteoarthritis, 199–205

Native protein structures, antibodies to, 160–1
Natural proteolysis of human link proteins, 53–4
Network
    characterization by molecular probes, 263–70
    fibrillar, pore size and hyaluronan mobility, 224
Non-human primates, human articular cartilage compared with, 248–51
Nucleus pulposus of intervertebral disc
    characterization of and sampling, 302–4
    measurement of pressure, 302–4
Number, cell, 235

Organization of cartilage constituents, 211–19
Oscillatory confined compression, electrokinetic transduction in, 291–2
Osmometer, new, 302–3
Osmotic pressure
 and glycosaminoglycan synthesis, 119–22
 measurement of, nucleus pulposus from intervertebral disc, 302–4
 measurement of, 298–301
 values of, using polyethylene glycol in human femoral head cartilage, 217
 see also Compression; Pressure
Osteoarthritis, 337–61
 changes in water content and tissue volume, 215
 and collagen gene mutations (type II), 199–205
 collagen markers in human urine, 348–52
 comparison with normal cartilage in sulfate uptake, 11–12
 low-temperature scanning, 64–5
 proteoglycan components in synovial fluid as markers of, 342–4
 in rhesus macaques as models for man, 341–2
 serum keratan sulfate measurement and proteoglycan metabolism, 345–7

Partition coefficients
 measured by gel chromatography, 251–5
 in solute transport, 243–5
 see also Coefficients
Perichondrial grafts, 316
Periosteal grafts, 316
Permeability, hydraulic
 and cartilage creep, 297–8
 in characterization of networks, 268–70
Phenotypic stability, and chondrocyte culture, 86–7
Physical properties of articular cartilage
 from uniaxial confined compression, 287–92
 from unconfined compression, 293–8

Physicochemical properties, 211 et seq., 241 et seq., 280
Plasma concentration of marker, 357
Polyacrylamide–agarose gel, recipe for, 41, 43
Polyclonal antibodies
 and immunochemical methods, 156–7
 to collagen, characterization and use of, 168–9
Polyethylene glycol solutions
 in osmotic pressure determination, 299
 in studies of intervertebral disc metabolism, 123–6
Pore size
 fibrillar network and hyaluronan mobility, 224
 and penetrability and globular protein, 223–4
Posttranslational events, analysis of, and biosynthesis of proteoglycans, 148–52
Potassium uptake in articular chondrocytes, 261–2
Precursor, see Radioisotopes
Preparation of specimens, 1–6
Preservation of samples for morphological studies, 19–23
Pressure
 contact, and deformation, 275–6
 measurement in human hip joint, 281–7
 tissue swelling, and matrix components, 225–6
 see also Compression; Osmotic pressure
Primates, articular cartilage composition, 248–51
Probes see Molecular probes
Protein
 complexes, large, electrophoresis of, 40–3
 globular, pore size and penetrability, 223–4
 link
  and radioimmunoassays, 157–60
  structure, 187
 precursor, proteoglycan core, pulse labeling and analysis of, 150–2
 structures, native or denatured, antibodies to, 160–1
Proteoglycans
 aggregates, age-related changes in stoichiometry of, 220–2
 binding region and radioimmunoassays, 157–60
 biosynthesis, analysis of post-translational events, 148–52
 in bovine articular cartilage explants, steady-state metabolism of, 108–12
 bovine and human, quantitation of keratan sulfate epitope in, 173–7
 characterization and immunochemical methods, 156–64
 components in synovial fluid as markers of osteoarthritis, 342–4
 connective-tissue, monoclonal antibodies against, 164–7
 domain structure and sequence homologies in, 187–90
 electrophoresis of
  agarose–acrylamide, 40–3
  monomers in agarose submerged gels, 44–6
 extraction from human articular cartilage, 36–9
 fragments
  gel filtration and affinity chromatography of, 174–5
  inhibitory capacity of, 175, 176
 metabolism, and serum keratan sulfate measurement and, 345–7
 osmotic pressure, 299–301
 radioimmunoassays, 93
 separation by centrifugal methodologies, 46–9
 synthesis and degradation, 113
 T-lymphocyte clones as new tool for research, 77–81
 turnover assessed using radioisotopes, 132–9, 142–54
Proteolysis of human link proteins, natural, 53–4
Pulse
 analyses of proteoglycan core protein precursor, 150–2
 -chase in assessment of turnover of proteoglycans in vivo, 138–9
 injection see Radioisotopes
 labeling and analysis of proteoglycan core protein precursor, 150–2
Purification see under Extraction, separation and analysis

Rabbits
  articular chondrocytes, immortalization of, 96–7
  collagen synthesis, 142
  patella, fluorescent-tracer labeling, 323
  proteoglycan turnover in cartilage of, 145–8
Radioimmunoassays, for proteoglycans binding region and, link protein, 157–60
Radioisotopes used to study metabolism of matrix molecules, 131–54
  biosynthesis of cartilage proteoglycan *in vitro*, 148–52
  collagen metabolism in cartilage and bone *in vivo*, measurement of, 140–2
  glycosaminoglycan synthesis rate, *in vitro* and *in vivo*, 143–8
  proteoglycan turnover assessed by pulse techniques *in vivo*, 137–9, 143–8
  proteoglycan turnover assessed by steady state techniques *in vivo*, 139
  radiolabeled glucosamine as precursor for measuring *in vitro* hyaluronan synthesis, 132–7
Rat
  growth-plate cartilage, 20–75
  ovarian granulosa cells, 133–6
Rate zonal sedimentation centrifugal method, 47
Recombinant DNA and cartilage matrix, 185–208
  collagen gene mutations and familial osteoarthritis, 199–205
  collagen type XII discovered, 190–4
  domain structure and sequence homologies in proteoglycans, 187–90
  lysozyme in chick embryo cartilage, 194–6
Regulation of chondrocyte gene expression, 196–9
Repair and remodeling, 313–35
  cultured chondrocytes as implants, 327–9
  fluorescent-tracer labeling for measuring, 322–4
  reflections on, 318–21

spongialization and healing in human, 324–7
Replication, low temperature, 65–6

Sampling of tissues
  for comparison between normal and osteoarthritic specimens, 12–13
  femoral head cartilage, 9–12
  general considerations, 1–9
  intervertebral disc, 17–19
  for morphological studies, 18–23
Scanning electron microscopy *see* Electron microscopy
Sedimentation
  centrifugal methods, 47
  macro- and micro-rate zonal, 48
Separation of matrix constituents *see* Extraction, separation and analysis
Sepharose CL-2B chromatography of proteoglycan aggregates, 37–8
Sequence homologies and domain structure in proteoglycans, 187–90
Serine residues, substitution of, 151
Serum
  fetal calf, and sulfate incorporation, 14–17
  human, analysis of, 175
  keratan sulfate measurement and proteoglycan metabolism, 345–7
  macromolecular substances cleared from, 352–7
Short-term culture of cartilage *see* Explant culture
Solute concentration profile in matrix as function of hydration, 218–19
Solute transport between tissue and environment, 241–73
  articular cartilage composition in primates, 248–51
  measurement of diffusion coefficients in biopolymer solutions and gels, 255–8
  measurement methods, 241–8
  measurement of partition coefficients by gel chromatography, 251–5

membrane transport, techniques for studying, 258–63
  network characterization by molecular probes, 263–70
Species and age influence on cartilage, 115
Stability, phenotypic, and chondrocyte culture, 86–7
Static methods of network characterization, 263–6
Steady-state
  conditions, continuous labeling under, 149–50
  label-chase in assessment of turnover of proteoglycans *in vivo*, 139
  metabolism of proteoglycans in bovine articular cartilage explants, 108–12
Stereological methods in articular cartilage research, 74–7
Stereoscopy, transmission electron microscopy, 73
Stoichiometry
  of human articular cartilage proteoglycan aggregates, age-related changes in, 220–2
  of type XII collagen, 54–5
Subchondral bone, perforation to, 316
Subpopulations of articular chondrocytes cultured in agarose gel, 90–2
Sulfate
  antibodies, anti-keratan, and quantitation of keratan sulfate epitope, 173–7
  chondroitin, monoclonal antibodies to, 161–2
  gradients cesium, 48
  incorporation
    age changes in, 13–14
    comparison between normal and osteoarthritic cartilage, 12–13
    and explant culture, 124–5
    in intervertebral disc, method for studying, 123–6
    and pressure, 121–2
    topographical and zonal variations in, 11–13
  radioactive, glycosaminoglycan synthesis rate traced, 143–8
Superficial zone *see* Articular surface
Suspension culture and chondrocyte culture, 87–8

Synovial fluid
  human, analysis of, 175
  macromolecular substances cleared from, 352–7
  proteoglycan components in as markers of osteoarthritis, 342–4
Synthesis
  of cartilage proteoglycans, 148–52
  collagen, 140–2
  decrease, enhanced by cytokine activity, 113–115
  glycosaminoglycan, rate traced by radioactive sulfate, 143–8
  hyaluronan, radiolabeled glucosamine used as precursor for measuring, 132–7
  of proteoglycans, 113
  also see Proteoglycan turnover; Sulphate incorporation
Synthetic matrix, implantation of, 317

Temperature, low, and scanning electron microscopy, 63–7
Thermodynamic molecular probes, 265–7

Thin cartilage slices, measurement of mechanical properties of, 304–8
Three-dimensional culture model for studying human chondrocytes, 93–5
T-lymphocyte clones as new tool in proteoglycan research, antigen-specific, 177–81
Topographical variations
  general considerations, 4–6, 61 *et seq.*
  human femoral head cartilage, 9–12, 14–5
  intervertebral disc, 17–9
Tracers *see* Radioisotopes
Transblotting, 43
Transmission electron microscopy stereoscopy, 73
Transport
  membrane, techniques for studying, 258–63
  between tissue and environment *see* Solute transport
Turnover, *see under* Proteoglycans; Collagen

Uptake studies
  of membrane transport, 260–2

of sulfate *see under* Sulfate incorporation
Urine, human, collagen markers of arthritis in, 348–52

Velocity sedimentation centrifugal method, 47
Vertical quadrat, 77
Volume, cartilage, function of hydration, 213–15

Water *see also under* Hydration
  cartilage, 213–15
  loss in tissue preparation, 64
Wharton's jelly, 222–3, 226–7

X-ray
  diffraction analysis of tissues, low-angle, 232–5
  scattering, collagen packing studied with, 227–32

Zonal sedimentation, macro- and micro-rate, 48